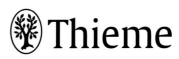

Muscle Injuries in Sports

Hans-Wilhelm Mueller-Wohlfahrt, MD
MW Center for Orthopedics and Sports Medicine
Munich, Germany

Peter Ueblacker, MD
MW Center for Orthopedics and Sports Medicine
Munich, Germany

Lutz Haensel, MD
MW Center for Orthopedics and Sports Medicine
Munich, Germany

William E. Garrett Jr., MD, PhD
Duke Sports Medicine Center
Durham, USA

With contributions by

Andreas Betthaeuser, Alfred Binder, Wilhelm Bloch,
Dieter Blottner, Johannes Boeck, Bernhard Brenner,
Klaus Eder, Jan Ekstrand, Martin Flueck, Lutz Haensel,
Helmut Hoffmann, J. Michael Hufnagl, Hans-Wilhelm
Mueller-Wohlfahrt, Peter Mundinger, Andreas Schlumberger,
Benedikt Schoser, Peter Ueblacker

Foreword by Jiri Dvorák, Zurich, Switzerland;
Chief Medical Officer, FIFA

505 illustrations

Thieme
Stuttgart · New York

Library of Congress Cataloging-in-Publication Data
is available from the publisher.

This book is an authorized translation of the German edition published and copyrighted 2010 by Georg Thieme Verlag, Stuttgart. Title of the German edition: Muskelverletzungen im Sport.

Translators: Terry Telger, Fort Worth, Texas, USA; Gertrud G. Champe, Surry, Maine, USA; Ruth Gutberlet, Chom, NCTMB, Hofbieber, Germany; Alexandra Kuhn-Thiel, MD, Wachenheim, Germany

Illustrators: Markus Voll, Munich, Germany; Andrea Schnitzler, Innsbruck, Austria

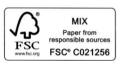

© 2013 Georg Thieme Verlag KG,
Rüdigerstrasse 14, 70469 Stuttgart, Germany
http://www.thieme.de
Thieme Medical Publishers, Inc., 333 Seventh Avenue,
New York, NY 10001, USA
http://www.thieme.com

Cover design: Thieme Publishing Group
Typesetting by Ziegler und Müller, Kirchentellinsfurt, Germany
Printed in China by Everbest Printing Ltd., Hong Kong

ISBN 978-3-13-162471-0

Also available as e-book:
eISBN 978-3-13-169661-8

Important note: Medicine is an ever-changing science undergoing continual development. Research and clinical experience are continually expanding our knowledge, in particular our knowledge of proper treatment and drug therapy. Insofar as this book mentions any dosage or application, readers may rest assured that the authors, editors, and publishers have made every effort to ensure that such references are in accordance with **the state of knowledge at the time of production of the book.**

Nevertheless, this does not involve, imply, or express any guarantee or responsibility on the part of the publishers in respect to any dosage instructions and forms of applications stated in the book. **Every user is requested to examine carefully** the manufacturers' leaflets accompanying each drug and to check, if necessary in consultation with a physician or specialist, whether the dosage schedules mentioned therein or the contraindications stated by the manufacturers differ from the statements made in the present book. Such examination is particularly important with drugs that are either rarely used or have been newly released on the market. Every dosage schedule or every form of application used is entirely at the user's own risk and responsibility. The authors and publishers request every user to report to the publishers any discrepancies or inaccuracies noticed. If errors in this work are found after publication, errata will be posted at www.thieme.com on the product description page.

To my dear wife Karin,
my daughter Maren and my son Kilian
for their support and understanding.

H.-W. Müller-Wohlfahrt

To my dear wife Anika,
and my children Malou, Elia, and Louis
for their love, *joie de vivre,* and understanding.

P. Ueblacker

To my dear wife Gloria
for her untiring support
and understanding.

L. Hänsel

Foreword

It is an undisputed scientific fact that sports not only promote the enhancement of physical fitness, regardless of age or gender, but are also the most effective way of preventing most cardiovascular diseases, diabetes, obesity, and many types of cancer (as outlined by Prof. Steven Blair in the *British Journal of Sports Medicine* 2009;43:1–2). Extensive promotion of recreational sports for all ages is the best way of improving public health and reducing healthcare costs.

If this health potential of competitive and recreational sports is to be fully exploited, the risk of injuries has to be reduced as much as possible. Particularly in sports that are widely popular, every effort has to be made to prevent injuries and their late sequelae. This should include adequate initial examinations, warm-up routines based on special exercises, and concepts of fair play, as well as optimal management of any injuries that are sustained.

Football (soccer) is unquestionably the most popular sport in the world. With almost 300 million players worldwide, any divergence from good practice is inevitably magnified on a tremendous scale.

On the basis of comprehensive epidemiologic studies conducted by the FIFA Medical Assessment and Research Center (F-MARC) of the International Federation of Association Football (FIFA), the average soccer player sustains approximately two injuries per year. Not only do these injuries incur primary treatment costs, but significant secondary costs also arise due to lost productivity and absence from work. The most common sports-related injuries involve the muscles, and even apparently minor injuries may have serious consequences when they occur on a repetitive basis. As the world's largest international sports association, FIFA has taken a keen interest in the prevention, diagnosis, and treatment of sports-related injuries. Trainers, physical therapists, and sports physicians at the recreational and amateur level must have sufficient knowledge to provide optimal diagnostic and therapeutic care.

The editors of this book, Hans-Wilhelm Müller-Wohlfahrt, Peter Ueblacker, Lutz Hänsel, and William Garrett, as well as the contributing authors, have had decades of practical experience in caring for thousands of professional and amateur athletes. As a result, *Muscle Injuries in Sports* offers state-of-the-art diagnostic and treatment information from the perspective of prominent sports physicians. The book includes a new system for the clinical classification of muscle injuries based on the history, physical examination, and imaging findings. The book's therapeutic focus is on conservative treatment, both in the setting of acute muscle injuries and in rehabilitation. As readers will see, the authors have gathered together the best and most useful information on the basis of decades of experience, with the goal of hastening the recovery of every injured athlete.

I personally know little about interference fields or energy emission analysis, but these chapters clearly warrant critical evaluation. This superbly illustrated book is completed by a chapter on preventive measures, which are definitely as important as treatment and may be far more important. Scientific studies with football players (Soligard et al., *BMJ* 2008;337:a2469) have shown that injuries can be reduced by 30–50% when preventive measures such as the 11+ exercise program, with proven efficacy, are applied as an integral part of warm-up routines before training and competition (http://f-marc.com).

In summary, everyone involved in the care of athletes should not only read this book but also implement the practical recommendations by seasoned experts that it offers on the prevention, diagnosis, treatment, and rehabilitation of sports-related muscle injuries.

Prof. Jiri Dvorák, MD
Chief Medical Officer, FIFA; Chairman, F-MARC

Preface

More than one-third of all injuries that occur in soccer involve the muscles; thigh muscle injuries represent the most common diagnosis in track and field athletes, American football, and basketball. However, muscle injuries are also common in recreational sports, where overlooked or misunderstood muscle injuries may lead to persistent problems.

It is also a fact that injuries to the skeletal muscles are often underestimated, misinterpreted, and improperly treated. The reasons for this include a lack of training and continuing education in this area, a lack of research, the absence—so far—of a practical, comprehensive, universal classification system for muscle injuries, and even a lack of uniform terminology. Moreover, guidelines for clinical or imaging diagnosis and treatment are lacking. For the sake of all injured athletes, this situation must change!

In the past, the specialized knowledge needed to diagnose and treat muscle injuries could only be obtained from individual publications, with considerable inconsistency in the use of muscle injury terminology. So far, there have been no textbooks providing a comprehensive, understandable description of the anatomy and physiology of the skeletal muscles or the clinical diagnosis, imaging, treatment, rehabilitation, and prevention of muscle injuries.

Having long planned a book on diagnosis and treatment, we felt it was time to undertake a comprehensive project of this type. The result is *Muscle Injuries in Sports*, which draws upon more than 35 years of practical experience in caring for professional soccer players and other top athletes from track and field and many other sports from all over the world.

The main problem in evaluating skeletal muscles is that they are so heterogeneous, from both the physiological and pathological standpoints. This makes it all the more difficult to establish a comprehensive classification that covers all injuries, as there are more borderline cases than in other types of injury such as fractures.

Only very few studies have been published on muscle injuries. Much of the information in this book—particularly the chapters on classification, clinical diagnosis, and treatment—is thus admittedly based more on empirical knowledge than on scientific data. But isn't it also true that other medical classifications are evidence-based only to a limited degree, due to a lack of scientific research? However, the empirical data used in this book are based on a large number of muscle injuries, as the authors and editors regularly see and treat competitive athletes.

Interestingly, while the musculature is the largest parenchymal organ in the human body, representing roughly 40% of the total body weight in adults, the muscles have been relegated to a secondary role in the past. It is only recently that they have become a focus of growing interest in research work, professional journals, and the press. More and more, the muscles are being recognized as a central organ that is responsible for numerous disorders and complaints and that is also accessible to treatment.

This textbook is being published at a time when greater attention is being given to the muscles in "musculoskeletal medicine"—the field that in the past dealt extensively with joints, ligaments, tendons, and bones. Our aim is to stimulate discussion about athletic muscle injuries in order to promote a new and improved understanding of the diagnosis, treatment, and prevention of these frequent and interesting disorders.

The original publication of this book in German in June 2010 was very successful, with a positive response from many physicians and therapists in the field of the diagnosis and treatment of muscle injuries who had been looking for a book like this for a long time. This led us to discuss the possibility of producing an English edition with the publishers.

The present English edition is a further development of the German one, based on the following events: In early 2011, we conducted a survey based on the hypothesis that the existing terminology for muscle injuries in the English language is highly inconsistent. Scientists and team doctors from national and first-division professional soccer teams, native English speakers, were asked to complete a questionnaire. The responses confirmed our hypothesis that there is marked variability in the use of medical terminology relating to muscle injury. The results emphasized the need for a more uniform terminology and classification system.

On the basis of these findings, we organized a consensus meeting of international sports medicine experts in Munich, Germany, on March 3, 2011. The following members took part in the meeting (in alphabetical order):

- Prof. Dieter Blottner (Associate Professor, Department of Vegetative Anatomy, Charité University Hospital, Berlin, Germany)
- Prof. Jan Ekstrand (Head of the UEFA Injury Study Group, Vice-Chairman of the UEFA Medical Committee, University of Linköping, Sweden)
- Dr. Bryan English (team physician of Chelsea Football Club, UK)

- Prof. William E. Garrett, Jr. (Duke Sports Medicine Center, Durham, North Carolina, USA)
- Dr. Lutz Hänsel (editor of this book, team physician of Bayern Munich Football Club, Germany)
- Dr. Gino M.M.J. Kerkhoffs (Department of Orthopedic Surgery, Orthopedic Research Center, Amsterdam, Netherlands)
- Dr. Steve McNally (team physician for Manchester United, UK)
- Dr. Kai Mithoefer (Harvard Vanguard Medical Associates, Harvard Medical School, US Soccer Federation, Boston, Massachusetts, USA)
- Dr. Hans-Wilhelm Müller-Wohlfahrt (editor of this book, team physician of Bayern Munich Football Club, Germany, and team physician of Germany's national football team)
- Dr. John Orchard, MD, PhD (Associate Professor, School of Public Health, University of Sydney; team physician of the Australian cricket team and Sydney Roosters rugby league team)
- Dr. Patrick Schamasch (Medical and Scientific Director of the International Olympic Committee, Lausanne, Switzerland)
- Dr. Leif Swaerd (Associate Professor, University of Göteborg, Sweden; team physician for Sweden's national football team and previously for England's national football team)
- PD Dr. Peter Ueblacker (editor of this book, team physician of Bayern Munich Football Club, Germany)
- Dr. Niek van Dijk (Head of the Orthopedics Department, Academic Medical Center, Amsterdam, Netherlands)

Practical and systematic terms for athletic muscle injuries were established at the conference.

It was decided not to recommend the use of the term *strain* anymore, as it is a biomechanical term that is not defined and is used indiscriminately for anatomically and functionally different muscle injuries. Instead of *strain*, the consensus panel proposed the use of the term *tear*, used for *structural muscle injuries*—i.e., injuries in which there is macroscopic evidence of muscle damage.

In addition, a comprehensive new classification system was developed that differentiates between:
- *Functional muscle disorders*—referring to disorders with no macroscopic evidence of fiber tear (type 1, overexertion-related; and type 2, neuromuscular muscle disorders)

and
- *Structural muscle injuries*—with macroscopic evidence of a fiber tear, i.e. structural damage (type 3, partial tears; and type 4, [sub]total tears/tendinous avulsions)

Subclassifications were defined for each type.

The aim of the new classification system is to improve the clarity of communication for both diagnostic and therapeutic purposes. This is intended to serve as the basis for future comparative studies to address the continued lack of systematic information on muscle injuries in the literature. The results of this consensus conference have been published in the *British Journal of Sports Medicine* (with open access on bjsm.com).

We are very proud that the classification has been included in the UEFA Champions League Injury Study. We hope that our work will stimulate research—based on the suggested terminology and classification—to prospectively evaluate the prognostic and therapeutic implications of the new classification system, which is based on clinical experience.

This book has been written for all sports physicians, sports scientists, physical therapists, and many others who are interested and involved in the care and treatment of competitive and recreational athletes. Our hope is that by describing our own experience, we may be able to advance the diagnosis and treatment of these frequent and interesting injuries.

Our special thanks go to Dr. Albrecht Hauff, CEO of the Thieme Publishing Group, for his enthusiastic response to our idea of writing a comprehensive textbook on skeletal muscle injuries. We are particularly grateful for his foresight and his support.

We are also very grateful to the staff at Thieme Publishers—particularly Angelika Findgott, for generous and professional planning; and to Anne Lamparter, Deborah Cecere, and Sophia Hengst, for their tireless help and support in seeing the project through to completion. Our thanks also go to Gertrud Champe, Ruth Gutberlet, Alexandra Kuhn-Thiel, and Terry Telger for the professional translations. The entire staff at the Thieme Publishing Group consistently looked after our needs with a great deal of effort and commitment and were able to find answers for our most challenging questions. They provided the high degree of collaboration that is essential for completing a project of this kind.

Our sincere thanks also go, of course, to all of our authors, whose contributions reflect the very highest level of technical competence and expertise. We are grateful to them for their dedicated and comprehensive work on the project, and particularly also in the translation and editing tasks needed for this English edition. We are proud to have worked with such an accomplished and experienced team of experts.

Hans-Wilhelm Müller-Wohlfahrt
Peter Ueblacker
Lutz Hänsel

Contributors

Andreas Betthäuser, MD
Schulter-Zentrum
Hamburg, Germany

Alfred Binder
FC Bayern München
Munich, Germany

Wilhelm Bloch, MD
Professor
German Sports University, Cologne
Cologne, Germany

Dieter Blottner, PhD
Associate Professor
Department of Vegetative Anatomy
Charité Berlin
Berlin, Germany

Johannes Böck, MD, MSc
Professor
Private Practice for Radiology and Nuclear Medicine
Munich, Germany

Bernhard Brenner, MD
Professor
Department of Molecular and Cell Physiology
Hanover Medical School
Hanover, Germany

Klaus Eder
EDEN Reha, Clinic for Sports and Trauma Injuries
Donaustauf, Germany

Jan Ekstrand, MD
Professor
UEFA Injury Study Group
Vice Chairman UEFA Medical Committee
Linköping, Sweden

Martin Flueck, MD
Professor
Institute for Biomedical Research
Manchester Metropolitan University
Manchester, UK

William E. Garrett, Jr., MD, PhD
Duke Sports Medicine Center
Durham, NC, USA

Lutz Hänsel, MD
MW Center for Orthopedics and Sports Medicine
Munich, Germany

Helmut Hoffmann
EDEN Reha, Clinic for Sports and Trauma Injuries
Donaustauf, Germany

J. Michael Hufnagl, MD
Bogenhausen Hospital, Munich
Clinic for Neuropsychology
Munich, Germany

Gerhard Luttke, MD
Private Practice for Radiology and Nuclear Medicine
Munich, Germany

Norbert Maassen, MD
Professor
Institute for Sports Medicine
Hanover Medical School
Hanover, Germany

Hans-Wilhelm Müller-Wohlfahrt, MD
MW Center for Orthopedics and Sports Medicine
Munich, Germany

Peter Mundinger, MD
Hessingpark Clinic
Augsburg, Germany

Andreas Schlumberger, PhD
Fitness Coach, Borussia Dortmund
Dortmund, Germany

Benedikt Schoser, MD
Professor
Friedrich Baur Institute
University of Munich
Munich, Germany

Peter Ueblacker, MD
MW Center for Orthopedics and Sports Medicine
Munich, Germany

Abbreviations

Ach	acetylcholine	IL-8	interleukin-8
AchR	acetylcholine receptor	IMP	inosine monophosphate
ADP	adenosine diphosphate	INR	international normalized ratio
AMP	adenosine monophosphate	IOC	International Olympic Committee
ASIS	anterior superior iliac spine	LIF	leukocyte inhibitory factor
ATP	adenosine triphosphate; Association of Tennis Professionals	MCP-1	monocyte chemoattractant protein-1
		MCSF	macrophage colony-stimulating factor
ATR	Achilles tendon reflex	MGF	macrophage growth factor
bFGF	basic fibroblast growth factor	MIF	macrophage inhibitory factor
BP	*Bereitschaftspotenzial,* readiness potential	MIP-1α	macrophage inflammatory protein-1α
CGRP	calcitonin gene-related peptide	Mn-SOD	manganese superoxide dismutase
CK-B	creatine kinase B	MRI	magnetic resonance imaging
CK-M	creatine kinase M	MTJ	muscle–tendon junction
CK-Mi	creatine kinase Mi	mTOR	mammalian target of rapamycin
CK-MM	muscle form of creatine kinase	MyHC	myosin heavy-chain
CNS	central nervous system	NADA	National Anti-Doping Agency
CPM	continuous passive motion	NADH	nicotinamide adenine dinucleotide
CPT	carnitine palmitoyltransferase	NADPH	nicotinamide adenine dinucleotide phosphate
CRP	C-reactive protein		
CRPS	complex regional pain syndrome	NFAT	nuclear factor of activated T cells
DM	myotonic dystrophy	NMJ	neuromuscular junction
DOMS	delayed-onset muscle soreness	NMT	neuromuscular technique
EEA	energy emission analysis	NO	nitric oxide
EEG	electroencephalography	NSAIDs	nonsteroidal anti-inflammatory drugs
EMG	electromyography	PDGF	platelet-derived growth factor
EPO	erythropoietin	PRP	platelet-rich plasma
EPSP	excitatory postsynaptic potential	REM	rapid eye movement
ER	endoplasmic reticulum	RICE	rest, ice, compression, and elevation
ESR	erythrocyte sedimentation rate	SR	sarcoplasmic reticulum
FDA	Food and Drug Administration	TB	triple burner
FGF	fibroblast growth factor	TENS	transcutaneous electrical nerve stimulation
FIFA	International Federation of Association Football	TGC	time gain compensation
		TGF	transforming growth factor
GABA	gamma-aminobutyric acid	TNF-β	tumor necrosis factor-β
GCSF	granulocyte colony-stimulating factor	TNF-α	tumor necrosis factor-α
GLUT	glucose transporter	UCL	UEFA Champions League
GTO	Golgi tendon organ	UEFA	Union of European Football Associations
HGF	hepatocyte growth factor	VBG	*Verwaltungs-Berufsgenossenschaft,* Administrative Professional Association
HIF-1α	hypoxia-inducible factor-1α		
IFN-γ	interferon-γ	VEGF	vascular endothelial growth factor
IGF	insulin-like growth factor	WADA	World Anti-Doping Agency
IL-6	interleukin-6		

Contents

1 Functional Anatomy of Skeletal Muscle ··· 1

D. Blottner

**Structure and Function of Skeletal Muscle
and the Locomotor System** ··· 2

Anatomic Terms in Skeletal Muscle ··· 3
  Nomenclature ··· 3
  Skeletal Muscle Fiber Types ··· 5

Functional Muscle Compartments
as a Structural Principle ··· 7

Muscle Compartments and Their Nerve and Vascular
Supply Relative to Injury Risks in Sports ··· 7
  Trunk Muscles ··· 9
  Muscles of the Anterior and Posterior
  Arm Compartments ··· 11
  Muscles of the Hip, Buttocks, and Leg ··· 14
  Intermuscular Septum,
  Rectus Sheath, and Iliotibial Tract ··· 23

Skeletal Muscles and
Their Typical Motion Patterns ··· 23
  Pennation Angle or Angulation
  of Fascicles in Skeletal Muscle ··· 24
  Anatomic versus Physiological Profile
  of Skeletal Muscle ··· 25
  Isotonic versus Isometric Contraction ··· 25

Functional Histology of Muscle Tissue ··· 26

Smooth Muscle ··· 26

Striated Muscle ··· 28
  Heart Muscle ··· 28
  Skeletal Muscle ··· 29

Molecular Architecture of
Skeletal Muscle Fibers (Sarcomeres) ··· 29
  Actin and Myosin Filaments ··· 29
  Striations ··· 30
  Sarcoplasmic Reticulum and Tubules ··· 30
  Regulatory Proteins, Tropomyosin,
  and Troponin ··· 30
  Accessory Proteins Titin and Nebulin ··· 31
  Muscle Fatigue ··· 31

Satellite Cells (Emergency Cells) ··· 32

Microvasculature and Capillaries ··· 32
  Ischemia ··· 33

Connective Tissue (Myofascial System) ··· 34

Principles of Skeletal Muscle Architecture ··· 35

Skeletal Muscle ··· 35
  Muscle Fascia and Intermuscular Septum ··· 36
  Secondary and Primary Bundles (Fascicles) ··· 36
  Muscle Fibers ··· 36

Muscle Tendons ··· 37
  Tendon Architecture ··· 37
  Tendon Function ··· 37

Muscle-Tendon Contacts
(Myotendinous Junction) ··· 38

Tendon–Bone Junction ··· 38

Support Structures in Skeletal Muscle ··· 38
  Tendon Sheaths, Bursa, and Retinaculum ··· 38
  Sesamoids ··· 40

Active versus Passive Muscle Insufficiency ··· 42

Innervation of Skeletal Muscle ··· 42

Motor Units and Neuromuscular Synapses ··· 43

Motor End Plate—Neuromuscular Junction ··· 43

Neuromuscular Spindle ··· 44
  Architecture ··· 44
  Neuromuscular Spindle Density ··· 45

Golgi Tendon Organ (GTO) ··· 45
  Architecture ··· 45
  Function of GTOs ··· 46

Functional Anatomic Principles
of Muscle Reflexes ··· 46
  Reflex Arcs ··· 46
  Rhythmic Movements in Sports ··· 47

The Innervated Locomotor Apparatus ··· 48

Brain and Spinal Cord ··· 48

Plexuses and Peripheral Nerves ··· 50
  Plexus ··· 50
  Spinal Syndromes ··· 53

Reference Muscles and Myotomes ··· 54

2 Basic Physiology and Aspects of Exercise ··· 59
B. Brenner, N. Maassen

Basic Physiology ··· 60

Sarcomere, Muscle Force,
and Muscle Shortening ··· 60

Basic Principles of Muscular
Contraction and its Regulation ··· 61
   Motor Unit ··· 61
   Neuromuscular End plate (Motor End plate) ··· 61
   Signal Transduction from the
   Motor Neuron to Skeletal Muscle Fibers ··· 62
   Initiating a Contraction
   (Electromechanical Coupling) ··· 62
   Production of Motile Forces
   by the Myosin Heads ··· 62
   Relaxation of Muscle ··· 65
   Time Course of Muscular Contraction
   (Mechanogram) ··· 65

Gradation of Muscle Force
during Voluntary Movements ··· 66

Types of Muscular Contraction ··· 67
   Passive Length–Tension Curve ··· 67
   Isotonic Contraction ··· 69
   Isometric Contraction ··· 69
   Auxotonic Contraction ··· 69
   Afterloaded Contraction
   and Contraction against a Stop ··· 69
   Muscular Work ··· 70
   Relationship between Lifted Load
   and Shortening Velocity of Muscle ··· 70
   Concentric and Eccentric Contractions ··· 70
   Adjusting Shortening Velocity
   to Changing Demands ··· 70

Neuromuscular Control Mechanisms ··· 71
   Hierarchical Organization
   of Voluntary Movements ··· 71

   Regulation of Muscle Length (Stretch Reflex) ··· 72
   Force and Tension Control in Muscles
   (Autogenous Inhibition) ··· 75
   Rhythmic Movement Patterns ··· 75
   Facilitation and Inhibition of Neuronal
   Circuits at the Spinal Cord Level ··· 75

Aspects of Exercise Physiology ··· 77

Types of Muscle Fiber ··· 77

Overview of Muscular Metabolism ··· 78
   Anaerobic Alactacid Energy Production ··· 78
   Activation of Phosphofructokinase ··· 78
   Activation of Glycogen Breakdown ··· 78
   Production of Lactate ··· 79
   Aerobic Metabolism ··· 79
   Fat or Carbohydrates? ··· 80

Warm-Up ··· 81
   Thermal Effects ··· 81
   Blood Flow ··· 81
   Excitability ··· 81
   Cooling Instead of Warm-Up ··· 82

Fatigue ··· 82
   Acidosis ··· 83
   ATP Resynthesis ··· 83
   Phosphate Effects ··· 84
   Excitability ··· 84
   Glycogen Deficiency ··· 84
   Free Radicals ··· 84
   Temperature ··· 86
   Central Fatigue ··· 86

Recovery ··· 86

Training Adaptations ··· 86
   Signal Chains ··· 87

3 Molecular and Cell Biology of Muscle Regeneration ··· 89
M. Flueck

Muscle Injury and Regeneration ··· 90

**Importance of Various Nutrient Additives
for Muscle Activity** ··· 92

Amino Acids ··· 92
   Essential Amino Acids ··· 92
   Amino Acid Demand in Athletes ··· 93

Metabolic Disturbance ··· 95
   pH Values ··· 95
   Creatine Kinase, Myoglobin, Uric Acid ··· 95
   Prevention and Therapy ··· 95

Antioxidants ··· 96
   Function ··· 96
   Intake ··· 96
   Importance of Antioxidants
   in Athletic Activity ··· 96

Minerals ··· 98
   Function in Muscle ··· 98
   Disturbances of Muscle Homeostasis ··· 98

Trace Elements ⋯ 99
  Function ⋯ 99
  Deficiencies ⋯ 100
  Intake ⋯ 100
  Importance of Trace Elements
  in Athletic Activity ⋯ 101

Vitamin D ⋯ 101
  Metabolism and Regulation ⋯ 101
  Intake ⋯ 102
  Importance of Vitamin D in Athletic Activity ⋯ 103

Conclusions ⋯ 103

4 Muscle Healing: Physiology and Adverse Factors ⋯ 105
W. Bloch

**Functional and Structural
Alterations in Muscle Tissue** ⋯ 106

Functional Muscle Disorders ⋯ 107

Minor Partial Muscle Tears ⋯ 107

**Moderate Partial Muscle Tear/
(Sub)Total Muscle Tear** ⋯ 108

Mechanisms of Muscle Damage ⋯ 108

Initial Damage Phase ⋯ 109
  Cellular Damage Mechanisms ⋯ 109
  Extracellular Damage Mechanisms ⋯ 109
  Dependence of Damage on Contraction
  and Fiber Types ⋯ 109
  Impaired Neuromuscular Regulation ⋯ 110

Secondary Phase of Injury ⋯ 110

**Regenerative Mechanisms
and Their Sequence** ⋯ 111

Destruction Phase ⋯ 111
  Migration of Macrophages ⋯ 112
  Migration of Neutrophils ⋯ 112

Repair Phase ⋯ 112
  Muscle Fiber Regeneration ⋯ 114
  Formation of Extracellular Matrix ⋯ 116
  Neovascularization ⋯ 118
  Reinnervation ⋯ 119

**Laboratory Markers
for Diagnosis and Healing** ⋯ 119

Factors Influencing Healing ⋯ 120

Nutrition ⋯ 120
  Antioxidants ⋯ 120
  Carbohydrates and Proteins ⋯ 120
  Carbohydrates ⋯ 120
  Protein ⋯ 120

Age ⋯ 120

Exercise ⋯ 122
  Approaches in Various Degrees
  of Muscle Injury ⋯ 122
  Effects of Exercise ⋯ 123

Drug-Based Therapy ⋯ 123
  Nonsteroidal Anti-Inflammatory Drugs ⋯ 123
  Glucocorticoids ⋯ 124
  New Treatment Approaches ⋯ 124

Physical Measures ⋯ 124
  Cryotherapy ⋯ 124
  Compression ⋯ 125
  Massage ⋯ 125
  Ultrasound and Electrotherapy ⋯ 125

5 Epidemiology of Muscle Injuries in Soccer ⋯ 127
J. Ekstrand

Consensus of Study Design ⋯ 128

Material ⋯ 129

Method ⋯ 129
  Definition: Injury ⋯ 129
  Definition: Injury Severity ⋯ 129
  Definition: Recurrent Injury ⋯ 129

Results ⋯ 129

Localization of Muscle Injuries in Soccer Players ⋯ 129

Injury Incidence ⋯ 130

Injury Risk ⋯ 131
  Muscle Injuries and Age ⋯ 131
  Variation in Injury Risk during Matches ⋯ 131
  Injuries Due to Contact Situations
  and Foul Play ⋯ 132

Injury Severity ⋯ 132

Recurrent Injuries ⋯ 132

Examination Procedures: MRI and Ultrasound ⋯ 132
  Hamstring Injuries ⋯ 133
  Quadriceps Injuries ⋯ 133

Evaluation of Data ⋯ 134

6 Terminology, Classification, Patient History, and Clinical Examination ··· 135
H.-W. Müller-Wohlfahrt, P. Ueblacker, A. Binder, L. Hänsel

Why a New Classification? ··· 136

Short Review of the Current Literature ··· 137

Terminology of Muscle Injuries ··· 137

Classification of Muscle Injuries ··· 137
    Fundamentals ··· 137
    Current Classification Systems ··· 138

Consensus Conference on Muscle Terminology
and Development of a New Comprehensive
Classification System ··· 139
    Terminology ··· 139
    New Classification System ··· 141

Type 1 and 2: Functional Muscle Disorders ··· 145
    Type 1: Overexertion-Related Muscle Disorder ··· 146
    Type 2: Neuromuscular Muscle Disorder ··· 147

Types 3 and 4: Structural Muscle Injuries ··· 149
    Type 3: Partial Muscle Tears ··· 149
    Type 4: Subtotal/Complete Muscle Tear
    or Tendinous Avulsion ··· 152

Contusion Injuries ··· 153

Patient History ··· 155

Examination of Muscle Injuries ··· 156

Examination Techniques ··· 156
    Palpation ··· 157
    Ultrasound Diagnosis ··· 159
    Magnetic Resonance Imaging (MRI) ··· 159
    Laboratory Diagnosis ··· 159

Typical Findings on Examination ··· 160

Type 1a: Fatigue-Induced Muscle Disorder ··· 160
Type 1b: Delayed-Onset Muscle Soreness
(DOMS) ··· 160
Type 2a: Spine-Related Neuromuscular
Muscle Disorder ··· 160
Type 2b: Muscle-Related Neuromuscular
Muscle Disorder ··· 160
Type 3a: Minor Partial Muscle Tear
(Intrafascicular/Bundle Tear) ··· 161
Type 3b: Moderate Partial Muscle Tear
(Interfascicular/Bundle Tear)
and Type 4: Subtotal/Complete Muscle
Tear or Tendinous Avulsion ··· 161

Other Muscle Injuries and Causes
of Muscle Symptoms ··· 162
    Functional Compartment Syndrome ··· 162
    Apophyseal Avulsion ··· 162
    Other Conditions ··· 163

Complications ··· 163

Post-Stress Muscle Imbalance ··· 163

Recurrence ··· 163

Seroma and Cyst ··· 163

Fibrosis/Scarring ··· 165

Traumatic Compartment Syndrome ··· 165

Myositis Ossificans and
Heterotopic Ossification ··· 165

Muscle Hernia ··· 165

7 Ultrasonography ··· 169
L. Hänsel, P. Ueblacker, A. Betthäuser

Introduction ··· 170

Relevant Physical Phenomena and Artifacts ··· 170

Absorption and Attenuation ··· 171

Reflection and Reflection Artifact ··· 171

Scatter ··· 171

Acoustic Shadow ··· 171

Acoustic Enhancement ··· 171

Reverberations ··· 172

Mirror-Image Artifact ··· 172

**Ultrasonographic Examination
of Skeletal Muscle** ··· 172

Ultrasonography of Normal Muscle
Tissue/Sonoanatomy ··· 174
    Factors that Affect Imaging ··· 175
    Examination Technique ··· 176
    Ultrasonographic Examination
    of the Lower Limbs ··· 177

Ultrasonography of Pathological Conditions ··· 185
    Fatigue-Induced Painful Muscle Disorder
    (Type 1a Lesion) ··· 185
    Delayed-Onset Muscle Soreness
    (Type 1b Lesion) ··· 185
    Spine-Related Neuromuscular
    Muscle Disorder (Type 2a Lesion) ··· 186

Muscle-Related Neuromuscular
Muscle Disorder (Type 2b Lesion) ⋯ 186
Minor Partial Muscle Tear (Type 3a Lesion) ⋯ 188
Moderate Partial Muscle Tear
(Type 3b Lesion) ⋯ 188
Subtotal or Complete Muscle Tear/
Tendinous Avulsion ⋯ 190
Contusion ⋯ 190

Ultrasonography of Complications ⋯ 195
Seroma, Cyst ⋯ 195
Fibrosis, Scar ⋯ 195
Myositis Ossificans ⋯ 197
Heterotopic Ossification ⋯ 198
Compartment Syndrome ⋯ 198

8 Magnetic Resonance Imaging ⋯ 203

J. Böck, P. Mundinger, G. Luttke

Relevant Anatomic Microstructure ⋯ 204

**MRI Examination Technique
and Normal Findings** ⋯ 204
Examination Technique ⋯ 204
MRI of Normal Muscle ⋯ 205

**MRI of Functional Muscle
Disorders and Structural Injuries** ⋯ 208
Fatigue-Induced Functional Muscle Disorder (Type 1a)
and Delayed-Onset Muscle Soreness (Type 1b) ⋯ 208
Spine-Related Neuromuscular Muscle Disorder
(Type 2a) ⋯ 208
Muscle-Related Neuromuscular Muscle Disorder
(Type 2b) ⋯ 208
Minor Partial Muscle Tear (Type 3a) ⋯ 209
Moderate Partial Muscle Tear (Type 3b) ⋯ 209
Subtotal or Complete Muscle Tear
and Tendinous Avulsion (Type 4) ⋯ 211
Muscle Contusion, Laceration ⋯ 211
Muscle Herniation ⋯ 213
Muscle Denervation ⋯ 213
Chronic Tendinosis, Tendon Rupture ⋯ 213

Complications ⋯ 215

Seroma/Cyst ⋯ 215
Fibrosis/Scar ⋯ 215
Myositis Ossificans ⋯ 215
Heterotopic Ossification ⋯ 215
Compartment Syndrome ⋯ 216

Differential Diagnosis ⋯ 216
Muscle Edema Pattern ⋯ 216
Fatty Atrophy Pattern ⋯ 216
Tumor, Hematoma, Bony Avulsion Pattern ⋯ 216

Prognostic Criteria ⋯ 217

**Risk Factors for
Recurrent Muscle Injury** ⋯ 217

Specific Muscle Injuries ⋯ 217
Quadriceps Muscle ⋯ 217
Hamstring Muscles ⋯ 220
Adductor Longus Muscle ⋯ 220
Gastrocnemius Muscle ⋯ 220
Less Frequently Involved Muscles ⋯ 220

Summary ⋯ 220

9 Differential Diagnosis of Muscle Pain ⋯ 227

B. Schoser

Special Diagnostic Issues ⋯ 228
Pain History in Myalgia ⋯ 228
Creatine Kinase ⋯ 228
  Macro-Creatine Kinase ⋯ 229
  Creatine Kinase in Healthy Individuals
  and Athletes ⋯ 229
  Rhabdomyolysis ⋯ 229
Indications for Muscle Biopsy ⋯ 229

Neurologic Disorders ⋯ 230
Clinical Symptoms and Lesion Location ⋯ 230
Lesions of the First or Second Motor Neuron ⋯ 232
Peripheral Nerve Lesions ⋯ 232
Muscle Cramps ⋯ 232

Hereditary Muscle Diseases with Myalgia ⋯ 233
Degenerative Myopathies ⋯ 233

Hereditary Metabolic Myopathies ··· 234
Glycogen Storage Diseases ··· 234
Fatty Acid Oxidation Disorders (β-Oxidation) ··· 234
Purine Metabolism Disorders,
Myoadenylate Deaminase Deficiency ··· 234
Mitochondrial Myopathies ··· 234

Nondystrophic and Dystrophic Myotonias ··· 235

Acquired Muscle Diseases with Myalgia ··· 235

Inflammatory Muscle Diseases with Myalgia ··· 235
Infectious Myositis ··· 235
Immunogenic Inflammatory Myopathies:
Dermatomyositis ··· 235

Endocrine Myopathies ··· 237

Toxic Myopathies with Myalgia ··· 237
Alcoholic Myopathy ··· 237
Steroid Myopathy ··· 238
Antilipemic-Associated Myopathy ··· 238

Rheumatologic Diseases ··· 238
Polymyalgia Rheumatica ··· 238

Myofascial Pain Syndrome ··· 239

Relationship of Myalgia to the Classification of Muscle Injuries ··· 242

Fatigue-Induced Muscle Disorder (Type 1a)
Differentiated from Myalgia ··· 242

Spine-Related Neuromuscular Muscle Disorder
(Type 2a) Differentiated from
a Myofascial Trigger Point ··· 242

Muscle-Related Neuromuscular Muscle Disorder
(Type 2b) Differentiated from
a Myofascial Trigger Point ··· 242

Partial Muscle Tears (Type 3) Differentiated
from a Myofascial Trigger Point ··· 242

10 Behavioral Neurology and Neuropsychology in Sports ··· 245
J. M. Hufnagl

The Brain's Influence on Muscles ··· 246

Interaction of Brain and Muscles ··· 246

Behavioral Neurology and Neuropsychology ··· 246

Time, Location, and Perspective
as Pivotal Elements of the World ··· 246

Brain Functions ··· 247

Attention ··· 248

Alertness ··· 249

Memory ··· 249
Declarative Memory ··· 249
Nondeclarative Memory ··· 250

Perception ··· 250

Thinking ··· 250

Language and Communication ··· 251

Autonomic Functions ··· 251

Affects and Emotions ··· 251
The Limbic System ··· 252
Anxiety ··· 252

Anticipation ··· 252

Goal Selection ··· 252

Planning ··· 252

Monitoring ··· 253

Drive and the Hierarchical Relativity
of Brain Functions ··· 253

Consciousness ··· 253

Motor Learning ··· 254

Motivation and Ambition ··· 254

Motives ··· 254

Intrinsic and Extrinsic Motivation ··· 255

Delivering and Optimizing Performance ··· 256

Increasing Demands Due
to Growing Complexity ··· 256

Team Sports ··· 257
The Team as a Unit ··· 258
Social Skills ··· 258
Effects of Muscle Injuries on the Team ··· 258

**Injuries and How the
Brain Deals with Them** ··· 258

Relaxation Techniques ··· 259

Certain and Possible Effects ··· 259

Requirements and Mechanisms Similar
in All Techniques ··· 259

Some Techniques in Detail ··· 260
Schultz Autogenic Training ··· 260
Jacobson Progressive Muscle Relaxation ··· 260
Yoga ··· 260
Tai Ji and Qi Gong ··· 260
Meditation ··· 261
Feldenkrais Technique ··· 261
Hypnosis ··· 261

Applicability of Techniques
in Different Situations ··· 261

Impact of Mental Training
on Athletic Performance ··· 262

Mental "Doping"? ··· 262

Examples from Soccer ··· 263

The Penalty in Soccer—
On the Field and in the Mind ··· 263

Cognition and Emotion as Reciprocal Processes ··· 264

11 Conservative Treatment of Muscle Injuries ··· 267
H.-W. Müller-Wohlfahrt, L. Hänsel, P. Ueblacker, A. Binder

Therapeutic Challenge of Muscle Injuries ··· 268

Primary Care ··· 268

Infiltration Therapy ··· 269

Therapeutic Agents (in Alphabetic Order) ··· 269
  Actovegin (Intramuscular) ··· 269
  Arnica, Trace Elements and Minerals
  (e.g., Enelbin Paste; Topical) ··· 269
  Discus Compositum (Epidural) ··· 270
  Escin (e.g., Reparil) and Bromelains (e.g.,
  Wobenzym, Phlogenzym, Traumanase; Oral) ··· 270
  Lactopurum (Intramuscular, Periligamentous) ··· 270
  Magnesium and Zinc (Oral, Intravenous) ··· 270
  Mepivacaine or Procaine
  (Intramuscular, Epidural, Perineural) ··· 270
  Nonsteroidal Anti-Inflammatory Drugs ··· 270
  Platelet-Rich Plasma (PRP) ··· 270
  Steroids ··· 271
  Traumeel S and Zeel (Intramuscular, Epidural) ··· 271
  Vitamins A, C, and E (Oral, Intravenous) ··· 271

Techniques ··· 271
  Muscle Infiltration Therapy ··· 271
  Spinal Infiltration Therapy ··· 272
  How Infiltration Therapy Works ··· 273
  Technique of Lumbar Infiltration Therapy ··· 274

Monitoring Blood Parameters in Athletes ··· 275

Physical Therapy and Physical Medicine ··· 278

**Treatment Plans for Different Types
of Muscle Injury** ··· 279
  Fatigue-Induced Painful Muscle Disorder
  (Type 1a) ··· 279
  Delayed-Onset Muscle Soreness
  (DOMS; Type 1b) ··· 279
  Neuromuscular Muscle Disorder—
  Spine-Related (Type 2a) ··· 279
  Neuromuscular Muscle Disorder—
  Muscle-Related (Type 2b) ··· 280

  Minor Partial Muscle Tear (Type 3a) ··· 281
  Moderate Partial Muscle Tear (Type 3b) ··· 282
  Subtotal or Complete Muscle Tear/
  Tendinous Avulsion (Type 4) ··· 283

Treatment of Other Muscular Injuries ··· 284
  Muscle Contusions ··· 284
  Functional Compartment Syndrome ··· 285

Treatment of Possible Complications ··· 285
  Myositis Ossificans ··· 285
  Recurrence ··· 286
  Intralesional Cyst Formation/Seroma ··· 286

Focal Toxicosis and Interference Fields ··· 286

Interference Fields ··· 286
  Definition ··· 286
  Otitis Media ··· 287
  Sinusitis ··· 287
  Tonsillitis ··· 287
  Temporomandibular Joint
  (Gnathologic Interference Field),
  Craniomandibular Dysfunction ··· 287
  Teeth ··· 287
  Appendicitis ··· 288
  Intestinal Dysbiosis or Mycosis ··· 288
  Cholecystitis ··· 288
  Chronically Inflamed Hemorrhoids ··· 288
  Genital Interference Fields ··· 288
  Scars ··· 288
  Material Intolerance ··· 288

Gleditsch Functional Circuits ··· 288

Mandel Energy Emission Analysis (EEA) ··· 289
  Lung/Lymph Coronas ··· 292
  Colon/Nerve Degeneration Corona ··· 292
  Triple Burner (TB)/Psyche Corona ··· 292
  Gallbladder/Fatty Degeneration Corona ··· 292
  Isolated Emissions below
  the Second and Third Toes ··· 292

12 Role of the Spine in Muscle Injuries and Muscle Disorders ··· 297
B. Schoser, P. Ueblacker, L. Hänsel, H.-W. Müller-Wohlfahrt

**Relationship between the Spine
and Skeletal Muscles** ··· 298

**Functional Spinal Causes
of Muscular Dysfunction** ··· 299

Hyperlordosis ··· 299

Locked Sacroiliac Joint ··· 299

Functional Leg Length Difference ··· 300

Joint Dysfunctions ··· 300

Sacrum Acutum or Highly Curved Sacrum ··· 300

**Structural Spinal Causes
of Muscular Dysfunction** ··· 301

Pelvic Obliquity, Leg Length Difference ··· 301

Spinal Stenosis ··· 302

Lateral Recess Stenosis, Foraminal Stenosis ··· 302

Disk Bulging and Herniation ··· 302

Spondylolysis, Spondylolisthesis ··· 303

Lumbosacral Ligament ··· 305

**Pseudoradicular Versus
Radicular Symptoms** ··· 305

Symptom Complex of
a Pseudoradicular Syndrome ··· 305

Symptom Complex of a Radicular Syndrome ··· 305

Differentiating between Pseudoradicular
and Radicular Syndromes ··· 306

13 Operative Treatment of Muscle Injuries ··· 307
W. E. Garrett, Jr.

Introduction ··· 308

Indirect Muscle Injuries—Muscle Tears ··· 308

Overview ··· 308

Injury Mechanisms ··· 308

Injury Resulting from Passive Stretch ··· 308

Injury Resulting from Active Stretch ··· 309

Muscle Tears—Hamstrings ··· 309

Distal Injuries ··· 309

Proximal Injuries ··· 309

Surgical Treatment
of Hamstring Avulsions ··· 311

Quadriceps Injuries ··· 312

Contusions of the Quadriceps ··· 312

Surgical Treatment of
Quadriceps Contusions ··· 312

Tears of the Quadriceps ··· 313

Surgical Treatment of Quadriceps Tears ··· 314

Results ··· 315

Muscle Lacerations ··· 316

Conclusions ··· 316

14 Physical Therapy and Rehabilitation ··· 319
K. Eder, H. Hoffmann

Requirements of the Care Team ··· 320

**Positive and Negative Influences
on the Myofascial System** ··· 321

Sport-Specific Changes and
Adaptations of the Musculoskeletal
System in Soccer Players ··· 321

Changes Caused by Contact
of the Kicking Leg with the Ball ··· 322

Support Leg Changes Caused by Kicking
Technique ··· 325

Adaptations of the Pelvic–Leg Axis ··· 326

Physical Therapy Implications
for the Myofascial System ··· 327

Treatment-Oriented Assessment Strategy ··· 327

Clinical Therapeutic Assessment ··· 328

Clinical Motion Analysis ··· 329

Kinesiologic Electromyography (EMG) ··· 329

Methods Used in Medical Training Therapy:
Rehabilitative Performance Testing ··· 330

Isokinetic Testing and Training Systems ··· 331

**Strategies for the Treatment
of Muscle Injuries** ··· 334

Immediate Measures ··· 334
Equipment ··· 334
Initial Inspection ··· 335
Further Treatment on the Sidelines
or in the Locker Room ··· 335
Establishing the Diagnosis ··· 336
Relieving Muscle Taping ··· 336

**General Aspects of Therapeutic Techniques
in the Treatment of Muscle Injuries** ··· 337
Adaptations and Changes
after Muscle Injuries ··· 337
Exaggerated Host Response ··· 339
Phases of Healing ··· 339
Complex Treatment Strategies
for Muscle Injuries ··· 339

Therapeutic Techniques ··· 340

Physical Modalities ··· 340
Electrotherapy ··· 340
Cryotherapy ··· 341

Manual Therapy ··· 343
Myofascial Release Techniques ··· 343
Cervical Fascia ··· 343
Strain–Counterstrain ··· 349
Spray and Stretch ··· 350
Muscle Release Techniques
(Neuromuscular Techniques 1–3) ··· 350
Tender Points and Trigger Points ··· 354

Elastic Taping (Kinesiotaping) ··· 356
Taping for Calf Muscle Inhibition ··· 357
Calf Muscle Taping Plus Lymphatic
Taping over the Achilles Tendon ··· 357
Combined Muscle Taping and Lymphatic Taping
on the Calf ··· 358

Medical Training Therapy ··· 358
Metabolically Oriented Forms of Training ··· 359
Tension-Oriented and Control-Oriented Forms
of Training ··· 360

15 Prevention of Muscle Injuries ··· 365

A. Schlumberger

Mechanisms of Muscle Injury ··· 366

Preventive Training Strategies ··· 367

**Training Measures for Preventive Optimization
of Neuromuscular Function** ··· 367
Flexibility and Stretching ··· 367
Concentric Muscle Function
and Concentric Training ··· 368
Eccentric Muscle Function
and Eccentric Training ··· 369

Force–Length Relationship ··· 370
Intermuscular Coordination ··· 371
Training to Improve Lumbopelvic
Control and Stability ··· 371

Optimizing Basic Fitness ··· 372
Endurance ··· 372
Coordination ··· 376
Warming Up: Importance and Techniques ··· 376

16 Special Case Reports from High-Performance Athletics ··· 381

P. Ueblacker, L. Hänsel, H.-W. Müller-Wohlfahrt

Introduction ··· 382

Cases 1 – 8 ··· 382

Subject Index ··· 405

1

Functional Anatomy
of Skeletal Muscle

D. Blottner

Structure and Function of Skeletal Muscle and the Locomotor System 2
Anatomic Terms in Skeletal Muscle 3
Functional Muscle Compartments as a Structural Principle 7
Muscle Compartments and Their Nerve and Vascular Supply Relative to Injury Risks in Sports 7
Skeletal Muscles and Their Typical Motion Patterns 23

Functional Histology of Muscle Tissue 26
Smooth Muscle 26
Striated Muscle 28
Molecular Architecture of Skeletal Muscle Fibers (Sarcomeres) 29
Satellite Cells (Emergency Cells) 32
Microvasculature and Capillaries 32
Connective Tissue (Myofascial System) 34

Principles of Skeletal Muscle Architecture 35
Skeletal Muscle 35
Muscle Tendons 37
Muscle–Tendon Contacts (Myotendinous Junction) 38
Tendon–Bone Junction 38
Support Structures in Skeletal Muscle 38
Active versus Passive Muscle Insufficiency 42

Innervation of Skeletal Muscle 42
Motor Units and Neuromuscular Synapses 43
Motor End Plate—Neuromuscular Junction 43
Neuromuscular Spindle 44
Golgi Tendon Organ (GTO) 45
Functional Anatomic Principles of Muscle Reflexes 46

The Innervated Locomotor Apparatus 48
Brain and Spinal Cord 48
Plexuses and Peripheral Nerves 50
Reference Muscles and Myotomes 54

Structure and Function of Skeletal Muscle and the Locomotor System

Skeletal muscles form the major part of the active locomotor system in humans (approximately 10% of body weight), alongside the passive locomotor system (the bony skeleton and joints). In male adults, ~40% of the muscle mass accounts for ~28 kg of normal body weight (70 kg). In newborns, the muscle mass amounts to ~20% of total body weight at birth. In athletes, however, the muscle mass may increase to up to 65% of normal body weight.

The human body contains ~640 individual skeletal muscles with ~220 specific muscles, with various sizes, shapes, and locations or fiber architecture (Kunsch and Kunsch 2005). Some muscles are quite long (e.g., the sartorius muscle at the thigh, 40 cm), while others are more broad (e.g., the latissimus dorsi on the back) or rather powerful and fleshy (e.g., the gluteus maximus at the hip). The smallest muscle in the body, the stapedius in the middle ear (< 1 mm), is attached to the stapes, the last of three small middle ear bones, which act as a cushioning or damping control unit to support the mechanical transfer of acoustic impulses from the eardrum (tympanum) to the inner ear structures (oval window of the cochlea). Some muscles are characterized by a high level of endurance and strength (e.g., the triceps surae and the masseter), while others are used for fine tuning of movements (e.g., the extraocular muscles and the palmar interossei and lumbrical muscles in the hand). In more region-specific muscles such as the facial expression muscles, the small fibers can be used for emotional expression and nonverbal communication. Along with the muscles of the tongue, throat, and diaphragm, the facial expression muscles do not primarily belong to the active locomotor apparatus, although in terms of type and origin they can be classified as skeletal muscle.

Note

In sports, defined muscle groups show an increase in muscle mass (hypertrophy) following heavy exercise and can therefore be used in various types of competition for short-duration power generation (e.g., sprinting, jumping, weightlifting) or else for endurance strength (e.g., middle-distance and long-distance running, marathons, swimming, soccer).

Together with the bones (levers) and joints (centers of rotation), the muscles are regarded as damping units in the lever system to help control performance in the weight-bearing musculoskeletal apparatus. For example, if you jump from a chair, the muscles in the thigh and calf that course over the ankles, knees, and hip joints are able to contract muscle by muscle in accordance with a typical pattern known as a "closed muscle chain" to cushion the gravitational load forces generated by the body's weight after the feet hit the floor. This coordinated motion mechanism makes it possible to stabilize the body's posture considerably and generally helps prevent injuries.

By definition, a muscle is attached by its tendon to the bone at its origin (usually proximal to the joint, known as the *origin*) and at its insertion point (usually distal to the same joint, known as the *insertion*). A muscle can run over a single joint, in which case it is known as a single-joint muscle (e.g., the brachialis), or over two or more joints, in which case it is known as a two-joint or multi-joint muscle (e.g., the biceps brachii). The human body contains more than 220 joints (Kunsch and Kunsch 2005) that can be moved by muscle contraction and are referred to as synovial joints, composed of two bony partners with an articular surface cartilage, cleft, and capsule; or as fibrous, cartilaginous, or bony joints, composed of sustainable jointlike structures in which the space between the bony partners (the cleft) is filled with either fibrous material (known as syndesmosis, interosseous ligament), fibrocartilage (known as synchondrosis, symphysis, intervertebral disks), or even bone material (known as synostosis, cranial sutures). Muscle contractions in freely mobile synovial joints result in either gliding, rotating, or angular movements, or combinations of these (diarthrodial function), depending on the design of the joint, whereas muscle contraction may only cause slight mobility in synarthrodial joints, which are mostly needed to support flexibility or stabilization in defined movement segments along the body axis (e.g., sternocostal joints, intervertebral disks, symphysis) or may be almost immobile, as in the cranial sutures.

Muscle contraction causes flexion or bending that brings the two bones closer together—for example, when bending the neck or trunk forward, a movement that is usually performed in the frontal plane (**Table 1.1**). For example, both arms and thighs are flexed when they are lifted anteriorly. The muscles doing so are usually known as flexors (e.g., the flexor carpi radialis). Extension is the reverse of flexion and brings the two bones back to their original position at the same joints. Straightening the fingers after making a fist (extensor digitorum) or straightening the knee during walking movements (quadriceps femoris) are examples of limb extensions. Extension usually moves the trunk into the erect position (erector spinae), or the upper limb (triceps brachii, brachioradialis) or lower limb (gluteus and hamstrings) posteriorly. The terms "supination" and "pronation" refer to movements of the radius around the ulna, resulting in a standard anatomic position of the hand (supination = back of the hand lying supine, supinator), or the reverse movement by showing the palm (pronation = hand lying prone, pronator teres). In the lower limbs, ankle movements resulting in swaying of the foot are usually referred to as inward (inversion) or outward (eversion) motions (**Table 1.1**).

Table 1.1 Orientation and directional terms, body axes

	Latin(-derived) term	Meaning			Latin(-derived) term	Meaning
Systematic arrangement	Anterior	In front of		**Motion terms**	Circumduction	Circular motion (arm, leg)
	Posterior	Behind			Elevation	Lifting body part superiorly
	Dexter	Right side				
	Sinister	Left side			Depression	Moving body part inferiorly
	Distal	Farther from				
	Proximal	Closer to			Opposition	Moving thumb to fingertips
	Dorsal	Toward back		**Planes versus axes of the body**	Median plane (midsagittal; Latin *sagitta*, arrow): median axis	
	Ventral	Toward front				
	External	Toward surface			Frontal (coronal) plane: frontal axis	
	Internal	Away from surface				
	Inferior	Below			Transverse plane: transverse axis	
	Superior	Above				
	Caudal	Toward tail				
	Cranial	Toward head				
	Lateral	Away from midline				
	Medial	Toward midline				
	Profundus	Deep				
	Superficial	Nearer the surface				
Motion terms	Abduction	Lateral raising				
	Adduction	Lateral lowering				
	Protraction	Forward motion				
	Retraction	Backward motion				
	Extension	Straightening				
	Flexion	Bending (flexion)				
	Plantar flexion	Pointing the toes (ankle flexion)				
	Dorsiflexion	Lifting the foot closer to the calf (ankle extension)				
	Pronation/ eversion	Radius rotates over ulna, palm faces posteriorly/turns sole laterally				
	Supination/ inversion	Turns radius and ulna back to parallel, palm faces anteriorly (the hand is lying supine)/ turns sole medially				
	Rotation	Rotational motion (joint)				

The anatomic names of the muscles thus often contain Latin-derived terms that describe the corresponding movements, which can therefore be used to help memorize the anatomic nomenclature of the skeletal muscle system (**Tables 1.1, 1.2**).

Anatomic Terms in Skeletal Muscle

Nomenclature

- *Location.* Some muscle names refer to the location of the muscle—for example, the brachialis muscle is located in the upper arm (Latin *brachium*, upper arm). The intercostales muscles are located between the ribs (Latin *costa*, rib). The flexor digitorum superficialis (superficial = close to the surface) is located above the flexor digitorum profundus (Latin *profundus*, deep).
- *Form and shape.* Some muscles are named after their form and shape. The deltoid muscle, for example, has a triangular shape (similar to the Greek capital letter delta). The left and right portions of the trapezius muscle form a trapeze. The gracilis (from the Latin word for "thin") at the inner thigh has a long, thin shape. The serratus anterior on the lateral thorax consists of fleshy jagged insertions on the ribs that look like a saw blade (Latin *serratus*, serrated). The platysma (from the Greek word for a flat plate) is a broad, thin muscle underneath the skin ("skinny muscle") in the frontal neck region.
- *Size.* The gluteus maximus (Latin *maximus*, largest), gluteus medius (*medius*, medium-sized), and gluteus minimus (Latin *minimus*, smallest) refer to the various muscle sizes. The peroneus longus (long) and brevis (short) on the side of the calf are named after their lengths relative to each other.

Table 1.2   Anatomic nomenclature and definitions (selected)

Latin	English	Latin	English	Latin	English
Angulus	Angle, edge	Fossa	Pit (e.g., armpit)	Planta	Sole of foot
Apertura	Opening	Humerus	Arm bone	Plexus	Network of nerve bundles
Aponeurosis	Flattened ligament/tendon	Incisura	Notch, indentation		
		Intermedius	Located between	Processus	Process
Ante-brachium	Forearm	Interosseus	Lying between bones (e.g., interosseus membrane)	Protrusio	Protrusion, shifting ventrally
Arcus	Arc, arch			Radius	Radius, spoke
Articulatio	Joint	Inter-vertebral	Between vertebrae (intervertebral disk)	Retinacu-lum	Straplike ligament
Axon	Long nerve extension propagating an impulse	Kyphosis	Thoracic curvature (convex) of spine	Scapula	Shoulder blade (pectoral girdle)
Brachium	Arm	Labrum	Liplike bone markings (glenoid lip of scapula)	Scoliosis	Lateral curvature of spine (pathologic)
Brevis	Short				
Bursa	Bursa, synovial "cushion"	Linea	Rimlike bone markings	Spina	Spikelike bony markings
		Longus	Long		
Calcaneus	Heel bone	Lordosis	Lumbar curvature (concave) of the spine	Sternum	Breast bone
Capitulum	Little head (of bone)			Sulcus	Furrow, groove
Carpus, -alis	Carpals, bony crescent at the wrist	Lumbus	Loin; lumbar region	Sustentac-ulum	Prop; bony support
		Margo	Margin of a bone		
Cervical	Belonging to the neck	Meniscus	Semicircular supportive joint structure (fibrous cartilage)	Syn-arthrosis	Articulation; slightly movable bone articulations lacking a synovial cavity
Collum	Neck				
Columna	Column (vertebral column)				
Condylus	Condyle, bone surface that forms joints	Malleolus	Knuckles (ankle joint)	Synchond-rosis	Cartilaginous joint (symphysis), with bones united by fibrous cartilage
		Musculus	Muscle		
Costae	Ribs	Neuron	Nerve cell body		
Cristae	Comblike bony ledges	Obliquus	Lying obliquely	Syndes-mosis	Fastening; fibrous joints, bones united by fibrous tissue (inter-osseous membrane)
Crus, -ris	Shank	Olecranon	Bony process of the ulna (elbow joint)		
Diarthro-ses	Synovial joints (with joint cavity)				
		Os	Bone	Talus	Ankle bone
Discus	Fibrous disklike structure (articular or intervertebral disk)	Palma	Inner surface of hand, palm	Tendo	Tendon
				Thoracic	Pectoral
		Pars	Part of	Thorax	Chest
Digitus	Finger or toe (digital bones)	Patella	Patella (small bone at the knee joint)	Trochanter	Massive lateral process on the proximal femur
Epi-condylus	Area between condyle and shaft of bone	Pecten	Comb; ridgelike bone markings (e.g., pec-tineal line of pubis)	Tuberculum	Hillocklike bony mark-ings
Facies	Plane area (surface)				
Fascia	Connective-tissue sheath (around a muscle)	Perforans	Perforating	Tuberositas	Bony asperity (bony markings)
		Perforatus	Perforated		
		Perios-teum	Connective-tissue ensheathment of bone	Ulna	Ulna
Fascicle	Larger fiber bundle			Vastus	Large, massive
Femur	Femoral bone, femur	Peritenon	Ensheathment of tendon	Venter	Belly (of muscle)
Fibula	Calf bone			Vertebra	Segment of the spinal column
Foramen	Hole (window)	Pelvis	Pelvis		

- *Direction of fibers.* The fibers of the rectus abdominis belly muscle (Latin *rectus*, straight) run parallel to the midline of the body (median), while the transversus abdominis and oblique muscle on the abdominal wall run at right and oblique angles to the midline, respectively.
- *Attachments.* Muscles are principally attached to bone at their origins and insertions. By convention, the origin is the less mobile attachment (Latin *origo*, source or fixed point), while the insertion is the more mobile attachment (Latin *insertio*, input or mobile point) in a normal body position. The origin is always located close to the body's midline (proximal), while the insertion is located away from the midline (distal). The origin of a muscle is always named first, followed by the insertion. For example, the brachioradialis originates from the bone of the forearm (humerus), and inserts on the radius bone more distally. By contrast, some muscles of the shoulder originate from the trunk or head and insert on the scapula (e.g., the trapezius). Muscles that move the head or trunk—for example, the erector spinae in the deep back or the sternocleidomastoid on the lateral neck—originate from lower attachment sites (caudal = from the tail) and insert on upper attachments (cranial = from the head). The muscles of the abdominal wall, the external and internal oblique, originate cranially and insert caudally. While the origin or insertion of a given muscle is always the same by anatomic convention, the fixed and mobile attachments of muscle may switch depending on body position or movements. For example, during dumbbell exercise, the brachialis and biceps brachii contract to lift the lower arm with a load (mobile attachment) closer to the humerus and shoulder (fixed attachments). During chin-ups, however, these muscles perform similarly to bring the body (now with mobile attachments) closer to the lower arm (now with fixed attachments) and bar.
- *Common attachments.* Some muscle groups originate with their overlapping tendons from common attachment sites at prominent bone structures (Latin *caput commune*, common head). Examples are the long extensors (epicondylus lateralis) and flexors (epicondylus medialis) in the forearm. Most of the adductors at the medial thigh originate from the symphysis area or around the frontal pelvic window (obturator foramen), and insert medially on a long ridge on the thigh bone known as the medial lip of the linea aspera of the femur (rough line of the femur).
- *Number of origins.* Muscles can have one or more heads at their origins (Latin *caput*, head), known as the biceps (two heads), triceps (three heads), or quadriceps (four heads). For example, the triceps of the calf has two individual heads (the lateral and medial heads) known as gastrocnemius (Greek *kneme*, calf), and one deep third head known as the soleus (Latin *solea*, sole). The term "vastus" (from the Latin word for "vast, huge") is used for powerful muscle heads such as the vastus lateralis.

- *Actions.* The primary action of a muscle is given with its name, such as flexor (flexion), extensor (extension), and adductor (drawing up) or abductor (drawing away). Examples of these are found in the anatomic names for the forearm and leg muscles (extensor digitorum, adductor hallucis, flexor digitorum), indicating the movements of the hand, foot, and digits.
- *Special descriptions.* Some names indicate special locations or functions of muscles that are related to each other. The extensor carpi radialis longus runs along the radius bone (see the radial group in the forearm muscle compartment) and acts as an extensor on the wrist (Latin *carpus*, wrist). The total length of this muscle is slightly greater than that of other wrist extensors such as the extensor carpi radialis brevis (Latin *brevis*, short), as it originates proximally from the lateral epicondyle of the forearm bone.

Note

The origin and insertion attachments of muscle are defined by anatomic nomenclature according to their more mobile or less mobile (fixed) attachment points. However, depending on performance control, the functional names for the attachments may be reversed, as in the example of the biceps and triceps forearm muscles during press-ups.

Skeletal Muscle Fiber Types

Type I and Type II Fibers

In adults, skeletal muscles are composed of a genetically determined pattern of muscle fiber types:
- Fast-twitch (oxidative-glycolytic and glycolytic) fibers, known as explosive-like power fibers (type II)
- Slow-twitch (oxidative) fibers, referred to as endurance fibers (type I)

In the embryo, early skeletal muscle dispositions are initially composed of cohorts of slow-twitch type I fibers. During development, the early type II fibers are then generated in fiber dispositions surrounding the type I fiber populations (known as cluster formation) due to the start of muscle use and its functional innervation around the time of birth. Thus, a unique distribution pattern of slow and fast fibers is generated during postnatal development, adolescence, and during adulthood in a muscle-specific way (**Fig. 1.1**). The quadriceps femoris, for example, represents a typical fast/slow mixed fiber type with an explosivelike power output (~60% type II versus 40% type I). As the deep part of the triceps surae, the soleus muscle represents a typically slow/fast mixed fiber type with strong postural or endurance capacity (~50% slow-type and 50% fast-type fibers).

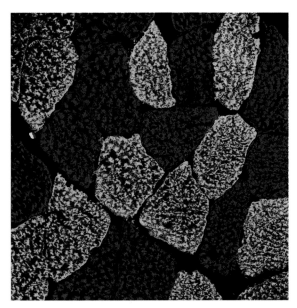

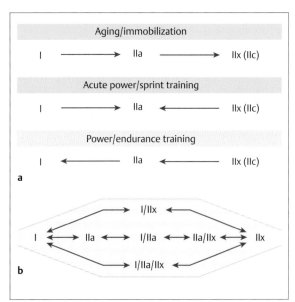

Fig. 1.1 The typical fiber distribution pattern in normal human skeletal muscle (soleus biopsy). Myosin heavy chain (MyHC) immunostaining for slow (type I, red) and fast (type II, green) MyHC in cross-sectional myofibers. Original image: M. Salanova, Charité Berlin, ZWMB, Germany.

Fig. 1.2a, b Muscle plasticity (fiber switching) following exercise or disuse.

a Skeletal muscle fiber types are classified according to their myosin heavy chain (MyHC) content into: type I (endurance), type IIa (fast-switch) or type IIx/IIc (high power output, but rapidly fatigable). The arrows indicate possible fiber adaptation (plasticity) following training or immobilization, which is reflected in MyHC fiber switching of the contractile apparatus of the muscle fiber in both directions.

b Altered amounts of hybrid fibers expressing variable slow and fast MyHCs (I/IIa; IIa/IIx; I/IIx) following a training pause or in the elderly may be signs of remodeling mechanisms.

Patterns of Transition

Human skeletal muscle also contains a certain number of fast fibers as transition forms (type IIa, IIb or IIc/IIx), depending on muscle activity. However, there is an overall distribution pattern in male and female skeletal muscle that shows heterogeneity of fiber types depending on everyday lifestyle, sports, activity status in childhood, adolescence, senescence (sedentary occupations versus athletes). The pattern of fiber types in skeletal muscle may therefore not be static or irreversible, and instead follows a continuum of change throughout life (**Fig. 1.2**).

> *Note*
>
> The fiber pattern of a muscle may not be permanently fixed, but may be significantly altered in either direction by intensive muscle training, long-duration intermittent training stops, or even by immobilization (**Fig. 1.2**).

The types of skeletal muscle fibers are based on the presence of myosin heavy-chain (MyHC) proteins, which are part of the contractile myofilament apparatus (sarcomere) in variable amounts in rapidly fatigable type IIa fibers or slowly fatigable type I fibers that are continuously used during performance control (gait, stance). In addition, another fiber type, IIc/x (with a high power output but very rapidly fatigable), is found in athletes and can be transformed from undisclosed reserve fibers of the type IIa fiber pool by intensive training protocols. In a given muscle, the IIx fiber pool allows the highest power output sporadically, such as during jumping. Exhausting training proto-

cols are likely to result in a fiber shift from type I to type IIa (in sprinters), while endurance exercises may shift the fiber pattern from type IIa to type I (in marathon and long-distance runners).

An increase in hybrid fiber formation (slow and fast MyHC expressed in one fiber, estimated at about 5–10% per muscle) is usually an indicator of intramuscular adaptation or a remodeling mechanism following intensive periods of training or after longer training intervals. Skeletal muscle plasticity may thus affect physiological functions, including endurance capacity, muscle fatigue, or power and force in a given muscle.

> *Note*
>
> The immunohistochemical MyHC type I fiber pattern shifts from type I to type IIa or IIc fibers in the elderly or following prolonged immobilization, which may seem paradoxical. However, this should be regarded as a maladaptation of intramuscular fiber type distribution mechanisms that lacks a normal translation of sarcomeric contractile proteins into force and power, as there will be a decline rather than an increase in muscle force and power following a disuse-induced fiber switch (Snobl et al. 1998).

Functional Muscle Compartments as a Structural Principle

From head to feet, the skeletal muscle apparatus of the human body is covered by a general fascia comparable to a whole-body stocking (cat suit). In this model, the skin—composed of hairs, sweat glands, vascular supply, and cutaneous nerves embedded in connective tissue—covers the general fascia and skeletal musculature and thus provides the final border layer between the body and the environment. However, the facial expression muscles are part of the skin layer without having a muscle fascia of their own. The actual skeletal muscles are located underneath the general body fascia (subfascially), embedded in special ensheathments such as muscle fascia and muscle compartments (**Fig. 1.3**).

The overall shapes of the typical muscle compartments in the upper and lower limbs resemble long tubes or longitudinally oriented spaces separated by fibrous connective-tissue sheets, known as septal walls or box fascia (**Fig. 1.4**). Muscle compartments contain one or more (mostly up to three) individual muscles with similar functions and are therefore termed flexor, extensor, or adductor compartments. Muscles in the same compartment usually work synergistically. Muscles from opposite compartments in the body work as antagonists, and are referred to as flexor compartments versus extensor compartments of the limbs, for example (see **Fig. 1.12**, p. 23).

Muscle compartments are classified and named according to their location in the trunk or extremities, such as the ventral and dorsal compartments of the forearm. Each compartment receives its own anatomically distinct vascular and nerve supply (afferent arteries, muscular nerves) that course via intermuscular fascicles or bundles to enter the target muscles in a given compartment. There, the nerves and arteries subdivide at the level of intramuscular connective tissue into smaller bundles that terminate in the microvascular capillary bed around smaller groups of myofibers and single fibers. The fascia of both the muscle compartment and the individual muscle belly may contain mechanosensors (mostly Pacini corpuscles), as well as pain sensors (nociceptors), which are responsible for local pain sensation and proprioceptive control (postural control) in the various motion segments of the musculoskeletal system.

Practical Tip

In this chapter, the classification of the muscle compartments is based on a functional anatomic perspective. The way in which the muscle compartments are presented can be used as a simple principle to help with general orientation, as well as for better understanding of the functional architecture of the human skeletal muscle system in sports. Understanding the general principles and more specific topographic relations between the muscle compartments and the nerve supply may be helpful in further understanding of performance control in individual body regions. It may also be helpful for finding easier ways of reaching a faster diagnosis for local muscle injuries and their possible effects on adjacent muscle groups that may result in compensatory movement patterns, in terms of protective postures.

Muscle Compartments and Their Nerve and Vascular Supply Relative to Injury Risks in Sports

For fast orientation, only those muscle compartments that may be associated with a special risk for injury in sports, for example, are described below with their individual muscle groups and their particular neurovascular supply (**Figs. 1.5** to **1.11**). Specifically, individual muscles have been selected from the muscle compartments of the trunk, forearm, pelvic girdle, and lower extremity and are listed by description, origin, insertion, action, and nerve supply in accordance with functional anatomic terminology (**Tables 1.3** to **1.11**).

Practical Tip

Following muscle injury, both muscle swelling and disruption of vascular structures in a muscle compartment may result in an acute compartment syndrome that has to be medically treated to prevent ischemia due to blood congestion. Otherwise, there will be a risk of more severe tissue damage—as typically seen, for example, in the anterior compartment of the lower leg. The treatment may thus include skin incision and transection of the affected muscle fascia (fasciotomy) as an acute method of relieving congestion pressure. A chronic compartment syndrome may occur in extensively trained athletes, for example. This symptom is associated with pain during exercise due to microtears in fibers and swelling, which increases intracompartmental pressure, while pain is usually relieved when the exercise is completed.

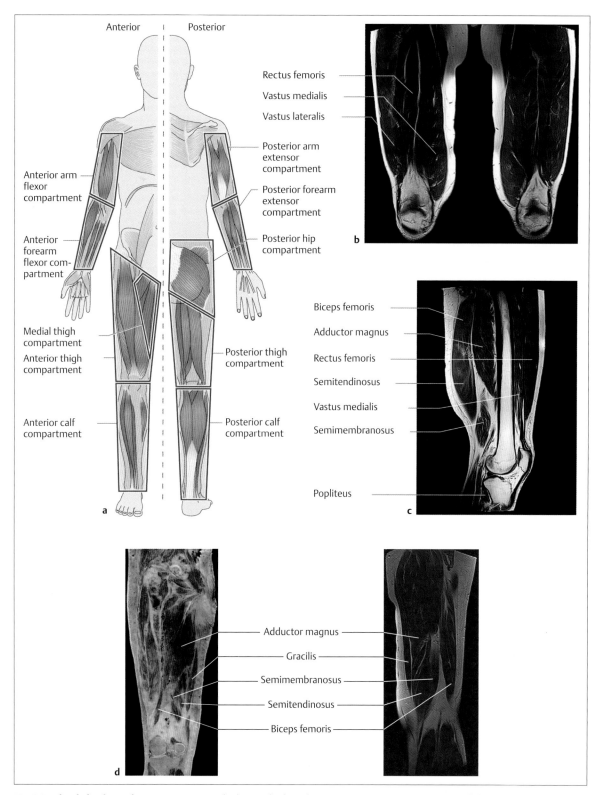

Fig. 1.3a–d Skeletal muscle compartments in the human body and magnetic resonance images (MRIs) of the thigh muscle compartments (examples).

a View from anterior (left) and from posterior (right), showing the anatomic location of the individual muscle compartments that are most relevant to sports injuries (for the intrinsic trunk muscles, see **Tables 1.3** and **1.4**).

b MRI. The anterior thigh muscle compartment (coronal view). 1, vastus lateralis; 2, rectus femoris; 3, vastus medialis.

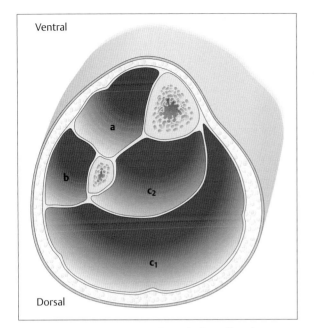

Fig. 1.4 Cross-sectional view through the calf, with "empty" muscle compartments. a, extensor calf muscle compartment; b, lateral calf muscle compartment (peroneus compartment); c_1, superficial flexor calf muscle compartment; c_2, deep flexor calf muscle compartment.

Trunk Muscles

Abdominal Wall Muscles

The sheetlike abdominal muscles (**Fig. 1.5** and **Table 1.3**), external oblique, internal oblique, transversus abdominis, and rectus abdominis span the lower thoracic cage to the pelvic girdle and compress the abdominal wall during heavy lifting. They receive their nerve supply via intercostal nerves (T7–T12) as well as from the iliocostal and ilioinguinal nerves coursing freely between the broad flat muscle sheets. The intercostal or subcostal arteries run in parallel to the abdominal wall and provide the blood supply.

The rectangular, fleshy quadratus lumborum in the deep lumbar region (**Fig. 1.5**) is supplied by the subcostal nerve (an extra intercostal nerve that has no intercostal space) and subcostal artery.

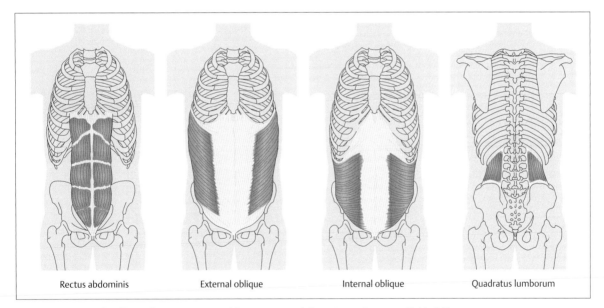

| Rectus abdominis | External oblique | Internal oblique | Quadratus lumborum |

Fig. 1.5 Abdominal wall muscle compartments (the transversus abdominis not shown; see **Table 1.3**).

Fig. 1.3a–d *continued*

c MRI. The anterior and posterior thigh muscle compartments (sagittal view). 1, adductor magnus; 2, semitendinosus; 3, semimembranosus; 4, biceps femoris; 5, popliteus; 6, rectus femoris; 7, vastus medialis.

d Anatomic dissection in comparison with MRI of the medial thigh muscle compartment (coronal views). *Left panel:* An anatomically dissected thigh from a 73-year-old man, showing a coronal view of the medial thigh muscles. The connective-tissue invasion (intramuscular and intermuscular adipose tissue) and slight re-

duction in muscle size due to aging should be noted. (Dissection and image courtesy of F. Glöckner and E. Heuckendorf, Department of Anatomy, Charité Berlin, Germany.) *Right panel:* An MRI image from a healthy 32-year-old man with well-trained medial thigh muscles using coronal view comparable to dissected thigh in the left panel. (MRI images in **Fig. 1.3b–d** courtesy of D. Belavý, Center for Bone and Muscle Research, Charité Berlin, Germany.)

Table 1.3   Abdominal wall muscle compartment—major actions: lumbar flexors, lateral flexors, lumbar rotators, and breathing assistance

	Muscle	Description (palpation)	Origin (O), insertion (I)	Innervation (segments)	Action
Lumbar flexors	Rectus abdominis (*rectus*, *straight*) Pyramidalis	Medial pair of flat muscles ensheathed by aponeurosis (rectus sheath) from lateral muscles; extends from ribs to pelvis, segmented by three tendinous intersections	O: Costal cartilages of ribs 5–7 I: Pubic crest and symphysis	Intercostal nerves T5–T12	• Flexes and rotates lumbar region • Stabilizes pelvis • Works against intra-abdominal pressure • Assists in forced expiration
Lateral flexors	External oblique	Most superficial flat muscle of abdominal wall, with fibers running downward obliquely from lateral to medial (like hands in pants pockets!)	O: Outer surfaces of ribs 5–12 I: Lateral aponeurosis of rectus sheath (outer sheet)	Intercostal nerves T5–T12 Iliohypogastric nerve	As for rectus abdominis • Lateral flexion (ipsilaterally) • Rotates trunk contralaterally
	Internal oblique	Flat middle muscle of abdominal wall, with fibers running obliquely from medial to lateral (opposite to external oblique)	O: Lumbar fascia (deep), iliac crest, inguinal ligament I: Costal margin, rectus sheath	Intercostal nerves T8–T12 Iliohypogastric and ilioinguinal nerves	As for external oblique • Rotates trunk ipsilaterally
	Transversus abdominis	Innermost flat muscle of abdominal wall, with horizontal fibers	O: Lumbar fascia (deep), iliac crest, anterior superior iliac spine (ASIS) I: Rectus sheath (inner sheet)	As internal oblique, plus genitofemoral nerve	• Abdominal pressure bilaterally • Rotation (ipsilateral)
Lumbar rotators	Quadratus lumborum	Fleshy deep muscle forming part of posterior abdominal wall	O: Iliac crest I: Costae 12 + transverse processes of lumbar vertebrae 1–4	12th intercostal nerve Subcostal nerve and upper lumbar nerves (ventral rami)	• Abdominal pressure bilaterally • Lateral flexion unilaterally • Assists in forced inspiration

Muscles of the Vertebral Column

The local intrinsic back muscles, known as the erector spinae (**Fig. 1.6** and **Table 1.4**) span the pelvis, vertebral column, and dorsal thoracic cage structures (ribs). The erector spinae is subdivided into three large columns located lateral to the vertebral column (lateral tract, straight system) and in the deeper back as a set of shorter columns medial to the vertebral column (medial tract, oblique system). The neck muscles are formed by a continuation of the two columns from the back to the head (e.g., the semispinalis and longissimus group). The intrinsic muscle groups are covered by a large fascia known as the thoracolumbar fascia, which runs from the pelvis to the head. The erector spinae is mostly covered by superficial muscles, the broad and flat latissimus dorsi and trapezius, the spinocostalis group, superior and inferior serratus, and the scapulospinal group of rhomboid muscles.

The erector spinae receives its nerve supply via the dorsal rami of the spinal nerves from each of the spinal cord segments, which thus penetrate the muscle in a segmental pattern. The deep neck muscles, rectus capitis and obliquus capitis, are innervated by the first dorsal ramus of spinal nerve C1, known as the suboccipital nerve. The intrinsic back muscles are supplied by dorsal rami of the intercostal arteries, and the deep neck muscles by the occipital artery.

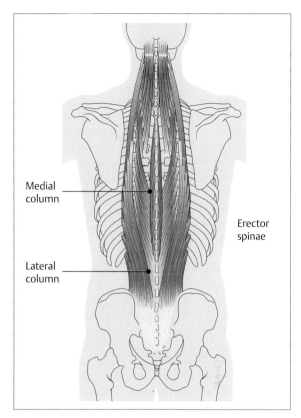

Fig. 1.6 Posterior trunk muscle compartment. The erector spinae, with lateral and medial columns (intrinsic back muscles).

Muscles of the Anterior and Posterior Arm Compartments

The anterior arm muscle compartment spans the shoulder, elbow joints, wrist, and finger joints (arm flexor compartment, **Fig. 1.7a** and **Table 1.5.**) and is supplied by the musculocutaneous nerve (humerus) or the medial and ulnar nerve (forearm). The posterior brachium and forearm muscle compartment (arm extensor compartment, **Fig. 1.7b** and **Table 1.5**) is supplied by the radial nerve. All of the arm muscle compartments are supplied by the subclavian artery (major afferent artery), brachial artery and

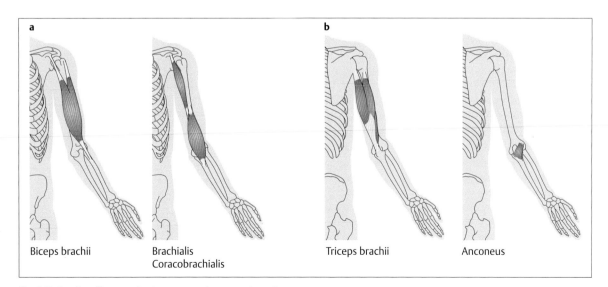

Fig. 1.7a, b Arm flexor and extensor muscle compartments.
a Arm flexor compartment (anterior view). **b** Arm extensor compartment (posterior view).

Table 1.4   Posterior trunk intrinsic muscle compartment—major actions: prime extensors of back and neck and lateral trunk flexors

	Muscle	Description (palpation)	Origin (O), insertion (I)	Innervation (segments)	Action
Prime extensors of back	Erector spinae	Composite intrinsic back muscle with two major columns (lateral and medial), running parallel to the spinal column	O: Sacrum, iliac crest, spine I: Via vertebrae, posterior ribs, and cervical column to occiput	Spinal nerves Lateral rami C1–L5	• Extension (bilateral) • Lateral trunk flexion and rotation (unilateral)
	Lateral column (LC) • Iliocostalis • Longissimus • Splenius	Long muscle strands extending from pelvis via thorax to neck, running more laterally to the spine (intermediate back muscle) Segmented muscle strands extending from the pelvis via thorax to the neck, running more medially to the spine (deepest back muscles)	O (Long.): Os sacrum, iliac crest I (Iliocost.): Costae 3–12, transverse processes of lumbar through cervical vertebrae (Long.) O. (Splenius): Spinal processes of thoracic vertebrae 3–6 I: Transverse processes cervical vertebrae 1–2 and mastoid		
	Medial column (MC) • Spinales • Semispinales • Rotators • Multifidus		O: Transverse processes of lumbar to cervical spine or sacrum (multifidus) I: Spinal processes from lumbar to cervical vertebrae and ligamentum nuchae and occiput		
Deep muscles of the neck	Major rectus capitis	Deep small muscles linking first and second cervical spine with occiput, used for fine adjustment for head and neck joints	O: Spinous process of axis (C2) I: Inferior nuchal line	Suboccipital nerve (C1), dorsal rami	• Head extension (bilateral) • Head rotation (ipsilateral)
	Minor rectus capitis		O: Superior tubercle of atlas (C1) I: Inferior nuchal line	Suboccipital nerve (C1), dorsal rami	As major rectus capitis
	Superior oblique capitis	Muscles closely linked to the vestibular system, head balance	O: Transverse process of atlas (C1) I: Inferior nuchal line	Suboccipital nerve (C1), dorsal rami	As major rectus capitis and • Lateral flexion (unilateral)
	Inferior oblique capitis		O: Spinous process of axis (C2) I: Transverse process of atlas (C1)	Suboccipital nerve (C1), dorsal rami	As major rectus capitis

Table 1.5 Posterior and anterior arm muscle compartment—major actions: extension and flexion of arm and forearm

	Muscle	Description (palpation)	Origin (O), insertion (I)	Innervation (segments)	Action
Posterior arm compartment	Triceps brachii (*triceps*, three-headed; *brachium*, arm) • Long head (LoH) • Lateral head (LH) • Medial head (MH)	Fleshy three-headed muscle of the posterior arm compartment; long and lateral heads lie superficial to medial head; inserts with common tendon to posterior elbow	O: • Infraglenoid tubercle of scapula (LoH) • Proximal part of humerus shaft (LH) • Distal third of humerus shaft (MH) I: Olecranon process of ulna (common tendon)	Radial nerve C6–C8	• Extension • Stabilization of shoulder • Adduction
	Anconeus (*ancon*, elbow)	Short triangular muscle located between posterior humerus and ulna; works mainly as stretcher of elbow capsule (protection)	O: Lateral epicondyle of humerus I: Lateral aspect of ulnar olecranon process	Radial nerve C6–C8	• Extension • Tensor (stretcher) of elbow capsule
Anterior arm compartment	Biceps brachii (*biceps*, two-headed; *brachium*, arm) • Long head (LH) • Short head (SH)	Fleshy two-headed (long and short head) muscle of anterior arm compartment with common tendon on the radius, and with superficial aponeurosis for medial taping of the common proximal heads of the forearm flexors	O: • Supraglenoid tubercle (LH) • Coracoid process of scapula (SH) I: Radial tuberosity	Musculocutaneous nerve C5–C7	Elbow: • Flexion • Supination (in flexed position) Shoulder: • Abduction • Medial rotation • Arm protraction
	Brachialis	Solid muscle belly, below brachialis on distal humerus	O: Distal front of humerus I: Ulnar tuberosity	Musculocutaneous nerve C5–C7	• Flexion
	Brachioradialis (*radius*, spoke of wheel)	Superficial muscle of lateral arm/forearm, extends from distal humerus via forearm to radial carpals	O: Lateral supracondylar ridge at distal humerus I: Styloid process of radius	Radial nerve C5–C7	• Flexion (extension) • Semipronation
	Coracobrachialis (*coracoides*, like a crow's beak)	Slender, cylindrical muscle of medial arm and armpit	O: Coracoid of scapula I: Medial third of humerus	Musculocutaneous nerve C6–C7	• Flexion • Adduction

their collaterals/branches (humerus), by branches of the radial and ulnar artery (forearm), and by an arterial circuit (palmar arc) and digital arteries in the hand for supply of the thenar, hypothenar, and palmar muscles.

Muscles of the Hip, Buttocks, and Leg

Muscle Compartment of the Hip and Buttocks

The anterior muscle compartment of the hip (**Fig. 1.8** and **Table 1.6**.) spans the hip joint and includes the iliopsoas, which is innervated by the femoral nerve, L2–L3, and the posterior hip muscle compartment, including the buttocks

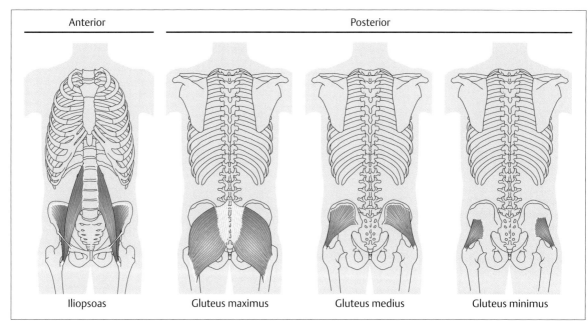

Anterior	Posterior
Iliopsoas	Gluteus maximus	Gluteus medius	Gluteus minimus

Fig. 1.8   The pelvic girdle muscles. The hip compartment (anterior view) and gluteus compartment (posterior view)

Table 1.6   Posterior hip and gluteus muscle compartments—major actions: flexors/extensors of thigh and leg rotators/abductors

	Muscle	Description (palpation)	Origin (O), insertion (I)	Innervation (segments)	Action
Hip muscles	Psoas major + minor (*psoa*, loin muscles)	Long and thick medial muscle, crossing the hip joint, long head of the iliopsoas	O: Transverse processes of lumbar spine incl. bodies and disks I: Lesser trochanter	Femoral nerve T12–L3 Direct branches of lumbar plexus	• Prime thigh flexion • Trunk flexion
	Iliacus (*ilium*, groin)	Fan-shaped more lateral muscle crossing the hip joint, flat head of the iliopsoas	O: Iliac fossa I: Lesser trochanter of femur	As for psoas	As for psoas
	Tensor fasciae latae (TFL) (*tensor*, stretcher; *latus*, wide, broad)	The TFL has its own fascia pocket located at lateral hip/thigh region to stretch the tendinous band of the iliotibial tract and the broad thigh fascia ensheathment (fascia lata), comparable to a support stocking for all thigh muscles	O: Anterior superior iliac spine (ASIP) I: Iliotibial tract	Superior gluteal nerve L4–S1	• Stretcher of fascia and iliotibial tract also • Hip abduction, hip flexion, medial rotation (thigh)

Table 1.6 Posterior hip and gluteus muscle compartments—major actions: flexors/extensors of thigh and leg rotators/abductors *(continued)*

	Muscle	Description (palpation)	Origin (O), insertion (I)	Innervation (segments)	Action
Gluteal muscles	Gluteus maximus (*glutos*, buttock)	Largest muscle of the gluteus compartment that forms bulk of buttock mass, covers all other gluteal muscles, ischial tuberosity and sciatic nerve	O: Sacrum, ilium, lumbar fascia, sacrotuberal ligament I: Iliotibial tract and gluteal tuberosity	Inferior gluteal nerve L5–S2	• Prime thigh extensor • Thigh abduction • Adduction
	Gluteus medius (*medius*, middle)	Thick muscle beneath gluteus max., site of i. m. injections	O: Lateral surface of ilium I: Greater trochanter top	Superior gluteal nerve L4–S1	• Thigh abduction • Hip stabilizer
	Gluteus minimus	Smallest and deepest muscle of the gluteus compartment	O: External surface of ilium I: Greater trochanter top	Superior gluteal nerve L4–S1	• Thigh abduction • Hip stabilizer
	Piriformis (*pirum*, pear; *forma*, shape)	Pyramidal muscle that spans the greater sciatic notch to insert at the greater trochanter	O: Sacrum (opposite greater sciatic notch) I: Trochanteric fossa	Sacral plexus sacralis L5–S2	• Abduction • Lateral rotation
	Gemellus superior and inferior (*Gemellus*, twin)	Pairs of small muscles with common insertions at trochanteric fossa of femur	O: Ischiadic spine and ischial tuberosity (inf.) I: Trochanteric fossa	Sacral plexus L5–S2	• As for piriformis
	Obturator internus	Deep muscle originating from inner pelvic foramen to insert on femur	O: Inner pelvic foramen I: Trochanteric fossa	Sacral plexus L5–S2	• As for piriformis
	Quadratus femoris	Short and thick muscle most inferior of lateral thigh rotators	O: Ischial tuberosity I: Intertrochanteric crest of femur	Inferior gluteal nerve L5–S2	• Lateral rotation • Hip stabilizer

(gluteus, tensor fasciae latae), which is innervated by the inferior or superior gluteal nerve, L5–S2 (sacral plexus). The deep muscles of the gluteal region (lateral rotators) are supplied directly by rami of the sacral plexus, L5–S2. The common iliac artery supplies the iliopsoas, and the superior and inferior gluteal arteries provide the blood supply to the gluteus and rotator muscles.

Anterior Muscle Compartment of the Thigh

The anterior muscle compartment of the thigh spans the hip and knee joints and contains the quadriceps femoris and sartorius (**Fig. 1.9a** and **Table 1.7**). The femoral nerve (lumbar plexus, L2–L4) and femoral artery (from the external iliac artery) provide the neurovascular support for this compartment.

Injury during sports or femoral nerve lesions in the quadriceps result in an extenuated knee extension. Thus, the ability to rise up from a seat or climb stairs is weakened but not fully prevented, as it can be compensated for by pressing the hand onto the knee during rising. Some patients are able to stabilize their upright position using the iliotibial tract (gluteus maximus, tensor fascia

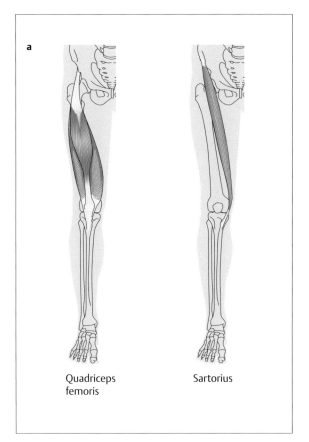

Quadriceps
femoris

Sartorius

lata) or by leaning forward slightly, as gravity simulates an extension force.

At major muscle tendon attachment sites to bone such as the patella, tibial tuberosity, and anterior superior iliac spine (ASIS), a condition known as painful insertion tendopathy may develop during excessive exercise training in sports. Atrophy of the anterior thigh muscles may result in partial luxation of the patella. This can be prevented by specific training of the vastus medialis to prevent the potential risk of lateral patellar luxation. In general, strengthening the quadriceps using specific training protocols may effectively counteract disturbed functioning (instability) in the knee joint.

Note

The sartorius has a major function as a guidance muscle for all the major movements of the thigh involving the hip and knee joint, such as when standing or even during the initial swaying phases of walking. The sartorius can therefore serve as a functional "global player" during thigh movements. However, it is rarely injured in sports.

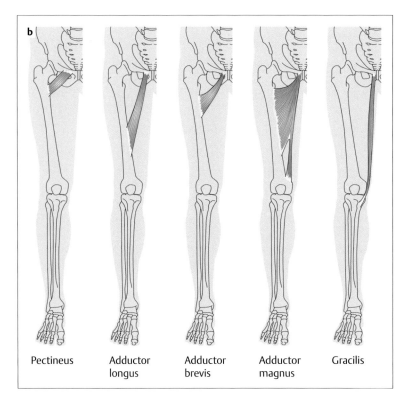

Pectineus

Adductor longus

Adductor brevis

Adductor magnus

Gracilis

Fig. 1.9a, b Thigh muscle compartment.

a Anterior thigh compartment (knee extensors).
b Medial thigh compartment (adductors).

Table 1.7 Anterior thigh muscle compartment—major actions: knee extension, hip flexion, and other leg motions (sartorius)

	Muscle	Description (palpation)	Origin (O), insertion (I)	Innervation (segments)	Action
Knee extensors	Quadriceps femoris: (*quadriceps*, four heads) • Rectus femoris (RF) (*rectus*, straight) • Vastus medialis (VM) (*vastus*, massive) • Vastus lateralis (VL) • Vastus intermedius (VI) • Articularis genus (*genu*, knee)	Massive superficial four-headed muscle of anterior thigh, runs straight down thigh (RF), with common tendon insertion via patella to the tibial tuberosity Quadriceps tone stabilizes knee function A small articularis genus muscle originates from distal intermedius fibers to serve as "capsule stretcher" of suprapatellar recessus of the proximal knee joint	O: • RF: anterior inferior iliac spine (AIIS) • VM: linea aspera (medial lip) • VL: linea aspera (lateral lip) • VI: frontal femur shaft I: (All) via patellar ligaments and tibial tuberosity (primary extensor apparatus); (VM, VL) via retinacular ligaments to supracondylar line of the tibia (secondary extensor apparatus)	Femoral nerve L2–L4	• Knee extension (prime movers) • Hip flexion (rectus femoris) • "Joint capsule stretcher" (articularis)
Sartorius	Sartorius (*sartor*, tailor)	A very long and slender muscle running obliquely across anterior thigh over medial knee joint, a two-joint muscle with variable actions. Muscle helps to produce cross-legged position	O: Anterior superior iliac spine (ASIP) I: Tibial tuberosity (medially)	Femoral nerve L2–L4	• Guidance muscle for producing fore-swing phase of walking • Hip flexion • Abduction/adduction • Knee flexion (weak)

Medial Muscle Compartment of the Thigh

The medial muscle compartment of the thigh spans the hip joint and contains the adductor muscles (adductor compartment of the thigh, **Fig. 1.9b** and **Table 1.8**) that are used in pelvic tilting movements and during walking or running. The adductor muscle compartment is supplied by the obturator nerve, L2–L4 (lumbar plexus), and by the obturator artery (a branch of the internal iliac artery). In sports, acute or chronic mechanical stress or stretching of the adductor tendon of origin (gracilis, adductor magnus and longus) often results in inguinal problems ("pulled groin") due to high load exercises, which may cause sharp pain originating in the thigh and radiating to the pubic or inguinal region. Alternatively, extensive tension on a muscle may result in local spindlelike pain, possibly induced by microlesions in intramuscular structures concentrated in the muscle belly that are regarded as being the weakest part of a muscle following mechanical overload, in comparison with its tougher tendinous endings or tendon–bone interfaces (see the note on entheses, p. 38).

Posterior Muscle Compartment of the Thigh

The posterior muscle compartment of the thigh spans the hip and knee joints and contains three fleshy muscles with variable architectures known as hamstrings, the biceps femoris, semitendinosus, and semimembranosus (**Fig. 1.10** and **Table 1.9**). The hamstrings are supplied by the tibial nerve, L5–S2 (a branch of the sciatic nerve), and by the deep femoral artery, which gives rise to at least three or four perforating arteries that pass through directly from the adductor magnus to the hamstring compartment. Following injury to the tibial nerve, walking and mounting stairs is weakened due to muscle atrophy, which may be partly compensated for by an intact gluteus maximus.

Lower Leg

The muscles of the anterior compartment of the lower leg cross the ankle and toe joints and consist of three powerful muscles, the tibialis anterior, extensor digitorum, and extensor hallucis longus, used for dorsiflexion of the foot (an extension by definition) (**Fig. 1.11a** and **Table 1.10**).

Table 1.8 Medial thigh muscle compartment—major action: thigh adduction

	Muscle	Description (palpation)	Origin (O), insertion (I)	Innervation (segments)	Function
Thigh adductors	Obturator externus (obturatus, congested; externus, outside)	Flat triangular muscle covering the outer aspect of the pelvic foramen deep in the medial thigh, fully covered by the pectineus	O: Obturator membrane I: Trochanteric fossa	Obturator nerve L2–L4	• Adduction • Lateral rotation • Pelvis stabilization
	Pectineus (pecten, comb)	Short and flat muscle on proximal thigh (groin) overlying adductor brevis	O: Pectineal line of pubis I: Pectineal line of posterior aspect of femur	Obturator nerve L2–L4 (femoral nerve, var.)	As for obturator externus
	Adductor longus (longus, long)	Most anterior of adductors; overlies middle part of adductor magnus	O: Pubis near symphysis I: Linea aspera (distal medial lip)	Obturator nerve L2–L4	As for adductor magnus
	Adductor brevis (brevis, short)	Short and deep muscle concealed by the adductor longus and pectineus	O: Pubis (inferior ramus) I: Linea aspera (proximal medial lip)	Obturator nerve L2–L4	As for adductor magnus
	Adductor magnus (adduco, bring toward; magnus, large)	Large, triangular muscle with broad insertions located more deeply in the medial thigh. Fleshy part inserts at linea aspera and tendinous part at supracondylar tuberosity to form adductor gap	O: Pubis (inferior ramus), ischiadic and ischial rami I: Linea aspera (deep); medial epicondyle (superficial) and adductor tubercle of femur	Obturator nerve L2–L4	• Adduction • Medial rotation • Hip extension • Pelvis stabilization
	Gracilis (gracilis, slender)	Straplike superficial muscle of medial thigh that runs straight from the symphysis down to the medial knee joint inferior to the medial condyle	O: Symphysis (ramus inferior) I: Medial tibial surface	Obturator nerve L2–L4	As for adductors, but also • Knee flexion

The anterior compartment of the lower leg is supplied by the deep peroneal (fibular) nerve, L5–S1 (lumbar plexus), and by an extension of the popliteal artery known as the anterior tibial artery. Muscle injury in this compartment may result in a typical clinical syndrome known as "compartment syndrome."

The muscles of the lateral muscle compartment of the lower leg cross the ankle and are reflected by two muscles, the peroneus fibularis longus and brevis, which are used for plantar flexion and eversion (lateral raising of the foot) and stabilization of the lateral ankle and longitudinal arch of the foot (mainly the peroneus longus) (**Fig. 1.11b**). The peroneus (fibularis) muscle compartment is innervated by the superficial peroneal nerve and supported by an extension of the deep tibial artery known as the peroneal or fibular artery.

There are two posterior muscle compartments in the lower leg: a superficial one contains the triceps surae, gastrocnemius and soleus, with a common strong tendon inserted to the calcaneus (heel) used for ankle flexion (**Fig. 1.11c**). The deep compartment contains three long muscles, the flexor digitorum, flexor hallucis longus, and tibialis posterior, that cross the ankle and toe joints and are used for plantar flexion of these structures. The small popliteus is located at the posterior knee and is used mainly to control movement in the lateral meniscus and for cushioning of the neurovascular structures during extensive knee motions.

Nerve lesions in the calf extensor compartment result in a typical clubfoot or equinus position (deep peroneal nerve), as the functional antagonists (flexors) may shift the foot to plantar flexion. Nerve lesions in the flexors

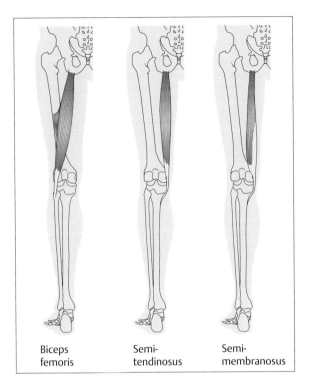

Biceps femoris   Semi-tendinosus   Semi-membranosus

may result in a typical "heel foot" position, as the antagonists (extensors) may shift the foot to dorsiflexion. To allow the foot to unroll properly while walking on the ground, the patient's thigh and knee in the free leg are typically moved slightly more upwards, like the walking pattern of a "cock on a dunghill." Injuries to the lateral ankle (lateral malleolus) may result in a dorsal tarsal syndrome, with pain just below the retinaculum and compression of the tibial nerve, as well as discomfort, with impaired sensation or blocked sweat secretion on the skin of the sole of the foot.

Fig. 1.10   The posterior thigh muscle compartment (back of the knee).

Table 1.9   Posterior thigh muscle compartment—major actions: hip extension and knee flexion

	Muscle	Description (palpation)	Origin (O), insertion (I)	Innervation (segments)	Actions
Hamstrings	Biceps femoris (*biceps,* two-headed)	Most lateral muscles of hamstrings (an old butcher's term for hanging hams for smoking), with a short and long head and common tendon marking the lateral proximal border of the popliteal fossa	O: • Ischial tuber (long head) and lateral lip of • Linea aspera (short head) I: Head of fibula and lateral tibia (both heads)	Tibial nerve L5–S2	• Hip extension • Knee flexion and • Stabilization of pelvis
	Semimembranosus (half-membranous)	Fleshy membranous muscle of hamstrings beneath the semitendinosus, located medial to the biceps, with strong tendon marking the medial proximal border of the popliteal fossa	O: Ischiadic tuber I: Medial tibial condyle	Tibial nerve L5–S2	As for biceps femoris and • Medial rotation (knee)
	Semitendinosus (half-tendinous)	Fleshy muscle of hamstrings running just above the semimembranosus, with longer tendon to insert at the medial tibial condyle; tendon marks the medial border of popliteal fossa	O: Ischiadic tuber I: Tibial tuberosity	Tibial nerve L5–S2	As for biceps and • Medial rotation (knee)
	Popliteus (*poples,* ham, posterior knee)	Small muscle running obliquely through the deep dorsal knee, fixes the lateral meniscus, supports neurovascular structures such as popliteal artery and tibial nerve	O: Lateral femoral condyle and lateral meniscus I: Proximal tibia (dorsally)	Tibial nerve L5–S2	• Knee flexion • Lateral rotation (knee)

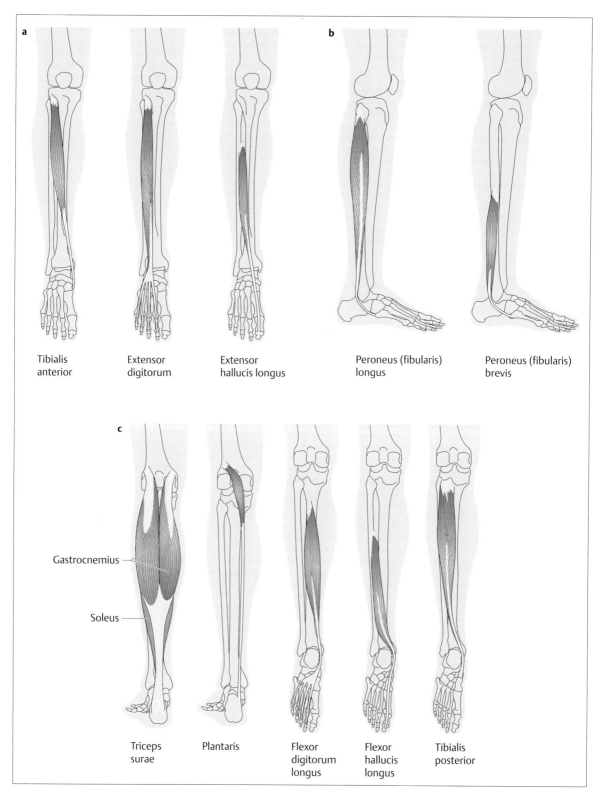

Fig. 1.11a–c Calf muscle compartments.

a Anterior calf muscle compartment (dorsiflexors, extensors).
b Lateral calf muscle compartment (pronators).
c Posterior calf muscle compartment (flexors).

Table 1.10 Anterior and lateral calf muscle compartments—major actions: ankle dorsiflexion (extensors) and foot swaying

	Muscle	Description (palpation)	Origin (O), insertion (I)	Innervation (segments)	Function
Extensors (Dorsiflexors)	Tibialis anterior (*anterius*, toward front)	Superficial muscle running parallel to the anterior margin of the tibia over ankle joints	O: Lateral tibia shaft, interosseous membrane I: First metatarsal (dorsally)	Deep peroneal nerve L4–S1	• Dorsiflexion (foot) • Inverts foot
	Extensor digitorum longus (digit = finger or toe)	Slender unipennate muscle with long tendons running lateral to the tibialis anterior over ankle joints to insert at distal toes 2–5	O: Lateral tibial condyle, interosseus membrane I: 4 partitioned tendons to dorsal aponeuroses of toes 2–5	Deep peroneal nerve L4–S1	• Dorsiflexion (foot) • Everts foot
	Extensor hallucis longus (hallux = great toe)	Deepest unipennate muscle with long tendon running between extensor digitorum and tibialis anterior to great toe	O: Anteromedial fibular shaft, interosseous membrane I: Distal phalanx of great toe	Deep peroneal nerve L4–S1	• Dorsiflexion (foot) • Inverts and everts foot • Extends great toe
Pronators	Peroneus (fibularis) longus (Greek *perone*, fibula)	Superficial lateral muscle that overlies fibula; long tendon curves under foot to support the medial foot arch	O: Head and upper portion of fibula I: First metatarsal and medial cuneiform (plantar)	Superficial peroneal nerve L5–S1	• Plantar flexion (foot) • Everts foot • Supports medial arch of foot
	Peroneus (fibularis) brevis (*brevis*, short)	Smaller muscle deep to peroneus longus, with tendon insertion at lateral border of foot	O: Shaft of fibula (distally) I: Fifth metatarsal (tuberosity)	Superficial peroneal nerve L5–S1	• Plantar flexion (foot) • Everts foot

Table 1.11 Posterior calf muscle box—major action: initiating ankle plantar flexion

	Muscle	Description (palpation)	Origin (O), insertion (I)	Innervation (segments)	Action
Calf flexors	Triceps surae (*triceps*, three-headed; *sura*, calf)	Powerful three-headed calf muscle with common strong tendon insertion at heel (Achilles tendon)	See below	Tibial nerve S1–S2	• Initiator of ankle plantar flexion
	Gastrocnemius (*gaster*, belly; *kneme*, leg)	Superficial muscle pair with two prominent heads (medial and lateral head) that shape the calf and form the distal borders of the popliteal fossa (two-joint muscle)	O: Medial and lateral epicondyle I: Calcaneal tuber via common calcaneal tendon	As for triceps surae	• Ankle flexion • Knee flexion
	Soleus (*solea*, sole)	Solelike flat muscle of posterior calf deep to the gastrocnemius; muscle origins form tendinous arch for passage of popliteal vessels and nerve (single-joint muscle)	O: Proximal tibia and fibula, interosseous membrane (tendinous arch) I: Calcaneal tuber via common tendon	As for triceps	• Initiator of ankle flexion • Strong postural capacity
	Plantaris (*planta*, sole)	A small and weak muscle deep in the popliteal fossa with very long and thin tendon into calcaneal tendon (may be absent)	O: Lateral epicondyle I: Calcaneal tuber	As for triceps	• Knee flexion • Unlocks knee from full extension
Deep calf flexors	Tibialis posterior	Strong and flat muscle deep to the soleus located between posterior flexors; tendon intersection by flexor digitorum long. before passing behind medial malleolus to the medial foot arch	O: Interosseous membrane, tibia and fibula I: Tarsal and metatarsal bones (plantar)	Tibial nerve L4–S1	• Initiator of ankle flexion and • Foot inversion • Supports medial and longitudinal arch
	Flexor digitorum longus (*digitus*, toe)	Strong bipennate muscle in deep medial calf, tendon intersection with tibialis posterior before passing behind medial malleolus through the longitudinal arch to individual toes	O: Posterior tibia surface and interosseous membrane I: Distal phalanges 2–5	Tibial nerve L5–S1	• As for tibialis anterior • Toe flexor at all joints
	Flexor hallucis longus (hallux = great toe)	Strong bipennate muscle lateral to tibialis post., with plantar tendon under crossing the flexor digitorum longus to insert at the hallux	O: Dorsal two-thirds of fibula shaft I: Distal phalanx of great toe (hallux)	Tibial nerve L5–S2	• As for tibialis anterior • Great toe (hallux) • Flexor; "push-off" muscle during walking

Intermuscular Septum, Rectus Sheath, and Iliotibial Tract

Some special connective-tissue structures allow better function during more complex movements of various muscle compartments with different actions (extensors versus flexors) located in the same motion segments. In the upper arm, for example, a special fascia reinforced by connective tissue, known as the intermuscular septum, separates the anterior compartment (flexors) from the posterior compartment (extensors) as it courses between the humerus shaft and the superficial fascia of the upper extremity, between the borders of the extensor and flexor muscle compartments (see **Fig. 1.23**, p. 36).

At the ventral abdominal wall, the rectus abdominis (see **Fig. 1.5**) reaches from the lower ribs to the pelvic girdle (pubic symphysis), lying with its three major bellies (cf. "six-packs") in a shell-like, tight fascia known as the rectus sheath. As there is no bony reinforcement in the abdominal wall, the rectus sheath functions as an "exoskeleton" (*exo-*, outer) serving as a mechanical abutment to support muscle contraction—for example, during crunches toward the knees.

A palpable reinforced fascia (aponeurosis) is typically found under the skin of the lateral thigh and extends from the iliac crest to the head of the fibula, known as the iliotibial tract and used for stretching of the fascia lata (Latin *latus*, broad) in the upper leg region. Like the rectus sheath, the iliotibial tract—along with the tensor fascia lata, a muscle located in a shell-like fascia at the upper thigh laterally—also acts as a mechanical abutment to the contracting vastus lateralis thigh muscle and thus helps generate muscle force directed toward the patella during knee extension.

Skeletal Muscles and Their Typical Motion Patterns

The motion patterns that take place in normal everyday life and in sports are quite complex and should really be studied and described using applied kinesiology methods. However, a more straightforward model assigns human movements to various motion segments along the body axis, such as the joints between the head and neck, between various segments of the vertebral column (e.g., cervical, thoracic, lumbar segments), and between the joints of the lower body or leg such as the hip, knee, and ankle joints. Normally, the skeletal muscles in the movement apparatus never act alone, but always as part of successfully linked motor units or segments that involve at least one agonist (e.g., biceps, brachialis) used for elbow joint/forearm flexion and one antagonist (e.g., triceps) used for elbow joint/forearm extension in the opposite direction (**Fig. 1.12**). It is known that in accordance with the routine biomechanics of the muscle system, an agonistically acting muscle or group always has to be damped by one or more antagonistically acting muscles or groups during a kinetically controlled motion. The damping process in muscle activity is usually a spontaneous one, controlled by proprioceptive sensors (muscle spindle or Golgi tendon organs) and is normally part of individually trained movement patterns in sports. However, the effect of spontaneous kinetic control by extensive muscle loading induced

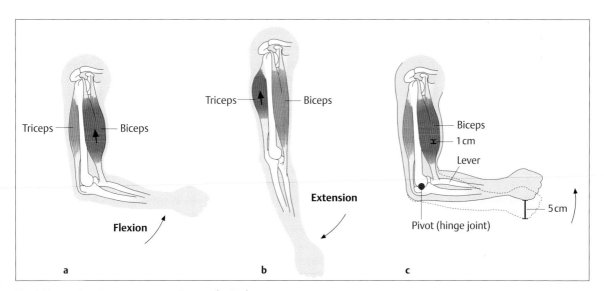

Fig. 1.12a–c   Agonist versus antagonist muscles in the arm.

a Elbow flexion: the biceps brachii (agonist) contracts, while the triceps brachii relaxes (antagonist).
b Elbow straightening: the triceps brachii (agonist) contracts, while the biceps brachii relaxes (antagonist).
c Lever arm: the biceps insertion point is close to the pivot joint; muscle shortening of ~ 1 cm may be sufficient to lift the forearm and hand for ~ 5 cm toward the arm and shoulder.

by prolonged periods of muscle damping can easily be perceived in the anterior leg muscle compartments (quadriceps, tibialis anterior), for example, during hiking in the mountains and walking downhill back to the valley—with the muscle stiffness and aches that develop afterward (see Chapter 6).

Functional muscle units may include two or more muscles that span one or two joints—during hammer throwing, for example, with the biceps, brachialis, and brachioradialis working together in the arm, forearm, and wrist. The hip and leg muscles at work during barbell squatting thus include the gluteus, quadriceps, and various calf muscles (triceps surae, tibialis anterior), and those at work during lunges include the gluteus maximus and quadriceps, as primary muscles. As mentioned earlier, muscles working in concert act in a closed muscle chain (kinematic chain) when the person is in weight-bearing, standing position, or act in an open muscle chain when the limb is moving freely, as during a swing phase in walking or knee extension on an isokinetic machine—that is, without the limbs directly touching the ground.

Note

A more theoretical approach to understanding the principles of redundant motions by their normal muscular actions in every day life style has been suggested by Richardson et al. (2004). In this model of body segmentation and stabilization, the skeletal muscles or groups are termed either "mobilizers," "stabilizers," or "locals," depending on their anatomic location and their actions during various motions. These muscles or muscle groups that are used in everyday motion may be integrated into other functional units or muscle chains in order to allow more specialized and complex motions, as in various sports.
However, this model can provide a basis for therapists, medical doctors, and even orthopedists to enable them to quickly grasp and interpret muscle injuries in sports or fitness training, allowing reliable diagnosis of functional impairments of the human skeletal muscle system.

- *Locals.* In normal everyday activity, local muscles in the trunk and particularly those located deep in the muscle system (close to bone and joints) in the lower body motion segments (hip, leg) work against gravitation and are therefore termed antigravity muscles or postural muscles. Typical locals include the erector spinae and the soleus, as examples for stabilization of segmental movements of the vertebral column (erector spinae) or lower leg and ankle (soleus) that in concert with other muscles allow an upright posture during sitting, standing, and walking.
- *Stabilizers.* Muscles that are located closer to joints or that spread across one or several joints (single or multijoint muscles) are mainly used for joint stabilization during movements. Because of their anatomic location

in the locomotor system (near joints) and their specific fiber orientation (pennation angle; see next section), some highly pennate muscles have relatively short contraction strokes—such as the short interossei and lumbricales in the hand or foot, or the long hamstring muscles (semitendinosus and semimembranosus) for exerting their maximum force (see below). Muscles with fibers running in parallel may have relatively long contraction strokes, such as the iliopsoas or adductor magnus, for producing maximum power and force output.

- *Mobilizers.* Some muscles in the shoulder girdle, arms, and legs in the human muscle system (deltoid, biceps, latissimus, quadriceps, sartorius) are used for actual mobilization of body segments in exercise and locomotion. Because of their anatomic orientation in the locomotor system and their often flat or spindle-shaped bellies with fibers that run in parallel—latissimus, biceps brachii, sartorius—they share long hoisting capacities that are necessary for actual mobilization of body segments or for sweeping motions of the arms and legs, and thus are used in sports for explosivelike motion patterns to generate fast and vigorous muscle torque and power, as in javelin throwing and sprinting, or for shooting in soccer.

In conclusion, all of the muscles and muscle groups in the sports locomotor apparatus can act in concert in a very complex way and in accordance with individually trained motion patterns that need to be analyzed in more detail. In general, motion patterns and the muscles included involve various predisposing factors such as genetics, success of training, and even nutrition. The motion patterns seen in competitive athletes, and the muscles involved, can thus generate either explosivelike powerful movements (as in sprinters and goal shooters), more endurance capacity (as in rowers and long-distance runners), or a mixture of various motion patterns (as in gymnastics and dancing).

Pennation Angle or Angulation of Fascicles in Skeletal Muscle

The orientation of the fascicles (bundles of fibers) in a muscle belly not only describes the intramuscular architecture but also determines the way in which muscle force is produced and the extent to which shortening of the belly is necessary to obtain full power and torque (lift capacity versus contraction strokes, as discussed above). As a rule, muscle shortening may be up to 40% of the initial length in a given muscle in normal physiological conditions (Kunsch and Kunsch 2005).

As mentioned, some muscles have a mostly parallel orientation in their fascicles, such as the biceps brachii in the anterior arm flexor compartment (**Fig. 1.12**), the sartorius in the anterior thigh/knee extensor compartment

(**Fig. 1.9a**), and the tibialis anterior in the anterior calf extensor compartment (**Fig. 1.11**). Some muscles have a unipennate arrangement of their fascicles—that is, the fibers in the belly run obliquely in one direction and insert at an acute angle to a lateral tendon, as seen in the semitendinosus, for example; or they may have a bipennate fiber arrangement—that is, the fibers in the belly run obliquely from both sides of the belly and insert at acute angles to a common central tendon, as seen in the hamstrings (semimembranosus and biceps femoris), (**Fig. 1.10**), extensor digitorum longus (**Fig. 1.11a**), and in the peroneus (fibularis) muscles of the lateral lower leg, for example (**Fig. 1.11b**). The deltoid at the shoulder joint has a complex fiber angulation pattern (pennation) in three major fascicle directions and is an example of a multipennate muscle with at least three different motion patterns .

Note

It is easy to picture the pennation or angulation fascicle arrangement in a given muscle by thinking of the structure of quills or bird feathers. The pennation angle or angulation plays an important role in determining contraction in a muscle belly, in its force development and in its power output, and should not be underestimated (Gans and de Vree 1987). For example, injuries to the semimembranosus hamstring muscle during soccer games often occur in close proximity to the myotendinous attachments and are possibly due to the complex angulation of the proximal short fibers and the distal long fascicles of the belly that merge in the flat aponeurosis-like muscle tendon. More importantly, angulation of fibers or fascicles may be significantly different in a normally active muscle in comparison with an extensively trained skeletal muscle, due to intramuscular adaptive changes in the fiber architecture, including fiber hypertrophy (Gans and de Vree 1987).

Single fibers or fascicles in some muscles are connected to each other via myomuscular junctions, which may also determine intramuscular force transmission (see multibelly muscle versus pennated muscle, in Chleboun et al. 2001). Earlier findings suggested that intramuscular junctions of this type between fibers may well support dynamic force transmission from the sarcomere to the intramuscular myoelastic connective-tissue structures (Laurent et al. 1991).

Practical Tip

Maladaptation of intramuscular angulation of single fibers or fiber bundles in highly trained muscles with angular complexity (hamstrings, adductors, triceps surae) may be a cause of the prevalence of injury in sports.

Anatomic versus Physiological Profile of Skeletal Muscle

The total number of myofibrils in a single muscle fiber determines its profile size. The number of fibers in a muscle also determines the profile size of a whole muscle belly. The cross-sectional area of a whole muscle is therefore a reliable measure of its physiological output (= force production). Usually, the torque per square centimeter of a muscle profile is ~5 kg or 50 N (Kunsch and Kunsch 2005). For example, the fusiform shape of the biceps brachii in the upper arm has a normal profile of ~ 10 cm^2 and a calculated maximum force production of ~ 500 Nm (Schünke 2000). The anatomic profile of a muscle is usually reflected by a cross-section through the mid-belly, which is thought to be the bulkiest portion of a muscle, in which most if not all fibers run rectangularly through the cross-sectional plane. In this model, the anatomic profile size should always be identical to the physiological profile size and the total number of fibers may directly reflect the magnitude of torque production in a muscle.

In pennate muscles, however, the anatomic profile may be completely different from the physiological profile, as the total number of individual fiber profiles that run through the cross-sectional plane in a rectangular direction may vary according to fiber angulation. For example, in a bipennate muscle (quill model) there are at least two virtual profiles with rectangularly cut fibers, which may easily double the total number of fibers per cross-sectional plane and likewise also increase the total output of muscle force accordingly (**Fig. 1.13**). As the pattern of angulation is responsible for muscle shortening and maximum force production, maximum force production is partly also reflected in some way by the physiological profile in a given muscle—that is, not merely by the anatomic size (caliber) of a belly. In conclusion, the physiological profile is always greater in size in pennate muscles in comparison with muscles with parallel fascicles.

Isotonic versus Isometric Contraction

Body movements are also determined by special contraction modes in skeletal muscle that allow holding, lifting, or lowering of loads (body, arms or legs, weights).

- *Isotonic contraction.* If you move a weight (dumbbell) by elbow flexion to your shoulder, you have performed muscle shortening using an "isotonic" contraction (from Greek *isotonos*, equally stretched) that has moved a load against gravity by force development (also termed dynamic contraction). If you then slowly lower your forearm with the same load in the opposite direction, you have performed a muscle elongation by an eccentric contraction. Both concentric and eccentric muscle activities are always accompanied by altered muscle length, known as isotonic force development (see resistive training, below).

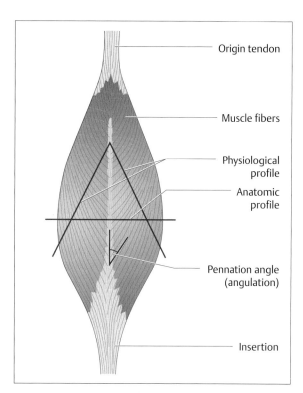

Origin tendon

Muscle fibers

Physiological profile

Anatomic profile

Pennation angle (angulation)

Insertion

Fig. 1.13 Anatomic versus physiological profiles during changes in skeletal muscle length, relative to torque capacity.

- *Isometric contraction.* If you hold a weight (load) with your arm outstretched in front of you, force development in the muscle is used to work against the gravity load, but no significant movement or muscle shortening is performed. This is known as an isometric contraction (from Greek *isometria,* equality of measure). Isometric contractions in a muscle produce force without significant muscle shortening. For example, if you tighten your buttock muscles during fitness training, you perform an isometric contraction of the gluteus muscles. This can be explained by mutual activation of the contractile elements (actin and myosin) of the contractile apparatus in series (sarcomeres) and power storage in the elastic molecular components (titin) of a single fiber, and also by power storage in the myoelastic elements of a muscle, such as intramuscular loose fibrous connective tissue around fascicles (perimysium, endomysium), their outer fascia layer (meshlike connective tissue), or even their tendons (parallel collagen mixed with elastic fibers).
- *Isokinetic contraction.* During coaching, isokinetic contractions (from Greek *iso-,* equal, and *kinetikos,* moving) are usually performed as consistent movements controlled by computer-assisted training devices that stipulate the rate of velocity during exercise, as they are used for controlled high load training protocols in competitive athletes.

- *Desmodromic contraction.* This mode of muscle contraction is performed on electronically controlled training devices that are used for maximum power output protocols (total exhaustion), also used only in high-performance sports.

In normal body posture and performance control, isometric and isotonic contractions may occur differently in local groups or muscle chains to develop and adjust muscle power as needed. In strength training, however, both eccentric and concentric muscle exercise, known as resistive exercise (resistance to gravity), such as controlled movements against gravity forces as in push-ups or squatting, is frequently used to increase muscle mass and strength—for example, by stimulating mechanosensitive molecular signaling pathways (see Chapters 2 and 3). Isometric contractions are successfully used in traditional Asian kinetics (such as *tai ji* and yoga) to strengthen postural muscle groups.

Note

Overloading in eccentric contractions (when muscle acts mainly as a "brake" during movement) may result in microtears in muscle cells. Following unaccustomed new exercises, intensity in a regular workout, or after extensive training protocols following a prolonged training pause, muscles may be overexerted—for example, as with an extensively working quadriceps and tibialis anterior in going down stairs, landing from a jump, or in downhill running. This mechanical overload, together with exhaustion of the metabolism, may develop into painful muscle aches (Böning 2002) with ultrastructurally confirmed microtrauma to single fibers (**Fig. 1.14**; see Chapters 6 and 7).

Functional Histology of Muscle Tissue

Smooth Muscle

Smooth muscle tissue consists of spindle-shaped (fusiform) and uninucleate single cells with pointed ends that do not have striations like skeletal muscle cells. In these cells, the actin and myosin fibrils are parts of an intracellular network, rather than being located in parallel series like the sarcomeres in striated muscle. Closely packed smooth muscle cells (like a shoal of fish) work together in sheets known as a "mechanical syncytium" (modern Latin, from Greek *syn-,* together, and *kytos,* cell). For example, the contraction of many single cells in multiunit muscles results in narrowing of the whole ringlike cell layer around the intestine. Smooth muscle layers are the major wall components of many organs, such as the stomach, intestine, bladder, and vessel walls (**Fig. 1.15a**). Contraction

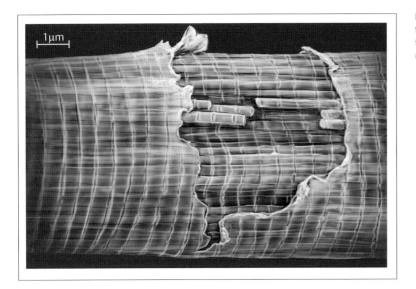

Fig. 1.14 A microtear in a single muscle fiber. A few ruptured microfibrils are visible through the torn outer cell membrane. (Scanning electron microscopy, modified.)

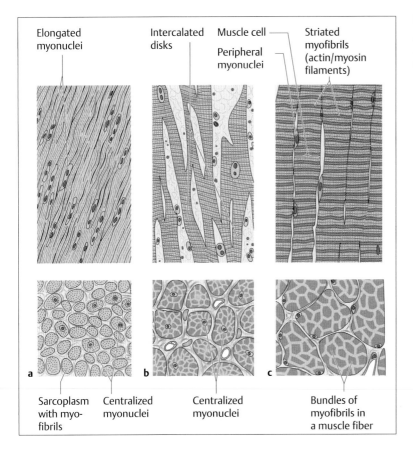

Fig. 1.15a–c Muscle histology

a Smooth muscle.
b Striated heart muscle.
c Striated skeletal muscle.

and relaxation of smooth muscle cells is spontaneously controlled by a network of autonomic nerve fibers that penetrate the muscle layers with either sympathetic or parasympathetic visceromotor terminals, which are also connected to intramural ganglia (see enteric nervous system).

Contraction and relaxation of smooth muscle cells occurs via neurotransmitters—for example, norepinephrine. Upon neural activation, the transmitters are released by autonomic nerve terminals known as varicosities (beaded axonal distensions) and bound for example to β-receptors (norepinephrine) on the muscle cells, followed by a calcium influx that results in a muscle cell contraction. The smooth muscle layer may also be modulated by endocrine hormones or even gaseous signals, such as nitric oxide (NO), known as a diffusible relaxation factor or as a potent vasodilatory agent derived from endothelial cells (NO released from nitroglycerol is vasodilatory). In sports, smooth muscle layers around blood vessels or in the tracheal wall, or around bronchi and bronchioli in the lungs, are used for wall tonus control and thus support breathing as well as blood perfusion as needed. In skeletal muscle, a similar mechanism of peripheral tonus control of the local microvascular bed with smooth muscle layers (arterioles, venules) allows blood perfusion as needed (see **Fig. 1.21a, b**).

Striated Muscle

Heart Muscle

Heart muscle is a special form of striated muscle tissue (**Fig. 1.15b**). The cardiomyocytes (heart muscle cells) are part of a three-dimensional network of branching single uninucleate cells, with a contractile apparatus of myofibrils and sarcomeres in series in each cell that gives them a striated pattern similar to skeletal muscle cells. The cardiomyocytes are joined together by specialized cell contacts (intercalated disks = disks inserted between) that

contain two distinct regions, one of desmosome-like structures needed for mechanical linkage during heart contractions, and another region of membrane accumulations of small tunnel-like channel proteins (gap junctions) used for intercellular ion transport, transmitting the contraction signal from one myocyte to the adjacent myocytes. The network of cardiomyocytes in the myocardium is therefore linked in both ways, mechanically and electrically, and works together almost simultaneously as a mechanoelectrically coupled merged cell system, known as a "mechanoelectrical syncytium." Notably, the regular neuromuscular junctions present in striated skeletal muscle are typically missing in cardiac muscle.

Practical Tip

Before a competition, the tone of the smooth muscle layer in the gastrointestinal tract and bladder may possibly increase due to sympathetic hyperactivity (stomach cramps, stress incontinence). Relaxation exercises such as autogenic training or going for a walk may therefore be helpful before the start of a contest or match.

Table 1.12 Terminology and definitions in myology

Commonly used term in cell biology	Definition used in myology
Muscle cell	Muscle fiber
Cell membrane	Sarcolemma
Cytoplasm, cytosol	Sarcoplasm, sarcosol
Endoplasmic reticulum (ER)	Sarcoplasmic reticulum (SR). Modification of the ER used for calcium storage in cell
Fingerlike membrane insertions	Transverse system (T tubules): for faster transmission of membrane potential to release intracellular calcium from the terminal cisternae (see below)
A network of tubulelike endoplasmic reticulum around myofibrils	Longitudinal system (L-tubules), identical to SR in the muscle fiber; calcium storage
Deep membrane insertions adjacent to the terminal cisternae of the ER	Triads, composed of a T tubule and two adjacent terminal cisternae of the SR (mostly located at the level of Z disks)
Nucleus	Myonucleus
Hemoglobin (erythrocyte)	Myoglobin (muscular O_2-binding protein)
Microfilaments	Myosin (myofilament)
Microfilament bundle	Myofibril (contractile)
Striated myofibrillar compartment between two Z disks	Sarcomere: smallest functional muscle unit confined by Z disks, comparable to miniaturized intracellular power chambers in series
Nerve contacts (synapses)	Neuromuscular synapse/junction

Skeletal Muscle

Skeletal muscle cells are long single cylinders with very obvious striations that contain many nuclei (multinucleate) and belong to the skeletal muscles attached to bones (or sometimes skin; see facial expression muscles). During development, single or mononucleate muscle cells (myoblasts) merge into larger multinucleate cells (myocytes) and are therefore regarded as a true "syncytium." The myocytes form elongated cell tubes, with their nuclei located in the periphery just beneath the outer membrane (**Fig. 1.15c**). Single muscle cells or fibers are covered with a fine sheath of loose connective tissue known as endomysium (= around the fiber). The muscle fibers are collected into larger units known as fascicles, covered by a more fibrous sheath known as perimysium (= around the fascicle). Larger fascicles are embedded in perimysial connective tissue to form primary or secondary fascicles that ultimately make up the muscle belly, covered with the general muscle fascia known as epimysium (= around the muscle). The epimysium is a fibrous membrane consisting of dense regular connective tissue with irregularly arranged collagen and elastic fibers and fibroblasts that serve as an overcoat for muscle (**Fig. 1.22a**).

Muscle fibers usually contain as many as 50–100 nuclei (Kunsch and Kunsch 2005) and have a total fiber length of ~ 20–40 cm. Like neurobiology, muscle biology (myology) has its own terminology, which uses "sarco-" and "myo-," for example, as typical prefixes (see **Table 1.12**). Each single skeletal muscle fiber is supplied by a synaptic contact of somatic motor nerves known as end plates or neuromuscular junctions (see **Fig. 1.30a, b**).

Molecular Architecture of Skeletal Muscle Fibers (Sarcomeres)

This section describes the general and more specific principles of the molecular architecture, to provide a better understanding of the subcellular compartmentalization and spatial ability of the contractile apparatus in skeletal muscle fibers. The precise physiological and molecular mechanisms of muscle contraction cycles are described in Chapter 2.

Actin and Myosin Filaments

A normal muscle fiber contains about a thousand or more myofibrils, which are bundled into several larger groups (myofibrillar bundles) inside the cell tube (**Fig. 1.16a**). The myofibrillar bundles of the contractile apparatus are the major part of the sarcoplasm in a fiber and do not leave much space for other organelles, mitochondria, nuclei, sarcoplasmic tubules, or glycosomes. Myofibrils consist of unbranched long cylinders with segmental repeats in series known as sarcomeres (= muscle segments). The sarcomeres are the basic contraction units in skeletal muscle. Each sarcomere consists of thin and thick myofilament proteins, actin and myosin, the regulatory proteins troponin and tropomyosin, and the accessory proteins titin and nebulin, which assist in the molecular and biochemical processes or biomechanics of the actomyosin motor proteins during myofilament sliding and contraction.

One thin actin myofilament consists of twisted G-actin globular proteins, and many of them are attached to a Z-shaped disk (Z line) that establishes the boundaries of a sarcomere. The actin filaments contain tropomyosin and troponin molecules, which can bind calcium (e.g., Tc = calcium receptor; see Chapter 2) as a prerequisite for actin-

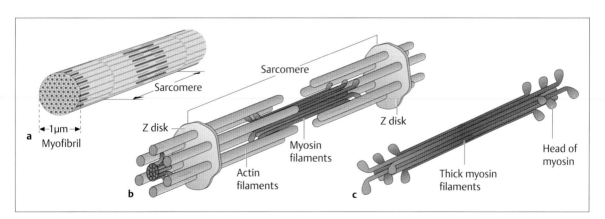

Fig. 1.16a–c Microarchitecture of a sarcomere.

a Myofibril with a sarcomere.
b Sarcomere (enlarged).
c Myosin filaments with heads.

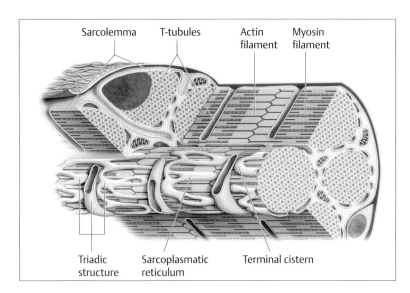

Fig. 1.17 Transverse tubules (T tubules) and sarcoplasmic reticulum (SR). The T tubules are invaginations of the outer fiber sarcolemma to direct membrane potentials toward inner muscle cell structures. The SR structure is used as an intracellular calcium store.

Labels in figure: Sarcolemma · T-tubules · Actin filament · Myosin filament · Triadic structure · Sarcoplasmatic reticulum · Terminal cistern

myosin unifying filament sliding (in the sliding filament theory). One thick myosin filament consists of ~ 250 single twisted myosin proteins capped with knoblike flexible proteins known as myosin heads, comparable to the head of a golf club. The thick myofilaments also contain ATPases to split adenosine triphosphate (ATP) into adenosine diphosphate (ADP) + P_i (for energy storage and release) during the contraction process (see Chapter 2). Several thick myosin filaments are located in the center of a sarcomere overlapping the actin filaments (**Fig. 1.16c**). Sliding of actin filaments past the myosin filaments (by calcium and ATP-driven flexible head movements) produces shortening of the sarcomeres in series in each myofibril in a muscle fiber, and finally of the skeletal muscle as a whole (**Fig. 1.16b**).

Striations

In light microscopy, the light and dark striations of longitudinally cut skeletal muscle fibers are readily visible in histological sections. They result from the parallel arrangement of the rod-shaped myofibrils with their sarcomeres of thick and thin myofilaments. Adjacent individual myofibrils in a muscle fiber line up perfectly and may not be distinguishable on hematoxylin–eosin-stained histological sections. The dark striations result from a central wide area in each sarcomere of thick myosin filaments overlapping thin actin filaments (A bands; A = anisotropic) and the most intensely stained Z lines, which represent the repeated boundaries of a sarcomere unit. The light striations in a sarcomere result from an area of overlapping thin actin filaments (I bands; I = isotropic) attached to the Z disks of adjacent sarcomeres. With a fiber length of ~ 10 cm, approximately 40 000 sarcomeres are consecutively linked to each other—that is, approximately 200 million sarcomeres can be found in a single muscle fiber (Tegtbur et al. 2009).

Sarcoplasmic Reticulum and Tubules

In a skeletal muscle fiber, each myofibril is supplied by a specialized endoplasmic tubular network known as the sarcoplasmic reticulum (SR), which serves as the main calcium storage organelle in a muscle fiber (**Fig. 1.17**). There are two sets of specialized tubular networks. Longitudinally oriented SR tubules adjacent to the myofibrils are known as L-tubules (L = longitudinal) and end with protrusions known as terminal cisterns ("end sacs"). Transversely oriented tubules are deeply invaginated continuations of the outer sarcolemma and are located at the level of the myofibrillar Z disks; they are known as T tubules (T = transverse). A complex of one T tubule flanked by two terminal cisterns located in the transition zone of the A–I band in each myofibril is known as a triad (group of three). The triads of adjacent sarcomeres are connected via short tubular networks in the SR. In general, the SR tubules express specialized channel proteins involved in intracellular calcium balance, such as the ATPase SERCA and IP_3 (Ca^{2+} influx into the SR is mostly at L-tubules), and the ryanodine receptors, RyR (for Ca^{2+} efflux from the SR) at the terminal cisterns, thus increasing the sarcosolic calcium concentration to support the contraction mechanism. In addition to the specialized SR surrounding the contractile apparatus, there is a small portion of endoplasmic reticulum (ER) used for housekeeping protein synthesis, mainly in the sarcosol as part of the myonuclear domain.

Regulatory Proteins, Tropomyosin, and Troponin

The thin actin myofilaments of each myofibril contain regulatory proteins called tropomyosin (Tm) and the triple-piece calcium receptor protein troponin (Tn, Ti, and Tc), which in the presence of calcium allows short-term local

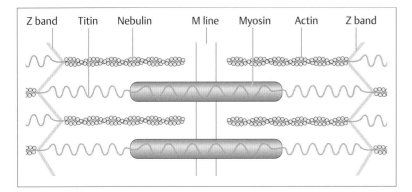

Fig. 1.18 Titin and nebulin accessory muscle proteins. Titin stabilizes the myosin filaments and allows myofibrillar elasticity, comparable to the functioning of a spring, during muscle relaxation. Nebulin serves to reinforce actin filaments during the muscle contraction–relaxation process.

binding of the myosin head to the actin filament (Tn switch on). After the myosin head pivots at its hinge, it lets go (with calcium released from the receptor), binds again to actin further along, and pivots again. This cycle is repeated several times during sliding for a single contraction. Shortening of the sarcomere thus allows concentric contractions by a progressive succession of actin–myosin interactions.

Note

Actin–myosin filament sliding is usually compared in textbooks to the equal impact of the paddling motions of eight or more occupants in a rowing boat. However, recent studies have suggested instead the presence of a mechanism comparable to the locomotion of a millipede on the ground (with many small legs that never lose contact while moving). Another model suggests the presence of Brownian molecular movements with similar motion stabilization mechanisms (studied by atomic force microscopy). We should therefore think of a continuation of actin–myosin bridging during muscle shortening and contraction.

Accessory Proteins Titin and Nebulin

The giant muscle accessory protein titin extends from the Z disk via myosin filaments to the M line at the sarcomere center (**Fig. 1.18**). Titin, the largest known polypeptide (3.6 MDa in size) in the human body, and its various isoforms are large, abundant proteins in skeletal muscle and may reflect the variable biodynamics in different muscle types (Labeit 1995). Titin thus stabilizes the location of the contractile sarcomeric proteins (resting tension) and allows for passive elasticity, so that the cassette of overlapping filaments returns to its starting position in the relaxed state of the muscle. In addition, titin interacts with several other sarcomeric proteins (telethonin, calpain, obscurin, MuRF1) involved in the sarcomeric integrity and viscoelasticity of muscle contractions.

Another giant muscle protein, nebulin (600–900 kDa in size), is a filamentous protein located in parallel to the thin actin filaments, fixed to the Z disk, and able to bind as many as 200 actin monomers (**Fig. 1.18**). Nebulin thus allows for sarcomeric stiffness and, like titin, also helps to maintain sarcomeric structural and functional integrity in myofibrils of skeletal muscle (Witt et al. 2006).

Note

In histology and ultrastructure, the patterns of striations of sarcomeres depend on the state of contraction in a skeletal muscle. In the relaxed state, the sarcomere is ~ 2.2 µm long and the actin–myosin filament overlap is relatively small. During maximum contraction, the sarcomere shortens to ~ 1.8 µm and maximum actin–myosin filament overlapping occurs. Following muscle stretching (passive or active), the sarcomere has a length of ~ 3.8 µm and there is minimal actin–myosin filament overlapping. As the lengths of the M line and A-bands do not change, the I bands and H zone have to change during sarcomere shortening (**Fig. 1.19**).

Muscle Fatigue

The term "muscle fatigue" means that an expected muscle power and force is no longer available or may not be maintained for a period of time. There are several reasons why muscle fatigue develops. There may be a central fatigue if psychological irritation or protective reflexes are located in the brain or spinal cord. Peripheral fatigue may weaken transmitter release from the neuromuscular junctions of somatomotor neurons (transmitter depletion). Similarly, the excitation–contraction coupling in myofibers may be reduced due to decreased membrane potentials. Finally, changes in calcium balance, loss of creatine phosphates, ATP, glycogen, or excess protons, phosphates or lactate in muscle can cause premature muscle fatigue during routine exercise regimens.

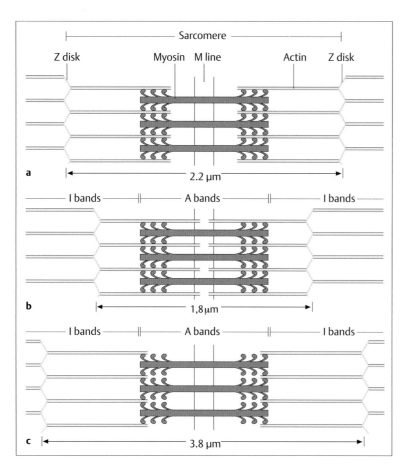

Fig. 1.19a–c   Alterations in the striated pattern of a sarcomere during the contraction–relaxation process in muscle.

a Relaxed state (resting tone).
b Maximum contraction state.
c Maximum stretching state.

Satellite Cells (Emergency Cells)

Satellite cells are considered as muscle-related stem cells that can be activated in conditions of regeneration and plasticity following effective exercise training. In development, satellite cells originate from a separate pool of myogenic progenitor cells that do not further differentiate into fused myoblasts, myocytes and myotubes, but instead persist as nonfused and quiescent (resident) single cells (satellites) adjacent to developing, growing, or adult muscle fibers in skeletal muscle (**Fig. 1.20**). Due to their location close to adult myofibers, the satellite cells (and their nuclei) should not be mistaken on light microscopy for peripheral myonuclei of muscle fibers. Notably, the satellite cell nuclei are always separated from the outer fiber sarcolemma by a basal lamina. In the case of a (partial) muscle tear, the resident satellite cells are thought to be activated by local tissue mediators such as cytokines/growth factors and start to proliferate. When they are activated in this way, the proliferating satellite cells may be able to replace lost myonuclei from the torn fiber periphery by a mechanism known as nucleus "donation" to the injured fiber (see **Fig. 1.14**). In rat muscle, satellite cells may also regulate the myofiber size in the developing rat soleus (Kawano et al. 2008). Because of their high capacity for regener-ation, satellite cells may be used in future stem cell therapy in humans (Wernig 2003). Indeed, satellite cells appear to stock up the number of myonuclei in muscle hypertrophy (Petrella et al. 2008). In senescence or in the elderly, the number of satellite cells in muscle is somewhat lessened (Sajko et al. 2004).

Microvasculature and Capillaries

The microvascular networks are important anatomic and physiological elements supporting metabolic requirements during muscle activity. The need for a regular supply of the muscle fibers with oxygen (O_2) and nutrients (glucose) and for evacuation of metabolites such as carbon dioxide (CO_2) and lactate when needed can be regarded as limiting factors during muscle activity. Together with the nerve fascicles, the arteries and veins enter a larger muscle compartment and branch into several feeder arteries (and veins) for individual muscle portions. At the level of the primary fascicles, they further divide up into arterioles (alternate vessels or valves), and finally into the capillary bed adjacent to single fibers. Normal adult skeletal muscle usually contains about three to five capillaries for each fiber (the capillary-to-fiber ratio), corresponding to ~ 300–

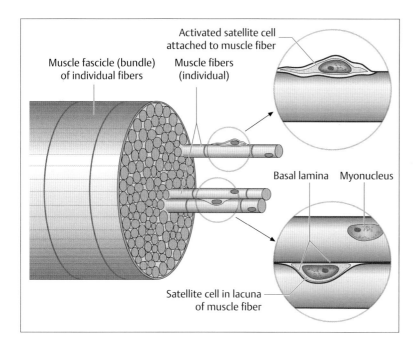

Fig. 1.20 Satellite cells in skeletal muscle. Following a microlesion, satellite cells that are present ("quiet cells") in small lacunae between the muscle fibers near a lesion site are stimulated by local tissue factors and start to proliferate. Activated satellite cells can fuse with the injured muscle fiber, helping to fill up the gap in lost myonuclei from the lesion site to support muscle fiber repair and regeneration.

400 capillary structures per square millimeter of muscle tissue—known as the capillary density in a given muscle.

In resting muscle, however, some spared sections of the microvascular network are only poorly perfused with blood (in a standby or saving mode). Following routine muscle activation, all sections of the microvascular network are then completely perfused with blood in order to optimally supply every single muscle fiber. The total volume of the microvascular bed may therefore increase simply by recruitment of restrained microvascular sections or, for example, by enhanced synthesis and diffusion of local vasoactive agents such as the vasodilator NO, which is known to be controlled by muscle activity. After several months of an exercise regimen, proper renewal of microvascular structures (by angiogenesis) may further enhance the capillary density in a muscle. Because of this adaptation mechanism, the blood perfusion rate may therefore improve in an effectively trained muscle to support physiological enhancement of the muscular metabolic supply among athletes (**Fig. 1.21**)

Ischemia

A muscle is usually well perfused in a relaxed state and slowly adapts to increased muscle activity. The blood perfusion rate is apparently proportional to the actual state of muscle activity during a workout (see "warming up" before start of exercise or "cooling down" thereafter). A slow gain in muscle activity therefore results in a moderate improvement in perfusion, whereas permanent muscle tension (like before or during a competition) may result, at least partly or regionally, in impaired perfusion rates. It should be noted that in principle, a muscle belly is only properly filled with blood during the relaxation phase, while the blood is distributed or "pressed out" in a muscle during its contraction phase. Together with sympathetic tone and stress, this mechanism may exacerbate a nonphysiological lack of blood (ischemia) in muscle shortly before or during a contest or a soccer match.

The diaphragm, the most important muscle in respiration, has a unique anatomic constriction on its blood supply. In addition to its minor blood supply through the thoracic cavity (from the pericardiacophrenic artery), two small arteries (the left and right phrenic artery) arise from the abdominal aorta very close to the aortic foramen, where they may be compressed by the flattened diaphragm muscle during powerful inspiration. This may further push down large organs such as the liver, stomach, and spleen that are located in the upper abdominal cavity, covered by the powerful muscle dome of the diaphragm (see lateral stitches in sports).

Note

During rhythmic respiration, temporally uncoordinated contractions of the diaphragm (often during middle-distance running) may result in impaired muscle perfusion rates. Permanently uncoordinated respiration during forced inspiration (with a basically low position of the contracting diaphragm) may result in painful ischemic provocation in the diaphragm, usually known as lateral stitches in sports.

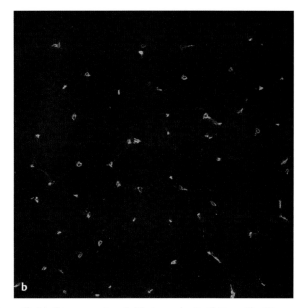

Fig. 1.21a, b   Microvascular bed in a human skeletal muscle, with capillaries (biopsy specimen). (Photographs: D. Blottner, Charité Berlin, Germany)

a Extensive microvascular networks (green) in a trained skeletal muscle.
b Weak to moderate microvascular networks (green) in an untrained skeletal muscle.

Connective Tissue (Myofascial System)

Skeletal muscle is covered with a strong and smooth collagenous surface fascia for sliding during movement. From the surface fascia, formed by dense irregular connective tissue and its supporting layer of loose connective tissue (epimysium), a network of loose connective tissue builds up more thin layers around the fascicles (perimysium) or around the individual muscle fibers (endomysium). In principle, the intramuscular connective tissue is made up of the following constituents (Laurent et al. 1991):

- Type I collagen fibers
- Fibroblasts, fibrocytes
- Extracellular matrix, as a gel-like ground substance

The intramuscular connective tissue wraps around the fascicles and fibers and carries the nerves and blood vessels for the neural and metabolic supply in muscle. However, the sheaths also provide much of the natural muscle elasticity and are in addition involved in inner and outer force transmission (lateral force transmission), which may affect the power output in a given muscle. The complex network of intramuscular collagenous fibers thus ensures adequate biomechanical qualities and appropriate shear stress and it is therefore an important component of the myofascial support mechanism for improving muscle function (Monti et al. 1999).

An increase in intramuscular connective tissue–related muscle stiffness has been documented in the tibialis in older rats, suggesting that lateral force transmission in muscle may be also impaired in the elderly (Gao et al. 2008). More rigid fascial structures have also been found in chronically disused leg muscle (60 days) in younger and middle-aged volunteers (aged 25–45) in bed rest immobilization studies, in a chronic muscle disuse control group without exercise countermeasures.

Note

Muscle activity may well control the microanatomic, biochemical, and molecular composition of the myofascial support system, which may possibly increase the power output of the muscles in sports. In the myofascial pain syndrome, muscle pain may be caused by tightened bands of fascicles that twitch following touching of the superficial skin (trigger points). The syndrome is often associated with overused postural muscle, and when the trigger point in a muscle is pressed, the pain is felt at more distant but predictable areas known as reference zones. Massage and exercise may lead to long-term recovery of the affected muscle.

Principles of Skeletal Muscle Architecture

Skeletal Muscle

A skeletal muscle (**Fig. 1.22**) generally consists of a belly with its end and side tendons.

Note

Note

As a rule, skeletal muscle fibers do not branch and do not merge into one another in the way that blood vessels may do, for example (as in vascular anastomoses). However, fascicles in the facial skin or tongue may branch before they course to the skin or mucosa. Isolated muscle fibers often have tapered endings. A spindle-shaped or fusiform muscle may therefore be explained by the shape of the individual fibers or fascicles, or may be due to larger numbers of fascicles in the bulky belly and fewer fascicles at the ends.

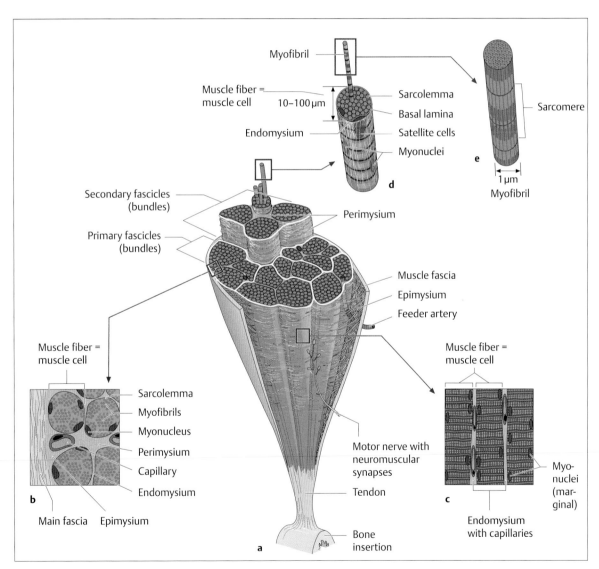

Fig. 1.22a–e   Structure of skeletal muscle.

a Overview.

b An enlarged fiber bundle (fascicle) with intramuscular connective-tissue ensheathments.

c An enlarged fiber bundle (fascicle; with three fibers) on a longitudinal plane.

d A single muscle fiber with myofibrillar bundles.

e A single myofibril, with sarcomere and actin–myosin microfilaments.

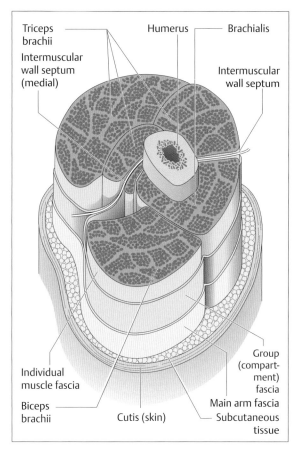

Fig. 1.23 **Structure of the outer and inner fascia of skeletal muscle.**

Muscle Fascia and Intermuscular Septum

In the human body, skeletal muscle may be covered by three different layers of fascia, with variable biomechanical properties. On the muscle belly itself, a thin muscle fascia consists of a "stretchy" collagenous, irregular connective tissue that securely encases the belly and serves as a boundary with adjacent tissues (fascia, bone, muscle, or peripheral nerves or blood vessels). The fibrous-elastic sheaths of this first layer also adapt to tone and shortening during muscle work and may add to overall force production. The body's regional muscles, such as those clearly present in the arms and legs, are functionally grouped by a more inelastic common group fascia (the second fascia layer) that forms the muscle compartments (see p. 7). Individual muscles may be located in an extra compartment or box (as in the sartorius). Intermuscular septal walls with a more rigid mechanical support for muscle are present, for example, where the deep second layer group fascia of the posterior and anterior muscle compartments meet (**Fig. 1.23**). Adjacent to bone, the fibrous septal walls are attached to the periosteum, and in the periphery the deep second fascia layer merges with the common super-ficial regional body fascia (the third fascia layer), as seen for example in the anterior, medial, and posterior thigh compartments covered with the broad fasciae latae of the upper leg, comparable to stockings or "leggings."

Secondary and Primary Bundles (Fascicles)

The muscle is subdivided into groups of fiber bundles (fascicles), with larger numbers of fibers known as secondary fascicles and smaller numbers of myofibers known as primary fascicles, wrapped in sheaths of loose connective tissue (external perimysium) carrying the nerves, blood, and lymphatic vessels. The secondary fascicles (sarcous fibers) are visible with the eye and in case of injury can be palpated as a single fascicle by an experienced examiner. The secondary fascicles are further subdivided by smaller bundles ensheathed by the internal perimysium, known as primary fascicles. They usually have a cross-sectional area of ~ 1 mm² and may contain ~ 50–250 individual muscle fibers (= muscle cells), depending on myofiber type distribution.

Muscle Fibers

An isolated single muscle fiber is a long, spindle-shaped, thin cell tube with a diameter ranging from ~ 0.2 mm up to a maximum of 0.5 mm, comparable to the size of a spider's thread. Its normal cross-sectional area is ~ 1000–7000 μm² in humans (Tipton 2008, Tegtbur et al. 2009). A muscle fiber is covered with a delicate connective-tissue layer (endomysium) that contains fibroblasts, capillaries, and nerves (see **Fig. 1.21**.). The fiber outer membrane itself is covered with a microscopically visible basal membrane mainly consisting of type 4 collagen and several other anchor matrix molecules (fibronectin, laminin) that provide mechanical support for adjacent fibers in a group, or to the perimysial sheaths of adjacent fascicles during a muscle workout.

Practical Tip

A partial muscle tear in sports often affects primary fascicles and not just a single muscle fiber (= muscle cell). As a result of a sudden tear in a fiber or bundle in either the primary or secondary fascicles, simultaneous injury to the microvascular network or even disruption of larger intramuscular vessels may produce a local hematoma with immediate local pain (see Chapters 4 and 6). It should be noted that a tear in only a single muscle fiber may occur acutely during exercise, but due to its minimal cell mass this not result in any pain sensation.

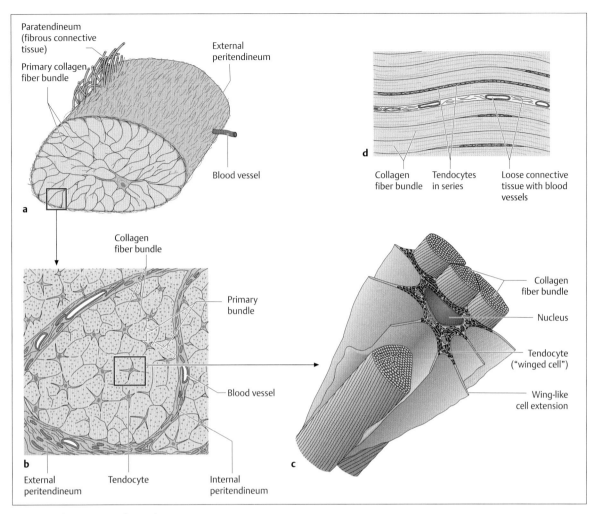

Fig. 1.24a–d   Structure of a tendon.

a Cross-section of a tendon.
b Detail of the cross-section of a tendon, with tendocytes.
c Spatial reconstruction of a tendocyte ("winged cell") "squeezed" between collagen fiber bundles.

d Histologically reconstructed tendon collagen fibers on a longitudinal plane.

Muscle Tendons

Tendon Architecture

Muscle tendons consist of dense regular connective tissue that is formed by parallel collagen fibers in bundles that are used for tensile strength, some elastic fibers used for preloading, fibrocytes (tendocytes), and a scant ground substance used as a supportive element for inner tendon biomechanical and metabolic properties. The tendon surface is wrapped in a thin fibrous layer of irregularly shaped connective tissue known as the external peritendineum (*peri*, around; *tendineum*, tendon) that carries some blood and lymphatic vessels and a few sensory nerve endings that may enter the inner tendon via bridges of loose connective tissue known as the internal peritendineum (**Fig. 1.24**). Flatter tendinous structures known as "aponeuroses" attach flat muscles to bone and have a denser irregular or meshlike connective structure. Due to the perpendicularly running fibers, the latter is more flexible relative to shear forces induced by shortening and relaxation of flat muscles from various angles (see abdominal wall muscles and latissimus dorsi).

Tendon Function

The stretch of a muscle tendon is limited to ~3–5% of its original length and the tensile forces amount to ~6 kg/mm² of tendon tissue. Given an average cross-sectional area of the human Achilles tendon (calcaneus tendon) of ~80–100 mm², a short maximum load-bearing capacity of 500 kg can be calculated for a jumper (jumping from a table 1 m high), resulting in a maximum peak force of ~50–100 N (Kunsch and Kunsch 2005). Pulling forces improve the total length of the Achilles tendon by ~3–5 mm (~0.1–0.2 inches). This means that the wavy pattern of the tendon fibers induced by preload forces of elastic elements (elastic fibers, adipocytes, or proteoglycans as sliding elements) in the relaxed tendon turns into a parallel, more regular fiber pattern during tensile forces following mechanical load. This biomechanical mechanism normally helps to properly transmit the pulling forces over the entire length of the tendon during acute loading without running the risk of the tendon rupturing. However, extremely high pulling forces that may result in an 8–10% increase in tendon length are regarded as a "point of no return," with irreversible rupturing of the tendon fibers.

Muscle exercise helps maintain the structural, biochemical, and biomechanical properties of tendons in athletes. However, an appropriate increase in the cross-sectional area of muscle tendon has not yet been clearly demonstrated following exercise protocols. Due to the weak metabolic input from the sparse blood supply, the process of renewing tendinocytes, fibers, and matrix molecules during exercise adaptation may be rather slow, in terms of a few months, following an intensive muscle workout regimen.

Note

The principal tendon architecture of rigid collagenous and elastic fiber bundles resembles a tow rope for cars, with some elastic elements woven into it. This biomechanical principle normally helps prevent tendon fibers from rupturing during normal exercise, as the pulling forces are transmitted to the rigid collagen fibers via elastic elements more slowly and appropriately. In kangaroos, for example, the tendons contain large amounts of elastic fibers that allow storage and release of kinetic energy and thus serve as springs during jumping.

Muscle–Tendon Contacts (Myotendinous Junction)

The muscle fascicles and their fibers terminate in finger-like protrusions (interdigitations) at the sites where they meet the unraveling fascicles of the muscle tendon (myotendinous junction). A network of protein microfibrils, such as intermediate-sized desmin fibers and collagen fibers, are attached to the basal lamina of the muscle fiber endings, where specialized anchor proteins such as tenascin (from Latin *tenere*, to hold) or fibronectin (from Latin *nexus*, interconnection) provide additional mechanical support for the muscle–tendon interface (**Fig. 1.25**).

Note

In skeletal muscle, fascicles and single fibers may be connected in series by specialized contacts known as myomuscular junctions (Hijikata and Ishikawa 1997). As the total length of a single muscle fiber may not exceed 20–25 cm, this principle allows anatomically and functionally longer contraction units that are, for example, present in the long sartorius (40–60 cm long) in the anterior thigh compartment.

The sartorius, for example, appears to consist of only ~ 30% of end-to-end fibers, while ~ 70% of the fibers are thought to be attached in series via myomuscular junctions (Harris et al. 2005). In the latissimus dorsi, abundant myomuscular and myotendinous junctions result in a more complex microarchitecture than was previously thought (Snobl et al. 1998).

Tendon–Bone Junction (Fig. 1.26)

Note

Insertion sites at the muscle–bone interface, fibrocartilage zones, or myofascial connective tissue structures, also known as myotendinous, myo-osseous, or myoligamentous junctions, have been recently collectively termed "entheses" (Benjamin et al. 2006). Enthesis structures, as sites of muscle or ligament attachment to bone (e.g., fibrous or fibrocartilaginous entheses) play a considerable biodynamic role in general muscle kinetics. They also may control the muscle tone or muscle stiffness. The myoelastic or visceroelastic elements in a muscle represent an estimated 5–20% of total muscle force production. Disorders of entheses, known as "enthesopathy" or "enthesitis" (mainly inflammatory) include many well-known disorders of the ligamentous or muscular attachments such as rotator cuff syndrome, elbow enthesopathy ("tennis elbow"), gluteal tendinitis, and enthesopathy of the knee (retinaculum and patella syndrome) or of the ankle, tarsus, and calcaneus.

Support Structures in Skeletal Muscle

The muscular support structures known as bursa, tendon sheath, and sesamoid bone play important roles in skeletal muscle function and performance control. The bursae or tendinous sheaths of the musculoskeletal system may reduce or even damp mechanical friction between muscle and bone or ligament structures. Sesamoid bones (such as the patella and pisiform bone) close to joints serve as elongated lever arms during joint movements, and according to biophysics save ~ 5–20% of the muscle force required. For example, resistive exercise in the quadriceps knee extensor would be considerably impaired following excision of the patella at the knee joint.

Tendon Sheaths, Bursa, and Retinaculum

Tendon sheaths are constructed as fibrous "slide tubes" that wrap around long muscle tendons at sites close to the joints of the wrist and hands, or ankles, feet, and toes (**Fig. 1.27a**). As in regular joints, the tendon sheath capsule is formed by an outer fibrous layer that is attached to adjacent bone. The tendon capsule and the gap are filled with a lubricant fluid known as the synovia, secreted by

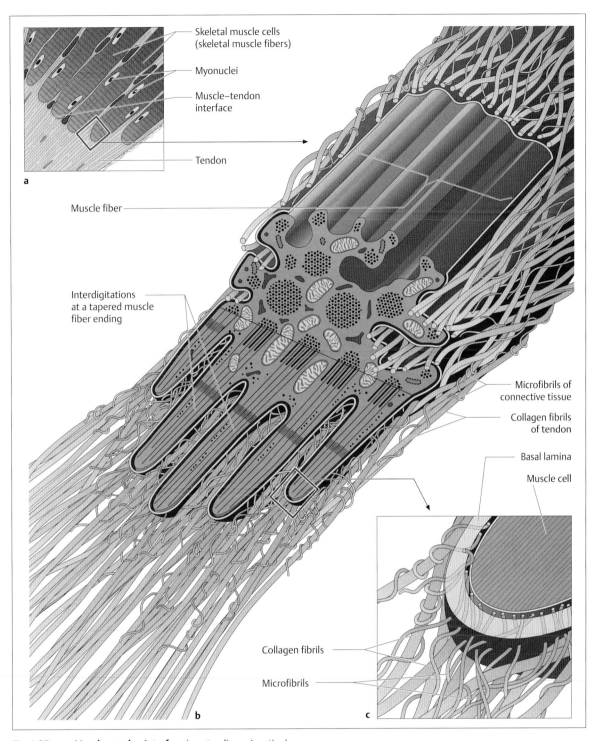

Skeletal muscle cells
(skeletal muscle fibers)

Myonuclei

Muscle–tendon
interface

Tendon

a

Muscle fiber

Interdigitations
at a tapered muscle
fiber ending

Microfibrils of
connective tissue

Collagen fibrils
of tendon

Basal lamina

Muscle cell

Collagen fibrils

Microfibrils

b

c

Fig. 1.25a–c   Muscle–tendon interface (myotendinous junction).

a Overview.
b Terminal muscle fibers merged to collagen fibers and microfibrils (drawing based on ultrastructural images).
c Detailed reconstruction showing tapered muscle fiber with terminal junction structures such as basal lamina, microfibrils, and collagenous tendon fibers.

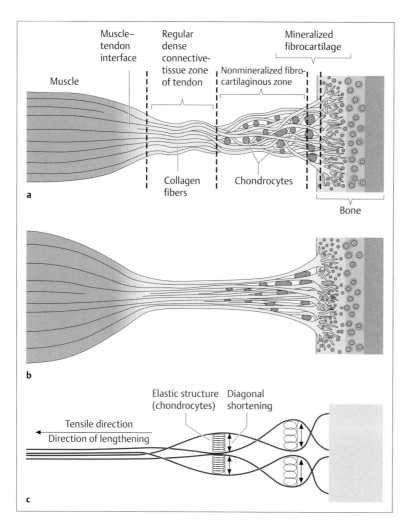

Fig. 1.26a–c Bone–tendon interface (tendo-osseous junction).

a Relaxed muscle–tendon–bone interface.
b Contracted muscle–tendon–bone interface.
c Diagram of the stretch-damping principle.

Figure labels: Muscle; Muscle–tendon interface; Regular dense connective-tissue zone of tendon; Mineralized fibrocartilage; Nonmineralized fibrocartilaginous zone; Collagen fibers; Chondrocytes; Bone.

Part c labels: Elastic structure (chondrocytes); Diagonal shortening; Tensile direction; Direction of lengthening.

the inner synovial layer of the tendon sheath wall. At both ends, the synovial gap is sealed with a flexible but tight membrane fold between the capsule and the tendon surface. For example, the long tendons of the forearm posterior extensor muscle compartment course over the wrist beneath the dorsal retinaculum, a girdlelike regular fibrous structure separated by up to six individual fibrous compartments (cassettes) each of which contains one of the six tendon sheaths of the forearm extensor muscles. By contrast, the long tendons of the anterior forearm flexor compartment are crowded together in a common tendon sheath that travels through the carpal tunnel to the palm, where the tendons split up again into the individual tendon sheaths of the five digits. In the lower leg, for example, comparable retinacular structures carry the long tendons of the anterior, posterior, and lateral calf muscle compartments in their respective tendon sheaths and compartments over the ankle joints to their final insertions at the phalangeal bones of the toes (**Fig. 1.27b**).

Mechanical friction between muscles or tendons and bone markings or overlying ligaments is reduced by bursa (the Latin word for purse), which functions as a local "glide cushion" to prevent rubbing between muscle, bone, and ligament structures during regular joint movements. A bursa is a flat fibrous sac lined with a synovial membrane and filled with synovial lubricant, as in a tendon sheath. The bursa and tendon sheaths are supplied by small vessels and sensory nerves (mostly pain sensation) via flexible suspensory ligaments (**Fig. 1.27a**).

Sesamoids

The best-known sesamoid is the patella in the knee joint, which is an integral bony part of the quadriceps tendon. The latter helps direct extension forces via the joint to the distal insertion point of the infrapatellar tendon at the tibia bone markings known as the tibial tuberosity (**Fig. 1.28**). As mentioned, the patella and other sesamoid

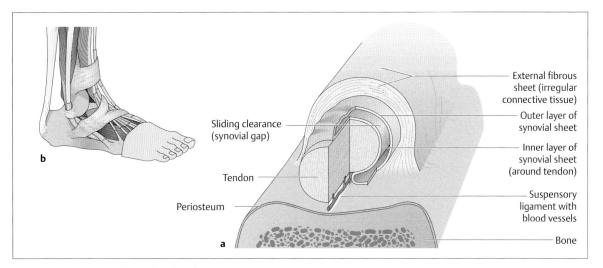

Fig. 1.27a, b   Structure of a tendon sheath.

a Histological reconstruction of a tendon sheath.
b Anatomic overview of tendon sheaths (blue) and retinacula (beltlike ligaments) in the foot and ankle (frontolateral view).

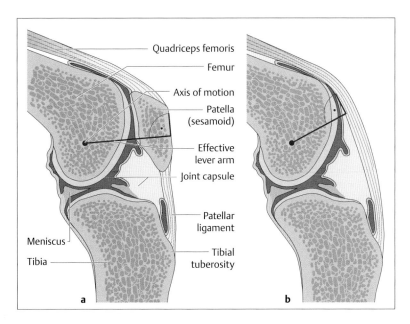

Fig. 1.28a, b   Sesamoids as functional levers, using the patella as an illustration.

a With the patella present, the lever arm (the virtual rectangular line between the quadriceps tendon and the joint axis) is longer.
b Without the patella, the lever arm is significantly shortened, resulting in reduced force (up to 20% in comparison with normal).

bones (e.g., in the thumb or great toe) serve as an elongated lever arm to optimize muscle forces. In addition, the inner cartilaginous surface of the patella has direct access to the knee joint capsule or gap, and the typical posterior surface marks on the patella help direct joint movements mechanically during knee extension versus flexion, as well as allowing final rotation in the joint closure position during terminal knee extension.

Caution

The anatomically recognized sesamoid bones should not be mistaken for cartilaginous or mineralized tissue nodes, which are usually referred to as ganglions in the musculoskeletal system. A ganglion node is sometimes palpable at tendinous or ligamental scar structures underneath skin that have been affected by overuse or chronic mechanical stress, as in the aponeuroses of the palm or foot soles (plantar ligaments) during various sports activities. These nodes may cause local pain, and particularly if they are mechanically activated during exercise they may induce foreign body sensations locally, impairing sports performance to some extent.

Active versus Passive Muscle Insufficiency

In general, the length and muscle shortening of a single-joint muscle allows optimal narrowing of the bone partners. Maximal shortening of the biceps brachii thus lifts the forearm to the humerus until the elbow joint is flexed to its final position. The following two features should be taken into account in multijoint muscles—for example, in the hamstrings, which course from the pelvic girdle ischium over the knee joint to insert at the lower leg (Schünke 2000):

- *Active muscle insufficiency* (insufficient shortening). Shortening of multijoint muscles that travel over several joints may not be sufficient to bring all of the joints to their final positions. For example, if the hip joint is in an extended position (in an upright posture), the hamstrings may not shorten enough to allow for the final flexion position of the knee joint. This feature can be appreciated after exercise if the quadriceps are stretched in an upright posture with knee flexion, when the hand can be placed on the ankle and careful pulling leads to a little more knee flexion and quadriceps stretching.
- *Passive muscle insufficiency* (insufficient stretching). If the knee is in its final position (final rotation joint closure), the hamstrings may not be stretched sufficiently to allow for full hip joint flexion. This problem can be easily appreciated during warming-up before exercise if the upper body is flexed at the hip joint to allow the fingertips to touch the ground in front.

Practical Tip

Problems with sufficient shortening of the biceps of the anterior upper arm muscle compartment during elbow flexion, or of the hamstrings in the posterior thigh muscle compartment versus the calf muscles in the lower leg during knee flexion, may also be due to increased muscle mass (hypertrophy) in the relevant muscle groups in extensively trained athletes. This type of insufficient muscle shortening can be termed soft/lean tissue-related inhibition.

Innervation of Skeletal Muscle

Muscle actions are driven by motor control from the central nervous system—that is, the brain and spinal cord, located in large bone cavities (the skull and spine) and by peripheral structures such as the spinal nerves (trunk) and plexus nerves (arm and legs) that course from the spine through the neural foramina (intervertebral foramina) to the peripheral muscles.

Note

The autonomic nervous system contributes in a more indirect way to motor control of muscle work, such as tonus control or muscle fatigue via sympathetic fibers located in the smooth muscle layer of microvessels, or via transmitter release of diffusible signals from special axonal swellings known as varicosities ("en passant" or "par distance" synapses—nerve–muscle contacts with a broad synaptic cleft). The precise mechanisms involved in the control of the somatic skeletal muscle system by the autonomic nervous system are as yet unknown.

The motor control of skeletal muscle is provided by efferent innervation starting from the premotor cortex of the brain, located in the precentral gyrus, via projection fibers known as the pyramidal tract to the ventral horn α-motor neurons in the spinal cord segments. In general, nerve entry points are located more proximally in most forearm muscles. The forearm muscles are mostly innervated by deep fascicles of the three main arm nerves, the median, ulnar and radial nerves, while the leg muscles are mostly innervated by ventral aspects of the lumbar plexus nerves, the obturator and femoral nerves, or dorsally by the sciatic nerve, which divides in the tibial and peroneal nerves to innervate all the other leg muscles.

Practical Tip

Motor points in normal skeletal muscle provide important anatomic landmarks for precise taping on of electrodes during functional electrostimulation of muscle. Usually, the motor points consist of nerve fascicles that enter the epimysium to split up inside the muscle into intramuscular branches. Some muscles in the arms or legs have multiple motor points, and this should be taken into account by the therapist. Initial anatomic maps of the motor points in the upper extremity are already available (Safwat and Abdel-Meguid 2007). It is generally agreed that the motor points need not be identical to the muscle trigger points mentioned above. Trigger points may be distributed over the entire muscle as either bandlike or pointlike palpable hypercontractions (see myofascial trigger points).

As in skeletal muscle, a peripheral nerve is also covered with a rigid outer sheet known as epineurium (from *epi-*, on, and neurium, the sheet layer around a whole nerve), the inner nerve fascicles are ensheathed by loose connective tissue known as the perineurium (*peri-*, around), and each nerve fiber or axon in a fascicle is wrapped in a delicate membrane known as the endoneurium (*endo-*, internal). The axon itself may either be wrapped from one node of Ranvier to the next with one typical Schwann cell with a myelin sheath (internodal segment) of varying thickness (strongly or moderately myelinated nerves), or may course without a myelin sheath (unmyelinated nerves)—for example, the postganglionic autonomic fibers, which

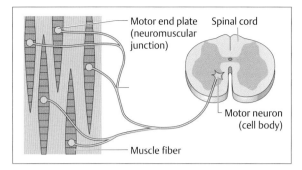

Fig. 1.29 **Motor units** in skeletal muscle and the spinal cord.

are embedded as a group with one Schwann cell along their fibers. As in muscle, the three main fascia sheets in a nerve contain blood and lymphatic vessels that supply or remove nutrients and blood gases.

Motor Units and Neuromuscular Synapses

Skeletal muscles may have relatively small motor units, such as the extraocular muscles in the orbits or interosseus muscles in the hand and foot (**Fig. 1.29**). In this case, each spinal motor neuron innervates ~ 5–10 individual muscle fibers. For example, each of the extraocular muscles is thought to contain ~ 1750 motor units (Kunsch and Kunsch 2005). Skeletal muscle with relatively large motor units, such as the biceps and quadriceps, may contain ~ 750 or even more than 1000 units per spinal motor neuron. The estimated maximum force production in a motor unit is ~ 0.001 Nm (Newton meter) in an extraocular muscle and ~ 0.5 Nm in the biceps (Kunsch and Kunsch 2005).

Note

A muscle's force production can be significantly increased through effective muscle exercise protocols, due to recruitment of additional motor units.

Motor End Plate— Neuromuscular Junction

Neuromuscular junctions represent highly specialized synaptic contacts between a somatic nerve terminal and a skeletal muscle fiber. In these locations, there are branched axon endings from α-motor neurons that are embedded in a system of deeply folded depressions in the muscle fiber outer membrane (sarcolemma), known as the postsynaptic membrane or subneural folded apparatus (**Fig. 1.30**). The main synaptic cleft is sometimes called the primary cleft, while the junctional folds are sometimes called secondary synaptic clefts. Unlike the central synapses, which have a narrow cleft of ~ 2 nm, the

neuromuscular synapse has a relatively broad cleft of ~ 5–10 nm that also has a synaptic basal lamina as part of the general basal lamina sheet of the fiber (**Fig. 1.30**). Both the axonal terminal and synaptic clefts are sealed by a terminal synaptic Schwann cell that covers these structures and thus separates the synaptic compartment from the extrasynaptic compartment to prevent lateral shifting of postsynaptic proteins or diffusion of transmitter signals to extrasynaptic sites (see the note on trigger points below).

Together with myotrophic and neurotrophic agents, the synaptic Schwann cell and basal lamina contribute to maintenance and regeneration of the neuromuscular synaptic microarchitecture throughout life (Hughes et al. 2006). This is seen in particular in the axonal sprouting mechanisms that occur after acute denervation (axotomy), supported by the terminal Schwann cell, as recently reported (Tam and Gordon 2003).

Practical Tip

In general, the neuromuscular junction is able to maintain a stable microarchitecture throughout life. In cases of muscle plasticity and adaptation, for example, due to regular muscle exercise protocols in athletes, or following extended disuse (bed rest), skeletal muscle fibers may show indirect or direct structural, biochemical, and physiological changes that can be also documented at the neuromuscular junction (Deschenes et al. 1994). Acute or chronic muscle stretching may also result in altered neuronal control (Dressler et al. 2005). Maps are currently being established to show the anatomic distribution of neuromuscular junctions in the body's individual muscle groups—for example, in the calf triceps (Parratte et al. 2002)—to identify more precise points for intramuscular needle injections in infiltration treatments (Laurent et al. 1991, Deschenes et al. 1994).

Note

The palpable and painful myofascial trigger points are thought to be reflected by morphological and physiological correlates of hypercontracted bands of individual fiber bundles. Although the precise molecular mechanisms are as yet unclear, it is evident that "painful trigger points," sometimes also known as "activated myofascial trigger points," may be induced by disproportionate local spillover of transmitters such as acetylcholine from overexcited or partially leaky motor end plates in an affected muscle fascicle (Mense 2003).

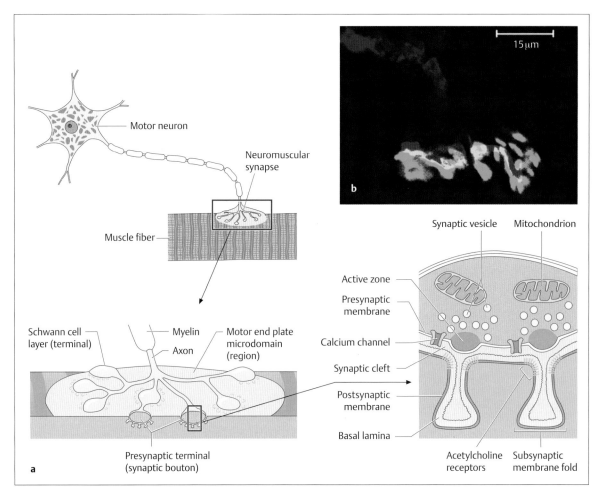

Fig. 1.30a, b   Neuromuscular synapses

a Diagrams showing the structure.
b Confocal laser scanning microscopy (D. Blottner, Charité Berlin, Germany). The motor nerve (immunostained in red) is in contact with a muscle fiber (unstained) via spliced nerve terminals that are deeply embedded in the postsynaptic membrane folds (green stain). Overlapping structures of the nerve and postsynaptic membrane are outlined in yellow.

Neuromuscular Spindle

Architecture

The neuromuscular spindle organs serve as encapsulated length sensors of a muscle and help to continuously monitor the position of limbs or the state of contraction of limb muscles. The neuromuscular spindle is mainly composed of the following structures:

- Intrafusal fibers (thin specialized fibers)
- Myelinated sensory terminals (Ia afferent components)
- Efferent axons (motor components)

Intrafusal fibers are specialized thin muscle fibers that run through a fusiform or spindle-shaped capsule and should be distinguished from the thicker extrafusal muscle fibers that make up the vast majority of normally contracting skeletal muscle fibers innervated by α-motor neurons of the ventral spinal cord. Due to the localization of their nuclei, there are two types of intrafusal fiber—one that has a bunch of central nuclei in a baglike region, called nuclear bag fibers, and a second type with the nuclei in series, known as nuclear chain fibers. Both fiber type endings have striated regions that are able to actively contract due to efferent input from ventral spinal cord γ-motor neurons. The neuromuscular spindles are located between muscle fibers in series and usually contain one nuclear bag fiber and a variable amount (usually up to five or more) of nuclear chain fibers (**Fig. 1.31a, b**).

The spindle organ receives sensory input via myelinated type Ia fiber terminals from dorsal root ganglion neurons that penetrate the capsule, where unmyelinated axons terminate in the form of spiral terminals at the nonstriated, noncontracting central portions (receptor region) of the intrafusal fibers. They are highly sensitive to length changes. For example, if the extrafusal fibers shorten during muscle contraction, the encapsulated neuromuscular spindle fibers oriented in parallel lose tension and become slack. At the same time, the striated poles of intrafusal fibers are activated via γ-motor neuron input and thus shorten (stretch) the fiber in a feedback control mechanism. This constant feedback control mechanism of the neuromuscular spindles is indispensable for normal performance control (Chalmers 2002, Windhorst 2007).

Neuromuscular Spindle Density

There is considerable variability in the neuromuscular spindles in muscles with regard to number, location, and even biochemical properties (Tegtbur et al. 2009). Notably, the number of spindles in a muscle (spindle density) varies depending on regional anatomic muscle groups. For example, axial muscle groups in the trunk, such as the erector spinae or neck muscles, have relatively large numbers of muscle spindles, while the muscles in the shoulder girdle have relatively small numbers. These differences are not seen in the spindle density of long or short muscles or in the postural versus stabilizing or mobilizing muscle groups of the human body (Richardson and Jull 1995). Proximal muscle groups in the arm have relatively smaller densities of spindles than distal groups such as those in the hand.

However, similar changes have not been found between leg and foot muscle groups (Banks 2006). This may reflect unique aspects of human evolution that resulted in adaptation of the hand as a fine coordinating and sensitive gripping tool, in contrast to the foot as a well-adapted anatomic tool for bipedal locomotion.

Golgi Tendon Organ (GTO)

Architecture

The Golgi tendon organs are considered to be regular muscle tension sensors in skeletal muscle that control muscle tone as needed, provide the nervous system with minute changes in muscle tensions, and help to control both muscle tone and biodynamics. In principle, GTOs are encapsulated structures ~1 mm long that are located at the muscle–tendon interface (**Fig. 1.31c**). Within the capsule, there is a network of longitudinal collagen fibers that is penetrated by myelinated and unmyelinated sensory group Ib fiber terminals. Stretching of the tendon during movement results in straightening of the collagen fibers and thus activation of the sensory terminals by fiber compression or by very small deformations in the GTO capsule. GTOs are readily activated by normal muscle contractions or during normal movements and thus also continuously measure force during muscle contraction, as

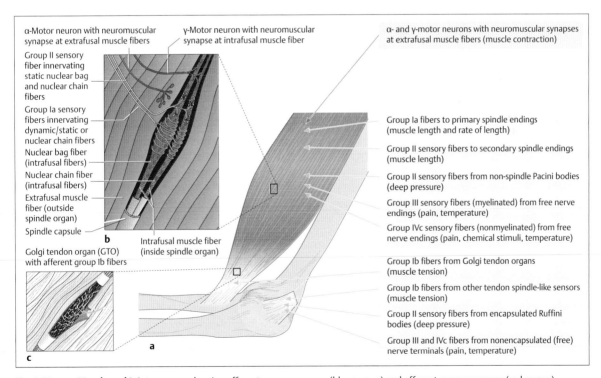

Fig. 1.31a–c Muscle and joint sensors, showing afferent nerves or axons (blue arrows) and efferent nerves or axons (red arrows).

a Anatomic distribution of musculoskeletal and joint sensors.
b Muscle spindle organ (intrafusal fiber) and nerve supply.
c Golgi tendon organs (GTOs) and nerve supply.

there is a positive correlation between the group Ib firing rate and force production.

Note

The precise position of GTOs is closer to the tendon–muscle interface, rather than in the tendon itself. GTOs are frequently found at attachments and insertion sites of muscles, in aponeuroses, and are more sparsely located in muscle compartment general fascia or muscular septum walls. GTOs are specialized sensory receptors known as tendon sensors and thus provide the basis for the tendon reflex necessary to reduce tension in a muscle—for example, during passive or active muscle stretching. Inhibition of the same muscle and excitation of the antagonist muscle in the tendon reflex is called the inverse myotatic reflex (that is, opposite to the stretch reflex = myotatic reflex).

Function of GTOs

Only a relatively small number of muscle fibers can activate a single GTO. Close to GTOs, there are other mechanosensors such as Pacini bodies and numerous nonencapsulated terminals. A single motor unit of extrafusal muscle fibers has at least one GTO in skeletal muscle (Jami 1988). It is well accepted that the GTOs located in series with the muscle fibers also form part of autogenic inhibition, as they measure and monitor muscle tension output from a single motor unit (force measurement)—for example, to maintain muscle power in sports (Chalmers 2002).

Functional Anatomic Principles of Muscle Reflexes

Note

Successful skeletal muscle actions are executed in a spatiotemporal manner and with a finely tuned production of force as needed. This is accomplished by coordinated interactions between agonist and antagonist muscles during performance (Figs. 1.31 and 1.32). In addition to vestibular and visuomotor mechanisms, spontaneous proprioceptive stimulation is an integral component needed to achieve the regular body posture necessary to support movements (in accordance with the principle that mobility depends on stability). This is ensured by two important mechanisms known as reflex-controlled movements and sensorimotor feedback control.

Muscle reflexes are essential and integral mechanisms for supporting motor activity and target control. A reflex is initiated by spontaneously and stereotypically executed muscle activation, which is relatively independent from the state of consciousness. The sensors relating to skeletal muscle control are as follows:

- Skin sensors (subcutaneous mechanosensors on the palms and soles)
- Muscle sensors (spindle organ)
- Tendon sensors (GTOs)
- Fascial and periosteal sensors (mechanosensors)
- Vestibular sensors (semicircular organs)

The stimulus responses in skeletal muscle behavior that are triggered include skeletomotor (muscle contraction), sensory (tone control, tension), and autonomic (vasomotor) responses.

Reflex Arcs

Reflexes are simple chains of one or more synaptically linked afferent and efferent neurons that are involuntarily and rapidly executed (automatically) on stimulation and may reflect the basic structural plan of the nervous system as one of the bases for skeletal muscular behavior. Usually, a sensor (receptor) or the terminal axon of a sensory neuron is located in the body's periphery, such as the skin or subcutaneous structures, while the neuronal soma is located in spinal ganglia close to the spine, for example.

Monosynaptic (Myotatic) Reflex

The simplest of all reflexes is the monosynaptic reflex arc or myotatic reflex, consisting of a circuit of one afferent and one efferent neuron with only one synaptic connection. This monosynaptic reflex is best illustrated by the patella tendon reflex in knee extension (**Fig. 1.32a**). The initial stimulus is provided by sudden muscle stretching (i.e., a length change in the intrafusal fibers of the muscle spindle in the quadriceps), triggered by a brief blow from a reflex hammer to the infrapatellar tendon, for example. The stimulus is then propagated to spinal α-motor neurons via fast-type Ia fibers, which in turn send back an axonal response for excitation of the rectus femoris (agonist) via the α1-fibers. Simultaneously, muscle tone in the dorsal hip flexors decreases by inhibition (i.e., reciprocal inhibition via spinal interneurons) of the α-motor neurons. Thus, contraction of the quadriceps and relaxation of the hamstrings result in unstretching or inactivation of the muscle spindle, causing reflex extension of the knee. The patella reflex circuit is often also called the extensor reflex.

Other examples of muscle reflexes relevant for clinically applied tests include:

- Biceps reflex (C5–C6)
- Brachioradialis reflex (C5–C6)
- Triceps brachii reflex (C7–C8)
- Adductor reflex (L2–L4)
- Quadriceps reflex (L2/3–L4)
- Tibialis posterior reflex (L5)
- Triceps surae reflex (S1–S2)

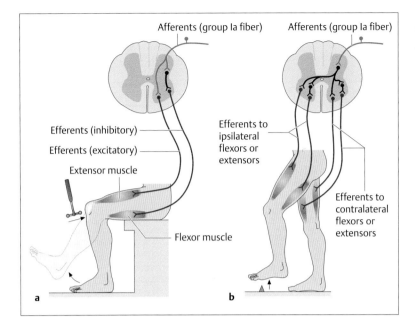

Fig. 1.32a, b Neuroanatomic organization of muscle reflex arcs.

a Monosynaptic reflex arc (with receptor and effector in the same organ). Example: patellar reflex.
b Polysynaptic reflex arc (the receptor and effector are spatially more distant from each other, not in the same organ). Example: withdrawing reflex in reflex pain avoidance.

Together with the extensor reflex, the flexor reflex helps restore the positioning of the joint from a fixed position mainly by stimulating the agonist muscle (quadriceps) while relaxing the antagonist muscle (hamstrings), maintaining control of the muscle length (**Fig. 1.32a, b**).

In skeletal muscle, mechanical loading is controlled via the muscle stretch reflex, including 1α muscle spindles (**Fig. 1.33a**) and GTOs (**Fig. 1.33b**), reducing the risk of muscle injury during heavy loading.

Withdrawal Reflex

This type of spinal reflex helps withdraw the limb from a harmful stimulus, with the contralateral limb being extended to take the body weight and prevent falling. In addition, several postural rearrangements of the trunk muscles and compensatory movements in the upper limbs may help maintain body support by reflexes that act without conscious control (**Fig. 1.32b**). The withdrawal reflex consists of polysynaptic circuits between an afferent Ia-neuron (dorsal root ganglia), one or more interneurons, and efferent neurons located as extensor or flexor neuron pools in the spinal cord, which project via the ventral roots to their respective extensor or flexor muscles in the periphery. The withdrawal reflex is therefore also known as a polysynaptic reflex arc. In general, spinal circuits control bipedal locomotion and coordinate several important neuroreflexive actions such as stepping patterns or alternating upper limb movements during gait or running (see quadruped locomotion). The polysynaptic circuits are controlled by hierarchical motor control from supraspinal and cortical brain areas (see p. 49, **Fig. 1.34**).

Note

More obvious examples of withdrawal reflexes are seen in cases of harmful stimuli on the hand or bare foot—for example, when touching a hot plate or stepping onto a piece of glass, or during reflex limb stretching (extension) when there is a risk of falling in sports activities. Other typical examples of polysynaptic reflex circuits include vegetative reflexes via sympathetic efferents to the vascular smooth muscle layer for vasomotor control.

Rhythmic Movements in Sports

Rhythmic movements, such as during walking or running in sports, consist of voluntary and also involuntary (reflex) elements. They are largely independent of the aim and purpose of an action and are controlled by supraspinal and cortical areas (brainstem, basal ganglia, motor cortex). The voluntary movements are reflected by primary and also learned actions derived from the higher sensorimotor centers such as the motor cortex, basal ganglia, and cerebellum.

In addition to the startle reflex, visual, acoustic, and vestibular sensory impressions, as well as feedback control mechanisms, have to be integrated in order to achieve a well-coordinated and fine-tuned performance. In competitive sports, such mechanisms may well determine the individual skill and agility of a talented athlete.

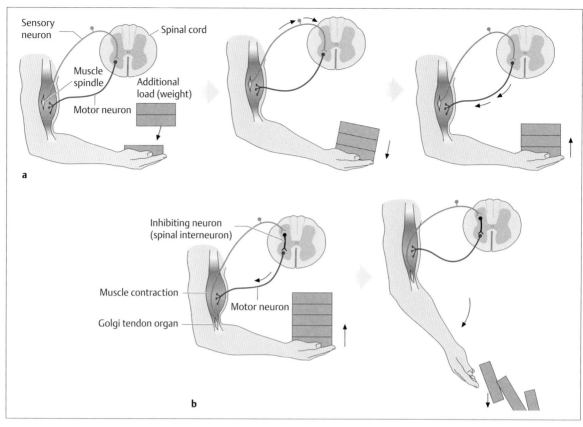

Fig. 1.33a, b Neuroanatomic organization of the stretch reflex (monosynaptic pathway).

a Muscle spindle reflex. As shown in the illustration, additional loading of the biceps results in stretching of intrafusal spindle fibers and slight lowering of the forearm. The afferent Ia fibers start to fire, resulting in reflex contraction of the extrafusal biceps fibers and thus reflex lifting of the forearm. Simultaneously, the Ia afferents also inhibit contraction of the antagonist muscle (triceps, not shown) via spinal interneurons. The antagonist remains in its relaxed state to allow appropriate flexion of the forearm during increasing loading.

b The Golgi tendon reflex. When there is more extensive loading of the forearm, the biceps has to contract more strongly. The Golgi tendon collagenous fibers are increasingly stretched, activating interwoven Ib terminal afferents of the tendon spindle via compression. As a result, the spinal motor neurons are increasingly inhibited by this type of afferent input from Golgi organs and—via spinal inhibitory Ia interneurons—the muscle suddenly relaxes, thus lowering the overloaded forearm (dropping the load) to prevent muscle injury.

Note

The complex regional pain syndrome (CRPS) is explained by a sympathetic reflex dystrophy that may result in a persistent burning pain sensation in the extremities following injury or other harmful stimuli. The pathogenetic mechanisms involved may include altered sensory, motor, or even autonomic mechanisms, but are at present unknown (Rohkamm 2000).

The Innervated Locomotor Apparatus

Brain and Spinal Cord

As mentioned above, voluntary movements are based on supraspinal input, as they are controlled by large motor neurons known as pyramidal cells (first neuron) located in cortical motor areas—for example, the primary motor cortex next to the precentral gyrus. The large pyramidal cells send their axon bundles via descending pathways, the corticospinal tract (also termed pyramidal tract), where they synapse to the second neuron (α-motor neuron) located in the ventral gray matter of the spinal cord. As the corticospinal tract runs through the brainstem,

~ 80% of the descending axons cross (or decussate) in the midline of the medulla just before entering the spinal cord (pyramidal decussation) and run contralaterally through the spinal white matter (lateral corticospinal tract) to reach their target α-motor neurons in the ventral horn. About 20% of corticospinal tract fibers run through the medulla and spinal white matter orthogradely (without crossing) and only cross as they enter each level of the spinal segment gray matter (anterior corticospinal tract) to make synaptic connections with the contralateral spinal α-motor neuron pool. However, stimulation of the left motor cortex results in movements on the right side of the body, and vice versa. The motor cortex shows an orderly pattern of defined regions in which, in principle, the cortical neurons of the most medial areas control the feet and legs, the intermediate parts control the trunk, arm and hand, and the lateral areas control the head and mouth—known as the somatotopic motor cortex organization.

The ventral spinal α-motor neurons project via the ventral roots to their peripheral target muscles, where they terminate at the motor end plates (neuromuscular junctions, NMJs) of the muscle fibers in a coordinated innervation pattern (see motor units). At the NMJ, the electrophysiological nerve impulse is translated into a chemical signal through exocytosis of the transmitter acetylcholine (ACh) from vesicles of the presynaptic membrane into the synaptic cleft. The transmitter ACh specifically binds to the postsynaptic membrane nicotinic ACh receptor (AChR), a sodium channel protein, and the sodium influx from the open AChR results in an excitatory postsynaptic potential (EPSP) that gives rise to a complex excitation contraction coupling mechanism, including calcium and ATP, and resulting in a muscle contraction (see Chapter 2). The bound ACh is restored via ACh-esterase, located at the synaptic basal lamina, and the choline residue is subsequently recycled by endocytotic reuptake mechanisms at the presynaptic nerve terminal.

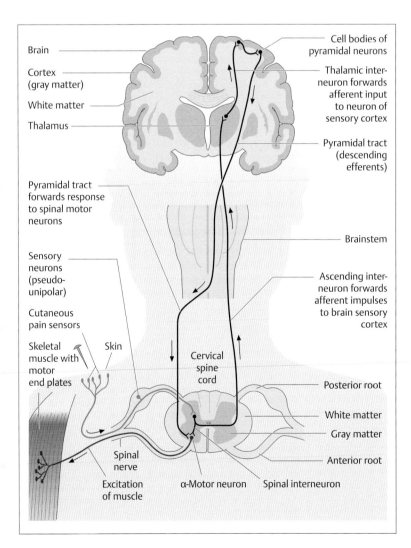

Fig. 1.34 Neuroanatomic structure of the skeletal muscle innervation, with efferent (red) and afferent (blue) neurons from the muscle or skin and vice versa, passing via central ascending (afferent) and descending (efferent) pathways (black) to cortical areas (motor cortex, sensory cortex), thalamus, brainstem, and spinal cord and back to their peripheral target organs.

Brain

Cortex (gray matter)

White matter

Thalamus

Pyramidal tract forwards response to spinal motor neurons

Sensory neurons (pseudo-unipolar)

Cutaneous pain sensors

Skeletal muscle with motor end plates

Skin

Cervical spine cord

Excitation of muscle

Spinal nerve

α-Motor neuron

Spinal interneuron

Cell bodies of pyramidal neurons

Thalamic inter-neuron forwards afferent input to neuron of sensory cortex

Pyramidal tract (descending efferents)

Brainstem

Ascending inter-neuron forwards afferent impulses to brain sensory cortex

Posterior root

White matter

Gray matter

Anterior root

The sensory cortex located in the brain's postsynaptic gyrus also receives input from peripheral sensors, such as the skin (mechano-, pain sensors) or proprioceptors from deeper tissues such as muscle spindles or GTOs, via sensory (afferent) pathways that, in principle, course from the pseudounipolar neurons of the dorsal root ganglia via the dorsal horn and ascending spinothalamic pathways to various interneurons in the thalamus. The thalamic neurons terminate with their ascending axons onto sensory neurons of the postcentral gyrus. From there, cortical interneurons close the anatomic and functional loop between the sensory and motor cortex as a major element of the sensorimotor system (**Fig. 1.34**). As in the motor cortex, the somatotopic organization of the sensory cortex provides a representation of the body's sensations, including touch, position, and pain as major feedback control mechanisms in the locomotor system. Other highly important areas of sensorimotor integration in terms of feedback control for motor output in the motor system are represented by the basal ganglia with the substantia nigra, cerebellum, or brainstem, which are discussed elsewhere in this book (see Chapter 2).

Plexuses and Peripheral Nerves

Plexus

> *Note*
>
> The term "plexus" refers to local networks of nerve fiber bundles located along the body's neuraxis that are composed exclusively of the anterior branches of the spinal nerves. More importantly, the nerve fibers (axons) of the spinal roots are "re-bundled"—that is, the nerve fibers from adjacent spinal segments are split up to form new fascicles in the periphery, so that each new fascicle now contains a mixed collection of nerve fibers from adjacent spinal segments. As a result of this division, "new" peripheral nerves are formed to innervate target muscle compartments in the extremities in general. This anatomic fiber division allows a better coordination between the central motor neuron column in the ventral spinal cord and the peripheral target muscle groups in the upper and lower limbs (**Fig. 1.35**).

In accordance with the basic structure of the vertebrate body, the human nervous system is organized with nerve structures (brain and spinal cord) that run from head to tail, sometimes known as the "neuraxis," during development. In the adult human body, the simple neuraxial structure is still seen in the segmentally structured innervation pattern, as each spinal cord segment gives rise to spinal nerves that run in the periphery to their target structures—for example, the deep axial muscle groups in the trunk (erector spinae). The intercostal nerves located in the intercostal spaces of the ribs, as well as the subcos-

tal, iliohypogastric, and ilioinguinal nerves that course "freely" (without intercostal space support) through the abdominal wall are also clear examples of the segmental innervation pattern in the trunk.

However, the upper and lower extremities have an alternative innervation pattern, known as plexus innervation. In the neck and shoulder region, there are two major plexuses that originate from the spine and spinal cord:

- The cervical plexus (C1–C4), which gives rise to smaller nerves in the infrahyoid muscles of the anterior neck, used for swallowing and speaking, and for some other intrinsic neck muscles, and the phrenic nerve of the diaphragm as the primary respiratory muscle (C4–C5)
- The brachial plexus (C5–T1), which gives rise to the three main peripheral nerves of the arm muscle compartments—the radial nerve (C5–C7), median nerve (C6–T1), and ulnar nerve (C7–T1)—as well as some muscles in the shoulder girdle (pectoralis, levator scapulae, rotator cuff)

In the lumbar and pelvic region, there are two other plexuses (the lumbosacral plexus) that arise from the spine and spinal cord:

- The lumbar plexus (L1–L5), which gives rise to the main nerves innervating the anterior hip (iliopsoas), anterior leg muscle compartment (T12–L4, femoral nerve, quadriceps, sartorius) and medial leg muscle compartment (L2–L4, obturator nerve, adductors).
- The sacral plexus (L4–S4), which gives rise to the gluteal nerves (L4–S1/2, superior and inferior gluteal nerves) innervating the posterior hip muscle compartment (gluteus, lateral rotators, including tensor fasciae latae); the sciatic nerve (S1–S4), innervating the posterior thigh (hamstrings), calf (triceps surae and deep muscles) and sole of the foot muscle compartments (L5–S2, tibial nerve); the deep fibular nerve (L5–S1) that innervates the anterior calf (long extensors), and the superficial fibular nerve (L5–S2) innervating the lateral calf muscle compartment (fibularis or peroneus group), or the dorsum of the foot muscle compartments, including the short toe extensors (**Fig. 1.35**).

Cervical Plexus

The cervical plexus (C1–C4) contains sensory nerves for the posterior regions of the skin of the head, behind the ear and the occiput, as well as for the anterior and lateral skin of the neck and shoulder (acromion). The superficial nerve fibers can be palpated in a lateral neck skin region known as the "punctum nervosum" (nerve point) just where the straplike omohyoid is covered by the anterior marking of the sternocleidomastoid. The motor nerve supply in the cervical plexus is represented by a deep slinglike nerve (ansa = sling) known as the deep cervical ansa (ansa cervicalis profunda), innervating the infrahyoids. The phrenic nerve (C4–C5) is a major portion of the cervical plexus and contains sensory and motor fibers

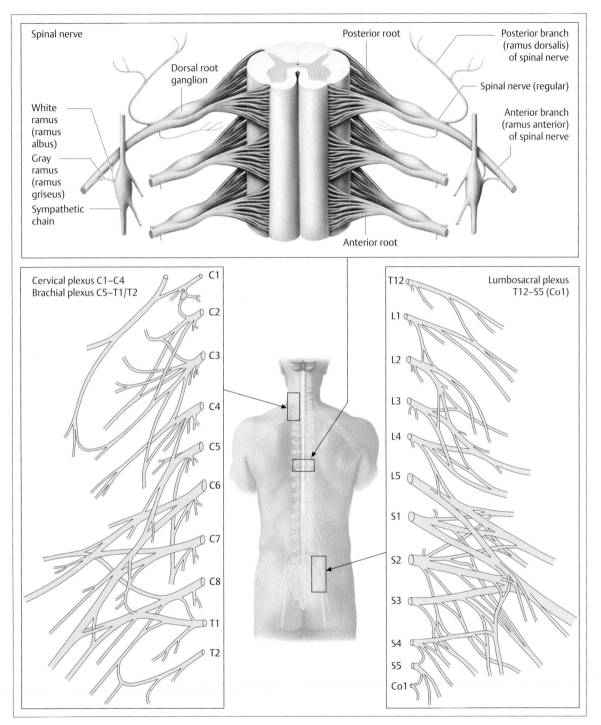

Fig. 1.35 Structure of the human neuraxis, with the spinal cord, spinal nerves (trunk), and nerve plexuses (arms and legs).

that pass through the chest to provide the mixed nerve supply for the diaphragm (the primary respiratory muscle).

Practical Tip

The mixed plexus nerves pass through a small gap between the medial and posterior scalenus known as the posterior scalene gap. This gap is largely covered by the sternocleidomastoid, and palpation of this portion of the cervical plexus is hardly possible. However, the superficial sensory nerves (the lesser occipital, great auricular, and transverse cervical nerves) are palpable at the lateral neck skin in a triangular pit close to the posterior margin of the sternocleidomastoid, known as the "punctum nervosum" (nerve point). The phrenic nerve runs more deeply, crossing the anterior scalenus to enter the upper thoracic aperture for the diaphragm. The phrenic nerve, however, is covered by the subclavian vein, which fills the space between the scalenus anterior and the clavicle known as the anterior scalene gap and is therefore not directly palpable (Reichert 2002).

Note

The unique innervation of the diaphragm by the phrenic nerve (C4–C5), supplied by the cervical plexus, may be explained by the fact that during the evolution of vertebrates with a well-developed pleural cavity (mammals), some muscle portions from the floor of the mouth were displaced caudally to the lower thoracic aperture along with their nervous supply from the cervical spine. The role of the floor of the mouth as a functional respiratory muscle can still be seen in some amphibians (frogs), which have oscillating mouth floor movements during air breathing (swallowing of air). Frogs do not have a real diaphragm and only have baglike lungs, without a pleural cavity.

Brachial Plexus

The brachial plexus (C5–T1) originates from the lower cervical spine via five to six individual roots that merge into three major nerve bundles known as the superior trunk (C5–C6), median trunk (C7), and inferior trunk (C8–T1). The three trunks divide up into three main fascicles—the lateral, posterior, and median fascicles. Due to axon rebundling at the level of the trunk divisions, each fascicle now contains axons from the adjacent spinal segments (C5–T1). In the armpit region, the nerve fascicles split up again into the main four nerves of the arm—the musculocutaneous nerve, originating mainly from the lateral fascicle; the radial nerve, originating mainly from the posterior fascicle; the median nerve, originating mainly from both the lateral and median fascicle; and the ulnar nerve, which receives its axon bundles mainly from the median fascicle.

The peripheral arm nerves supply the following muscle compartments (overview below):

- Upper arm (brachium):
  - Musculocutaneus nerve (C5–C7)—anterior arm muscle compartment (flexors)
  - Radial nerve (C5–T1)—posterior arm muscle compartment (extensors)
- Forearm:
  - Median (C8–T1) and ulnar (C7–T1) nerve—anterior arm muscle compartment (flexors)
  - Radial nerve (C5–C7)—posterior arm muscle box (extensors)
- Hand:
  - Median nerve (C6–C7)—thenar muscles (thenar = palm) in the ball of the thumb
  - Ulnar nerve (C8–T1)—hypothenar (hypothenar = beneath the palm) muscles in the ball of the little finger, and midpalmar muscles (lumbricales and interossei)

Note

Occasionally, the median and ulnar nerves have co-innervation from some thenar muscles (flexor pollicis brevis, opponens pollicis) and some midpalmar muscles (radial lumbricales and interossei) in the hand.

Most of the shoulder girdle muscles for movements of the upper arm—for example, the pectoralis, deltoid, latissimus dorsi, and muscles of the rotator cuff—are innervated by individually named branches of the brachial plexus (see the list of muscles in **Table 1.1**). The trapezius and parts of the sternocleidomastoid are, however, innervated by the accessory nerve (cranial nerve XI).

Practical Tip

- The solid nerve bundles from the trunks of the brachial plexus that leave the deep scalene gap at the lateral neck can be palpated in vivo through the flat platysma by their divisions in a triangular skinny pit just behind the clavicle, known as the lateral cervical triangle.
- The median and ulnar fascicle may be palpable in the armpit at the level of the axillary artery.
- Both the median and ulnar nerve may be palpable together with the brachial artery (pulsation) in a medial groove of the arm between the anterior and posterior muscle compartments.
- The radial nerve is palpable in the upper arm at its most sensitive superficial portion, called the radial groove of the humerus, about two fingerbreadths below the deltoid insertion (deltoid tuberosity)—the location of the radial nerve compression point.
- In the proximal forearm, only the radial nerve is palpable close to the lateral epicondyle of the elbow, beneath the brachioradialis (pressure point). Due to their deep passages through the anterior forearm muscle compartments, both the median and ulnar nerves are hardly palpable. A superficial branch of

the ulnar nerve runs beneath the skin of the wrist and may be palpable there (ulnar nerve compartment), while the median nerve runs more deeply together with the long forearm flexor tendons through a narrow bony groove known as the carpal tunnel, covered with a strong transversely coursing fascia (the flexor retinaculum).

Lumbosacral Plexus

The lumbosacral plexus originates from the lumbar spine, mainly in two overlapping portions known as the lumbar plexus (L1–L5) and sacral plexus (L4–S4). The spinal roots of these two portions originate from the most distal part of the spinal cord, from the medullary cone (conus medullaris) at vertebral levels L2–L3 (the end of the medullary spinal cord). From there, the roots run in a horse's tail shape (cauda equina) through the saclike spinal dura mater caudally to leave the spinal canal via the intervertebral windows (L5–S5), where they are united with the major lumbosacral plexus nerves of the lower body, the femoral nerve (L2–L4), the obturator nerve (L2–L4), the sciatic nerve with the tibial nerve (L4–S2), and the common peroneal (fibular) nerve (L5–S3). The upper plexus (T12–L2) also gives rise to the various freely coursing abdominal wall nerves—the subcostal, iliohypogastric, ilioinguinal, and genitofemoral nerve—that innervate abdominal wall muscles as well as some skin areas in the groin and genital region. In addition, the lateral cutaneous nerve of the thigh arises from L2–L3 as another subcutaneous plexus branch, mainly for the thigh.

Note

In the spinal canal, the medullary spinal cord terminates with a conelike ending at the L2–L3 vertebra level. However, the spinal roots that emerge from this cone continue as a fiber bundle shaped like a horse's tail (cauda equina) into the spinal dura mater sac caudally to leave the spinal canal at the intervertebral windows T12–S4. The length of the spinal cord does not fully match the length of the spinal canal. This is important, since in the lower thoracic and lumbar spine there is a clear shift between the origins of the roots from the spinal segments and their exits from the spine at the neuroforamina. For example, the ventral motor neurons located in spinal segment L1 are actually located at the level of the tenth vertebrate body, but their axon roots leave the spinal canal at intervertebral window L1 between the first and second lumbar vertebrae, which is about 10 cm further down the spine from their neuronal cell bodies in the spinal cord.

Practical Tip

- The femoral nerve leaves the pelvis together with the iliopsoas through a narrow exit site beneath the groin ligament known as the muscular lacuna (lacuna = hollow space). The nerve may be palpable together with the femoral artery (pressure point) passing through the "vascular lacuna" at the femoral triangle of the groin, which is bounded by the sartorius and gracilis muscles and the inguinal ligament.
- The obturator nerve leaves the pelvis through the obturator canal of the obturator membrane, which covers the ventral pelvic hole and thus runs deep through the medial leg adductor compartment, covered by muscle bellies, and therefore may not be palpable at the thigh.
- The sciatic nerve leaves the pelvis dorsally via the greater sciatic notch and passes through a gap between the deep rotator muscles, the piriformis and superior gemellus (infrapiriform gap), in the deep gluteus muscle compartment. The sciatic nerve is thus covered by the gluteus maximus and may not be palpable in the posterior hip region.
- The tibial nerve runs together with the popliteal artery through the popliteal pit and may be palpable underneath the popliteal fascia. The continuation of the tibial nerve through the posterior calf compartment between the superficial and deep calf flexors may not allow palpation. At the ankle joint, the tibial nerve together with the posterior tibial artery curves behind the medial malleolar canal, covered by the flexor retinaculum, to the foot, where it splits up into two or three plantar nerves of the sole. Palpation of the tibial nerve and artery (pressure point) is therefore possible at the medial ankle joint.
- The superficial peroneal (fibular) nerve winds around the proximal head of the fibula and runs through the lateral calf compartment. The nerve may be palpable beneath the skin more distally from the fibular head (but there is a risk of injury) (Reichert 2002).

Spinal Syndromes

Lesions in the spinal cord may result in various syndromes that can affect the functioning of the skeletal musculature:
- *Epiconus syndrome.* The following syndromes are distinguished according to the level of the lesion (L4–S2) (Duus 1990):
  - Paresis (palsy) of the hip muscles, including lack of lateral rotation
  - Paresis of hip extension
  - Paresis of knee flexion
  - Paresis of dorsal extension and plantar flexion (including digits)
  - Lack of an Achilles tendon reflex (ATR)

- *Conus syndrome* (S3–C1). Palsy of muscles of the lower extremity is mostly absent, but the pelvic organs are often affected, resulting in:
  - Incontinence
  - Impotence
  - Lack of anal reflexes
- *Cauda syndrome* (L4–S1). Distal intervertebral disk protrusions at L4–L5 and S1 may partly compress the cauda equina bundle, resulting in sensorimotor failures affecting the following target skeletal muscles (Duus 1990, Rohkamm 2000):
  - Quadriceps (L3)
  - Tibialis anterior (L4)
  - Extensor hallucis longus (L4)
  - Extensor hallucis brevis, lacking the tibialis posterior reflex (L5)
  - Peroneus, lacking the triceps surae reflex

Reference Muscles and Myotomes

Reference muscles are regarded as skeletal muscles that typically respond, depending on the extent of an injury to their nerve supply, with comparable gradual changes in normal muscle function. For example, different grades of nerve lesions may result in muscle tremor/facilitation, loss of reflex control, weakness, or complete palsy in an affected muscle. In the trunk, the reference muscles are almost always located in the same anatomic regions where the motor nerve supply usually originates (the segmental innervation pattern). In the shoulder girdle and the extremities, however, the anatomic location of the reference muscles is shifted distally or caudally from the original nerve supply from more proximal plexuses (**Table 1.13**).

The term "myotome" is used in functional anatomy to identify all of the skeletal muscles that receive their nerve supply from common spinal roots or their dorsal or ventral branches. The myotomes are innervated by ventral branches of the spinal nerves, which originate from adjacent spinal cord levels or segments of the spine. The dorsal branches of the spinal nerves support the axial (paravertebral) musculature located very close to the spine, such as the erector spinae. In clinical practice, the reference muscle paradigm is often used to narrow down or identify the precise anatomic level of root lesions or avulsions, as myotomes with their respective muscles are mostly innervated by one or two adjacent spinal segments.

The most important reference muscles in the human body are listed below in **Table 1.13** and **Table 1.14**. The most important human myotome locations with their segmental levels are illustrated in **Fig. 1.36**. More elaborate illustrations of the segmental innervation pattern and their movement patterns are available elsewhere (Duus 1990, Rohen 2000).

The anatomic location of the myotomes in the trunk corresponds well with the dermatomes (i.e., skin areas innervated by common spinal segments) in the trunk—that is, the myotome and dermatome areas mostly overlap with each other. In contrast with the myotomes, however, the dermatomes of the extremities are shifted distally from their proximal spinal nerve origins, as seen in regional dermatome maps of the lower extremity (**Fig. 1.37**).

Table 1.13 Selected list of reference muscles and their motor nerve roots (segments) (adapted from McKinnon and Morris)

Segment/ root	Reference muscles
C4	Diaphragm
C5	Rhomboid muscles, supraspinatus, infraspinatus, deltoid
C6	Biceps brachii, brachioradialis
C7	Triceps brachii, extensor carpi radialis, pectoralis, flexor carpi radialis, pronator teres
C8	Adductor pollicis brevis, abductor digiti minimi, flexor carpi ulnaris, flexor pollicis brevis
L3	Quadriceps, iliopsoas, adductors
L4	Quadriceps (vastus lateralis)
L5	Extensor hallucis longus, tibialis anterior, tibialis posterior, gluteus medius
S1	Gastrocnemius, gluteus maximus

Table 1.14 Segmental innervation patterns and movements in the human leg (adapted from McKinnon and Morris)

Joint	Movement	Root
Hip	Flexion	L1, L2, L3
	Adduction	
	Medial rotation	
	Extension	L4, I5, S1
	Adduction	
	Lateral rotation	
Knee	Extension	L3, L4
	Flexion	L5, S1
Superior ankle	Extension (dorsally)	L4, L5
	Flexion (plantar)	S1, S2
Inferior ankle	Inversion	L4, L5
	Eversion	L5, S1
Foot	Toe extension	L5, S1
	Muscles of foot sole	S3

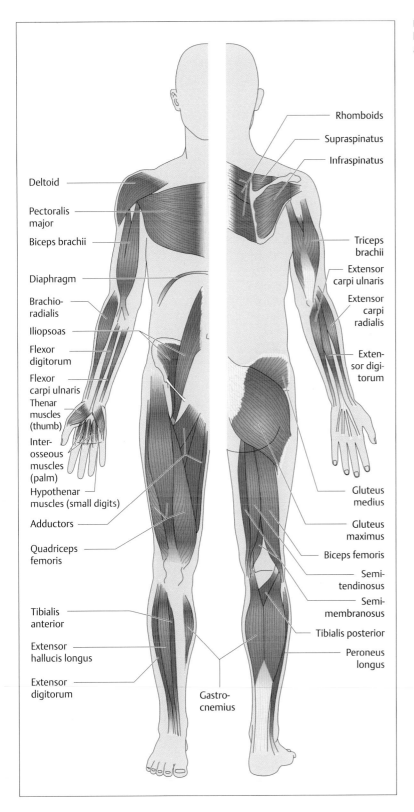

Rhomboids

Supraspinatus

Infraspinatus

Deltoid

Pectoralis major

Biceps brachii

Triceps brachii

Diaphragm

Extensor carpi ulnaris

Brachio-radialis

Extensor carpi radialis

Iliopsoas

Flexor digitorum

Exten-sor digi-torum

Flexor carpi ulnaris

Thenar muscles (thumb)

Inter-osseous muscles (palm)

Hypothenar muscles (small digits)

Gluteus medius

Adductors

Gluteus maximus

Quadriceps femoris

Biceps femoris

Semi-tendinosus

Semi-membranosus

Tibialis anterior

Tibialis posterior

Extensor hallucis longus

Peroneus longus

Extensor digitorum

Gastro-cnemius

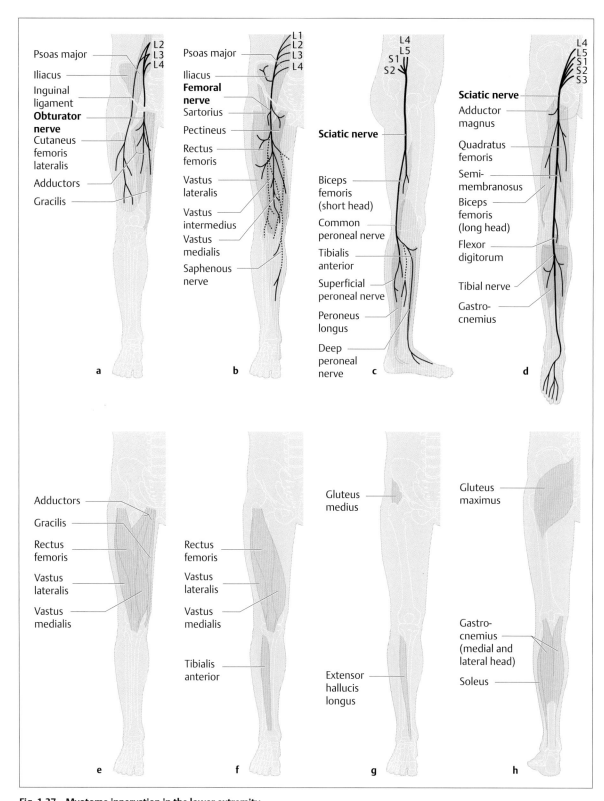

Fig. 1.37 Myotome innervation in the lower extremity.
Muscle and skin nerve supply (upper panel, **a–d**), with reference muscles and affected muscles (lower panel, **e–h**).

References

Banks RW. An allometric analysis of the number of muscle spindles in mammalian skeletal muscles. J Anat 2006; 208(6): 753–768

Benjamin M, Toumi H, Ralphs JR, Bydder G, Best TM, Milz S. Where tendons and ligaments meet bone: attachment sites ('entheses') in relation to exercise and/or mechanical load. J Anat 2006; 208(4): 471–490

Böning D. Muskelkater – Ursachen, Prophylaxe und Therapie. Dtsch Arztebl 2002; 99: A372–A375

Chalmers G. Do Golgi tendon organs really inhibit muscle activity at high force levels to save muscles from injury, and adapt with strength training? Sports Biomech 2002; 1(2): 239–249

Chleboun GS, France AR, Crill MT, Braddock HK, Howell JN. In vivo measurement of fascicle length and pennation angle of the human biceps femoris muscle. Cells Tissues Organs 2001; 169(4): 401–409

Deschenes MR, Covault J, Kraemer WJ, Maresh CM. The neuromuscular junction. Muscle fibre type differences, plasticity and adaptability to increased and decreased activity. Sports Med 1994; 17(6): 358–372

Dressler D, Saberi FA, Barbosa ER. Botulinum toxin: mechanisms of action. Arq Neuropsiquiatr 2005; 63(1): 180–185

Duus P. Neurologisch-topische Diagnostik. Anatomie, Physiologie, Klinik. Stuttgart: Thieme; 1990

Gans C, de Vree F. Functional bases of fiber length and angulation in muscle. J Morphol 1987; 192(1): 63–85

Gao Y, Kostrominova TY, Faulkner JA, Wineman AS. Age-related changes in the mechanical properties of the epimysium in skeletal muscles of rats. J Biomech 2008; 41(2): 465–469

Harris AJ, Duxson MJ, Butler JE, Hodges PW, Taylor JL, Gandevia SC. Muscle fiber and motor unit behavior in the longest human skeletal muscle. J Neurosci 2005; 25(37): 8528–8533

Hijikata T, Ishikawa H. Functional morphology of serially linked skeletal muscle fibers. Acta Anat (Basel) 1997; 159(2–3): 99–107

Hughes BW, Kusner LL, Kaminski HJ. Molecular architecture of the neuromuscular junction. Muscle Nerve 2006; 33(4): 445–461

Jami L. Functional properties of the Golgi tendon organs. [Article in French]. Arch Int Physiol Biochim 1988; 96(4): A363–A378

Kawano F, Takeno Y, Nakai N, et al. Essential role of satellite cells in the growth of rat soleus muscle fibers. Am J Physiol Cell Physiol 2008; 295(2): C458–C467

Kunsch K, Kunsch S. Der Mensch in Zahlen. Heidelberg: Spektrum Akademischer Verlag; 2005

Labeit S, Kolmerer B. Titins: giant proteins in charge of muscle ultrastructure and elasticity. Science 1995; 270(5234): 293–296

Laurent C, Johnson-Wells G, Hellström S, Engström-Laurent A, Wells AF. Localization of hyaluronan in various muscular tissues. A morphological study in the rat. Cell Tissue Res 1991; 263(2): 201–205

Mense S. The pathogenesis of muscle pain. Curr Pain Headache Rep 2003; 7(6): 419–425

Monti RJ, Roy RR, Hodgson JA, Edgerton VR. Transmission of forces within mammalian skeletal muscles. J Biomech 1999; 32(4): 371–380

Parratte B, Tatu L, Vuillier F, Diop M, Monnier G. Intramuscular distribution of nerves in the human triceps surae muscle: anatomical bases for treatment of spastic drop foot with botulinum toxin. Surg Radiol Anat 2002; 24(2): 91–96

Petrella JK, Kim JS, Mayhew DL, Cross JM, Bamman MM. Potent myofiber hypertrophy during resistance training in humans is associated with satellite cell-mediated myonuclear addition: a cluster analysis. J Appl Physiol 2008; 104(6): 1736–1742

Reichert B. Palpation Techniques. Surface Anatomy for Physical Therapists. Stuttgart–New York: Thieme Publishers; 2010

Richardson CA, Jull GA. Muscle control-pain control. What exercises would you prescribe? Man Ther 1995; 1(1): 2–10

Richardson CA, Hodges P, Hides J. Therapeutic exercise for lumbopelvic stabilization. A motor control approach for the treatment and prevention of low back pain. 2nd ed. Edinburgh: Churchill Livingstone; 2004

Rohen JW. Topographische Anatomie – Lehrbuch mit besonderer Berücksichtigung der klinischen Aspekte und der bildgebenden Verfahren. Stuttgart: Schattauer; 2000

Rohkamm R. Taschenatlas der Neurologie. Stuttgart: Thieme; 2000: 32–37

Safwat MD, Abdel-Meguid EM. Distribution of terminal nerve entry points to the flexor and extensor groups of forearm muscles: an anatomical study. Folia Morphol (Warsz) 2007; 66(2): 83–93

Sajko S, Kubínová L, Cvetko E, Kreft M, Wernig A, Erzen I. Frequency of M-cadherin-stained satellite cells declines in human muscles during aging. J Histochem Cytochem 2004; 52 (2): 179–185

Schünke M. Funktionelle Anatomie – Topographie und Funktion des Bewegungssystems. Stuttgart: Thieme; 2000

Snobl D, Binaghi LE, Zenker W. Microarchitecture and innervation of the human latissimus dorsi muscle. J Reconstr Microsurg 1998; 14(3): 171–177

Tam SL, Gordon T. Mechanisms controlling axonal sprouting at the neuromuscular junction. J Neurocytol 2003; 32(5–8): 961–974

Tegtbur U, Busse MW, Kubis HP. Exercise and cellular adaptation of muscle. [Article in German] Unfallchirurg 2009; 112(4): 365–372

Tipton CM. Historical perspective: the antiquity of exercise, exercise physiology and the exercise prescription for health. World Rev Nutr Diet 2008; 98: 198–245

Wernig A. Regeneration capacity of skeletal muscle. [Article in German] Ther Umsch 2003; 60(7): 383–389

Windhorst U. Muscle proprioceptive feedback and spinal networks. Brain Res Bull 2007; 73(4–6): 155–202

Witt CC, Olivieri N, Centner T, Kolmerer B, Millevoi S, Morell J, Labeit D, Labeit S, Jockusch H, Pastore A. A survey of the primary structure and the interspecies conservation of I-band titin's elastic elements in vertebrates. J Struct Biol 1998; 122 (1–2): 206–215

Further Reading

Bettinzoli F. Anatomie und Radiologie. DVD-ROM WIN/MAC. Montagnola: Bio Media SA; 2005

Fucci S, Michna H, eds. Atlas der Sportanatomie des Bewegungsapparates. Wiesbaden: Ullstein Medical; 1997

Hüter-Becker A, Dölken M, eds. Biomechanik, Bewegungslehre, Leistungsphysiologie, Trainingslehre. Stuttgart: Thieme; 2004

Kandel ER, Schwartz JE, Jessell TM. Principles of neural sciences. 4th ed. New York: McGraw-Hill; 2000

Lim EC, Seet RC. Botulinum toxin: description of injection techniques and examination of controversies surrounding toxin diffusion. Acta Neurol Scand 2008; 117(2): 73–84

McKinnon P, Morris J. Oxford Lehrbuch der klinischen Anatomie. Bern: Hans Huber;1997

Möller TB, Reif E. MR-Atlas des muskuloskelettalen Systems. Berlin: Blackwell Wissenschaft; 1993

Netter FH, Ciba Geigy Corporation. (Ardsley, NY). The Ciba collection of medical illustrations. Vol 5: Krämer G, ed. Nervensystem I, Neuroanatomie und Physiologie. Stuttgart: Thieme; 1987

Netter FH. Atlas der Anatomie des Menschen. Basel: Ciba-Geigy AG; 1995

Platzer W. Color Atlas of Human Anatomy. Vol. 1: Locomotor System. Stuttgart–New York: Thieme Publishers; 2008

Schünke M, Schulte E, Schumacher U. Thieme Atlas of Anatomy: General Anatomy and Musculoskeletal System. Stuttgart–New York: Thieme Publishers; 2010

Weineck J. Sportanatomie. Balingen: Spitta; 2008: 84

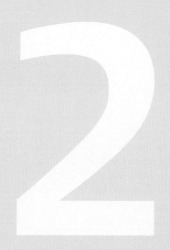

2 Basic Physiology and Aspects of Exercise

B. Brenner, N. Maassen

Translated by Terry Telger

Basic Physiology   60
Sarcomere, Muscle Force,
and Muscle Shortening   60
Basic Principles of Muscular
Contraction and Its Regulation   61
Gradation of Muscle Force
during Voluntary Movements   66
Types of Muscular Contraction   67
Neuromuscular Control Mechanisms   71

Aspects of Exercise Physiology   77
Types of Muscle Fiber   77
Overview of Muscular Metabolism   78
Warm-Up   81
Fatigue   82
Recovery   86
Training Adaptations   86

Basic Physiology

B. Brenner

Sarcomere, Muscle Force, and Muscle Shortening

Active forces and the shortening of muscle are the result of repetitive, cyclic interactions of myosin molecules with actin filaments. To generate the highest possible forces per cross-sectional area, filaments of actin and myosin form a close-packed arrangement within the basic contractile unit of muscle, the sarcomere (**Fig. 2.1a**; see also **Figs. 1.16** and **1.18**). The sarcomere is the segment of a myofibril of muscle fiber located between two adjacent Z disks. Macroscopic forces are generated by the parallel arrangement of myofibrils in the muscle fibers and by the parallel arrangement of myriad muscle fibers in a muscle. Numerous sarcomeres are arranged in series (approximately 500 per millimeter of fiber length), so that the microscopic shortening of individual sarcomeres adds up to macroscopic changes in muscle length.

Each myosin molecule (**Fig. 2.1b**) is composed of two intertwined heavy chains. Each heavy chain consists of a globular head domain and a threadlike tail. The tails of the two heavy chains are coiled around each other to form the rod of the myosin molecule. Each head domain is associated with two light chains. Several hundred myosin molecules associate at their rod parts to form the bipolar myosin filaments (**Fig. 2.1c**). Titin molecules are springlike structures associated with the myosin filaments and keep the myosin filaments centered in the sarcomere. The globular actin molecules associate into two strands twisted together to form the helical actin filaments. Wrapped around the actin filaments are the regulatory proteins troponin and tropomyosin (**Fig. 2.1 d**), which regulate the activity of the muscle fibers (see below). The actin filaments are anchored to the Z disks and interdigitate between the myosin filaments. Each sarcomere is divided at its center by the M line. This structure is responsible for the hexagonal, closely packed arrangement of myosin and actin filaments that appears in the cross-section of a sarcomere (see **Fig. 2.1a**, inset).

During their cyclic interactions with actin filaments, the myosin heads exert forces that pull the actin filaments along the myosin filaments in a telescopelike movement, thus driving active shortening of muscle. When a muscle is stretched, on the other hand, the actin filaments are pulled out of the spaces between the myosin filaments. During active shortening or passive stretching of muscle, actin filaments are pulled along the myosin filaments, while the lengths of both actin and myosin filaments themselves remain unchanged. When external conditions

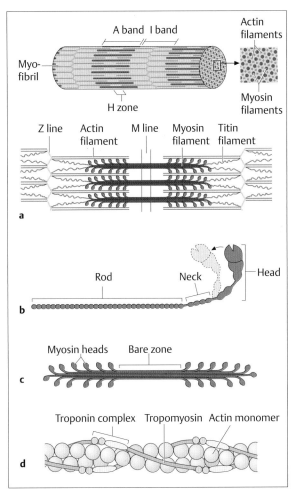

Fig. 2.1a–d Structure of myosin and actin filaments and their arrangement in the sarcomere.

a Diagram of a myofibril. The arrangement of myosin and actin filaments in the sarcomere illustrates how these structures form the striation pattern—the A band, I band, Z line, and H zone—that is seen on light microscopy. The elastic tension in the titin filaments keeps the myosin filaments centered in the sarcomere. The cross-section illustrates the hexagonal arrangement of the myosin and actin filaments.

b Myosin molecule with rod, neck, and two globular head domains. Each head domain has two light chains close to the head–neck junction. This segment functions as a lever arm.

c A myosin filament, showing the staggered arrangement of the head pairs and the central bare zone.

d An actin filament, with actin monomers arranged in a long-pitch double helix wrapped by tropomyosin and troponin molecules.

(e.g., a heavy lifting load or a fixed joint) prevent the actin filaments from moving relative to the myosin filaments, the motile forces of the individual myosin heads add up to muscle forces.

Basic Principles of Muscular Contraction and its Regulation

Motor Unit

For a skeletal muscle to contract, it must receive a stimulus from a neuron, called the α-motor neuron. Located in the spinal cord, the α-motor neurons distribute axons via the peripheral nerves to the muscles, where the axons divide into terminal branches before reaching the surface of the muscle fibers. Accordingly, one motor neuron innervates multiple muscle fibers. That group of muscle fibers is called a "motor unit."

> *Note*
>
> The axons of the motor neurons divide into terminal branches in the associated muscle. The muscle fibers innervated by one motor neuron constitute a "motor unit."

Neuromuscular End plate (Motor End plate)

At the surface of the muscle fibers, the terminal branches of the axons form synapticlike contacts called motor (or neuromuscular) end plates (**Fig. 2.2a**). Synaptic vesicles in the bulblike terminals of an axon contain acetylcholine, the transmitter of the neuromuscular end plate. The membrane of the axon terminals (presynaptic membrane) and the surface membrane of the muscle fiber (subsynaptic membrane) are separated from each other by a small gap called the synaptic cleft. The subsynaptic part of the surface membrane of the muscle fiber forms subsynaptic folds to increase the surface area available for signal transduction from the axon terminals to the skeletal muscle fiber.

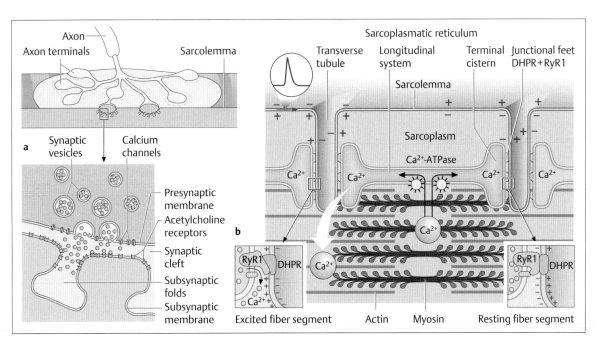

Fig. 2.2a, b Neuromuscular signal transduction and changes in intracellular calcium concentration during excitation of a muscle fiber.

a Neuromuscular end plate, with presynaptic terminals and folds in the subsynaptic membrane of the muscle fiber for increasing the surface area. The high-powered view shows how presynaptic vesicles containing acetylcholine release the neurotransmitter into the synaptic cleft (adapted from Kandel et al. 1995).

b Release of calcium ions from the sarcoplasmic reticulum during excitation and removal from the sarcoplasm by active transport back into the longitudinal tubules of the sarcoplasmic reticulum.

Left side: excited fiber segment. A change in the conformation of the dihydropyridine receptors (DHPR) during depolarization opens the ryanodine receptors (RyR1), allowing release of calcium ions from the terminal cisterns of the sarcoplasmic reticulum (inset at left).

Right side: unexcited fiber segment. With the RyR1 closed, calcium ions are actively transported from the sarcoplasm into the sarcoplasmic reticulum by calcium ATPase (adapted from Alberts et al. 2002).

Signal Transduction from the Motor Neuron to Skeletal Muscle Fibers

When an action potential reaches the motor end plate, calcium channels open in the axon terminals (**Fig. 2.2a**). The influx of calcium ions induces synaptic vesicles to fuse with the presynaptic membrane of the axon terminal facing the subgraphic area of the muscle fiber. In this process, the vesicles release the neurotransmitter acetylcholine into the synaptic cleft. The acetylcholine diffuses across the synaptic cleft to the subsynaptic membrane of the skeletal muscle fiber. At their ridges, the subsynaptic folds bear numerous receptors for acetylcholine, which are channel proteins with specific binding sites for acetylcholine (nicotinic acetylcholine receptors). When acetylcholine molecules bind to their specific sites, the channel proteins are opened. The influx of sodium ions depolarizes the surface membrane in the area of the synaptic cleft. Usually, the depolarization of the subsynaptic and postsynaptic membranes goes beyond the threshold for triggering an action potential at the muscle-fiber surface membrane outside the synapse. Once initiated, the action potential spreads throughout the membrane of the entire skeletal muscle fiber. Accordingly, every acetylcholine-mediated action potential that arrives at the motor end plate gives rise to an action potential, which is conducted throughout the entire innervated skeletal muscle fiber.

Acetylcholine that is released in the synaptic cleft is cleaved by the enzyme acetylcholinesterase. This stops the depolarization of the muscle fiber membrane in the synaptic cleft, causing the membrane to return to its resting state. The cleavage product choline is available for re-uptake into the axon terminal, where it can be reused for acetylcholine synthesis.

> *Note*
>
> The neurotransmitter acetylcholine mediates signal transduction at the motor end plate. Acetylcholine is released at the neuromuscular junction between the motor nerve fiber and muscle fiber. Acetylcholine excites skeletal muscle by binding to its receptor in the muscle fiber membrane.

Initiating a Contraction (Electromechanical Coupling)

Rise of Calcium Ion Concentration in the Sarcoplasm

When an action potential spreads across the surface membrane of a muscle fiber, it also travels deep into the interior of the muscle fiber through tubular invaginations of the surface membrane. These tubular invaginations, called the transverse tubules (T-tubules), are present in each sarcomere at the ends of the myosin filaments (see **Fig. 2.2b**). Inside the muscle fibers, the T-tubules are in close contact

with the terminal cisterns of a branched, tubular membrane system called the sarcoplasmic reticulum. Two proteins that are incorporated into both membranes interact directly with each other at these contact sites. The proteins in the membrane of the terminal cisterns are specialized calcium channels (ryanodine receptors, RyR1) that can be directly opened by dihydropyridine receptors in the membrane of the T-tubules (see **Fig. 2.2b**, insets). When an action potential reaches the contact site via the T-tubules, it alters the conformation of the dihydropyridine receptors, causing them to open up ryanodine receptors in the membrane of the terminal cisterns. The calcium ions accumulated in the terminal cisterns of the sarcoplasmic reticulum can then flow through these release channels into the sarcoplasm (see **Fig. 2.2b**, left inset), where they eventually reach the actin filaments. Because the T-tubules extend into the innermost regions of skeletal muscle fibers, the concentration of calcium ions in the sarcoplasm rises in synchrony throughout the fiber cross-section.

Control of Myosin Docking Sites by Regulatory Proteins

The calcium ions released from the sarcoplasmic reticulum can bind to calcium binding sites on the troponin molecules. The troponin molecules, along with the filiform tropomyosin molecules, are wrapped around the actin filaments along their entire length (**Fig. 2.3**). The tropomyosin molecules regulate high-affinity binding sites on the surface of the actin monomers. The heads of the myosin molecules can dock to the high affinity binding sites only in the presence of calcium. When no calcium ions are bound to the troponin molecules, the tropomyosin molecules block the high-affinity docking sites (**Fig. 2.3b**, top). But when calcium ions bind to the troponin molecules, the troponin–tropomyosin complex moves away from the high-affinity binding sites, making them accessible to the myosin head (**Fig. 2.3b**, center).

> *Note*
>
> Muscle contraction is triggered by a rise in the calcium ion concentration in the sarcoplasm. The binding of calcium ions to troponin unlocks the tropomyosin, giving the myosin heads access to high-affinity docking sites on the actin filaments.

Production of Motile Forces by the Myosin Heads

The Myosin Head in Relaxed and Activated Muscle

When the high-affinity sites for the docking of myosin to the actin filaments are blocked by tropomyosin, the myosin heads can undergo only weak, transient interactions with actin. Although adenosine triphosphate (ATP) is already split into adenosine diphosphate (ADP) and P_i at

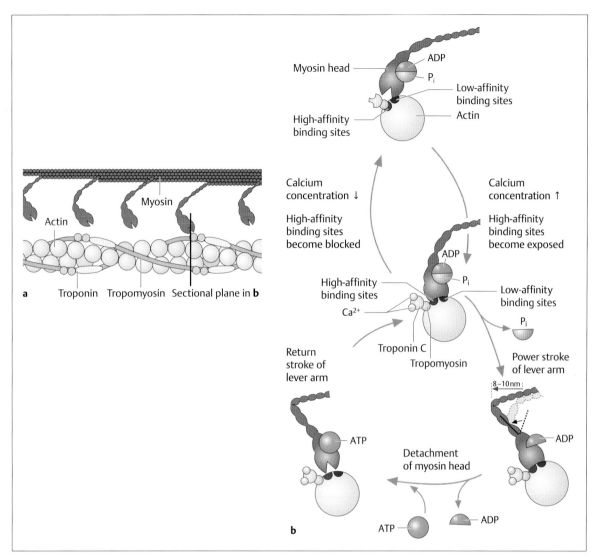

Fig. 2.3a, b   Calcium-dependent activation and inhibition of muscle contraction.

a The arrangement of the myosin heads in the sarcomere relative to actin filaments, with the regulatory proteins troponin and tropomyosin.

b Calcium-dependent movement of tropomyosin relative to the low-affinity and high-affinity docking sites for myosin heads on the actin filament (adapted from Vibert et al. 1997). This movement enables cyclic interaction between the myosin heads and the actin filament.

Low calcium ion concentration: The myosin heads have bound ADP and P_i at their catalytic center and can attach only to low-affinity actin binding sites.

High calcium ion concentration: In this state, the myosin heads with ADP and P_i can also bind to high-affinity docking sites. As P_i is lost from the active center, the high-affinity docking unlocks the power stroke of the lever arm (dotted and solid lines indicate the lever arm axis before and after the stroke). This causes the actin and myosin filaments to slide 8–10 nm relative to each other. If the filaments cannot slide, the lever arm undergoes elastic deformation (shaded configuration). The resulting elastic recoil is manifested as muscular force. After the dissociation of ADP and binding of a new ATP molecule, the myosin head detaches from the actin filament. When the ATP molecule is hydrolyzed into ADP and P_i, the lever arm tilts back to its initial position and the cycle is ready to repeat.

the catalytic center of the myosin heads, the cleavage products cannot leave the active center (see **Fig. 2.3b**, top). Accordingly, the muscle cannot generate active forces and the muscle fibers offer little resistance to stretch; the muscle is relaxed. The forces that develop in response to passive stretch are mostly generated by stretching of the titin molecules in the sarcomeres (see **Fig. 2.1a**).

When the troponin–tropomyosin complexes change their conformation and expose the high-affinity binding sites on the actin filaments (see **Fig. 2.3b**, center), myosin heads can firmly dock to those sites. This high-affinity binding displaces the P_i from the catalytic center and "unlocks" the power stroke of the lever arm domains of the myosin heads. The power stroke of the lever arm generates motile forces that can pull the actin filament approximately 10 nm toward the center of the sarcomere. When the lever arm has completed its stroke, the remaining ADP can leave the catalytic center on the myosin head. With the active center empty, a new ATP molecule can bind to it. This occurs in only a few milliseconds at physiologic ATP concentrations of 1–5 mM/L. When ATP binds to the catalytic center, it disrupts the high-affinity docking of the myosin head to actin, causing the myosin head to detach from the actin filament (**Fig. 2.3b**, lower left). When the ATP molecule is subsequently hydrolyzed into ADP and P_i at the catalytic center, the lever arm domain swings back to its initial position. Since the myosin head is released from the actin, it exerts no reverse forces on the actin filament when the lever arm swings back. The myosin head can bind to the high-affinity sites on actin, with the displacement of P_i from the catalytic center, only after ATP hydrolysis has taken place and the lever arm has returned to its initial position (**Fig. 2.3b**, center).

Production of Macroscopic Muscle Shortening

During each of these cycles, one molecule of ATP is consumed and the actin filament slides approximately 10 nm toward the center of the sarcomere. This results in an overall shortening of about 1% of the initial length of each sarcomere and consequently of the muscle as a whole. Multiple cycles are needed to produce greater filament shifts that cause macroscopic shortening of more than 10% of the initial muscle length. This does not mean that each individual myosin head must complete several cycles of binding and releasing actin. When the high-affinity docking sites are exposed, the numerous myosin heads on even a single myosin filament do not synchronize their cycles like the rowers in a boat. Instead, the heads cycle at random, so that at any given time different myosin heads are at different stages of their cyclic activity. Accordingly, other myosin heads may continue to pull an actin filament as soon as the first heads have bound a new ATP molecule and detached from the actin filament. On completing its power stroke, however, the myosin head must detach from the actin filament fast enough that it does not hamper the efforts of other myosin heads to keep the filament sliding. As a result, myosin filaments in fast-twitch mus-

cles are characterized by a very rapid dissociation of ADP and especially by the rapid binding of a new ATP molecule.

Production of Muscle Force

When its power stroke is "unlocked," the lever arm domain cannot always pull the actin filament approximately 10 nm toward the center of the sarcomere. For example, when a muscle is trying to lift a load that is too heavy, the muscle will maintain a constant length despite the active myosin heads (isometric contraction, see p. 69). In this situation, the lever arm cannot freely execute a power stroke; instead, it undergoes an elastic deformation (dotted shape; lower right panel in **Fig. 2.3b**) when the lever arm moves at its anchoring site in the catalytic domain from the dotted line to the solid line (**Fig. 2.3b**) As a result, the myosin head tightens like a coiled spring and exerts an elastic recoil force on the actin filaments. So instead of shortening the muscle, the myosin heads generate muscular force.

In the absence of unrestrained movement of the lever arm domains, it is more difficult for the remaining ADP to leave the catalytic center, and so its dissociation is delayed. This is advantageous, however, in that it prolongs the highly strained state of the force-generating myosin head. In this way, a highly strained myosin head contributes longer to force production than a myosin head which shortens the muscle by pulling the actin filament toward the M line in a power stroke. The greater the delay of ADP dissociation in the strained myosin head, the less ATP is consumed to develop a sustained force like that required in postural muscles, for example.

Different types of myosin (slow and fast isoforms) differ from one another in this very property, among others. Postural muscles are distinguished by the fact that they express slow isoforms of myosin and therefore can generate force more economically (with low ATP consumption) for a prolonged period of time. This high "postural economy" is gained at the cost of an impaired, slower shortening velocity. The delayed dissociation of ADP that precedes the binding of a new ATP molecule also delays the disruption of the high-affinity bond after the lever arm domain has completed its power stroke, and this hampers further sliding of the actin filaments by other myosin heads. As a result, the myosin in the postural muscles is less suitable for fast movements.

Note

The same molecular process—the cyclic interaction of myosin heads with actin filaments—is responsible for both muscle force development and muscle shortening.

Relaxation of Muscle

Calcium ions are actively transported by calcium pumps from the sarcoplasm into the tubules of the sarcoplasmic reticulum that run longitudinally along the muscle fibers (longitudinal system, see **Fig. 2.2b**). These calcium pumps are built into the membrane of the sarcoplasmic reticulum and are powered by the hydrolysis of ATP. They are therefore also known as calcium adenosine triphosphatases (Ca^{2+}-ATPases). When a muscle fiber is no longer stimulated by the associated motor neuron, calcium ions cease to flow from the sarcoplasmic reticulum into the sarcoplasm through open ryanodine receptors. The dominant process at this time is the active reuptake of calcium ions into the sarcoplasmic reticulum, leading to a fall in the sarcoplasmic concentration of free calcium ions. As a result, calcium ions are released from their binding sites on the troponin molecules, and the troponin–tropomyosin complexes move back to a position that blocks the high-affinity docking sites for myosin heads on the actin filaments. At this point, the myosin heads can no longer perform their cyclic interaction with actin filaments and can no longer contribute to active force production and shortening. The muscle relaxes.

Time Course of Muscular Contraction (Mechanogram)

Single Twitch

The time course of a muscle contraction is described in a mechanogram (**Fig. 2.4a**). A contraction that is triggered by a single action potential is called a single twitch. The time course of a single twitch consists of three phases:

- *Latent period:* the period between the start of the muscle action potential and the onset of force development or muscle shortening. This period includes the processes of electromechanical coupling described above. It extends from excitation of the muscle fiber surface membrane and release of the myosin docking sites to flexion of the lever arm. The duration of the latent period is several milliseconds.
- *Time to peak force:* the period in which maximum active force or maximum active shortening is achieved.
- *Relaxation time:* the period in which the force declines from the peak value to complete relaxation or the time required for the muscle to return from maximum shortening back to its initial length. The relaxation time depends mainly on the rate at which calcium ions can be eliminated from the sarcoplasm and by the rate of ADP dissociation from the myosin head. Generally, the relaxation phase is of longer duration than the time to peak tension (see **Fig. 2.4a**).

Fast- and slow-twitch fiber types can be distinguished in almost all skeletal muscles on the basis of the time course of the single twitch in the mechanogram (see **Fig. 2.4a** and p. 77):

- *Slow-twitch muscle fibers* (e.g., in the soleus): These fibers are rich in myoglobin ("red muscle"), express slow myosin isoforms with high postural economy, and produce ATP by the aerobic pathway via oxidative enzymes.
- *Fast-twitch muscle fibers* (e.g., in the gastrocnemius): These fibers have much less myoglobin ("white muscle") and express fast myosin isoforms with low postural economy but a high muscle-shortening velocity. They produce ATP mainly by the anaerobic pathway via glycolytic enzymes.

Superposition

The action potential of skeletal muscle is of much shorter duration (a few milliseconds) than a single twitch (50–500 ms; see **Fig. 2.4a**). For this reason, a second action potential can be transmitted to the muscle during a single twitch. If the interval between the two action potentials is shorter than the duration of a single twitch, the mechanical response will be amplified due to superposition (**Fig. 2.4b**, double stimulus). Series of action potentials evoke repetitive mechanical responses. The individual responses may be partially or completely fused together (see **Fig. 2.4b**), depending on the frequency of the action potentials. Accordingly, the resulting responses are known as "incomplete" or "complete tetanic contractions" (fused tetonic contraction). Normally only a partial superposition is achieved in individual motor units, even during maximal voluntary contractions.

Pronounced superposition or fused tetonic contraction (e.g., in response to electrical stimulation at a high impulse frequency) leads to rapidly progressive inhomogeneities of the sarcomeres. This is the result of the structural arrangement of the myosin filaments at the center of the sarcomeres. Minute differences in the forces produced by active myosin heads in the two halves of the sarcomere will shift the myosin filaments out of their centered position. The elastic recoil forces of the titin molecules are too weak to counteract this disparity of active forces. Complete relaxation must occur before the titin molecules can recenter the myosin filaments in the sarcomere. The same applies to slight differences in the active forces produced by different sarcomeres within a muscle fiber. Weaker sarcomeres become stretched. This allows fewer myosin heads to interact with the actin filaments, further reducing the active forces produced by those sarcomeres. Again, the increase in passive forces caused by stretching (passive stretch curve) is too small to compensate for differences in the active forces, and developing inhomogeneities from sarcomere to sarcomere are equalized only when the muscle is completely relaxed.

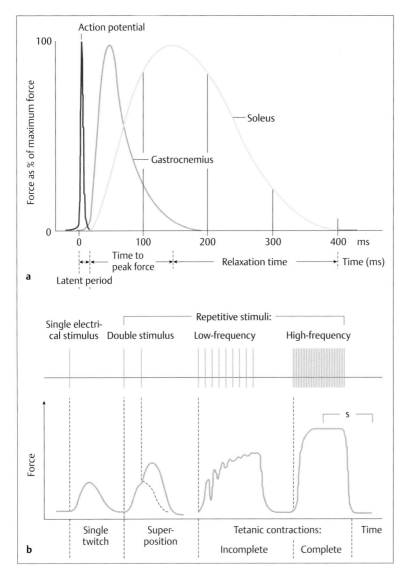

a Mechanograms of fast-twitch (gastrocnemius) and slow-twitch skeletal muscle
fibers (soleus) in comparison with the
time course of the action potential.
b Mechanical response of a skeletal muscle
fiber to direct electrical stimulation. Single stimulus, double stimulus, and serial
stimuli, with increasing superposition of
the mechanical responses with frequency of stimuli.

Caution

**Skeletal muscle fibers may be stimulated at such a
high frequency that the single twitches evoked by
individual action potentials are superimposed. The
resulting sustained contractions carry a risk of aggra-
vating structural inhomogeneities in muscle fibers due
to local overstretching and overcontraction.**

Gradation of Muscle Force during Voluntary Movements

The amplitude of a single twitch in a motor unit is practically constant in skeletal muscle. Every action potential
from a motor neuron triggers the excitation of all muscle
fibers innervated by that motor neuron. Moreover, each
individual fiber almost invariably responds to excitation
with the same contractile amplitude. Accordingly, the single twitch of motor units obeys the all-or-none law.

Nevertheless, different magnitudes of muscle force and
muscle shortening can be achieved during voluntary
movements. For weak voluntary movements, the motor
neurons transmit action potentials at frequencies of 6–
8 Hz, evoking corresponding repetitive contractions in individual fibers or individual motor units. Because the individual motor units are driven asynchronously by their
motor neurons, their individual responses are superimposed to yield a reasonably smooth contraction even
when the individual motor units respond only with a series of single twitches. Increasing the firing rate of the motor neurons triggers more frequent contractions of the individual motor units, leading to an increased net force
produced by the muscle as a whole and smoothing the
overall time course of the contraction (temporal summa-

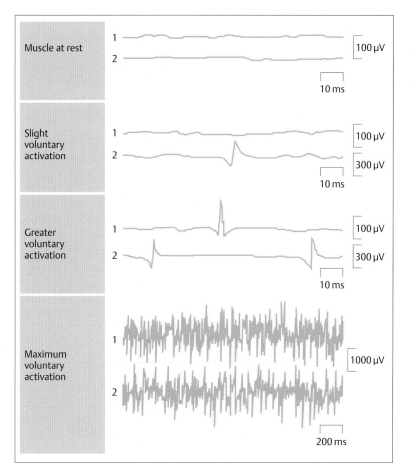

Fig. 2.5 Electromyography at rest and during voluntary muscle activation. Signals from two motor units recorded with two needle electrodes. When the muscle is at rest, no action potentials are recorded. As the intensity of voluntary activation is increased, a second motor unit is recruited and the frequency of the action potentials increases in both motor units.

tion). The developed muscular force and the speed of lifting a load can be further increased by the activation of additional motor units (recruitment or spatial summation). The smaller the motor units are (i.e., the smaller the additional force contribution from the individual motor unit), the greater the ability to achieve fine gradations of muscle function.

The activity of motor units can be recorded by electromyography. The activity of individual motor units can be traced with needle electrodes inserted directly into the muscle (**Fig. 2.5**).

Caution

Besides increasing the frequency of action potentials (temporal summation), voluntary muscle force can also be increased by the recruitment of additional motor units (spatial summation). At high action potential frequencies, there is a risk that the increasing superposition of individual responses (temporal summation) will cause progressive structural inhomogeneities in the individual skeletal muscle fibers.

Types of Muscular Contraction

The behavior of muscle force and muscle shortening at various initial muscle lengths is described by the length–force or length–tension diagram (**Fig. 2.6**).

Passive Length–Tension Curve

An isolated, unstimulated muscle assumes its equilibrium length. Usually, this length is somewhat shorter than the length of the same muscle inside the body at rest (the resting length of the muscle). When the muscle is stretched past its equilibrium length, passive recoil forces develop that increase roughly exponentially as the muscle is stretched further. These passive forces originate mainly from the titin molecules in the sarcomeres (see **Fig. 2.1a**). The passive forces are described by the passive length–tension curve (see **Fig. 2.6a**).

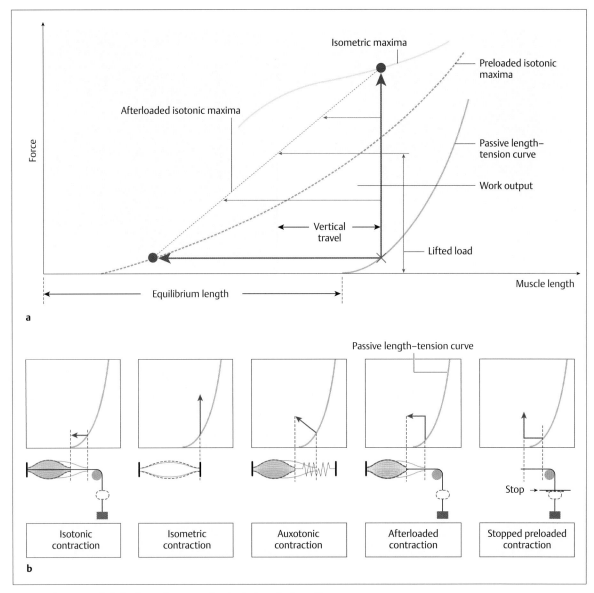

Fig. 2.6a, b   Types of skeletal muscle contraction in the length–force diagram.

a Length–force diagram with length–tension curve of resting muscle together with the curves of isometric and isotonic maxima. The curve of afterloaded maxima is also plotted for one working point (x). The isometric and isotonic contractions are also plotted for that point, in addition to afterloaded contractions for three different loads. Physical work is also shown for one of the afterloaded contractions. It represents the product of lifted load and vertical travel, and is expressed by the area enclosed by both quantities (shaded yellow).

b Length–force relations plotted for isotonic, isometric, positive auxotonic, afterloaded contraction, and preloaded contraction against a stop.

Isotonic Contraction

In an isotonic contraction, the muscle shortens under a constant load while developing a constant force (see **Fig. 2.6b**). This type of contraction occurs, for example, when a weight (preload) is suspended from a relaxed, isolated skeletal muscle (preloaded contraction). Initially, the weight passively stretches the muscle until the passive forces generated by titin molecules equal the gravitational force of the suspended weight. Lifting the weight during stimulation of the muscle is effected by an isotonic contraction, since the load remains constant during active shortening and the muscle lifting the weight must always develop a total force that equals the load to be lifted but acts in the opposite direction.

If we start from the passive length–tension curve and plot the maximum possible shortening for a given initial length horizontally (isotonic) and to the left (shortening), we can connect the end points to obtain the curve of preloaded isotonic maxima (see **Fig. 2.6a**).

Isometric Contraction

In an isometric contraction, the ends of the muscle are fixed (see **Fig. 2.6b**) so that the muscle length cannot change. An example is the function of the postural muscles. In this type of contraction, the length of the sarcomeres remains constant, provided there is negligible stretching of the tendons. When the lever arm of the myosin head executes a power stroke after high-affinity docking, the myosin heads (and to a lesser degree the actin and myosin filaments) come under elastic tension. The resulting elastic recoil forces can be measured externally as an active muscle force. The maximum muscle force depends on the number of myosin heads arranged in parallel. Consequently, the greater the total cross-section of all the fibers in the muscle, the greater the maximum muscle force.

The initial length of the muscle influences the passive forces that develop in the muscle (passive length–tension curve) as well as the active isometric force that is additionally developed during stimulation (see **Fig. 2.6a**). The active and passive forces for each initial length add together to yield the maximum isometric force. The reason for this lies in the parallel arrangement of the titin and actin filaments, which generate passive forces (titin filaments) and also transmit the active forces produced by the myosin heads (actin filaments). The active isometric force is maximal near the equilibrium length and declines both with increasing length above the maximum and with decreasing muscle length. If we plot the actively developed isometric force vertically upward from the passive length–tension curve (isometric contraction), the line connecting the end points will define the curve of the isometric maxima (see **Fig. 2.6a**).

Auxotonic Contraction

An auxotonic contraction is characterized by a simultaneous change in length and force (see **Fig. 2.6b**). Movements of joints often affect the length of the effective lever arm. Thus, even when a constant weight is being lifted, the load acting on the muscle will change as the muscle shortens. In a positive auxotonic contraction, the load increases with shortening (see **Fig. 2.6b**). In a negative auxotonic contraction, the load decreases.

> *Note*
>
> **Isotonic, isometric, and auxotonic contractions are the basic types of muscular contraction.**

Afterloaded Contraction and Contraction against a Stop

Afterloaded Contraction

An afterloaded contraction is a composite type of contraction. A common example is lifting an object (see **Fig. 2.6b**). The contraction consists of two phases:

- *Phase 1:* First the muscle must develop a level of force commensurate with the weight of the object to be lifted. The active force increases, while the muscle length remains constant (isometric phase).
- *Phase 2:* In the second phase, the object is lifted while the muscle shortens (afterloaded isotonic phase). When afterloaded contractions occur in an intact organism, the second phase is often more auxotonic than isotonic, due to the change in the effective lever arms.

The smaller the load to be lifted, the greater the vertical travel in an afterloaded contraction (see **Fig. 2.6a**). The vertical travel is described by the curve of the afterloaded maxima. The end points of the curve are defined by the purely isometric and purely isotonic contractions that are possible for the given initial resting length. The curve roughly follows a straight line connecting the end points of the corresponding isometric and isotonic contractions. The curve of the afterloaded maxima must be redetermined for each initial resting muscle length, starting from the corresponding point on the passive length–tension curve.

Preloaded Contraction against a Stop

Preloaded contractions against a stop are another type of composite contraction. A typical example is a chewing motion, in which the jaws close with each excursion (see **Fig. 2.6b**).

- *Phase 1:* In the first, preloaded isotonic phase of the contraction, the muscle shortens until it encounters a firm end point (jaw closure).

- *Phase 2:* In the second, isometric phase of the contraction, the muscle develops force (masticatory pressure) without changing its length.

Note

Afterloaded contractions and preloaded contractions against a stop are composite types of contraction that include an isometric phase and a preloaded or afterloaded isotonic or auxotonic phase.

Muscular Work

The physical work produced by muscle in lifting a load is the product of lifted load times amplitude of the lift (vertical travel in **Fig. 2.6a**). Because the force developed by the muscle must equal the load to be lifted, the physical work done by the muscle during an afterloaded contraction is represented in the force–length diagram by the area of the rectangle whose sides are the vertical travel and the lifted load (see **Fig. 2.6a**). The work is maximal in the intermediate load range and diminishes at lower and higher loads. For loads that correspond to the maximum isometric force (vertical travel = 0) or with shortening without a load (load = 0), no physical work is done because one of the factors in the work equation is zero. Nevertheless, ATP consumption still occurs in the cross-bridge cycle in both types of contraction. But in this situation, all of the chemical energy released by the hydrolysis of ATP is given off in the form of heat.

Relationship between Lifted Load and Shortening Velocity of Muscle

When the shortening velocity of a muscle measured in the isotonic phase of an afterloaded contraction is plotted against the lifted load or the muscle force needed to lift the load, we obtain the load–velocity or force–velocity relationship (**Fig. 2.7**). In the absence of an external load, the muscle shortens at its maximum possible speed, the maximum unloaded shortening velocity. The shortening velocity decreases hyperbolically as the load increases. If the load is just equal to the maximum isometric force, the shortening velocity is equal to 0—i.e., the muscle can no longer shorten by lifting the load (isometric contraction).

The same applies to stretching forces that act on a muscle. As the stretching forces increase, the shortening velocity dwindles. When the stretching forces exceed the maximum isometric force, the muscle is lengthened or stretched while actively contracting. This functional range is of major importance in deceleration movements (e.g., during downhill walking) and in the fine-tuning of movements by antagonists. While lengthening or stretching, the actively contracting muscle generates forces that may be up to twice the maximum isometric force (see **Fig. 2.7**).

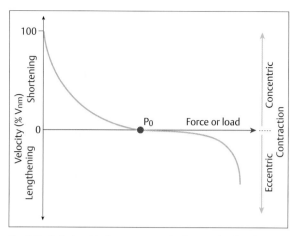

Fig. 2.7 Relationship between muscle force or load and velocity of shortening or lengthening of a skeletal muscle. If the external loads are smaller than the maximum isometric force, the muscle shortens (concentric contraction). In the absence of an external load, the maximum shortening velocity (V_{max}) is attained. As the load increases, the velocity in the isotonic shortening phase declines. When the load equals the maximum isometric force (P_0), the muscle undergoes isometric contraction without shortening or lengthening. With external forces or loads greater than P_0, the contracting muscle is lengthened (eccentric contraction).

Concentric and Eccentric Contractions

All contractions in which the muscle shortens are classified as concentric. They include afterloaded contractions in which the load is smaller than the maximum isometric force, so that the muscle shortens when lifting the load (see **Fig. 2.6a, b** and **Fig. 2.7**). When a muscle is lengthened (stretched) during a contraction, the contraction is described as eccentric (see **Fig. 2.7**, range of lengthening).

Caution

The active (tensed) muscle performing an eccentric contraction is lengthened by external forces (loads, braking movements, antagonists). The high forces that develop during the lengthening may cause microlesions, and the repair of those lesions may cause muscle soreness (delayed-onset muscle soreness, DOMS).

Adjusting Shortening Velocity to Changing Demands

When an object is to be lifted, the total active muscle force can be increased by increasing the action potential frequency with which the motor units are driven (temporal summation) and by the recruitment of additional motor units (spatial summation). Both processes reduce relative load on individual fibers, while the lifted weight remains constant. Thus, the object can be lifted faster in accordance with the force–velocity relationship. Similarly, the speed of movements of agonists can be precisely controlled by lengthening and the consequent braking action of coactivated antagonistic muscles—that is, by changing the load acting on the agonists.

The speed at which the object is lifted is also determined partly by the type of muscle fibers that are activated. Most skeletal muscles contain both slow-twitch and fast-twitch fibers, but in varying proportions. This means that the lifting speed can be adjusted to demands not only by recruitment and summation in the agonist, or by activation of antagonists, but also by the selective activation of fast or slow motor units.

Neuromuscular Control Mechanisms

All movements of the skeletal system, including the most complex movement patterns, are attributable to changes in the force and length of muscle fibers. The precise spatial and temporal coordination of numerous muscle actions enables complex movements to be performed. Motor activity, then, results from the very precisely coordinated innervation of motor units in various muscle groups by the corresponding α-motor neurons. Motor activity encompasses more than just movement; it also includes the control of body posture. Thus, precise voluntary movement (target oriented motor activity) also calls for simultaneous and coordinated adjustments in body position (postural motor activity). Fine adjustments in body posture result from the precisely coordinated activity of motor units in the postural muscles.

Hierarchical Organization of Voluntary Movements

The execution of a voluntary, target-oriented movement is accomplished through a "hierarchical cascade." This chain of events ranges from intention, planning, and programming to execution of the movement, which is effected by the selective activation of muscles by a complex activity pattern of the α-motor neurons that supply the participating motor units.

The motor intention, or the intent to perform a specific movement, arises in the cortical (e.g., frontal cortex) and subcortical motor areas (e.g., limbic system) of the brain. The motor intention is transformed into a motor plan (decision) in the motor association cortex. The program for executing the movement is generated jointly in the motor cortex, basal ganglia, motor thalamus, and cerebellum. The execution is initiated and guided by the motor cortex. To execute the planned movement, central efferents retrieve movement patterns that are preprogrammed via neuronal circuits at the spinal cord level.

Note

Voluntary movements are centrally initiated and monitored. They are executed by retrieving movement patterns that have been preprogrammed at the spinal cord level.

Fine Control of Motor Activity (Voluntary and Postural Motor Activity)

The fine control of motor activity requires the precise monitoring of body posture and of the planned movement. To accomplish this, the body posture as well as the tone and length of the various active muscle fibers must be constantly tailored to momentary demands by changing the activity pattern of the participating α-motor neurons. This involves the precisely coordinated activation of agonists and antagonists in order to, say, purposefully slow the speed of a movement by the antagonists (see p. 70). Another example is maintaining or adjusting the tone of the postural muscles in response to postural changes during the course of a movement. Both of these functions also serve to prevent unwanted braking forces that would otherwise counteract the voluntary movements.

This complex monitoring and control is carried out by phylogenetically old areas of the cerebellum and motor centers in the brainstem. They update the activity of the neuronal circuits at the spinal cord level and the resulting movement patterns (spinal reflexes). Sensory afferents from sensors for muscle length, muscle force, joint position, and touch, along with afferents from the visual or vestibular system, transmit information on the current progress of the planned movement to higher centers. If any discrepancy is found between the plan and its execution, the movement patterns programmed at the spinal cord level are modulated via efferent pathways until the plan and its execution coincide.

Note

Mediated by sensory afferents, the execution of voluntary movements is monitored by higher motor centers. The selection and activity of the movement patterns preprogrammed at the spinal level are adjusted via efferent pathways.

Preprogrammed Movement Patterns

Complex voluntary movements always include involuntary components. These components, which can be tested individually, are called "spinal reflexes." They represent a collection of postural and movement patterns, such as controlling muscle length and force, along with more complex patterns such as swallowing, breathing, walking, and running. During voluntary movements, these basic patterns are so intimately integrated into complex movements that they are no longer identifiable as separate patterns. Meanwhile, higher control levels no longer need to be accessed for each individual step in the execution of these basic patterns. The higher control levels serve only to monitor and correct the overall execution.

Note

Spinal reflexes such as the monosynaptic stretch reflex, and polysynaptic reflexes like the crossed extensor reflex, are examples of movement patterns that are preprogrammed at the spinal level. Some of these movement patterns can be clinically assessed.

Regulation or Control?

For very fast movements, the constant fine-tuning of motor activity via closed-loop feedback with sensory afferents (regulation) can be bypassed in order to save time. Following the principle of an open-loop control system, habitual "ingrained" activity patterns can be retrieved without having to go through a time-consuming, moment-by-moment closed-loop feedback process to match the actual movement to the intended movement. This type of control results in motions that are less precise and less reproducible, but it allows the movement to be executed more quickly. A potential disadvantage is the risk of dysregulation, such as an undesired high tone of antagonists. This is particularly common with actions that have not become fully patterned (see Chapter 6).

Motor Units as the Target Organ for Neuromuscular Regulation or Control

The target organ for even the most complex voluntary and postural motor actions is the motor unit of skeletal muscle. Every movement pattern, no matter how complex, is ultimately based on a combination of isometric, isotonic, and auxotonic contractions involving a fixed muscle length or a given length change at a precisely controlled speed. The precise control of muscle force, muscle length, and the rate of length change must be ensured even when the loads change during the course of the movement. Examples are changes in joint position, which directly influence effective lever arms.

In addition, two basic neuronal circuits are established at the spinal cord level which unconsciously and very rapidly (like a reflex) maintain a constant muscle length or muscle force, or adjust those variables to match a preset program. Each circuit functions as a feedback loop. Both of these feedback loops (one for muscle length, the other for muscle force) regulate the activity of the motor neurons of the individual motor units in skeletal muscle and drive them to execute voluntary movements via motor efferents.

Regulation of Muscle Length (Stretch Reflex)

Muscle length is regulated according to the requirements of postural function and voluntary movement. Specifically, the activity pattern of the α-motor neurons is adjusted so that muscle length is maintained or adjusted to an appropriate new length. For this purpose, the length of the muscle must be measured (actual value) and compared with the desired target value. If the actual and target values differ, the activity pattern of the α-motor neurons must be modulated until the values coincide.

Muscle Spindles

Muscle spindles are the sensors for muscle length. They consist of a group of short, specialized muscle fibers, the intrafusal fibers, that are separated by a connective-tissue capsule from the other fibers in skeletal muscle, the extrafusal muscle fibers (**Fig. 2.8a**, inset; see also Chapter 1). Muscle spindles are aligned parallel to the extrafusal fibers and are attached to their perimysium.

Length changes in the extrafusal muscle fibers lead to corresponding length changes in the intrafusal fibers. This allows the muscle spindles to measure the momentary length of the extrafusal fibers. The intrafusal fibers are noncontractile in their central region. The two adjacent contractile fiber segments are innervated by γ-motor neurons. The noncontractile region of both types of intrafusal fiber—the nuclear bag fibers and nuclear chain fibers—is wrapped by annulospiral endings. These are the sensory endings formed by afferent Ia fibers, known also as the "primary sensory endings." Peripheral to them on the nuclear chain fibers are other sensory endings, the secondary sensory endings of the group II fibers (see **Fig. 2.8a**, inset).

Efferent Innervation of Muscle Spindles

The contractile ends of the intrafusal fibers receive motor innervation like the extrafusal muscle (see **Fig. 2.8a**, inset). The efferents originate from γ-motor neurons, which are located along with α-motor neurons in the anterior horn of the spinal cord. While nuclear bag fibers are chiefly activated on a short-term phasic basis, nuclear chain fibers can undergo sustained tonic contractions. The discharge frequency of the gamma efferents alters the tone of the contractile ends of the intrafusal fibers to set the threshold and sensitivity of the muscle spindles.

Discharge Pattern of Muscle Spindles

Muscle spindles are stimulated by the length or changing length of the noncontractile central regions of the nuclear chain and nuclear bag fibers. Even when a muscle is at resting length, action potentials are still being transmitted through the Ia and II afferents to the spinal cord. When a muscle is stretched from its resting length, the noncontractile central regions of the nuclear chain and nuclear bag fibers are also stretched. The receptive membrane of the Ia and II axons is positioned such that it is stretched in turn, causing mechanosensory ion channels to open. The resultant change in the membrane potential has the effect of increasing the frequency of afferent action potentials. As the stretch is relieved, the afferent frequency declines. The discharge rate of Ia afferents is proportional to

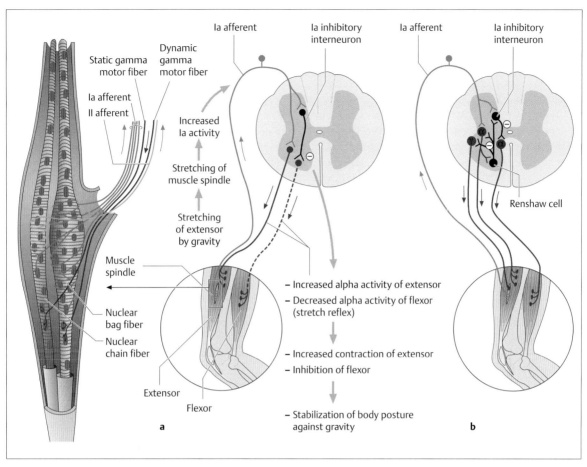

Fig. 2.8a, b   Muscle spindles in the control of skeletal muscle length. Innervation of the spindles, reciprocal inhibition, and Renshaw inhibition.

a Diagrammatic representation of the length-stabilizing feedback loop (muscle stretch reflex), with reciprocal inhibition of antagonistic motor neurons via inhibitory Ia interneurons.
Inset: Afferent and efferent innervation of the muscle spindle for nuclear chain and nuclear bag fibers. There are two types of sensory afferents and motor efferents; the majority are dynamic type Ia afferents and static type II afferents from the noncontractile central regions of the intrafusal fibers. Static and dynamic gamma efferents lead to the contractile segments of the intrafusal fibers.

b Renshaw inhibition in the functional unit consisting of α- and γ-motor neurons and the associated Ia interneuron. The Renshaw cell monitors the activity of this functional unit and is influenced by both excitatory and inhibitory central efferents. Central efferents also have direct access to α- and γ-motor neurons and to the Ia interneuron.

the length (stretch) of the sensory segment. It also undergoes short-term exaggerated changes in response to stretch or unstretch (dynamic differential response). The discharge rate of the secondary endings is proportional only to length.

With constant gamma efferent input to the contractile ends of the intrafusal fibers, the muscle spindles increase their discharge rate in response to the stretching of relaxed as well as activated muscle (eccentric contraction). The discharge pattern remains practically unchanged during an isometric contraction, and the discharge rate declines during isotonic shortening.

Afferents and their Connections

Both types of afferents (Ia and II) enter the spinal cord via the dorsal roots (see **Fig. 2.8a**). Passing through the posterior horn, they project directly or via interneurons to the motor neurons in the anterior horn (α-motor neurons) of the extrafusal fibers of the associated homonymous muscle (stretch reflex).

When the type Ia afferents enter the spinal cord, they pass directly to the α-motor neurons of the associated muscle, where they form excitatory synapses. Type II afferents from the secondary endings also connect to α-motor neurons of the associated muscle, but usually do so by way of an interneuron. They also send impulses to the α-motor neurons of synergistic muscles via other interneurons. As a result, the stretching of a muscle increases the depolarization of the α-motor neurons of its extrafusal fibers. This increases the frequency of the efferent action potentials, stimulating the stretched muscle to contract (see **Fig. 2.8a**). The overall effect of the type Ia and type II afferents is to counteract stretch. The opposite occurs during the unstretching or shortening of a muscle. In this way, the muscle length is stabilized at a level predetermined by the activity of gamma efferents passing to the contractile ends of the intrafusal muscle fibers.

Reciprocal Inhibition

As described above, the Ia afferents enter the spinal cord and synapse on the α-motor neurons of the associated muscle (homonymous α-motor neurons). However, branches from the afferents also stimulate interneurons in the spinal cord that act via inhibitory synapses on the α-motor neurons of antagonistic muscles (see **Fig. 2.8a**). When a muscle is stretched, therefore, increased activation of its α-motor neurons is not the only mechanism that counters the stretch. Simultaneous inhibition of the α-motor neurons to antagonistic muscles (reciprocal inhibition) limits the ability of the antagonists to counteract the corrective shortening of the agonist.

Because the Ia afferents from antagonistic muscles have corresponding connections, a total of four processes may occur in response to passive (gravity-induced) changes in the position of a joint—all of which serve to counteract the change in joint position:

- Stretching of the muscle spindles in extensors leads to increased excitation of the extensor motor neurons.
- This is combined with decreased excitation of the flexor motor neurons through reciprocal inhibition.
- As the stretch on the flexor muscle spindles is relieved, the flexor motor neurons become less active.
- The same process also reduces reciprocal inhibition of the extensor motor neurons (disinhibition).

As a result of these processes, the overall excitation of the extensor motor neurons increases, that of the flexor motor neurons decreases, and the upright body posture is stabilized against gravity.

Renshaw Inhibition

The α-motor neurons have recurrent axon collaterals in the spinal cord that form excitatory synapses with interneurons called Renshaw cells. The Renshaw cells in turn synapse with the original α-motor neurons. They secrete the inhibitory transmitter glycine or gamma-aminobutyric acid (GABA) at their synapses, causing inhibition of the original α-motor neurons. This simple negative feedback loop to the same α-motor neuron serves to limit its activity.

Besides the α-motor neurons, the Renshaw cells also inhibit the associated γ-motor neurons and the corresponding Ia interneurons that mediate the reciprocal inhibition of antagonistic muscles. In this way, the Renshaw cells influence the degree of counterregulation to muscle stretch, for example, both by limiting counterregulation of the homonymous muscle and its agonists and by limiting the reciprocal inhibition of the antagonists. From a control systems standpoint, Renshaw inhibition dampens the mechanisms that regulate muscle length. Descending pathways can act on the Renshaw cells to modulate the degree of inhibition. The cells, then, make up part of the "functional units" that coordinate the activation and inhibition of the agonists and antagonists acting on a common joint (see **Fig. 2.8b**).

The depression of Renshaw cell activity can adversely affect the fine control of motor actions. This may result in excessive counterregulation or excessive tone of the antagonists. This condition may compromise the "looseness" of an athlete, making it more difficult to perform target tasks or movements that require an explosive force. The increased tone of the antagonists must be overcome during movements. This makes it necessary to recruit additional motor units and also increase the efferent discharge rates to the individual motor units. The latter results in greater superposition, causing an abnormally high tone in the individual motor units. This could be a potential cause of muscle-related neuromuscular muscle disorder as a sign of neuromuscular dysregulation (see Chapter 6). If coordination problems continue, the increase in sarcomere inhomogeneities due to greater superposition (see p. 65) may lead to irreversible structural damage, with progression from "muscle stress" to tearing of muscle fibers.

Gamma Loop and Alpha–Gamma Coactivation

The muscle spindles and their circuits stabilize the muscle length at a level that is predetermined by the initial tension on the noncontractile central region of the intrafusal fibers. Extensive or prolonged changes in muscle length require a resetting of the target value of the noncontractile central region of the intrafusal muscle fibers. This reset is accomplished by the efferent gamma innervation to the contractile ends of the intrafusal muscle fibers. If only gamma innervation were altered by central efferents, the activation of α-motor neurons would be slaved to feedback signals from the spindle afferents (gamma loop). But central efferents act simultaneously on α- and γ-motor neurons (alpha–gamma coactivation), with the result that the lengths of the extrafusal fibers and the contractile ends of the intrafusal fibers are changed simultaneously. Feedback via the muscle spindles can then be used for the final stabilization and fine control of movements.

Note

Muscle length is controlled by comparing the desired length of a muscle with its actual length via muscle spindles. Spinal circuits then act to adjust the muscle length to the desired value. This process involves the reciprocal activation of muscular agonists and antagonists. The degree of counterregulation and reciprocal inhibition of the antagonists is limited by the Renshaw cells. α-motor neurons of one agonist and the corresponding γ- and α-motor neurons of the antagonists and their Ia interneurons form functional units with the associated Renshaw cells. These units coordinate the activation and inhibition of the agonists and antagonists that act on a common joint.

Force and Tension Control in Muscles (Autogenous Inhibition)

Golgi Tendon Organs

Golgi tendon organs consist of unmyelinated nerve endings, enclosed in a fibrous capsule, that branch between the collagen fibers of tendons near the muscle–tendon junction (**Fig. 2.9a**, inset; see also Chapter 1). The unmyelinated nerve endings are stimulated by tension on the collagen fibers. Due to their location, the tendon organs sense the forces (tensions) acting on multiple extrafusal muscle fibers. The unmyelinated endings are the terminal branches of myelinated nerve fibers, the Ib afferents.

For a relaxed muscle at its resting length, the Ib afferents from the tendon organs are silent. They increase their firing rate only in response to passive stretch and passive recoil forces or to the active generation of muscle force, as in an isometric contraction. Accordingly, the tendon organs are sensors for active and passive muscle force (tension).

Afferents and Their Connections

The Ib afferents enter the spinal cord through the dorsal root and synapse with inhibitory interneurons (Ib interneurons), which in turn synapse with α-motor neurons of the homonymous muscle (see **Fig. 2.9a**). Accordingly, increased muscle force leads to increasing inhibition of the homonymous α-motor neurons ("autogenous inhibition"), while diminishing muscle force causes decreased inhibition (disinhibition) of the homonymous muscle. Thus, the tendon organs do more than protect against overloads. Through disinhibition, they can also compensate for a decline in muscle force due to fatigue, for example. In this way, the tendon organs and their circuits act to maintain a constant degree of muscle force (tension) in response to external changes. The resulting maintenance of constant force is essential in isotonic contractions, for example.

Note

Active muscle force (tension) can also be precisely regulated via a feedback loop when necessary (e.g., during isotonic contraction). The sensor for muscle force (tension) is the Golgi tendon organ.

Rhythmic Movement Patterns

Neuronal circuits at the spinal cord level are feedback loops that regulate not only muscle length and force, but also rhythmic activities such as walking and running. Spinal circuits produce rhythmic activity patterns (rhythm generator). Every limb has a half-center that has reciprocal connections with the half-centers in the other limbs. The basic element of the rhythm generator is the flexor reflex with the crossed extensor reflex. Afferents (e.g., for touch or pain) are wired at the spinal cord level in such a way that they produce coordinated activation of the flexors at the same side, while inhibiting the extensors. Conversely, the extensors are activated on the opposite side, while the flexors are inhibited. When a painful stimulus is encountered (e.g., stepping on a rock), the flexors are activated to move the affected leg away from the painful stimulus. This movement is supported by concomitant extension of the opposite leg (flexor withdrawal reflex).

Integrated into the rhythm generator, this neuronal circuit mediates rhythmic walking or running with alternating stance and swing phases—that is, alternating activation of the extensors (stance phase) and flexors (swing phase). Thus, their coordinated, alternating, rhythmic activation does not require rhythmic input from higher centers, but is preprogrammed at the spinal cord level. The task of the central efferents is to turn the rhythm generator on or off.

Note

Even complex movement patterns such as walking, with its alternating stance and swing phases, are preprogrammed at the spinal level. The task of higher centers is to "switch" this movement pattern on or off and correct any discrepancy between the desired movement and the actual execution of the movement.

Facilitation and Inhibition of Neuronal Circuits at the Spinal Cord Level

The Ia interneurons that mediate reciprocal inhibition are excited not only by Ia afferents from the muscle spindles. They also receive inputs from other primary peripheral afferents and from multiple descending pathways. In principle, all afferents and descending pathways to the motor neurons also act on the corresponding Ia interneurons. This ensures that whenever a motor neuron population needed for a certain motor program is activated, the cor-

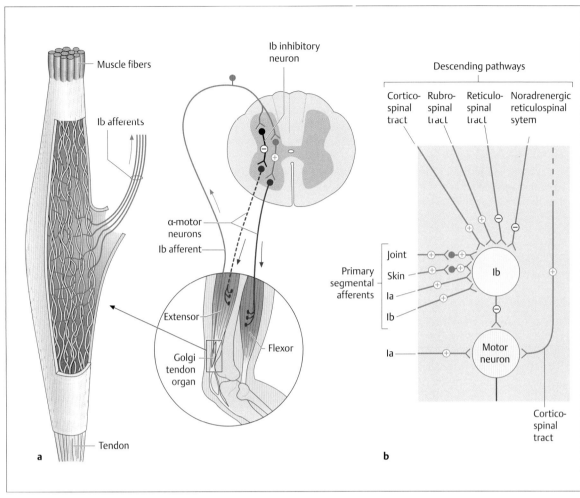

Fig. 2.9a, b   Golgi tendon organ and Ib interneuron in the control of skeletal muscle tension.

a Diagrammatic representation of the feedback loop for muscle force (mechanical muscle tension). Autogenous inhibition of the agonist (and synergistic muscles) via an inhibitory Ib interneuron and the activation of antagonistic muscles via activating interneurons. A decline in muscle force (active muscle tension) due to fatigue, for example, decreases the inhibition of the agonist and synergistic muscles with less activation of antagonists. This results in greater efferent input to the agonist and to synergistic muscles. In this way muscle force can be maintained despite fatigue.
Inset: Golgi tendon organ with arrangement of the free endings of the Ib afferents between the collagen fibers of the tendon.

b Arrangement of the inhibitory Ib interneuron with convergence of four descending pathways and four different peripheral receptor types. Primary afferents have an excitatory action; descending pathways have a combination of excitatory and inhibitory actions. The circuits shown provide a basis for the multimodal integration of different afferents and central efferents by the Ib interneuron. Activation of the inhibitory Ib interneuron leads to inhibition and disinhibition of the associated motor neurons. Motor neurons are also excited directly by corticospinal pathways and Ia spindle afferents, without interposed interneurons.

responding Ia interneurons will be activated as well. This is done to ensure the concomitant reciprocal activation of the antagonists.

Similarly, the Ib interneurons are excited not only by Ib afferents from the Golgi tendon organs, but also by primary afferents from the muscle spindles and from receptors in the skin and joints. In addition, various descending, excitatory, or inhibitory pathways also converge on the Ib

interneurons (see **Fig. 2.9b**). Their excitatory or inhibitory action opens or closes neuronal feedback loops (gating) just as needed to perform the planned movement. By presynaptic inhibition, certain primary afferents to the Ib interneurons can be selectively suppressed. In this way, the Ib interneurons provide for the multimodal integration of various afferents and central efferents.

One task of the descending pathways is to select the population of interneurons involved in a specific motor program, along with their associated motor neurons, through facilitation and inhibition (disfacilitation). The descending pathways also select the feedback loops (e.g., for length or force control) that are necessary for the desired movement by opening or closing primary afferents through presynaptic inhibition. Together with corticospinal pathways and the Ia afferents from muscle spindles that synapse directly on α-motor neurons, the Ib interneurons specifically activate the pool of active motor neurons needed for the particular motor task and adjust the moment-to-moment motor actions to match the planned movement.

Note

The Ib interneurons are central relay stations that receive inputs from peripheral primary sensory afferents and from excitatory and inhibitory descending pathways. Central efferents act via Ib interneurons to open or close feedback loops and the corresponding motor units ("gating") as required for the planned movements. Presynaptic inhibition at the inputs to the Ib interneurons provides a mechanism for selecting the feedback loops and associated sensory afferents (e.g., muscle spindles for length control, Golgi tendon organs for force control) that are necessary for the specific task.

Practical Tip

Given the complex circuits that exist at the spinal level and their targeted selection and modulation by central efferents and primary afferents from the periphery, we can understand why disturbances in higher centers and even in peripheral afferents (e.g., due to a change of playing surface) can impact on voluntary and postural motor activity (see Chapter 6). This can result in significant impairment of normal muscle tone, precise coordinated motor sequences (target tasks), or maximum explosive strength (explosive capability).
At the same time, disturbances of reciprocal inhibition (see p. 74) or Renshaw inhibition (see p. 74) can compromise the functional units that coordinate the agonists and antagonists. The results may include increased resistance to voluntary movements, making it necessary to increase the tone of the agonist muscles by increased activity of their individual motor units and the recruitment of additional motor units. Increasing fatigue with a decline in muscle force will further increase the activity of the α-motor neurons of the agonists through Ib disinhibition (see above). On the whole, the rising activity of the α-motor neurons will result in increasing superposition (see p. 75) or even painful contraction of the individual motor units. We suspect from clinical experience (see Chapter 6) that functional failure of neuromuscular control mechanisms may form the basis of "muscle-related neuromuscular muscle disorders" and could account for their fusiform pattern. This could also help us understand the transition to a structural injury (e.g., partial muscle tear) based on progressive inhomogeneity in the fine structure of the muscle fibers. Explosive movements such as cutting maneuvers and maximal forces that bypass the feedback loops (see p. 65) could promote the loss of fine coordination and contribute to the pathogenesis of the muscle-related form of neuromuscular muscle disorders.

Aspects of Exercise Physiology

N. Maassen

Types of Muscle Fiber

The two main types of muscle fiber are classified as red (slow-twitch) and white (fast-twitch) fibers. Muscle fibers can also be classified as oxidative or glycolytic, on the basis of their enzyme pattern for energy production. Another way to distinguish muscle fibers is on the basis of heavy myosin chains, resulting in the designation of type I and type II muscle fibers. Type II fibers are further subdivided into types IIa, IIb, and IIx. The type IIb heavy myosin chains permit the fastest contractions. The varying properties of muscle fibers are summarized in **Table 2.1**.

The type IIb fiber is even faster than type IIx, but is either absent or very rare in humans. Type IIx was formerly classified as type IIb.

Besides the differences noted above, there are other structural and functional differences between the fiber types. For example, sodium channels are more abundant in the sarcolemma of fast-twitch fibers than that of slow-twitch fibers. The volume of the T system is twice as large in the fast-twitch fibers, and the volume of the sarcoplasmic reticulum is approximately 50% greater. These fibers are optimally adapted for fast contractions, owing to rapid impulse conduction, rapid calcium release, and short diffusion paths to the regulatory proteins. Actomyosin ATPase activity is approximately three times higher. Taken together, these properties mean that the time to reach maximum force amplitude is only about 25% of that in slow-twitch muscles (see p. 62). Fast-twitch fibers also have a higher relaxation speed. The half-time to relaxation is approximately 80% faster than in slow-twitch muscles, due in part to the more than three times faster uptake rate of calcium ions into the sarcoplasmic reticulum.

Table 2.1 Types of muscle fiber

Fiber type	Type I	Type II a	Type II x
Contraction speed	Low	High	Very high
Mitochondrial density	High	High	Moderate
Capillary density	High	Moderate	Low
Oxidative capacity	High	High	Moderate
Glycolytic capacity	Low	High	High
Fatigability	Low	Moderate	High
Maximal power	Low	Moderate	High

Overview of Muscular Metabolism

Anaerobic Alactacid Energy Production

As noted earlier, the cross-bridge cycle in muscular contraction consumes energy in the form of ATP. But sodium-potassium ATPase and the transport of calcium ions back into the sarcoplasmic reticulum also require ATP. The signal for this rise in energy metabolism is the action potential that precedes calcium release. Calcium initiates the cross-bridge cycle, in which ATP is hydrolyzed. Because the ATP concentration in the cytosol is relatively low (only about 7 mmol/L) and is sufficient only for brief periods of work, a mechanism must be available for the immediate resynthesis of ATP. This can be accomplished through a number of metabolic pathways:

- *Myokinase reaction.* The most direct pathway is the myokinase reaction. Catalyzed by the enzyme myokinase (adenylate kinase), it supplies ATP and adenosine monophosphate (AMP) from two molecules of ADP. The ATP is again available for energy supply, while the newly formed AMP is partially broken down by AMP deaminase to inosine monophosphate (IMP) and ammonia.
- *Creatine kinase reaction.* In this reaction, the enzyme creatine kinase transfers the phosphate group from creatine phosphate to ADP, yielding ATP, creatine, and P_i from the cleavage of ATP.

Both of the above reactions fall under the heading of "anaerobic alactacid energy production." Because the creatine phosphate concentration in the cytosol is only about four times higher than the ATP concentration, the net energy yield from both of these reactions is small.

> *Note*
>
> The intramuscular creatine phosphate concentration can be increased by creatine supplementation as a means of improving sprint performance and maximum force. Creatine supplementation does not affect maximum oxygen uptake, but it can adversely affect endurance.

Activation of Phosphofructokinase

The importance of the above metabolic pathways goes beyond pure energy production. Changes in the concentrations of the metabolites involved have effects on other energy-yielding metabolic pathways. Phosphofructokinase, the key enzyme of glycolysis, is activated by a fall in the levels of ATP and creatine phosphate. Increased levels of free ADP, free AMP, and probably ammonia have even greater effects. This means that changes in the concentrations of metabolites from the anaerobic alactacid metabolic pathways activate anaerobic glycolysis.

Another reaction should be emphasized: protons are eliminated from the cytosol during the breakdown of creatine phosphate. As a result, the breakdown of this compound functions as a metabolic hydrogen ion buffer, causing a rise in pH. This is another factor that contributes to the activation of phosphofructokinase (**Fig. 2.10**). It is particularly important at the start of exercise, because whenever the ATP turnover rate rises, the creatine phosphate concentration falls. Thus, the proton concentration also falls until the creatine phosphate concentration reaches a new equilibrium state. The fall in creatine phosphate parallels the percentage maximum oxygen uptake well into the range of high exercise intensities.

> *Note*
>
> The breakdown of high-energy phosphates (anaerobic alactacid metabolism) activates phosphofructokinase.

Activation of Glycogen Breakdown

The initial substrate must be provided in order for activated glycolysis to supply energy. The substrate for activated phosphofructokinase is fructose-6-phosphate. It may be obtained from glucose absorbed from the blood (important in McArdle's disease), or it may be formed from intramuscular glycogen. The breakdown of this intracellular storage compound is regulated by phosphorylase. This enzyme is activated by calcium ions (via calmodulin), meaning that the signal to contract also initiates the immediate

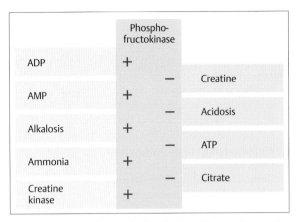

Fig. 2.10 The regulation of phosphofructokinase. See text for details.

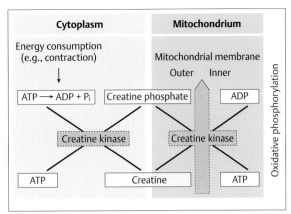

Fig. 2.11 Diagrammatic representation of the phosphocreatine shuttle (Bessman cycle). ADP, adenosine diphosphate; AMP, adenosine monophosphate; ATP, adenosine triphosphate; CK, creatine kinase; P_i = inorganic phosphate.

breakdown of glycogen to provide a substrate for anaerobic glycolysis. Phosphorylase is activated by lower calcium ion concentrations than the cross-bridge cycle. Calcium plays a significant role only at the start of exercise, and metabolites from the breakdown of high-energy phosphates provide a further stimulus for phosphorylase. Epinephrine also activates glycogen breakdown during intensive exercise (Watt et al. 2001).

Production of Lactate

The end product of phosphorylase and phosphofructokinase activation is pyruvate. The further pathway for pyruvate metabolism depends on the ability to utilize the citric acid cycle and respiratory chain, or aerobic metabolism. If this capacity is lacking, so that the accumulation of pyruvate is greater than its breakdown in mitochondrial metabolic pathways, lactate is formed. Accordingly, a lack of oxygen is not necessarily the cause of lactate production (anaerobic lactacid energy metabolism—yields a proton in addition to lactate, resulting in lactic acid). It may also result from an imbalance of flow rates (activations) in the cytosolic and mitochondrial metabolic pathways. The key enzyme in this regard is pyruvate dehydrogenase. Through decarboxylation, it yields activated acetic acid (acetyl-CoA), the initial substrate for the citric acid cycle. Pyruvate dehydrogenase is activated by calcium, but is also stimulated by exercise-induced changes in the metabolites of high-energy phosphates, the falling pH, and a rising pyruvate concentration (Parolin et al. 1999).

Because lactate is converted back to pyruvate by lactate dehydrogenase, it also serves as a "pyruvate reservoir" for oxidative metabolism. This takes place inside the lactate-producing fiber, because diffusion from the fiber is limited. When lactate is released by the muscle fibers, principally type II fibers, it is absorbed by adjacent type I fibers and undergoes oxidative breakdown. Lactate in this case functions as a substrate for oxidative metabolism (lactate shuttle).

Note

Lactate production not only allows direct energy production by the anaerobic pathway, but is also important for oxidative metabolism.

Aerobic Metabolism

The utilization of aerobic (mitochondrial) metabolic pathways, which involve mitochondrial ATP production, must be adjusted to exercise demands. Again, the breakdown of creatine phosphate plays a role. This process is directly proportional to exercise intensity, and so the creatine concentration also rises in proportion to intensity. Creatine can diffuse to the mitochondria from its site of formation. The mitochondrial double membrane contains additional creatine kinase. The creatine kinase reaction is reversed at this location, in that a phosphate group is transferred to creatine from intramitochondrial ATP. The newly formed creatine phosphate is again available for energy-consuming processes in the cytosol. The concentration of ADP, the most potent stimulator of the respiratory chain, rises within the mitochondrium. This process is known as the phosphocreatine shuttle, or Bessman cycle (Bessman and Carpenter 1985; **Fig. 2.11**).

This concept is supported by the parallel nature of the time course (kinetics) of creatine phosphate breakdown and oxygen uptake, which is noted during the transition from rest to exercise and also after exercise (Whipp et al. 1999). The Bessman cycle cannot fully explain the activation of oxidative phosphorylation, however. The turnover of ATP may be increased even with the concomitant inhibition of creatine kinase. It has also been shown that oxygen uptake kinetics can be accelerated by the preliminary activation of pyruvate dehydrogenase (Parolin et al. 1999). Other factors that regulate aerobic metabolism include:

- Calcium
- Cytosolic free ADP
- P_i
- pH

The net result is as follows: when glycogen is metabolized by the anaerobic route alone, 3 moles of ATP are produced from one subunit (glycosyl unit). When the glycosyl unit is broken down to carbon dioxide and water, a total of 31 or 33 moles of ATP are produced, depending on the fiber type.

Note

Aerobic and anaerobic metabolism cannot be separated or viewed as alternatives. In fact, anaerobic alactacid metabolism and anaerobic lactacid metabolism (ultimately the oxygen deficit, **Fig. 2.12**) are both necessary in order to activate and optimize aerobic metabolism.

Fat or Carbohydrates?

Either carbohydrate metabolism or beta oxidation (part of fat metabolism) may be the source of the acetyl-CoA that is broken down in aerobic metabolism. Free fatty acids are the substrate for beta oxidation. They may be transported from the blood through the sarcolemma by fatty acid–binding proteins, or they may be formed within the cytosol by the action of a hormone-sensitive lipase. It is likely that the hormone-sensitive lipase is swiftly activated by calcium ions, so that fat breakdown as well as carbohydrate breakdown begin immediately at the start of exercise.

The quantitative relationship between the two is determined by the supply of carbohydrates and free fatty acids. How this interaction takes place is not fully understood. Several possibilities have been discussed (Spriet and Watt 2003):

- *Randle cycle.* This process appears to play a role in skeletal muscle at rest. Its importance during exercise is disputed, however, because the concentrations of the critical metabolites (acetyl-CoA, citrate, glucose-6-phosphate) show little if any increase when the fat supply is increased.
- With an abundance of free fatty acids:
  - Reduced nicotinamide adenine dinucleotide (NADH) increases, and it inhibits pyruvate dehydrogenase.
  - The free fatty acids up-regulate pyruvate dehydrogenase kinase, thereby inhibiting pyruvate dehydrogenase.
- With an abundance of carbohydrates:
  - The availability of free fatty acids, and thus their transport into the mitochondria, is reduced in an insulin-dependent manner.
  - Glucose or glycogen activate phosphorylase. This results in the increased activation of pyruvate dehydrogenase by pyruvate and a fall in pH.

Another interaction has been discovered in recent years: interleukin-6 (IL-6) is released from muscle during prolonged exercise (Febbraio et al. 2003). This stimulates lipolysis in adipose tissue and also provides indirectly for increased fat breakdown by the release of cortisol. If this breakdown continues for a prolonged period, protein breakdown will also increase.

The metabolic pathways described above are basically operative in both types of muscle. However, they differ in their quantity and speed in red and white muscle fibers.

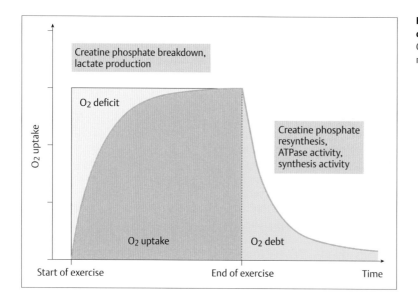

Fig. 2.12 Oxygen deficit and oxygen debt during moderate muscular exercise. Only quantitatively significant processes are represented in the graph.

Warm-Up

Warm-up is done to prepare the muscle or organism for exercise, optimize performance, and also prevent injuries. Warm-ups can be classified as active or passive.

- *Passive methods:* warm bath, sauna, etc. Static stretching can also be considered a passive method, since it does not actively work the muscle.
- *Active methods:* active warm-up is produced by muscle contractions—for example, dynamic stretching/stretching exercises (see Chapter 15).

In evaluating the effects of warm-up, it is helpful to distinguish between pure thermal effects and exercise effects.

Thermal Effects

Raising the temperature in a muscle (from approximately 33°C to over 37°C) by external means such as a sauna is sufficient to increase metabolic activity, on the basis of the reaction speed–temperature rule. The viscosity of the muscle is decreased. The resting membrane potential is hyperpolarized, while the amplitude of the action potentials is increased and their duration shortened. This is accompanied by a faster propagation speed of the action potentials, and the contraction velocity is increased. The thermally induced right shift in the oxygen binding curve in itself will facilitate oxygen delivery to the muscles.

Blood Flow

The effects of active warm-up go beyond those of passive methods. Blood flow increases at once with the onset of exercise. Because the muscle temperature is generally lower than the core temperature, the muscle is warmed by the influx of blood. A certain amount of time is needed for significant metabolic heat production to occur. Once the muscle temperature exceeds the core temperature, the body core is warmed by the muscles. When exercise is started, blood flow to the muscle increases as rapidly as oxygen uptake by the muscle, resulting in almost constant oxygenation during this transition (Grassi et al. 2003). Consequently, the oxygen deficit does not result from a deficiency of oxygen in the working muscle.

The rapid increase in blood flow is mediated by factors that are released from the working muscle and red blood cells. The relationships are not yet fully understood. Metabolites from energy metabolism, nitric oxide and probably potassium, whose concentration in the interstitium rises immediately at the start of exercise, are known to play a role. This interaction closely links energy consumption to the oxygen and nutrient supply at the start of exercise and during exercise. Because blood flow remains elevated for some time after exercise ceases, the supply situation is also improved for some time after the completion of an active warm-up (**Fig. 2.13**).

Excitability

Warm-up also influences the electrical properties of muscle. In addition to raising temperature, the electrolyte shift from the action potential leads to the activation of sodium-potassium ATPase. Because this enzyme is electrogenic, it causes hyperpolarization of the membrane, resulting in an increased amplitude of the action potentials. They spread electrotonically through the muscle fibers, and the propagation speed increases due to the stronger currents (see **Fig. 2.13**). The complete activation of sodium-potassium ATPase by muscular activity appears to take 15–20 minutes. Continuous exercise does not need to be maintained during that time; short, vigorous bouts will also suffice. Sodium-potassium ATPase can also be stimulated by epinephrine.

Some of the muscular effects of active warm-up are shown in **Fig. 2.13**.

Warm-up has effects that go beyond muscle-specific changes. Raising the skin temperature heightens the sensitivity of free nerve endings and skin receptors. The function of the muscle spindles is also optimized. The flow of information from the above receptors to the central nervous system (CNS) is important for coordination and thus for the precise execution of movements.

Simple passive stretching does not affect blood flow, nor does it produce any of the warm-up effects described above. Stretching does not appear to change the viscoelastic properties of muscle and only increases its stretch tolerance (Thacker et al. 2004). There is no evidence of positive effects in terms of immediate injury prevention (Thacker et al. 2004). It is possible, however, that passive stretching may be a beneficial training aid, with positive long-term effects when applied in conjunction with other measures (e.g., eccentric training; see also the remarks on stretching in Chapter 15).

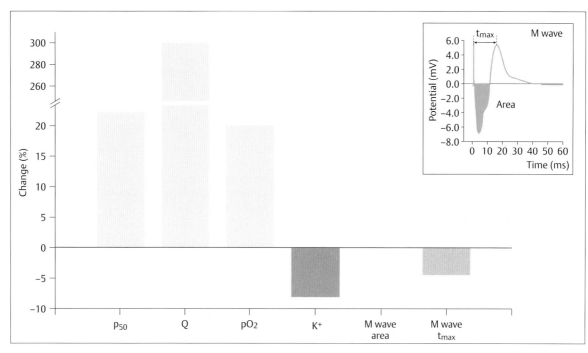

Fig. 2.13   Effects of muscle warm-up. The quantities were recorded in forearm muscles 5 minutes after active warm-up. The graph indicates percentage changes relative to rest. The warm-up intensity was 50% of the maximal incremental exercise intensity.

p_{50} = Half-saturation pressure of the oxygen binding curve
Q   = Muscle blood flow
pO_2 = Oxygen tension in venous blood from muscle
K^+ = Potassium concentration measured in venous blood
          (the falling concentration results from the activation of
          sodium-potassium ATPase)

M wave = Area of the compound action potential
t_{max} = Time of maximum M wave amplitude (t_{max} is an indicator
          of propagation speed; as t_{max} falls, the propagation speed
          rises)

Inset: compound action potential of the muscles.

Note

Simple, passive stretching during warm-up does not affect blood flow. Stretching does increase the stretch tolerance of muscle, but does not acutely change the viscoelastic properties of muscle.

Note

Warm-up enhances performance by reducing muscle viscosity, raising temperature, increasing the supply of oxygen and nutrients, activating energy metabolism, stabilizing excitability, and improving coordination. Problems may result from warm-up that causes an excessive temperature rise or an excessive consumption of resources.

Cooling Instead of Warm-Up

As early as the 1980s, it was shown that cooling, which lowers the core body temperature, can improve exercise performance. The most likely explanation is that water, which makes up approximately 60% of the human body, has a high heat capacity. Cooling that lowers the core body temperature delays the point at which critical temperatures are reached during any given exercise. Performance enhancement has been observed only in cyclic exercises that do not involve a high degree of coordination, however. Recent studies also document positive effects from partial body cooling.

Fatigue

There are two fundamentally different definitions for fatigue:
- Fatigue is the *point in time* at which a desired exercise can no longer be performed.
- Fatigue is a *process* that begins at the start of exercise and eventually leads to an inability to continue the exercise.

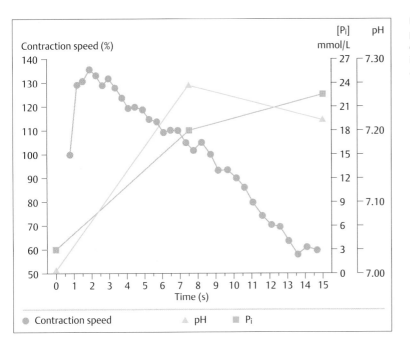

Fig. 2.14 Intracellular measurement of phosphate concentration and pH in the calf muscle during maximal exercise lasting 15 seconds (NMR phosphate spectroscopy). See text for details.

Regardless of these differences, a distinction is still made between central and peripheral fatigue:

- *Central fatigue:* includes processes extending from the CNS to the motor neuron level.
- *Peripheral fatigue:* applies to muscular processes.

This chapter deals primarily with muscular processes.

The mechanisms that lead to fatigue depend on the type, intensity, and duration of the exercise. They may also differ from one type of fiber to the next. The principal causes of fatigue are as follows:

- Intracellular acidosis
- Inhibition of energy production (substrate deficiency)
- Inhibition of the cross-bridge cycle by phosphates
- Reduction of excitability
- Effects of free radicals
- Temperature

Acidosis

It is widely agreed that the acidosis that develops during intensive exercise (though its cause remains controversial; Böning et al. 2008) adversely affects metabolism and the mechanism of muscular contraction. Massive intracellular acidosis occurs only during exercises that induce exhaustion within a period of approximately 40 seconds to 4 minutes. Thus, it is only in this type of exercise that the fall in pH becomes a significant factor.

The metabolic effects are explained largely by phosphofructokinase inhibition. In vitro studies have indeed shown that the activity of this enzyme declines with a fall in pH, but this decline is not observed in vivo. Kraft et al.

(2000) were able to identify the cause: as the pH falls, phosphofructokinase binds to actin and thus maintains its ability to function (see above). Many in vitro experiments do show a decrease in contractile force with increasing acidosis, but most of these experiments were done at temperatures below 30°C. When the temperature is raised to a physiologic 35°C in the muscles of warm-blooded animals, pH-related manifestations of fatigue are no longer observed (Westerblad et al. 1997).

ATP Resynthesis

Acidosis does not occur during short bouts of maximal exercise (lasting less than 20 seconds), but intracellular alkalosis does occur (Zange et al. 2008). Even so, the contraction speed of the muscle undergoes a linear decline (**Fig. 2.14**). Low ATP synthesis leading to a fall in the ATP concentration is often cited as the cause. The ATP concentration does fall to approximately 50% of the initial values. However, in individuals with an AMP deaminase deficiency, the ATP concentration does not fall even during maximal exercise, although their performance is comparable to that of normal individuals (Norman et al. 2001). On the one hand, these studies show that a high ATP concentration does not prevent fatigue. They also show that a fall in the ATP concentration, even at very high ATP turnover rates, is not caused by a lack of resynthesis during exercise, but that its cause is related to the activity of AMP deaminase.

Phosphate Effects

The concentrations of P_i and free ADP rise sharply at maximal exercise levels (see above). It has been suggested that these two metabolites may cause fatigue by interfering with the cross-bridge cycle. The effect of P_i on contractile force is similar to that of pH in that, as the temperature rises, the fatigue-producing effects of P_i decline. When we extrapolate the data of Coupland et al. (2001) from 30°C to 37°C, we find that the phosphates in fast-twitch muscle fibers appear to have a negligible effect.

Another effect of P_i was demonstrated by Westerblad et al. (1997). When present in high cytosolic concentrations, P_i enters the sarcoplasmic reticulum and forms a complex with calcium ions, thereby reducing calcium release as well as contractile force. It is questionable whether this process plays a role during exercise lasting less than 1 minute, as some time is needed for P_i to enter the sarcoplasmic reticulum.

Excitability

A decrease in muscle excitability could be another potential cause of fatigue during maximal exercise. The concentration of extracellular potassium rises sharply at these exercise levels, due to the high frequency of the action potentials. The result is a depolarization and consequent reduction of the action potential amplitude, which may lead to a decrease in contractile force (Harrison and Flatman 1999). Decreased amplitude of the action potentials during intensive exercise is also seen in humans (**Fig. 2.15a**). But if exercise is preceded by active warm-up of the muscles (see p. 81), the compound action potential (M wave) does not fall below the resting values. Without an adequate warm-up, the decrease in excitability at high exercise levels may be a cause of fatigue. This is unlikely when exercise is preceded by active warm-up, however, due to the resulting increase in the action potential and propagation speed (see **Fig. 2.15**).

Glycogen Deficiency

During prolonged exercise in which acidosis and phosphate accumulation are not very high, glycogen deficiency becomes a potential cause of fatigue. The relationship between the duration of continuous exercise and intramuscular glycogen content has been described by Bergström et al. (1972) and other authors. The mechanism for this relationship is unknown, however. If there were a substrate deficiency for ATP resynthesis, we would expect the ATP concentration to fall during continuous exercise. But this is not the case. Again, a decrease in excitability is postulated as the cause of muscular fatigue. With each action potential, potassium leaves the cell and is partially eliminated in the blood. As the duration of exercise continues, therefore, the intracellular potassium concentration falls. It declines further as a result of concomitant water uptake

in the muscle. As a result, the membrane is depolarized and the amplitude of the action potential is diminished. This decrease in action potential amplitudes during prolonged exercise has been demonstrated in experimental animals and in humans. It was found that glucose supplementation or sodium lactate infusion could limit or prevent depression of the M wave. Loss of muscle force was simultaneously reduced (Karelis et al. 2004, Stewart et al. 2007). It is still uncertain whether a causal relationship exists between action potential and force. A similar effect is seen with bicarbonate administration (Sostaric et al. 2006).

Glycogen deficiency or processes associated with that deficiency have a limiting effect not only in prolonged exercise, but also in very intense continuous exercise and in interval exercises such as those occurring in many types of sport. Maximal power in incremental performance tests is also adversely affected.

Free Radicals

The action of free radicals is a mechanism that can induce fatigue in many types of exercise. These highly reactive species are formed during energy metabolism and nitric oxide metabolism and can act on a variety of structures. For example, free radicals can damage membrane lipids, affect contractile proteins, hamper calcium reuptake into the sarcoplasmic reticulum, and inhibit the sodium-potassium pump. Free radicals are formed at all levels of exercise, but they form in greatest abundance during very intensive exercise with a high aerobic component (Bailey et al. 2003). Endurance training increases the antioxidative capacity of muscle. An artificial increase induced by the massive infusion of *N*-acetylcysteine was found to improve individuals' endurance capacity during intensive exercise (McKenna et al. 2006). The oral administration of antioxidants was not found to produce a definite, acute performance-increasing effect, however.

Caution

Antioxidants should be used with caution, because free radicals are necessary in signal chains that allow for training adaptations. Free radicals not only express genes that increase antioxidative capacity, but also influence other signal chains.

Note

The etiology of muscle fatigue in vivo is not yet fully understood. There are definitely no "either/or" mechanisms that underlie fatigue. The involvement of specific factors in peripheral fatigue is determined by the intensity, duration, and nature of the exercise.

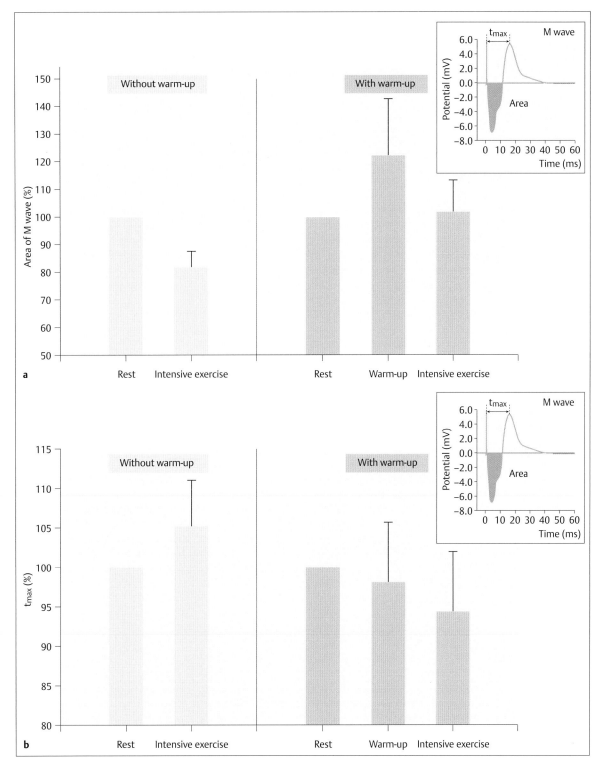

Fig. 2.15a, b Behavior of the compound action potential (M wave) during very intensive exercise, with and without warm-up of the muscle. The graphs show that, with adequate warm-up, the decline in excitability does not significantly affect fatigue during vigorous exercise.

a Area of the compound action potential. The area is almost 20% smaller immediately after exercise without warm-up. When exercise is preceded by warm-up, however, it differs very little from the resting value.

b The t_{max} of the compound action potential. The increase in t_{max} indicates a decline in propagation speed during intensive exercise without warm-up. When exercise is preceded by warm-up, the propagation speed increases even during maximal exercise.

Temperature

The body core temperature is also a significant limiting factor in "whole-body exercise." The upper limit is 39–40°C. Temperatures in that range do not appear to be a problem for muscle. Raising the temperature from 37°C to 43°C did not impair the performance of red muscles in mice. The effect of temperature is probably linked to central mechanisms. To a degree, the same may be said of the effects of partial body cooling, described above (see p. 82).

Central Fatigue

Our current understanding of central fatigue mechanisms can be summarized as follows. Central structures collect and process information from all organs. Information from working muscles (including respiratory muscles) is carried centrally to the brain by neural afferents and the bloodstream. When a certain (stress) level is reached during processing of the information, the performance level is lowered. This is evidenced by a reduction in the activity of motor neurons. The specific factors that trigger the information relayed to the brain are still unknown (Amann et al. 2009).

Recovery

An important task after exercise is to eliminate fatigue factors. Conditions must be established that make it possible to replenish muscle stores, stop breakdown processes, and initiate repairs. The stores that are replenished most quickly and easily after exercise are the ATP and creatine phosphate stores. This occurs in aerobic processes that cause oxygen uptake by the muscles to remain elevated for some time after the cessation of exercise. These processes create a portion of the oxygen debt (see **Fig. 2.12**). Creatine phosphate is resynthesized from aerobically produced ATP by the creatine kinase reaction. Because sufficient energy reserves are generally still present in the muscles at the end of exercise, the muscles need only an adequate oxygen supply. This requires that the blood flow to the muscles remain elevated for a considerable time after exercise. This is ensured "automatically" by a persistent post-exercise rise in the interstitial concentration of lactate and protons and other metabolites of energy metabolism. On the other hand, the sweat-induced increase in viscosity due to water loss tends to compromise muscular blood flow. This underscores the importance of fluid intake after exercise.

Although sodium is not considered a true deficiency element, sodium chloride replacement after exercise may be beneficial. On the one hand, it supports the rehydration of the body and stabilizes the blood volume. Additionally, sodium intake can improve the absorption of glucose in the bowel. This can support the effect of glucose replacement, which is beneficial after prolonged intensive exercise. Because type 4 glucose transport proteins in the mus-

cle fiber membrane are more active after exercise, increased amounts of glucose are transported into the muscles. This effect is amplified by the increased insulin concentration. Glucose is used during the recovery phase less for energy production than to replenish glycogen stores. Insulin simultaneously stimulates amino acid uptake by the muscles and has an anabolic effect on protein metabolism. It is beneficial, therefore, to combine carbohydrate administration with protein replacement.

Besides glucose and amino acid uptake, potassium uptake into the muscle is also increased after exercise, especially when the insulin concentration is increased, since insulin stimulates sodium-potassium ATPase. Thus, intracellular potassium stores are replenished concurrently with glycogen stores. The necessary transport and synthesis functions of the muscle consume energy, which is produced aerobically. As a result, oxygen uptake remains high and the oxygen debt is greater than the oxygen deficit, especially after prolonged and intensive exercise.

Practical Tip

"Normal" nutrition is best for supporting the regeneration phase, as it provides the broadest range of nutrients and is most effective in preventing deficiency states. Support by supplementation is recommended following prolonged, intensive exercise and/or if the following regeneration period is short. This is because supplementation provides a greater nutrient density and often leads to faster absorption of the supplements.

Exercising during the recovery phase (i.e., active recovery) consumes resources. It consequently slows the muscular regeneration processes described above and delays the return of optimum muscular performance capacity. During this phase after exercise, a trade-off must be made between muscular requirements and other factors such as circulatory regulation and psychological preferences. Passive measures such as massage can be effective in supporting recovery.

Training Adaptations

Training effects require a certain adaptability (plasticity) of the musculature. Studies on the effects of switching motor neurons between red and white muscle have established the fact that any muscle fiber can develop into either type. Experiments with electrical stimulation (Pette 1999) have shown that nearly all the structures in muscle fibers are changeable. Continuous stimulation can induce the development of a red fiber phenotype with:
- Increased capillarization
- Increased mitochondrial mass, with an increased capacity for oxidative metabolism
- A reduction in glycolytic enzymes
- A decrease in fiber cross-section

- An increased concentration of sodium-potassium ATPase in the sarcolemma
- An increase in slow calcium ATPase in the sarcoplasmic reticulum
- An increase in type I myosin heavy chains

When the constant stimulus is withdrawn, the muscle fibers tend to revert to their previous phenotype, developing back in the direction of type II fibers. It is not surprising, then, that the paralyzed muscles of paraplegics have an extremely high percentage of fast-twitch fibers, with a negligible proportion of type I fibers.

Training, too, can alter the spectrum of muscle fiber types by increasing the proportion of fast-twitch fibers. However, it is more difficult to effect this change in humans than to increase the proportion of slow-twitch fibers. Dawson et al. (1998) found that short sprint training could increase the proportion of type II fibers at the expense of type I fibers. Similar effects were achieved with certain forms of strength training (review in Friedmann 2007). The intracellular signals leading to these changes have been the subject of long and extensive research.

Signal Chains

The direction in which muscle fibers develop with training depends on four factors:
- Metabolic status (energy status of the muscle)
- Innervation patterns
- Mechanical loads
- Nutrition (substrate supply)

The signal chains that initiate the effects in the cell act via:
- AMP-activated protein kinase
- Hypoxia-inducible factor-1α (HIF-1α; a transcription factor)
- Calcineurin/nuclear factor of activated T cells (NFAT), calmodulin
- Mammalian target of rapamycin (mTOR)
- Macrophage growth factor (MGF)/insulin-like growth factor (IGF)
- Hormones

AMP-activated protein kinase and HIF act on mitochondrial development. AMP-activated protein kinase functions as the energy sensor of the cell, responsible for shifting the enzyme pattern in the direction of red fibers. On the other hand, there are findings indicating that AMP-activated protein kinase is unnecessary for this transformation. HIF is the oxygen sensor and tends to shift the enzyme pattern toward glycolytic metabolism.

Calcineurin/NFAT serves as a sensor for muscular activity. It is represented by changes in the calcium ion concentration in the muscle fiber. With a prolonged rise in the calcium concentration, the heavy chain pattern in myosin is shifted toward the type I fiber and mitochondrial enzymes are expressed.

mTOR is activated by mechanical stresses and provides for increased protein synthesis, leading to hypertrophy.

Protein synthesis is supported by the growth factors MGF and IGF and by hormones. They are responsive to mechanical stresses (by MGF) as well as nutritional status.

The signal chains are interconnected with each other and with other still unnamed chains. As research in this area is still in its early stages and is proceeding very rapidly, the picture should change considerably in the future. Currently we are still far from a point where we could confidently derive training guidelines from a knowledge of signal chains. Today, we are mainly studying different forms of training in an effort to derive clues as to the signal chains that are involved in various effects. In the long term, this type of research is certain to improve the effectiveness of training in competitive sports and in rehabilitation.

References

Basic Physiology
Alberts B. Johnson A, Lewis J, et al. Molecular biology of the cell. 4th ed. New York: Garland Science; 2002
Kandel E, Schwartz J, Jessel T. Neurowissenschaften. Heidelberg: Spektrum; 1995
Vibert P, Craig R, Lehman W. Steric-model for activation of muscle thin filaments. J Mol Biol 1997; 266(1): 8–14

Aspects of Exercise Physiology
Amann M, Proctor LT, Sebranek JJ, Pegelow DF, Dempsey JA. Opioid-mediated muscle afferents inhibit central motor drive and limit peripheral muscle fatigue development in humans. J Physiol 2009; 587(Pt 1): 271–283
Bailey DM, Davies B, Young IS, et al. EPR spectroscopic detection of free radical outflow from an isolated muscle bed in exercising humans. J Appl Physiol 2003; 94(5): 1714–1718
Bergström J, Hultman E, Roch-Norlund AE. Muscle glycogen synthetase in normal subjects. Basal values, effect of glycogen depletion by exercise and of a carbohydrate-rich diet following exercise. Scand J Clin Lab Invest 1972; 29(2): 231–236
Bessman SP, Carpenter CL. The creatine-creatine phosphate energy shuttle. Annu Rev Biochem 1985; 54: 831–862
Böning D, Maassen N, Lindinger MI, et al. Point: Lactic acid is the only physicochemical contributor to the acidosis of exercise. J Appl Physiol 2008; 105: 358–359
Coupland ME, Puchert E, Ranatunga KW. Temperature dependence of active tension in mammalian (rabbit psoas) muscle fibres: effect of inorganic phosphate. J Physiol 2001; 536(Pt 3): 879–891
Dawson B, Fitzsimons M, Green S, Goodman C, Carey M, Cole K. Changes in performance, muscle metabolites, enzymes and fibre types after short sprint training. Eur J Appl Physiol Occup Physiol 1998; 78(2): 163–169
Febbraio MA, Steensberg A, Keller C, et al. Glucose ingestion attenuates interleukin-6 release from contracting skeletal muscle in humans. J Physiol 2003; 549(Pt 2): 607–612
Friedmann B. Neuere Entwicklungen im Krafttraining. Muskuläre Anpassungsreaktionen bei verschiedenen Krafttrainingsmethoden. Dtsch Z Sportmed 2007; 58(1): 12–18

Grassi B, Pogliaghi S, Rampichini S, et al. Muscle oxygenation and pulmonary gas exchange kinetics during cycling exercise on-transitions in humans. J Appl Physiol 2003; 95(1): 149–158

Harrison AP, Flatman JA. Measurement of force and both surface and deep M wave properties in isolated rat soleus muscles. Am J Physiol 1999; 277(6 Pt 2):R1646–R1653

Karelis AD, Marcil M, Péronnet F, Gardiner PF. Effect of lactate infusion on M-wave characteristics and force in the rat plantaris muscle during repeated stimulation in situ. J Appl Physiol 2004; 96(6): 2133–2138

Kraft T, Hornemann T, Stolz M, Nier V, Wallimann T. Coupling of creatine kinase to glycolytic enzymes at the sarcomeric I-band of skeletal muscle: a biochemical study in situ. J Muscle Res Cell Motil 2000; 21(7): 691–703

McKenna MJ, Medved I, Goodman CA, et al. N-acetylcysteine attenuates the decline in muscle Na+,K+-pump activity and delays fatigue during prolonged exercise in humans. J Physiol 2006; 576(Pt 1): 279–288

Norman B, Sabina RL, Jansson E. Regulation of skeletal muscle ATP catabolism by AMPD1 genotype during sprint exercise in asymptomatic subjects. J Appl Physiol 2001; 91(1): 258–264

Parolin ML, Chesley A, Matsos MP, Spriet LL, Jones NL, Heigenhauser GJ. Regulation of skeletal muscle glycogen phosphorylase and PDH during maximal intermittent exercise. Am J Physiol 1999; 277(5 Pt 1):E890–E900

Pette D. Das adaptive Potential des Skelettmuskels. Dtsch Z Sportmed 1999; 50(9): 262–271

Sostaric SM, Skinner SL, Brown MJ, et al. Alkalosis increases muscle K+ release, but lowers plasma [K+] and delays fatigue during dynamic forearm exercise. J Physiol 2006; 570(Pt 1): 185–205

Spriet LL, Watt MJ. Regulatory mechanisms in the interaction between carbohydrate and lipid oxidation during exercise. Acta Physiol Scand 2003; 178(4): 443–452

Stewart RD, Duhamel TA, Foley KP, Ouyang J, Smith IC, Green HJ. Protection of muscle membrane excitability during prolonged cycle exercise with glucose supplementation. J Appl Physiol 2007; 103(1): 331–339

Thacker SB, Gilchrist J, Stroup DF, Kimsey CD Jr. The impact of stretching on sports injury risk: a systematic review of the literature. Med Sci Sports Exerc 2004; 36(3): 371–378

Watt MJ, Howlett KF, Febbraio MA, Spriet LL, Hargreaves M. Adrenaline increases skeletal muscle glycogenolysis, pyruvate dehydrogenase activation and carbohydrate oxidation during moderate exercise in humans. J Physiol 2001; 534(Pt 1): 269–278

Westerblad H, Bruton JD, Lännergren J. The effect of intracellular pH on contractile function of intact, single fibres of mouse muscle declines with increasing temperature. J Physiol 1997; 500(Pt 1): 193–204

Whipp BJ, Rossiter HB, Ward SA, et al. Simultaneous determination of muscle 31P and O2 uptake kinetics during whole body NMR spectroscopy. J Appl Physiol 1999; 86(2): 742–747

Zange J, Beisteiner M, Müller K, Shushakov V, Maassen N. Energy metabolism in intensively exercising calf muscle under a simulated orthostasis. Pflugers Arch 2008; 455(6): 1153–1163

Further Reading

Bierbaumer N, Schmidt RF. Biologische Psychologie. 6th ed. Heidelberg: Springer; 2006

Buchthal F. An introduction to electromyography. Copenhagen: Gyldendel; 1957

Carlson FD, Wilkie DF. Muscle Physiology. Eaglewood Cliffs: Prentice-Hall; 1974

Jankowska E, Lundberg A. Interneurones in the spinal cord. Trends Neurosci 1981; 4: 230–233

Klinke R, Pape H-C, Kurtz A, et al. Physiologie. Stuttgart: Thieme; 2009

Squire J. The structural basis of muscular contraction. New York: Plenum Press; 1981

Wilkie DR. Muscle. London: Arnold; 1968

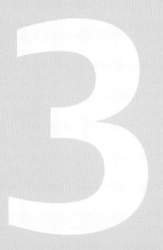

3

Molecular and Cell Biology of Muscle Regeneration

M. Flueck

Muscle Injury and Regeneration   90

Importance of Various Nutrient
Additives for Muscle Activity   92
Amino Acids   92
Metabolic Disturbance   95
Antioxidants   96
Minerals   98
Trace Elements   99
Vitamin D   101

Conclusions   103

Muscle Injury and Regeneration

Skeletal muscles are exposed to a range of motion-dependent phenomena. Impacting forces have a major influence on the energy demand from the stressed muscle tissue. This is particularly important for the buildup of muscle for sports performance. The load-dependent processes in muscles are closely associated with the conditioning of skeletal muscle during training and competition.

The known consequences of muscle loading reflect a continuum of cellular disturbances, ranging from transient metabolic fatigue and microtrauma in muscle cells (the muscle fiber) up to macroscopic tear of muscle fibers and muscle fiber bundles (fascicles) (**Table 3.1**). These disturbances trigger catabolic and anabolic reactions that promote tissue healing by renewing damaged cellular components. The regeneration process can be specifically accelerated through supplementation with selected nutrients and local therapy. This chapter explores the molecular and physiological mechanisms underlying this type of adjuvant treatment.

The biological material of skeletal muscle undergoes continuous renewal. On the basis of labeling experiments in rodents, it appears that up to 1% of muscle's nuclear material is turned over in 1 week (Schmalbruch and Lewis 2000). The organic elements required for renewing muscle cell material are provided through the recycling of degraded cell material and the consumption of food

(**Fig. 3.1**). In this process, the composition and quantity of nutrient intake determine the speed and quality of the muscle tissue being formed.

Note

The basal metabolic rate in skeletal muscle increases markedly with regular physical activity. Because of this relation, active athletes are more dependent on an adequate intake of general and essential nutrients. This becomes strikingly apparent during the treatment of muscle injuries that involve occlusion of the affected muscle (which cuts it off from much-needed nutrients).

It is important to bear in mind that stimuli to muscle that increase the turnover of muscle material are often related to damage to the muscle cells (**Table 3.1**). It has now been confirmed that transient rupture of the cell border of muscle fibers (the sarcolemma) occurs with everyday mechanical loading of muscle fibers (McNeil and Khakee 1992, Mackey et al. 2008). This leads to significant local disturbance of the compartmentalization of the affected fibers (Allen et al. 2005, Appell et al. 1992). Depending on the degree of muscle trauma with muscle overload (see Chapter 6), the associated structural disintegration may affect the entire muscle. The resulting mixing of electrolytes leads to the elimination of intracellular gradients. Many biochemical reactions are inhibited and muscle power decreases as a consequence (Milne 1988). The biochemical alterations in injured muscle are followed by a disturbance of local metabolism; a hypermetabolism, with increased proteolysis and possibly inflammation, develops (**Fig. 3.2**; Belcastro et al. 1998, Sorichter et al. 1998, Smith et al. 2008). The ensuing damage may reduce the excitability of whole muscle groups through afferent mechanisms (**Fig. 3.3**; Komi 2000).

Minerals and organic compounds with a high redox potential and proteinogenic materials are essential for muscle recovery (Meyer et al. 1994). This applies in particular to trace elements, antioxidants, and vitamins (**Fig. 3.4**). Their essential role as cofactors critically influences the rate of protein and energy metabolism. This characteristic provides targets for therapeutic (and partly prophylactic) muscle regeneration through oral or local administration.

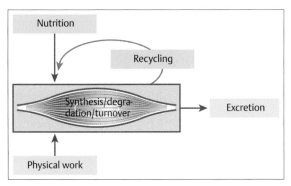

Fig. 3.1 Homeostasis in skeletal muscle. The development and breakdown of skeletal muscle are influenced by the physical work carried out relative to the nutrient supply.

Table 3.1 Continuum of muscle injury. Cellular causes of muscular injury and its grading

Term	Cause
Fatigue-induced muscle disorder	Microtear in a muscle fiber
Minor partial muscle tear (intrafascicular/bundle tear)	Tear in a primary to secondary bundle
Moderate partial muscle tear (interfascicular/bundle tear)	Tear in several secondary bundles
Muscle tear	Tear in the entire muscle

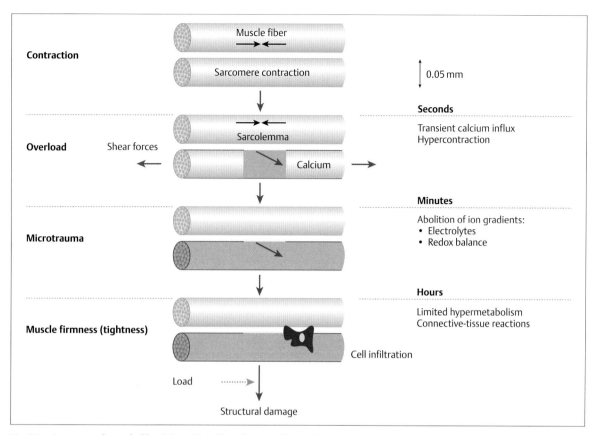

Fig. 3.2 Sequence of muscle fiber injury. The affected muscle fiber is shown in gray.

Biological effects therefore often oscillate within a narrow range between deficiency and toxic overdose (**Fig. 3.5**). Optimal treatment can therefore only be provided if accurate individual reference values exist. Ideally, these would be derived from exhaustive laboratory testing of blood serum and long-term symptoms.

In the following section, general and specific issues involved in the prevention and treatment of muscle injury by nutrient intake are discussed. The cellular regeneration processes discussed here were selected on the basis of a literature search using public databases (www.pubmed.gov).

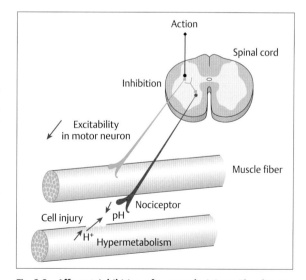

Fig. 3.3 Afferent inhibition after muscle injury. The diagram shows the peripheral mechanisms involved in muscle inhibition after injury. An increase in the extracellular concentration of hydrogen ions (and lactate) leads, via the activation of metabolism-sensitive nociceptors and neuronal connections, to desensitization of α-motor neurons. The excitability of the affected muscle group decreases.

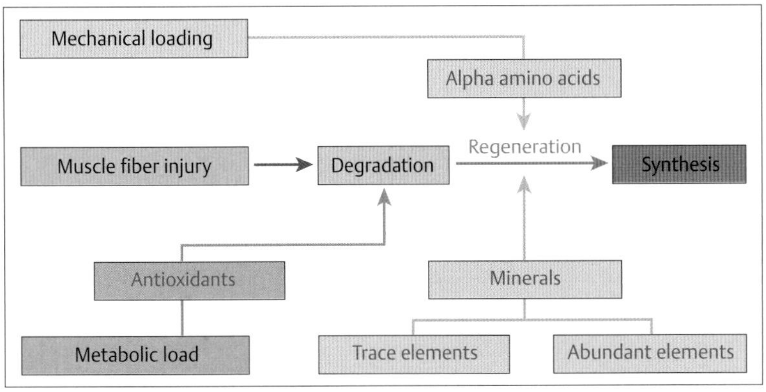

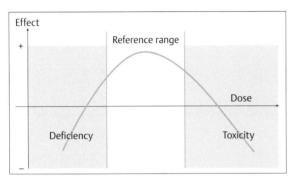

Fig. 3.4 Elements involved in muscle regeneration. The diagram shows the entry point of natural nutrients in muscle regeneration.

Fig. 3.5 Pharmacological spectrum. The dose–response relationship of a pharmacological intervention.

Importance of Various Nutrient Additives for Muscle Activity

Amino Acids

Amino acids are a class of organic compounds with a carboxyl group in the vicinity of an amino group. The subclass of α-amino acids provides the building blocks for protein buildup. Twenty proteinogenic α-amino acids are known (**Table 3.2**). They are incorporated into new polypeptides during gene-mediated protein synthesis (**Fig. 3.6**). Other amino acids that are found in humans appear through recoding of genetic material (e.g., selenocysteine) and posttranslational modification of proteins (e.g., proline to hydroxyproline, serine to *O*-phosphoserine). Apart from their anabolic role, proteinogenic and nonproteinogenic amino acids and their metabolites also regulate metabolic reactions in muscle. Their main role in this context appears to be related to the biosynthesis of the dipeptides and tripeptides creatine, carnitine, and carnosine, which are involved in energy supply. Also involved in this process are the amino acid derivates taurine, β-alanine, and glycine and tryptophan-derived neurotransmitters.

In the nonfasting state, amino acids are mainly derived from proteolytic breakdown of protein sources in ingested foods. They are further processed in the liver: amino acids derived from protein degradation are recycled, or excreted by deamination and decarboxylation in the uric acid cycle. This involves removal in the form of urea by the kidney (**Fig. 3.7**; see also **Fig. 3.6**).

Essential Amino Acids

In addition, new amino acids can be synthesized from existing amino acids. There are eight vital (essential) α-amino acids that cannot be produced by the human body:

- Valine
- Methionine
- Leucine
- Isoleucine
- Phenylalanine
- Tryptophan
- Threonine
- Lysine

Note

In a situation in which there are high metabolic rates, such as during development and following injury, it is necessary to increase the intake of other proteinogenic building materials as well.

This includes the semi-essential amino acids α-arginine, cysteine, histidine, tyrosine, and taurine. Reference values are given in **Table 3.2**.

Owing to the dynamic dependence between proteinogenic components, organisms normally prefer a balanced mix of α-amino acids in their diet. If an amino acid is only present in small amounts, the use of other amino acids for protein synthesis may be reduced as well. Amino acid ratios thus determine the biological value of food. All essential amino acids can be found in plants. An appropriate combination of vegetarian products can therefore in principle constitute a sufficient source for amino acids.

Table 3.2 Amino acids in skeletal muscle (source: FAO et al. 1985)

Class	Substance	Source	Recommended intake (mg/kg body weight/day)	Indication for increased dose
α-Amino acid	Isoleucine	Essential	10	Rhabdomyolysis
	Leucine		14	
	Lysine		12	
	Methionine		13	
	Phenylalanine		14	
	Threonine		7	
	Tryptophan		3	
	Valine		10	
	Arginine	Semi-essential	In protein	
	Cysteine			
	Histidine			
	Tyrosine			
	Alanine	Nonessential		
	Asparagine			
	Aspartic acid			
	Glutamine			
	Glutamic acid			
	Glycine			
	Proline			
	Serine			
β-Amino acid	β-alanine			
Sulfonic acid	Taurine	Derivative of cysteine	40–400	High-intensity exercise
Dipeptide	Carnitine	Biosynthesis from lysine and methionine		Endurance sports
	Carnosine	Biosynthesis from β-alanine and L-histidine		
Tripeptide	Creatine	Synthesis from arginine, glycine, and methionine		High-intensity exercise

Amino Acid Demand in Athletes

The relationship between amino acid uptake and muscle activity has been documented since the work of Justus von Liebig and Edward Smith 150 years ago. Contrary to the initial assumptions, amino acids are not essential, but optional, in providing energy for muscle work. Oxidation of amino acids normally only provides a fraction of energy production (10%). During intense physical exertion, however, amino acid combustion is probably not negligi-

ble in maintaining the high mechanical output of contracting skeletal muscle. Amino acid metabolism is important for covering the increasing energy demands during periods of intense exercise (Wagenmakers 1998). This partly explains the increased reliance of physically active people on increased protein intake. Today's recommendations are that athletes should consume 1.8–2.0 g protein/kg body weight per day. This is twice the amount for a person who is not physically active (**Table 3.2**; Lemon et al. 1984).

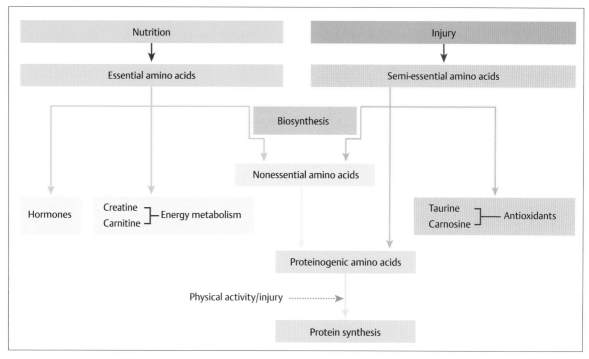

Fig. 3.6   Amino acid metabolism. The diagram shows the metabolic pathway for proteinogenic amino acids and their derivatives in skeletal muscle.

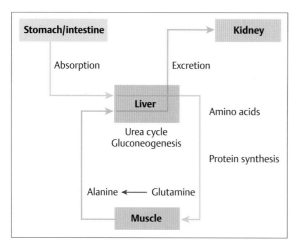

Fig. 3.7   Cycle of amino acid metabolism. The cycle of amino acid metabolism in muscle in the context of the organ system.

Glutamine

Conversion of a proportion of the most abundant amino acid, glutamine, to alanine results in a negative nitrogen balance. Release of alanine from muscle cells into the blood increases glycogen production in the liver through stimulation of the urea cycle (**Fig. 3.7**). Skeletal muscle can lose considerable amounts of amino acids with repetitive phases of high-intensity exercise, which drives con-

tinued stimulation of glycogen production in the liver. The replenishment of glutamine is mainly driven by the three essential branched-chain amino acids leucine, isoleucine, and valine. In this regard, it is noteworthy that leucine intake also increases growth hormone and insulin levels, which have a direct anabolic effect on protein synthesis in exercised muscles.

Creatine

The products of amino acid metabolism also influence the recovery of energetic processes in muscle. It has been shown that supplementation of the dipeptide creatine improves muscle performance in repeated sprints (Tarnopolsky and MacLennan 2000, Hespel et al. 2006). This is particularly indicated by studies on soccer training.

Creatine supplementation is not always indicated for elite athletes, due to the occasional formation of edema and possible increases in muscle tonus (editors' observations).

Taurine, Alanine, and Carnosine

The same case can be made for supplementation with taurine, which has been shown in animal experiments to result in an increase in muscle force production in fast contractile muscle fibers (Goodman et al. 2009). This effect is related to the antioxidative capacity of taurine, which maintains the gradients of the electrolytes potassium and magnesium over the sarcolemma of muscle fibers. This is essential to drive contraction and relaxation of excited muscle fibers. A similar positive effect on muscle strength has been described for the β-amino acid alanine and the dipeptide carnosine (Van Thienen et al. 2009).

Metabolic Disturbance

pH Values

The high demand on energy stores during hard physical work leads to increased concentration of hydrogen ions (H^+, protons). This reflects the accelerated splitting of protons during adenosine triphosphate (ATP) hydrolysis. At times of increased metabolic flux through the anaerobic degradation of glucose (glycolysis), the rate of ATP hydrolysis exceeds the capacity of internal buffers and proton pumps (**Fig. 3.8**; Robergs et al. 2004). The subsequent drop in pH below the range of 7.35–7.45 leads to metabolic acidosis. This can be detected by blood gas analysis. Lowering of intracellular pH acutely affects the biochemical reactions inside the cell by altering the redox environment of proton-dependent processes.

Creatine Kinase, Myoglobin, Uric Acid

Depending on its anatomic location, skeletal muscle is exposed to a variable degree of mechanical stress. This may increase the risk of injury to a considerable degree in fatigued muscle groups, as evident in the release of muscle material from injured muscle fibers into the blood serum. In high-performance athletes, this relationship is reflected in increased activity of the muscle form of creatine kinase (CK-MM) and myoglobin concentration in blood serum above reference values (Armstrong 1986).

In addition, an increase in the level of uric acid above 6 mg/dL (> 350 mmol/L), a result of nucleic acid degradation, and a rise in serum urea levels above 50 mg/dL (8 mmol/L), indicate the extent of muscle injury (Neumayr et al. 2003, Ascensão et al. 2008). In this context, it is important to bear in mind that estimates of muscle damage based on urea measurement alone may be ambiguous. The elevation in urea may also reflect an increase in protein metabolism to drive gluconeogenesis in the liver, increased protein intake, or dehydration. Serum levels of muscle cell proteins provide the best diagnostic tool for grading muscle cell damage that reduces muscle power (see **Figs. 3.1** and **3.2**).

Note

The laboratory values for injury markers in athletes after a training load usually exceed normal levels even in the absence of injury. In athletes, laboratory diagnosis, unlike functional characterization, is therefore not relevant for assessing muscle injury.

Hypercontraction of skeletal muscle can be observed when there is major muscle fiber injury, resulting from an influx of calcium from the calcium-rich extracellular

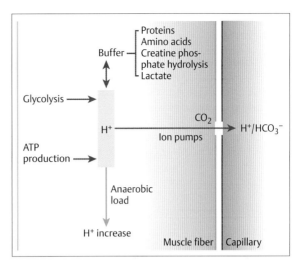

Fig. 3.8 Origin of metabolic acidosis. The energy provided by ATP hydrolysis during muscle contraction produces hydrogen ions, which are neutralized by buffering systems (mainly mediated by carbonic acid) and proton pumps at an equilibrium level of pH 7.35–7.45. Physical exercise to exhaustion leads to overloading of the myocellular buffers and export capacity. This leads to an increased proton concentration, and the pH falls. In untrained individuals, this occurs at 400 W on a bicycle ergometer, for example.

space surrounding muscle fibers. This leads to the induction of calcium-dependent proteases, which degrade the damaged tissue. Muscle components and mediators/cytokines are then released, which trigger an inflow of immune cells and inflammation (see **Fig. 3.2**; Allen et al. 2005). The time course of events is illustrated by a mild increase in the injury markers myoglobin, creatine kinase, and urea in the blood plasma 30 minutes after an intensive soccer game (editors' observations; Ascensão et al. 2008). This is accompanied by a reduced sprinting capacity and the infiltration of phagocytes and neutrophil activation in exercised muscle within the first few hours. Changes in the levels of acute-phase proteins after severe muscle activity have been measured in the context of ultra-endurance events. It was shown that there is a massive increase in C-reactive protein (+300%) after a 160-km multi-sport triathlon (Taylor et al. 1987). The increased level of this liver protein is closely related to an increase in body temperature (fever) following the release of cytokines.

Prevention and Therapy

An improved training status in muscle and the intake of amino acid metabolites can prevent load-induced muscle injury (Armstrong et al. 1991). Recent studies have shown that creatine supplementation produces a striking reduction in muscle damage and inflammation following a 30-km race (Santos et al. 2004). Research has also shown a slight performance increase and hypertrophy after creatine supplementation (Watsford 2003). This highlights the role of energetic processes in the development of stress injuries in muscle.

Practical Tip

Good physical preparation and short-term creatine supplementation reduce the extent of muscle injury after intense muscle activity.

In cases of extreme indirect muscle injury or traumatic external influences, the extent of muscle injury can escalate into a severe medical incident (Bolgiano 1994). The high level of muscle protein breakdown (rhabdomyolysis) observed in such cases can lead to serious metabolic problems. In rare cases, when the filtration capacity of the kidney for urea and amino acids is exceeded, this can result in kidney damage. With increasing severity of injury to the musculoskeletal system, the need for amino acids can rise dramatically. Amino acid supplements are therefore an important component of postoperative therapy (DeBiasse and Wilmore 1994). As amino acid uptake is strongly dependent on the perfusion and mechanical loading of muscle, a diet with amino acids is relatively inefficient in immobilized muscle (**Fig. 3.9**). These deficiencies in amino acid supply in bedridden patients can be overcome with passive stretching of muscle.

Practical Tip

Research findings support the effectiveness of physical measures such as ultrasound, massage, and movement therapy in the immobilized muscle after wound closure has taken place (Järvinen and Lehto 1993). Motor neuron inhibition of contraction in injured muscle has a protective function (see Fig. 3.3) and should not be challenged on the first day after an insult with physical measures that may cause stress to the affected muscle.

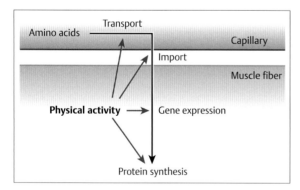

Fig. 3.9 Load dependence of the amino acid supply. The diagram illustrates amino acid transport in skeletal muscle. The uptake of nutrients into muscle fibers is substantially reduced in immobilized muscles. Physical exercise increases the blood supply and stimulates amino acid import through mechanical activation of the channels. This promotes muscle anabolism.

Antioxidants

Function

Antioxidants are a heterogeneous class of predominantly organic substances that inhibit oxidation. Their supplementation prevents the loss of negative charge from organic molecules and inorganic substances. Antioxidants thus protect cell proteins, lipids, and ribonucleic acids against irreversible modifications that might alter their reactivity (**Fig. 3.10**). However, antioxidants can also prevent the progression of biological chain reactions, through their action as radical scavengers.

Reactive oxygen species are the main source of radical formation in biological systems. They result primarily from cellular respiration in mitochondria or the action of reduced nicotinamide adenine dinucleotide phosphate (NADPH) oxidase in the phagocytes of inflamed tissue. Through their significant control over reactive processes, antioxidants can exert important effects on cell metabolism and on the functioning of the organism.

The most important antioxidants in muscle are:
- Sulfur-containing proteins:
  - Glutathione
  - Thioredoxin
- Enzymes:
  - Catalase
  - Superoxide dismutase
  - Peroxidase

Research has also indicated that the redox-active amino acid metabolites taurine and carnosine, as well as vitamin C (ascorbic acid) and vitamin E (α-tocopherol), play important roles (McDonough 1999).

Intake

Antioxidant levels are primarily maintained by a balanced diet. Fresh fruit and vegetables are the main sources of antioxidants. They also provide a good source of vitamins and minerals, which are required for the synthesis of enzymatic antioxidants. Appropriate guidelines have been developed (**Table 3.3**).

In addition to these natural antioxidants, antioxidative substances are now increasingly being supplied through artificial food additives.

Importance of Antioxidants in Athletic Activity

Despite their high biological potency, the use of oxidation inhibitors is often still ignored. Positive effects are often dismissed as a simple consequence of improved hygiene. Over the years, however, evidence has accumulated that demonstrates the important influence of antioxidants on

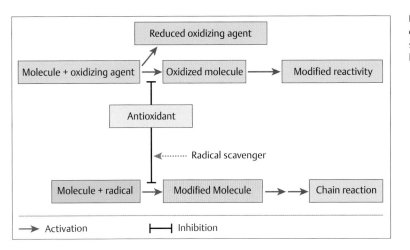

Fig. 3.10 Mechanisms of action of antioxidants. The diagram shows the main sites of action for oxidation inhibitors in biochemical processes.

Table 3.3   Important antioxidants of skeletal muscle (source: WHO Expert Committee 1973)

Substance	Source	Normal intake (mg/day)	Therapeutic indication	Therapeutic dose (mg/day)
Glutathione	Protein synthesis			
Thioredoxin				
Catalase				
Superoxide dismutase				
Peroxidase				
Taurine	Biosynthesis from cysteine			
L-carnosine	Biosynthesis from β-alanine and L-histidine	250–750	High-intensity exercise	
Vitamin C	Essential, no biosynthesis, must be contained in diet	60	Injury	> 500
Vitamin E		15	Intensive exercise/injury	100–200

the regulation and function of the muscle cell (Powers and Jackson 2008).

The role of antioxidants is especially pronounced with intense physical activity. This is explained by high metabolic flux rates, which increase the formation of oxygen radicals as a consequence of augmented cellular respiration. This may result in subclinical muscle damage (Shepard and Shek 1996). Nutrients that are rich in the antioxidants vitamin E and coenzyme Q_{10} appear to strongly reduce cell defects related to oxygen radicals, such as lipid oxidation. The importance of the role of antioxidants in muscle is underlined by the observation that deficiencies in vitamin E or vitamin C reduce endurance capacity (Witt et al. 1992). This is due on the one hand to the role of ascorbic acid in the synthesis of collagen and connective-tissue components; on the other, it reflects the protective effect of α-tocopherol against peroxidation of lip-

ids and cell membranes. This view is supported by the fact that prolonged vitamin C supplementation, but not acute vitamin C intake, results in positive effects on muscle damage after intensive sports (Thompson et al. 2003, Thompson et al. 2001). Positive effects on endurance performance have been attributed to the antioxidative amino acids taurine and carnosine, which are abundant in muscle (Van Thienen et al. 2009).

Paradoxically, increased intake of only a few antioxidant substances is known to produce robust effects on macroscopic parameters for athletic performance in well-nourished populations (Witt et al. 1992). The absence of overall physiological effects of common antioxidants is probably related to the suppression of biochemical signaling processes, which are driven by radical reactions but are inhibited with antioxidant supplementation (Jackson et al. 2004). It has now been shown that molecular adaptations of skeletal muscle to a hard training unit no longer occur with intake of vitamin C and E (Thompson et al. 2001, Jackson et al. 2004, Gomez-Cabrera et al. 2008). However, the amounts used were well beyond the daily recommendations for vitamin C (16-fold) and vitamin E (26-fold). Negative effects of therapeutic doses of vitamin C on muscular adaptations to training appear to occur after prolonged periods of treatment (Thompson et al. 2003). These observations indicate that antioxidants play a subtle role in the prevention and treatment of muscle injuries.

Caution

With prolonged therapeutic overdoses, the positive effects of vitamin supplementation can reverse into their opposite.

The functional implications of the changes in heat-shock proteins (Jackson et al. 2004) and mitochondrial proteins (Gomez-Cabrera et al. 2008) observed during these processes are not understood.

The complexity of the metabolism of vitamins and oxygen radicals explains why vitamin therapy is not necessarily always successful in healthy individuals (Steinhubl 2008). It should be noted that the effects show widely varying time courses due to the different reactivity and pharmacokinetics of antioxidants (Chen 1989). Vitamin E is also highly reactive and produces free radicals with their own toxic effects (Tafazoli et al. 2005). An increased mortality rate has been reported in individuals receiving long-term supplementation with high doses of antioxidative vitamins (Steinhubl 2008). The threshold that should not be exceeded for vitamin E is 400 IU/day (267 mg; Miller et al. 2005). The (toxic) effects of vitamin E are partly offset by other antioxidants such as vitamin C (Chen 1989). Because of its lipid solubility, it can also be stored to a certain extent and released during increased lipolysis with exercise. By contrast, there is almost no retention of vitamin C, which is water-soluble, and it is rapidly excreted through the kidneys.

Practical Tip

Moderate doses of antioxidants can assist muscle regeneration in periods of increased physical activity. After traumatic events with signs of inflammation, regular intake of vitamins C and E is indicated in order to maintain the immune status and support the reconstruction of connective tissue (Shepard and Shek 1996).

Minerals

Function in Muscle

Several minerals are particularly important for the body's electrolyte balance and for muscle excitation phenomena. These elements include the cations calcium, sodium, potassium, and magnesium, and the anions chloride and phosphorus. Differences in the concentration of electrolytes along the cell membranes of the motor neuron and sarcolemma have a decisive influence on the excitability of muscles. This is associated with a voltage potential across the sarcolemma caused by differences in the charge of sodium and potassium ions (Na^+ and K^+) between the inside and outside of muscle fibers. The opening of acetylcholine-dependent ion channels in the sarcolemma after stimulation of the motor neuron results in the partial elimination of ion gradients. Electromechanical coupling of this depolarization increases the myocellular concentration of calcium by emptying calcium stores. The resulting calcium-induced structural change in myosin motors triggers the contraction of muscle fibers within ~ 20 milliseconds after neuron excitation.

The speed and amplitude of the muscle tension produced in this way are graduated by the myosin type and the frequency of neuromuscular signal propagation along the motor neuron. Typical contractions result from high-frequency and repetitive stimulation of muscle fibers by the motor neuron. This leads to a summation of the force of a single muscle stimulation, which keeps the power at a constant high level like a tetanus. The reestablishment of ion gradients by energy-dependent ion pumps is essential for relaxing the contracted muscle fiber. This allows subsequent muscle contraction, which is the basis for dynamic movements. This process is usually complete within 20–40 milliseconds.

Disturbances of Muscle Homeostasis

Spasms

Note

In extreme cases, a major electrolyte imbalance can lead to serious malfunction of electrical processes in the heart and nervous system. Electrolyte disturbances resulting from genetic defects or long-term malnutrition can also lead to muscle-specific disorders such as convulsions and paralysis.

In the context of sports, spasms are a specific issue. These persistent muscle contractions reflect an increased neurogenic excitability caused by problems in the depolarization and repolarization of the muscle fiber (Jerusalem and Zierz 2003). It is important to distinguish whether this affection occurs at rest or during exercise:

- *At rest.* A disturbance in the resting state is seen after a period of intense stress. These spasms reflect unbalanced electrolyte deficiencies resulting from loss of sodium chloride and magnesium due to a long-term increases in perspiration (Buchman et al. 1998).
- *During exercise.* Convulsions can also arise in the context of increased muscle loading with extensive exercise. Known as tetanus, this is caused by slower reestablishment of the electrolyte balance due to increased extracellular potassium. It is thought that the slowing of the relaxation phase after the contraction of fatigued muscle increases the likelihood of tetanus after subliminal neural stimulation (Bentley 1996). With continued high-intensity exercise, the affected muscle enters a vicious circle from which only stopping and stretching the antagonists provides relief.

The latter symptoms, as well as clinical studies, indicate a close interaction between electrolyte deficiencies and strain-induced reflexes of proprioception (Schwellnus et al. 1997). This view is supported by the therapeutic effects of plyometric training, which includes high eccentric torques and an explosive contraction phase (Bentley 1996).

Therapy

Restoring the electrolyte balance and reestablishing normal neurotransmission are extremely important in a situation of muscle spasm.

> #### Caution
> It should be noted that acute symptoms of muscle spasm are not always corrected by an increased intake of sodium and potassium.

This is because adequate amounts of these minerals are already present in the basic diet. The restoration of normal electrolyte gradients across the plasma membrane of muscle and nerve fibers is therefore not accelerated by sodium and potassium supplementation. Instead, the importance of magnesium needs to be mentioned in connection with the release of muscle from tetanus. This effect is explained by the way in which the mineral reduces the extent of membrane depolarization. The block counteracts the aberrant triggering of muscle excitation caused by disturbed electrolyte levels. Magnesium also plays an active role in general muscle metabolism. It should be mentioned here that magnesium supplementation does not increase maximum performance (Lukaski 2000).

In the context of electrolyte supplementation, it should be noted that increased mineral intake may lead to stronger regulation of the water balance by the kidney. This is the body's way of protecting itself against changes in osmolarity that might seriously disrupt the blood volume.

> #### Note
> Magnesium supplementation should be limited to situations in which there is an imbalance in the electrolyte metabolism.

Trace Elements

Trace elements are minerals that occur at levels of less than 50 mg/kg in the human body. This is considerably lower than the highly abundant minerals sodium, potassium, chlorine, calcium, phosphorus, and magnesium. The list of trace elements includes:
- Metals:
  - Chromium
  - Cobalt
  - Iron
  - Copper
  - Manganese
  - Molybdenum
  - Selenium
  - Vanadium
  - Zinc
- Semimetals:
  - Silicon
- Halogens:
  - Fluorine
  - Iodine

Trace elements can appear in ionized forms, with markedly increased reactivity (**Table 3.4**).

Function

Trace elements act as inorganic cofactors in the reaction center of enzymes. Redox-dependent changes in the valence (charge) of enzyme-bound trace elements are crucial in catalyzing biochemical reactions. Examples include manganese superoxide dismutase (Mn-SOD) in the mitochondria, the iron-containing cytochromes myoglobin and hemoglobin, glutathione peroxidase, which contains selenium, and the zinc-binding matrix metalloproteinases in connective tissue. On the other hand, charge-dependent properties of essential trace elements are involved in the folding of enzymes. This includes the zinc-dependent three-dimensional structure of DNA-binding enzymes, for example.

The essential involvement of known trace elements in catalytic processes has a special role in maintaining the mechanical and metabolic performance of skeletal muscle. This is explained by the increasing requirement for buffering of oxidative stress with elevated respiration during hard muscular work and the activation of gene transcription during the subsequent recovery period. This is particularly evident in larger partial muscle tears with subsequent fibrosis and activation of metalloproteinases (Rullman et al. 2009). During this phase of hypermetabo-

Table 3.4 Trace elements in skeletal muscle (WHO Expert Committee 1973)

Substance	Effect	Intake/day		Therapeutic indication
Iron	Cytochrome, myoglobin, and hemoglobin	10–15	mg	Intensive exercise
Fluorine	Seed crystal for calcium storage	3–4	mg	
Copper	Redox enzymes	1.0–1.5	mg	Intense exercise/hypoxia
Manganese	Superoxide dismutase	2–5	mg	Intense exercise/hypoxia
Silicon	Connective tissue	30	mg	
Zinc	Transcription factors, matrix metalloproteinases	7–10	mg	Muscle injury/connective tissue inflammation
Chrome	Glucose tolerance factor	30–100	µg	
Cobalt	Vitamin B_{12}	0.2	µg	
Iodine	Thyroid hormone	150	µg	
Molybdenum	Unexplained	50–100	µg	
Selenium	Glutathione peroxidase	30–70	µg	Muscle injury
Vanadium	Unexplained	10	µg	

lism, an increased supply of the trace elements zinc, iron, selenium, and manganese is indicated in order to improve the stress responses in the affected muscle (König et al. 1998). It is also advisable in individuals with a regular intensive physical workload, since in this context the muscle is deprived of water-soluble trace elements and more abundant magnesium in muscle (Buchman et al. 1998).

Deficiencies

Recommendations for the daily dose of trace elements have been developed on the basis of epidemiological and cell-biological evidence (**Table 3.4**). A lack of essential trace elements can result in a significant reduction in exercise capacity via metabolic disturbances.

Iron

Chronic iron deficiency (anemia) becomes manifest through a marked reduction in physical performance due to reduced oxygen-transport capacity in the red blood cells.

Zinc

Zinc deficiency can suppress glandular function and lead to growth disorders and anemia, especially in young people. This is seen in decreased immune function, hair loss, dry skin, and brittle nails.

For active athletes, it is relevant in this context that zinc has a marked influence on muscle performance. It has been shown that dynamic isokinetic strength and isometric endurance are increased after supplementation with zinc (Lukaski 2000). Accordingly, deficiencies in zinc are associated with a decrease in muscle growth. These observations are related to the leakage of zinc from injured

muscle fiber with acute muscle damage. Serum zinc levels are thus acutely increased as a result of endurance activity, whereas they are reduced with chronic endurance training (Lukaski 2000).

Practical Tip

This suggests the need for long-term zinc substitution of endurance athletes. However, because of the negative effects of zinc on the copper balance and high-density lipoprotein levels, it is recommended that the intake of zinc should be limited to 15 mg/day intravenously (or 100 mg orally) (Lukaski 2000).

Silicium

Silicium is a nontoxic semimetal that occurs in concentrations of up to 200 mg/kg in the human body. It directly affects the synthesis and elasticity of collagen and plays an important part in the development of connective tissues. Silicium is crucial for the formation and maturation of bone (Carlisle 1970, Charnot and Pérès 1972). Research into skeletal growth disorders in rodents has suggested that a daily intake of 30 mg of silicium is required in order to maintain the structure of connective tissue in humans.

Intake

It is conceivable in this context that a subclinical reduction in regenerative capacity in individuals with an increased metabolic rate may be associated with a deficiency in vitamin-bound trace elements. An adequate supply of trace elements is usually achieved by increasing the nutrient intake.

It should be noted that balanced amounts from vegetable and meat sources should be consumed in order to compensate for seasonal deficiencies.

Depending on geographic location, however, overdosage of minerals may develop, sometimes involving serious levels of toxicity. This has been documented for the trace elements selenium and arsenic in particular. An individual's trace element status can be assessed using whole-blood analysis, but the muscle values that are actually relevant cannot be routinely measured.

Importance of Trace Elements in Athletic Activity

The demand for trace elements in skeletal muscle increases due to the enzyme consumption associated with increased energy expenditure during physical work. The essential involvement of trace elements in catalytic processes means that they have a special role in maintaining the mechanical and metabolic performance of muscle. This is explained by the need to buffer the oxidative stress caused by an increase in cellular respiration during hard muscular work and the increased protein turnover during recovery from exercise. This is characterized by up-regulation of gene transcription for several factors whose activity depends on binding of the trace element zinc during the recovery period after a workout—particularly transcription factors and metalloproteinases (Schmutz et al. 2006). This is particularly important in muscle cell injuries with subsequent fibrosis (Rullman et al. 2009). Increasing the levels of the trace elements zinc, iron, selenium, and manganese is indicated during this phase of hypermetabolism in order to improve the muscle's stress responses (König et al. 1998). In addition, major losses in trace elements can result from regular physical activity, as these water-soluble elements may leave the body through the skin as a result of sweating (Buchman et al. 1998). From this perspective, the appropriateness of the calculations generally used for the supply of trace elements in elite athletes must be regarded with caution.

Practical Tip

Special attention should be given to the recommended dosage of certain trace elements (particularly zinc and iron for preventive purposes) in individuals exercising at maximal work capacity for longer periods and when signs of muscle injury become apparent. It is best to collaborate with a nutritionist to develop an appropriate dietary protocol.

Vitamin D

Vitamin D is a fat-soluble chemical messenger in the calcium phosphate metabolism (Dusso et al. 2005). There are several subtypes of vitamin D. Vitamin D_3 (calciol, cholecalciferol) is the physiologically important vitamin D metabolite in humans. It regulates ossification and is essential for morphogenesis of the musculoskeletal system. Chronic vitamin D_3 deficiency becomes manifest in the form of impaired bone mineralization and disorganized bone growth. This may lead to pathological conditions such as rickets in children and osteomalacia in adults.

Metabolism and Regulation

Vitamin D_3 (calciol, cholecalciferol) is produced during the light-dependent synthesis of the cholesterol derivative of 7-dehydrocholesterol (a provitamin) in the skin (**Fig. 3.11**). It is also taken up from food. The biologically active form of vitamin D_3 (calcitriol) is generated via two steps: hydroxylation of vitamin D_3 at the C_{25} position in the liver to calcidiol (25-hydroxycholecalciferol) and a second hydroxylation in the kidneys by 25-hydroxyvitamin D-1α-hydroxylase to 1,25-dihydroxyvitamin D_3, abbreviated as $1,25(OH)_2D_3$. Many other tissues also have a 25-hydroxyvitamin D 1α-hydroxylase (1-OHase) capacity and can locally convert 25-hydroxyvitamin D_3 to the active form.

Vitamin D_3 variants are transported in the blood by vitamin D-binding proteins. When it enters target cells (such as osteoblasts), vitamin D_3 has effects similar to those of a steroid hormone, with activation of gene expression in the nucleus by the vitamin D receptor.

Serum calcitriol levels are strictly regulated. Low calcium and phosphate in serum increase the activity of 1α-hydroxylase via a parathyroid hormone–mediated feedback mechanism (**Fig. 3.11**). Conversely, high calcitriol and glucocorticoid levels inhibit 1α-hydroxylase activity and increase the inactivation of calcitriol via 24R-hydroxylase. In contrast, the amounts of vitamin D_3 and calcidiol remain in steady-state equilibrium because conversion is not subject to any significant regulation. A new balance in vitamin D_3 levels is often only reached after a period of months, due to the kinetics of partial retention of vitamin D_3 and its precursors in adipose tissue. Serum levels of calcidiol (25-hydroxycholecalciferol) thus reflect the vitamin D_3 supply during the previous 2–4 months. Vitamin D_3 levels, on the other hand, indicate the supply within the previous few hours or days.

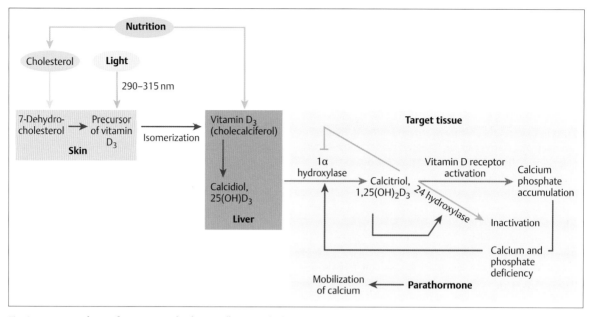

Fig. 3.11   Biosynthesis of vitamin D₃. The diagram illustrates the biosynthesis of vitamin D₃ in the skin, liver, and target tissues, as well as its effects on calcium phosphate homeostasis and regulatory feedback mechanisms.

Practical Tip

Measuring calcidiol (25-hydroxycholecalciferol) has the greatest practical relevance, as this vitamin metabolite reflects the vitamin D supply during the previous 2–4 months.

In this context, assessment of the individual's levels of calcium, phosphate, parathormone, and creatinine should be considered in order to exclude the possibility of primary hyperparathyroidism or kidney disease.

Intake

Vitamin D insufficiency is present at values below 30 ng/mL and vitamin D deficiency at values below 20 ng/mL in blood. The contribution made by light-bound and food-related vitamin D₃ synthesis varies widely due to seasonal and geographic conditions and eating habits. This is explained by the dependence of vitamin D₃ synthesis on ultraviolet B radiation, with wavelengths of 290–315 nm. At higher altitudes, lower altitudes, and with skin tanning, skin-bound biosynthesis declines, making dietary supplementation essential. On the basis of current studies, it is thought that a daily intake of 2000 IU of vitamin D is safe and covers everyday needs without additional light exposure.

It appears that the current recommendations are a conservative underestimate for vitamin D substitution. The most reasonable approach here is to measure serum levels of 25–hydroxycholecalciferol (calcidiol) and start long-term supplementation until levels > 30 ng/mL, or prefera-

bly around 50 ng/mL are reached. This can be achieved with supervised individual care if needed.

Instead of the daily vitamin D intake, higher doses of vitamin D can also be administered over longer periods, as the cholecalciferol administered is stored in the form of vitamin D before hydroxylation in the kidney to produce active 1,25(OH)₂D₃. Good compliance on the part of the patient is important here.

Calcium supplementation is not considered to be necessary in individuals with a normal diet including milk, cheese, yoghurt, and mineral water. If calcium supplementation is administered, it should be limited to avoid cardiovascular side effects.

Note

Vitamin D intake should be enhanced during the winter months, and in individuals with a confirmed deficiency, using oral supplementation and ultraviolet or sun exposure and appropriate dietary supplementation. However, data show that during October to March in the northern hemisphere, ultraviolet B radiation at latitudes north of 42° (the level of Rome) is not sufficient for vitamin D synthesis in the skin. There are also studies showing that even in summer, a large proportion of the population are not supplied with adequate amounts of vitamin D.

Vitamin D values are currently a matter of active debate. It is now clear that many diseases involving lifestyle factors, such as colon cancer, breast cancer, osteopenia and osteoporosis, and cardiovascular diseases are associated with low vitamin D$_3$ levels (Spina et al. 2006). These relationships are of particular importance, given that epidemiological studies show significant deficiencies of vitamin D in a large proportion of the population.

Note

There have been frequent warnings about the possible toxicity of vitamin D. However, very high doses of vitamin D have to be administered intentionally or very negligently in order to cause negative effects. The critical dosage for adult humans probably starts at a chronic daily consumption of around 40,000 IU (Vieth 1999). The therapeutic index for vitamin D is thus generally very large (Vieth 1999).

The mechanism causing vitamin D toxicity involves unbridled expression of 1,25(OH)$_2$D-like activity. Whether 1,25(OH)$_2$D$_3$ or 25(OH)D$_3$ is the main signaling molecule causing vitamin D toxicity is still a matter of debate (Vieth 1999).

Importance of Vitamin D in Athletic Activity

The effects of vitamin D$_3$ in the regulation of the musculoskeletal system are modulated depending on muscle loading. Thus, simultaneous vitamin D$_3$ and calcium supplementation reduces the risk of bone fracture by 25% (Holick 2006b). Vitamin levels below 30 ng/L (75 nmol/L) are associated with low muscle strength and power (Holick 2006a, Pfeifer et al. 2002). This suggests that vitamin D is involved in the conditioning of muscle strength via mechanical phenomena that involve moment arms. Vitamin D substitution is specifically indicated in high-performance athletes, who are often undersupplied with it (Bischoff-Ferrari et al. 2004).

Note

Vitamin D is currently a topic of widespread research interest, with investigations focusing on its numerous modes of action and its influence on coordination skills. It is being successfully used as part of measures to prevent falls in the elderly population.

Conclusions

The increased energy load during exercise alters metabolic demand in muscle. In addition to increased requirements for minerals and amino acids, athletes also need an increased intake of vitamins and antioxidative elements in order to promote the development and regeneration of the musculoskeletal system, and skeletal muscle in particular. Interdependencies between the implicated biological components and their different spectra of activity have only been studied in the context of intensive-care medicine (DeBiasse and Wilmore 1994). For healthy individuals, it is therefore advisable to seek advice from a dietitian, with recommendations based on laboratory tests and symptoms, before fundamental changes in diet and physical activity are introduced.

References

Allen DG, Whitehead NP, Yeung EW. Mechanisms of stretch-induced muscle damage in normal and dystrophic muscle: role of ionic changes. J Physiol 2005; 567(Pt 3): 723–735

Appell HJ, Soares JM, Duarte JA. Exercise, muscle damage and fatigue. Sports Med 1992; 13(2): 108–115

Armstrong RB. Muscle damage and endurance events. Sports Med 1986; 3(5): 370–381

Armstrong RB, Warren GL, Warren JA. Mechanisms of exercise-induced muscle fibre injury. Sports Med 1991; 12(3): 184–207

Ascensão A, Rebelo A, Oliveira E, Marques F, Pereira L, Magalhães J. Biochemical impact of a soccer match – analysis of oxidative stress and muscle damage markers throughout recovery. Clin Biochem 2008; 41(10–11): 841–851

Belcastro AN, Shewchuk LD, Raj DA. Exercise-induced muscle injury: a calpain hypothesis. Mol Cell Biochem 1998; 179(1–2): 135–145

Bentley S. Exercise-induced muscle cramp. Proposed mechanisms and management. Sports Med 1996; 21(6): 409–420

Bischoff-Ferrari HA, Dawson-Hughes B, Willett WC, et al. Effect of Vitamin D on falls: a meta-analysis. JAMA 2004; 291(16): 1999–2006

Bolgiano EB. Acute rhabdomyolysis due to body building exercise. Report of a case. J Sports Med Phys Fitness 1994; 34(1): 76–78

Buchman AL, Keen C, Commisso J, et al. The effect of a marathon run on plasma and urine mineral and metal concentrations. J Am Coll Nutr 1998; 17(2): 124–127

Carlisle EM. Silicon: a possible factor in bone calcification. Science 1970; 167(916): 279–280

Charnot Y, Pérès G. Comparative research on silica metabolism in soft and calcified tissues in mammals. [Article in French] J Physiol (Paris) 1972; 65(Suppl. 3): 3, 376A

Chen LH. Interaction of vitamin E and ascorbic acid (review). In Vivo 1989; 3(3): 199–209

DeBiasse MA, Wilmore DW. What is optimal nutritional support? New Horiz 1994; 2(2): 122–130

Dusso AS, Brown AJ, Slatopolsky E. Vitamin D. Am J Physiol Renal Physiol 2005; 289(1):F8–F28

FAO et al. Energy and protein requirements. Report of a joint FAO/WHO/UNU Expert Consultation. World Health Organ Tech Rep Ser 1985; 724: 1–206

Gomez-Cabrera MC, Domenech E, Romagnoli M, et al. Oral administration of vitamin C decreases muscle mitochondrial biogenesis and hampers training-induced adaptations in endurance performance. Am J Clin Nutr 2008; 87(1): 142–149

Goodman CA, Horvath D, Stathis C, et al. Taurine supplementation increases skeletal muscle force production and protects muscle function during and after high-frequency in vitro stimulation. J Appl Physiol 2009; 107(1): 144–154

Hespel P, Maughan RJ, Greenhaff PL. Dietary supplements for football. J Sports Sci 2006; 24(7): 749–761

Holick MF. High prevalence of vitamin D inadequacy and implications for health. Mayo Clin Proc 2006a;81(3): 353–373

Holick MF. The role of vitamin D for bone health and fracture prevention. Curr Osteoporos Rep 2006b;4(3): 96–102

Jackson MJ, Khassaf M, Vasilaki A, McArdle F, McArdle A. Vitamin E and the oxidative stress of exercise. Ann N Y Acad Sci 2004; 1031: 158–168

Järvinen MJ, Lehto MU. The effects of early mobilisation and immobilisation on the healing process following muscle injuries. Sports Med 1993; 15(2): 78–89

Jerusalem F, Zierz S. Muskelerkrankungen. Stuttgart: Thieme; 2003

Komi PV. Stretch-shortening cycle: a powerful model to study normal and fatigued muscle. J Biomech 2000; 33(10): 1197–1206

König D, Weinstock C, Keul J, Northoff H, Berg A. Zinc, iron, and magnesium status in athletes—influence on the regulation of exercise-induced stress and immune function. Exerc Immunol Rev 1998; 4: 2–21

Lemon PW, Yarasheski KE, Dolny DG. The importance of protein for athletes. Sports Med 1984; 1(6): 474–484

Lukaski HC. Magnesium, zinc, and chromium nutriture and physical activity. Am J Clin Nutr 2000; 72 (2, Suppl): 585S–593S

McDonough KH. The role of alcohol in the oxidant antioxidant balance in heart. Front Biosci 1999; 4: D601–D606

Mackey AL, Bojsen-Moller J, Qvortrup K, et al. Evidence of skeletal muscle damage following electrically stimulated isometric muscle contractions in humans. J Appl Physiol 2008; 105 (5): 1620–1627

McNeil PL, Khakee R. Disruptions of muscle fiber plasma membranes. Role in exercise-induced damage. Am J Pathol 1992; 140(5): 1097–1109

Meyer NA, Muller MJ, Herndon DN. Nutrient support of the healing wound. New Horiz 1994; 2(2): 202–214

Miller ER III, Pastor-Barriuso R, Dalal D, Riemersma RA, Appel LJ, Guallar E. Meta-analysis: high-dosage vitamin E supplementation may increase all-cause mortality. Ann Intern Med 2005; 142(1): 37–46

Milne CJ. Rhabdomyolysis, myoglobinuria and exercise. Sports Med 1988; 6(2): 93–106

Neumayr G, Pfister R, Hoertnagl H, et al. The effect of marathon cycling on renal function. Int J Sports Med 2003; 24(2): 131–137

Pfeifer M, Begerow B, Minne HW. Vitamin D and muscle function. Osteoporos Int 2002; 13(3): 187–194

Powers SK, Jackson MJ. Exercise-induced oxidative stress: cellular mechanisms and impact on muscle force production. Physiol Rev 2008; 88(4): 1243–1276

Robergs RA, Ghiasvand F, Parker D. Biochemistry of exercise-induced metabolic acidosis. Am J Physiol Regul Integr Comp Physiol 2004; 287(3):R502–R516

Rullman E, Norrbom J, Strömberg A, et al. Endurance exercise activates matrix metalloproteinases in human skeletal muscle. J Appl Physiol 2009; 106(3): 804–812

Santos RV, Bassit RA, Caperuto EC, Costa Rosa LF. The effect of creatine supplementation upon inflammatory and muscle soreness markers after a 30 km race. Life Sci 2004; 75(16): 1917–1924

Schmalbruch H, Lewis DM. Dynamics of nuclei of muscle fibers and connective tissue cells in normal and denervated rat muscles. Muscle Nerve 2000; 23(4): 617–626

Schmutz S, Däpp C, Wittwer M, Vogt M, Hoppeler H, Flück M. Endurance training modulates the muscular transcriptome response to acute exercise. Pflugers Arch 2006; 451(5): 678–687

Schwellnus MP, Derman EW, Noakes TD. Aetiology of skeletal muscle 'cramps' during exercise: a novel hypothesis. J Sports Sci 1997; 15(3): 277–285

Shepard RJ, Shek PN. Impact of physical activity and sport on the immune system. Rev Environ Health 1996; 11(3): 133–147

Smith C, Kruger MJ, Smith RM, Myburgh KH. The inflammatory response to skeletal muscle injury: illuminating complexities. Sports Med 2008; 38(11): 947–969

Sorichter S, Mair J, Koller A, Pelsers MM, Puschendorf B, Glatz JF. Early assessment of exercise induced skeletal muscle injury using plasma fatty acid binding protein. Br J Sports Med 1998; 32(2): 121–124

Spina CS, Tangpricha V, Uskokovic M, Adorinic L, Maehr H, Holick MF. Vitamin D and cancer. Anticancer Res 2006; 26(4A): 2515–2524

Steinhubl SR. Why have antioxidants failed in clinical trials? Am J Cardiol 2008; 101(10A): 14D–19D

Tafazoli S, Wright JS, O'Brien PJ. Prooxidant and antioxidant activity of vitamin E analogues and troglitazone. Chem Res Toxicol 2005; 18(10): 1567–1574

Tarnopolsky MA, MacLennan DP. Creatine monohydrate supplementation enhances high-intensity exercise performance in males and females. Int J Sport Nutr Exerc Metab 2000; 10(4): 452–463

Taylor C, Rogers G, Goodman C, et al. Hematologic, iron-related, and acute-phase protein responses to sustained strenuous exercise. J Appl Physiol 1987; 62(2): 464–469

Thompson D, Williams C, McGregor SJ, et al. Prolonged vitamin C supplementation and recovery from demanding exercise. Int J Sport Nutr Exerc Metab 2001; 11(4): 466–481

Thompson D, Williams C, Garcia-Roves P, McGregor SJ, McArdle F, Jackson MJ. Post-exercise vitamin C supplementation and recovery from demanding exercise. Eur J Appl Physiol 2003; 89(3–4): 393–400

Van Thienen R, Van Proeyen K, Vanden Eynde B, Puype J, Lefere T, Hespel P. Beta-alanine improves sprint performance in endurance cycling. Med Sci Sports Exerc 2009; 41(4): 898–903

Vieth R. Vitamin D supplementation, 25-hydroxyvitamin D concentrations, and safety. Am J Clin Nutr 1999; 69(5): 842–856

Wagenmakers AJ. Muscle amino acid metabolism at rest and during exercise: role in human physiology and metabolism. Exerc Sport Sci Rev 1998; 26: 287–314

Watsford ML, Murphy AJ, Spinks WL, Walshe AD. Creatine supplementation and its effect on musculotendinous stiffness and performance. J Strength Cond Res 2003; 17: 26–33

WHO expert committee on Trace elements in human nutrition. World Health Organ Tech Rep Ser 1973; 532: 1–65

Witt EH, Reznick AZ, Viguie CA, Starke-Reed P, Packer L. Exercise, oxidative damage and effects of antioxidant manipulation. J Nutr 1992; 122(3, Suppl) 766–773

Further Reading

Linus Pauling Institute, Oregon State University. (http://lpi.oregonstate.edu/infocenter/)

Medics Labor AG. Bern (http://www.medics-labor.ch)

4

Muscle Healing: Physiology and Adverse Factors

W. Bloch

Translated by Alexandra Kuhn-Thiel

**Functional and Structural
Alterations in Muscle Tissue** *106*
Functional Muscle Disorders *107*
Minor Partial Muscle Tears *107*
Moderate Partial Muscle Tear/
(Sub)Total Muscle Tear *108*

Mechanisms of Muscle Damage *108*
Initial Damage Phase *109*
Secondary Phase of Injury *110*

**Regenerative Mechanisms
and Their Sequence** *111*
Destruction Phase *111*
Repair Phase *112*

**Laboratory Markers
for Diagnosis and Healing** *119*

Factors Influencing Healing *120*
Nutrition *120*
Age *120*
Exercise *122*
Drug-Based Therapy *123*
Physical Measures *124*

Functional and Structural Alterations in Muscle Tissue

Muscle injuries are characterized by functional and structural changes in the muscle tissue. Whereas in clinical terms a certain number of muscle injuries only become manifest in the form of functional limitation and pain, in pathobiological terms a functional impairment is always associated with ultrastructural damage. The clinical and pathobiological approaches to injury diverge in some cases of severe muscle injury as well. This chapter attempts to do justice to both points of view, projecting the pathobiological view onto the clinical one. In this way the mechanisms of muscle regeneration as well as current therapeutic approaches can be more clearly understood and perhaps optimized, and approaches for new treatment options can be found based on a fuller awareness of the mechanisms involved.

Muscle injuries are usually classified clinically into three or four groups, depending on their severity (see also Chapter 6)—ranging from functional muscle disorders to a complete muscle tear (**Fig. 4.1**). In this classification

system, clinically manifest ultrastructural damage is not detectable before it reaches the level of a functional muscle disorder, but this does not apply to injuries starting at the level of a torn muscle fiber. From the pathobiological point of view, all muscle injuries involve structural changes, but in some instances these can only be observed using microstructural tissue analysis. In a broader definition, structural damage already starts before an actual injury can be spoken of, and it represents an aspect of the load-dependent adaptation that takes place in muscle tissue. In this chapter, the transition from "physiological" to "pathophysiological/pathobiological" structural alterations in muscles must therefore be regarded as a gradual one—making it clear that it is difficult to distinguish precisely between mild muscle injury and physiological processes of adaptation.

A distinction also has to be made between direct and indirect traumas causing damage to muscles (Best and Hunter 2000, Järvinen et al. 2005; see also Chapter 6):

- *Direct muscle trauma* mainly involves contusions and lacerations.
- *Indirect muscle trauma* can be caused by muscle activity during physical exercise, external traction, and ischemic reperfusion.

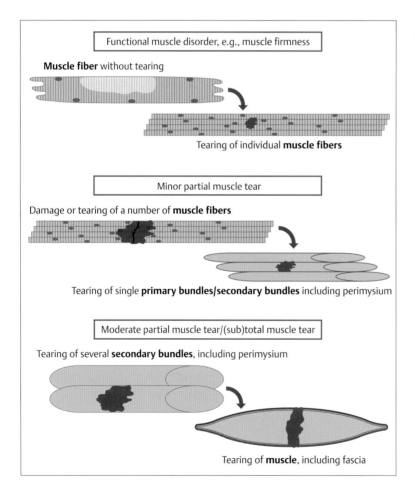

Fig. 4.1   Pathobiological classification of muscle injuries.

Functional muscle disorder, e.g., muscle firmness

Muscle fiber without tearing

Tearing of individual **muscle fibers**

Minor partial muscle tear

Damage or tearing of a number of **muscle fibers**

Tearing of single **primary bundles/secondary bundles** including perimysium

Moderate partial muscle tear/(sub)total muscle tear

Tearing of several **secondary bundles**, including perimysium

Tearing of **muscle**, including fascia

The type of trauma involved is an essential factor in relation to the effects of the injury and the course of recovery. The patterns of damage and the process of repair are considered here, in addition to factors influencing the repair process, mainly on the basis of indirect trauma due to muscle activity during physical exertion. An attempt is also made to identify possible differences in damage patterns depending on the type of trauma, as these may be important for repair and treatment.

In addition to acute muscle injuries, there are chronic injuries, which are not directly discussed in this chapter. These should not be overlooked, however, and the approaches based on mechanism of effect offered here may be relevant to them as well. Before we go on to consider acute muscle injuries and muscle repair in more detail, the clinical grades of injury need to be assigned to the corresponding patterns of pathobiological damage.

Functional Muscle Disorders

These are injuries characterized clinically by functional limitations and pain, which are closely associated with a more or less pronounced increase in muscle tone. Particularly in connection with cases of muscle firmness, they do not necessarily have to occur immediately after physical exertion and may appear after a delay of several hours to a full day.

In pathobiological terms, however, structural or ultrastructural changes are at the root of functional muscle disorders; these are referred to as microlesions and can only be depicted histologically. Microstructural alterations are already present in the sarcomere structure, especially in the region of the Z line; the extracellular matrix only shows biochemically recognizable restructuring processes, and increased amounts of proinflammatory cytokines and vasoactive substances are released. These give rise to an inflammation-like situation in the muscle, which may be associated with a mild degree of activation and migration of inflammatory cells (macrophages and neutrophils), causing changes in vessel permeability (Clarkson and Hubal 2002, Tidball 2005). Deterioration of muscle fibers may take place in some cases. When accompanying injuries to the vessels are present, bleeding occurs, which may also lead to microbleeding. During this phase, the damaged fibers and cells die due to necrosis. This in turn intensifies the local inflammatory reaction, although it is not induced solely by the necrotic cells and fibers. The increased muscle tone is in most cases a consequence of altered vessel permeability and interstitial fluid accumulation resulting from this condition, which leads to a tight elastic consistency within the connective-tissue sheath structures (perimysium and epimysium) of the damaged muscle. A state of hypercontractility can also contribute to firmness, due to altered calcium homeostasis in the muscle fibers.

Note

The transition between physiological muscle reactions and functional muscle disorders is considered to be gradual, as proinflammatory factors and vasoactive substances are also released in association with physiological load, depending on intensity, duration, and type.

Reversible structural alterations in the region of the myofilaments may also ensue, in this case in the Z line and in the costameres, which anchor the myofilaments to the sarcolemma (Hurme et al. 1991, Best and Hunter 2000, Järvinen et al. 2005). These changes represent triggers for restructuring processes in the muscle that give rise to functional and structural adaptations in it (**Table 4.1**).

Minor Partial Muscle Tears

Note

Tears in numerous muscle fibers are injuries that become manifest clinically as structural lesions.

As a rule, a minor partial muscle tear is characterized in pathobiological terms by further destruction of muscle fibers and results in defects in the muscle fiber, associated with a loss of the myosin–actin connection in the sarcomere in part of the myofilament. In these cases, the passive cytoskeleton may remain intact, or may already be ruptured. At this point, single fibers may be torn as well, and these die due to necrotic processes. This also results in damage to the cell membrane, which in turn induces secondary damage mechanisms, as described in the following section (Clarkson and Hubal 2002).

Clinically detectable (partial) muscle tears, according to the pathobiological definition, involve tearing of numerous muscle fibers, anatomically known as the primary fascicle (bundle), or tearing of several primary bundles or secondary fascicles (see also Chapters 1 and 6). In most instances, secondary fascicles (bundles) are already affected as well, and the tear may measure several millimeters.

In muscle injuries starting at the level of minor partial muscle tears, extensive structural and morphologically recognizable damage to additional cellular and extracellular components of the muscle tissue occurs. Consequently, an increasing number of capillary and connective-tissue sheaths (which surround and organize the primary and secondary bundles) become damaged, such as the endomysium and perimysium (see **Table 4.1**), (Best and Hunter 2000, Clarkson and Hubal 2002).

Table 4.1 Comparison of clinical and pathobiological approaches to muscle injuries, relative to the degree of injury

Causes of injury and location	Functional muscle disorder (types 1 and 2)	Minor partial muscle tear (type 3a)	Moderate and severe (partial) muscle tear (type 3b–4)
Clinical approach	• Minor injury • Functional • Macroscopically, no structural changes • Increase in muscle tone • Location: muscle fascicle (bundle) in its entire length, to the entire muscle	• Minor injury • Structural and mechanical • Longitudinal extension beyond the elasticity limit • Location: usually musculo-tendinous junction • Rupture of muscle fibers	• Major injury • Structural and mechanical • (Partial) loss of continuity in the muscle due to rupture of structures ranging from muscle fascicles (bundles) to the entire muscle • Damage to accompanying structures: fascia, vessels, nerves
Pathobiological approach	• Microlesions • Ultrastructural damage in fibers ranging to tearing of single fibers • Lesion in the vicinity of the myofilaments and the sarcoplasmic reticulum • Disturbances in calcium metabolism • Capillary damage • Displacement of interstitial fluid • Migration of inflammatory cells	• Further destruction of muscle fibers • Tearing of several muscle fibers ranging to rupture of primary or secondary bundles • Blood vessel damage, bleeding, edema • Damage to endomysium and perimysium • Inflammatory reaction	• Tearing that already affects larger muscle bundles up to several centimeters, or the entire muscle cross-section • Massive defects in practically all structures found in the muscle (blood vessels and connective-tissue sheaths, including the fascia and nerves) • Hematoma, edema • Inflammation

Moderate Partial Muscle Tear/ (Sub)Total Muscle Tear

In these injuries, loss of continuity in the muscle is clinically palpable and can be depicted using imaging techniques. Defects present in the muscle fascia can also be diagnosed at an early stage using these methods.

Pathobiologically, tearing already affects larger muscle bundles measuring several millimeters to centimeters, causing partial to almost complete destruction of the muscle fascia. Due to the massive defects involved, virtually all of the structures comprising the muscle are damaged; this includes blood vessels (not only capillaries, but also arteries and veins), axon endings and their synapses, all connective-tissue sheath structures, endomysium, perimysium, and epimysium, as well as the muscle fascia (see **Table 4.1**).

Mechanisms of Muscle Damage

Muscle damage can be caused by longitudinal distraction beyond the limits of the muscle's elasticity, with eccentric loading while the muscle is tensed, or directly by contusions or lacerations. Contusions do not usually give rise to longitudinal disruption of the structure, but cause displacement of the muscle fibers.

- *Muscle contusions.* These *direct* injuries arise when the muscle is exposed to sudden compressive forces, as in high-contact sports, which frequently involve hard blows directly to the muscle.
- Muscle injuries resulting from *longitudinal distraction.* Indirect injuries of this type tend to occur in connection with sports in which high tensile forces are generated and inflicted on the muscles; these forces in turn place an eccentric load on the muscle, resulting in tears in the vicinity of the myotendinous junctions in the muscle fibers.
- *Overexertion-related muscle injuries.* These can occur in the context of activities such as marathon running, for example, and primarily lead to microinjuries in the muscle, which quite often cannot be diagnosed on the basis of clinically manifest structural defects.

- *Ischemia with subsequent reperfusion.* This type of damage is less sport-specific.

While the damage mechanisms associated with direct trauma such as contusions or lacerations are obvious, injuries induced by longitudinal distraction also appear to be comprehensible on the basis of the mechanism of the effects, as the muscle is subjected to tractional forces that exceed the maximum load capacity—in most cases in the region of the myotendinous junctions. A tense or firm muscle is particularly vulnerable here, due to the pretensed state of the relevant structures (Best and Hunter 2000, Järvinen et al. 2005).

At this point, the question arises of why muscle is able to tolerate certain loads at certain times, whereas the same load can cause the very same muscle structures to tear at a different point in time. In addressing this question, it appears important to consider precisely where the initial muscle damage arises. The damage starts in the muscle fibers in the region of the myofilaments, where eccentric stress is inflicted at the level of the sarcomeres—stress that is caused either by external tensile forces or is induced by the muscle contraction itself.

Note

Eccentric stress on a precontracted or firm muscle (bundle) is particularly likely to result in injury to the muscle.

Initial Damage Phase

Cellular Damage Mechanisms

During the course of contraction, homogeneous and synchronized muscle contractions do not lead to this type of eccentric stress at the level of individual sarcomeres; it is only when unsynchronized, heterogeneous contractions take place that greater eccentric forces are inflicted on single sarcomeres, resulting in overextension of the individual sarcomeres. Directly connected with this is the loss of the overlapping structure of the actin and myosin filaments that necessarily occurs, in turn causing overextension of the neighboring sarcolemma. In cases of more extensive stretching and tearing of passive structures such as the titin filaments, direct tearing of the muscle fiber is the result. In such cases, the tears occur in the region of the Z line, where the sarcomere's passive support structures are anchored.

Damage to the sarcolemma that does not involve tears in the passive structures apparently does not lead to direct and complete destruction of myofilament continuity and thus of the muscle fiber as a whole, but does trigger various intrinsic autodegenerative and proteolytic mechanisms via an increased calcium flow from outside (Best and Hunter 2000, Howatson and van Someren 2008). It is this unregulated entry of calcium that activates calcium-dependent proteases, which in turn break down the cellular structure proteins—for example, myofibrillary and other cytoskeletal proteins. Rupture of desmin and sarcomere filaments then ensues. The proteases have the overall effect of inducing self-digestion of the muscle fiber or at least of parts of the muscle fiber, resulting in primary loss of the myofilament architecture and subsequent damage to the mitochondria and loss of muscle glycogen. This process in turn induces an inflammatory reaction involving the migration of neutrophils and macrophages.

This process of protease-induced muscle destruction can also be explained as being due to metabolic overload in the muscle fiber, during which the adenosine triphosphate (ATP) demand exceeds the supply, rendering the ATP-dependent calcium transport mechanism defective, with subsequent cytosolic calcium overload and activation of the above-mentioned proteases. Type II fibers appear to be more susceptible to such damage (Tee et al. 2007).

Extracellular Damage Mechanisms

In addition to the muscle fibers themselves, the surrounding extracellular matrix is also subject to change. It appears that a major portion of the extracellular matrix around the muscle fibers is lost and that the intercellular space between the muscle fibers increases. Typical plasma proteins such as fibrinogen and albumin are deposited in this widened intercellular space, an indication that the integrity of the capillaries has been disturbed, followed by loss of the endothelial barrier function in the muscle. These changes would also explain the appearance of tissue edema, since in addition to the extravasation of plasma proteins, water is displaced into the intercellular space. The ensuing space-occupying mass, causing an increase in pressure in the muscle when the connective-tissue sheaths (perimysium and epimysium) are still intact, becomes evident during clinical examinations as a tight or stiff muscle (Smith et al. 2008).

Dependence of Damage on Contraction and Fiber Types

The question arises of what types of muscle contraction are likely to lead to the macrolesions and microlesions in the muscle described above and which mechanisms are involved.

Note

There appears to be sufficient evidence to confirm that eccentric contractions cause more muscle damage than concentric and static contractions.

The forces generated during eccentric contractions are 1.5–1.9 times greater than those generated during isometric contractions (Byrne et al. 2004). When the mechanisms involved at the subcellular level in muscle fibers are considered, the fundamental question arises of whether or not virtually all skeletal muscle injuries that occur due to contractions result from eccentric contractions, as some authors have suggested (Howatson and van Someren 2008).

The mechanisms described are helpful for understanding the ways in which different levels of stress tolerance can exist in muscles, depending on the state of muscle loading. Changes in the calcium metabolism or the metabolic situation in the muscle fibers at the subcellular level can cause the sarcomeres to be in different states of contraction (Best and Hunter 2000). Subcellular differences in the calcium concentration can therefore result in inhomogeneous states of contraction in neighboring sarcomeres. It may be speculated that during prolonged periods of stress in particular, metabolic changes can occur in the muscle fibers that also lead to local ATP deficits and disturbed calcium homeostasis (Tee et al. 2007). As a consequence of these changes, it is possible for there to be heterogeneous states of contraction between and within the fibers that cause the overextension of the sarcomeres described above.

Further research is needed to determine the extent to which this is also the reason why type II fibers, which consume larger amounts of energy and thus more ATP, are more likely to suffer microlesions. Another explanation for the propensity of type II fibers to suffer injury may be their more inefficient Z line architecture; these fibers have narrower Z lines, which may be less stable. Another topic for further research is the extent to which the heterogeneous arrangement of myosin filament types that have differing contraction characteristics inside a single muscle fiber may play a role here. Our own research has demonstrated not only the well-known phenomenon of fiber chimerism, with the expression of slow and fast heavy myosin chains in a single fiber, but has also confirmed that key signal pathways responsible for regulating the contraction and metabolism of muscle fibers involve subcellular differences in the muscle fibers. This might have an impact on the function of muscle fibers and might lead to inhomogeneity in their metabolism, as well as in the regulation of contractions in the muscle fibers.

Impaired Neuromuscular Regulation

Neuromuscular regulation is centrally important both for regulating contraction and for muscle fiber metabolism, and exercise-related changes in neuromuscular regulation have also been described (Byrne et al. 2004). However, the mechanical significance of impaired neuromuscular regulation in muscle fibers, for example, has not yet been defined in relation to the occurrence of muscle injuries. It may be speculated that unsynchronized activation of muscle fibers results in a high tensile and extensive load on muscle fibers. This could also represent an important mechanism during the second phase of injury following the initial damage, as already-damaged muscle fibers

with reduced stability would then be particularly susceptible to further injury. The extent to which reported changes in proprioception in the damaged muscle may have a mechanical influence on neuromuscular regulation has also not yet been explained.

Secondary Phase of Injury

In general, the secondary phase of injury appears to be vitally important in determining the extent of the injury. Secondary injury arises in the muscle fiber as a result of disturbed calcium homeostasis, which becomes manifest in the form of an increase in the cytosolic calcium concentration. As outlined above, this leads to hypercontractility in individual sarcomeres and muscle fibers, which increase their pulling force on already damaged sarcomeres or muscle fibers and on the passive skeleton in the muscle fibers. The onset of the hypercontractions is delayed, following an initial phase of tension reduction in the muscle, and is terminated after more extensive destruction of the muscle fiber through a second phase of muscle relaxation. The influx of calcium also promotes "autodigestion" of the muscle fibers and their cellular and extracellular environments through the activation of proteolytic enzymes. In addition, the damaged muscle fibers release proinflammatory cytokines and vasoactive substances such as interleukin-8 (IL-8), tumor necrosis factor-α (TNF-α), and TNF-β. This in turn leads to intensified migration of neutrophils and macrophages, which in turn release additional proinflammatory cytokines and in particular oxygen radicals, which lead to further damage to cellular and extracellular structures in the damaged areas through what is known as an "oxidative burst."

Another mechanism responsible for increasing the inflammatory reaction in muscle, as well as vessel permeability, is activation of the complement system and thrombocytes, which migrate to the wounded area. In addition to this migration of inflammatory cells and the accompanying secondary effects, the development of edema in the tissue results in a decrease in the local nutritional supply to the tissue, thus intensifying cell damage. It is therefore logical for primary treatment measures following muscle injury to be aimed at reducing bleeding, the inflammatory reaction, and edema formation, as well as reducing the contracted state of the muscle, in order to keep secondary damage at an absolute minimum (Howatson and van Someren 2008).

Practical Tip

Muscle injuries occur in two phases: the primary phase is the actual injury, and the secondary phase involves damage caused by reactions to the primary injury. The second phase is the starting point for measures taken to reduce the extent of the injury.

Regenerative Mechanisms and Their Sequence

To understand the process of muscle regeneration after acute injury, it is necessary to examine the different phases that make up the regenerative process (**Fig. 4.2**). These generally follow a basic, constant pattern, regardless of whether the muscle has undergone damage due to direct or indirect trauma. However, the differing causes of the damage may lead to variations in the process.

- *Destruction phase.* The initial reaction is known as the destruction phase and is characterized by rupturing of tissue structures, which may range from individual intracellular filaments to total rupture of the entire muscle. Depending on the degree of damage, the corresponding connective-tissue structures, blood vessels, and nerves may also undergo destructive damage to varying degrees of severity. If the damage results in accompanying injury to the blood vessels, bleeding takes place, which may result in hematoma formation. During this phase, the damaged fibers and cells die as a result of necrosis, leading in turn to an amplified local inflammatory reaction, although this is not induced solely by the necrotic cells. Migration of inflammatory cells in connection with the local inflammation occurs during this phase. It is also during this phase that the secondary damage described above occurs, directly after the primary injury, and this has the effect of intensifying the injury.
- *Repair phase.* The second phase, which starts gradually over a few days, is known as the repair phase. It is characterized primarily by phagocytosis of destroyed cellular and extracellular material. During this phase, mac-

rophages also migrate into the tissue. Muscle fibers are repaired and new muscle fibers form. The extracellular matrix is increased due to incipient collagen synthesis, and fresh capillaries begin to sprout and grow. Processes are coordinated during this phase in order to close the defect as quickly as possible. The original tissue quality and structure are therefore not yet reached, and functionally inferior cellular and extracellular material is used to close the defect.

- *Remodeling phase.* The third phase is referred to as the remodeling phase and is characterized by focused restructuring of the tissue, involving retraction and reorganization of scar tissue and reestablishment of the muscle tissues' functional capacity (Järvinen et al. 2007).

Note

Muscle repair takes place in three phases:
- *Destruction phase,* **with removal of destroyed structures**
- *Repair phase,* **with formation of immature tissue to close the defect quickly**
- *Remodeling phase,* **with maturation of the tissue to restore the original stability and functionality**

The individual repair mechanisms are discussed in more detail below.

Destruction Phase

The actual repair mechanism starts with disintegration of damaged cellular and extracellular components by proteases that are activated and released into the tissues from the local cells and from their extracellular matrix bonds, as well as by enzymes released from the infiltrating neu-

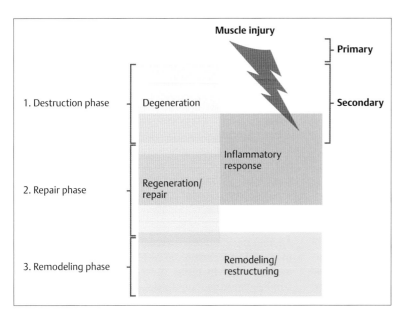

1. Destruction phase — Degeneration

Muscle injury
— Primary
— Secondary

Inflammatory response

2. Repair phase — Regeneration/ repair

3. Remodeling phase — Remodeling/ restructuring

Fig. 4.2 Fluid transitions in the processes responsible for muscle repair during the three phases of muscle reconstruction. Occurrence of primary and secondary damage during the phases of muscle repair.

trophils and macrophages. The neutrophils, and particularly the macrophages, then phagocytose the disintegrated tissue components.

An adequate blood supply is a prerequisite for this initial wound-cleaning process. Impairment of the local circulation, especially in connection with more complex injuries to muscle, leads to a delay in the healing process even at this early stage, as subsequent repair processes are impeded and their onset is delayed.

Migration of Macrophages

The migration of macrophages, which are needed for the breakdown of damaged tissue, forms part of the inflammatory reaction. As already discussed above, the influence this has on muscle injury is not purely positive, as the initial inflammatory reaction also plays a major role in the secondary tissue damage mentioned above. The course of events and the extent of the inflammatory reaction are therefore of critical importance and have to be seen in the context of treatment measures involving nonsteroidal anti-inflammatory drugs (see p. 123).

The initiation of inflammation and subsequent infiltration by circulating immune cells, important for this phase of healing, are induced by local factors such as cytokines or growth factors (**Table 4.2**), which are produced by the injured muscle fibers, endothelial cells, and fibrocytes. The local factors released during muscle injuries also include vasoactive substances, which on the one hand dilate the blood vessels and on the other increase vessel permeability. This enhances circulation and facilitates diapedesis of the immune cells (neutrophils, macrophages, monocytes, basophils, eosinophils, and natural killer cells) into the damaged tissues. The release of vasoactive substances, particularly nitrogen monoxide, as well as the vessel reaction itself, can be induced by the released cytokines and growth factors, on the one hand, and by local metabolic factors (hypoxia, lactate, adenosine, oxidative stress) on the other, as well as by the platelets activated in connection with bleeding incidents and the factors released by the platelets (for example, serotonin, histamine, and thromboxane A_2).

Another as yet little-investigated mechanism involved in muscle injury is the activation of proteases, which break down the extracellular matrix and in the process make it easier for nonspecific immune cells (macrophages and neutrophils) to enter. It is known that matrix metalloproteinases are released, probably even in a fiber-specific way, during the destruction phase. We have demonstrated that this type of release already takes place during intensive exercise-related stress. However, there has been practically no research on the significance of this for immune cell infiltration and the destruction phase in general. Information obtained from other tissue types, including cardiac muscle, suggests that it is extremely important, and this has also been suggested by our own studies on heart muscle following acute injury, which indicate initial pro-

cessing of the extracellular matrix following ischemia or reperfusion damage.

In addition to these mechanisms, the activation of the complement system associated with bleeding into tissue also plays a role in the chemoattraction of immune cells in the context of muscle injury.

Migration of Neutrophils

The migration of neutrophils in particular leads to further intensification of the inflammatory response. If it becomes excessive, there is a risk of the secondary damage described above developing. In principle, an inflammatory response involving the release of IL-6 and TNF-α is an important process that makes a "successful" destruction phase possible, as it leads to temporally differentiated migration of various types of immune cell from the nonspecific immune system into the tissues. These mainly consist of the different macrophage subtypes, which appear in a temporally staggered sequence. It can also be assumed that the macrophages are responsible not only for phagocytosis, but also initially influence the subsequent repair phase. Although immune cell infiltration is dependent to some extent on the extent of the muscle injury, it has been observed that following an initial predominance of neutrophils, the number of macrophages starts to increase after approximately 2 days, while the number of neutrophils declines (Best and Hunter 2000, Clarkson and Hubal 2002, Järvinen et al. 2005, Smith et al. 2008).

> ### Caution
>
> An adequate blood supply is necessary for the initial removal of destroyed tissue structures and for migration of immune cells, particularly macrophages. Bleeding and an excessive inflammatory response, however, both have a negative influence on this initial "cleaning-up process."

Repair Phase

The inflammatory situation in the muscle involving the release of various cytokines and growth factors, as well as protease-dependent breakdown of the extracellular matrix, creates a growth-promoting environment for fast muscle tissue regeneration. A distinction has to be made here between three different types of regeneration process:

- Muscle fiber regeneration
- Neovascularization
- Formation of extracellular matrix

Another repair process involves axon growth, with the formation of new motor end plates for reinnervation of the muscle fibers. In terms of its timing, however, this is strongly dependent on the degree of muscle injury and is also more likely to take place during the remodeling

Table 4.2 Cytokine release and releasing cells in various phases of muscle injury

	Destruction	Repair	Remodeling
Cell types	Injured muscle fiber	Injured muscle fiber	Injured muscle fiber
	Endothelial cells	Endothelial cells	Endothelial cells
	Fibroblasts	Fibroblasts	Neutrophils
	Neutrophils	Neutrophils	Natural killer cells
	Natural killer cells	Natural killer cells	Macrophages
		Macrophages	T lymphocytes
		Muscle precursor cells and new muscle fibers	B lymphocytes
			Muscle precursor cells and new muscle fibers
Cytokines	TNF-α	TNF-α	TNF-β
	IL-1β	IL-1β	IL-1β
	IL-1α	IL-1α	IL-2
	IL-6	IL-6	IL-6
	FGF-2	IL-8	IL-15
		VEGF	VEGF
		IFN-γ	PDGF
		G-CSF	IFN-γ
		M-CSF	MCP-1
		MIP-1α	IGF-1
		MCP-1	IGF-2
			HGF
			FGF-1
			FGF-2
			TGF-β
			LIF
			MIF
			HMGP
			CNTF

CNTF	ciliary neurotrophic factor	MCP	monocyte chemoattractant protein
FGF	fibroblast growth factor	M-CSF	macrophage colony-stimulating factor
G-CSF	granulocyte colony-stimulating factor	MIF	macrophage migration inhibitory factor
HGF	hepatocyte growth factor	MIP	macrophage inflammatory protein
HMGP	high mobility group protein	PDGF	platelet-derived growth factor
IFN	interferon	TGF	transforming growth factor
IGF	insulin-like growth factor	TNF	tumor necrosis factor
LIF	leukocyte inhibitory factor	VEGF	vascular endothelial growth factor

phase. The processes taking place during this phase, in addition to being quite complex, also interact with each other. The optimal balance between such processes during this phase is one of the decisive factors, if not *the* decisive factor, for complete structural and functional regeneration of the muscle tissue (Best and Hunter 2000, Järvinen et al. 2005).

Note

During the repair phase, muscle fibers are regenerated, blood vessels newly formed, and the extracellular matrix restructured. When there is more extensive muscle injury, reinnervation becomes necessary.

Muscle Fiber Regeneration

Satellite Cell Division

Muscle fiber regeneration originates primarily in the satellite cells (**Fig. 4.3**), located between the basal membrane and the sarcolemma (Chargé and Rudnicki 2004, Grefte et al. 2007, Gayraud-Morel et al. 2009, Le Grand et al. 2009).

Following the initial expansion of the satellite cell pool, satellite cells fuse together, in some cases with the portion of muscle fiber still remaining, while in others they fuse together to form myotubes (**Fig. 4.4**). The basal membranes, or their components, are essential for activating satellite cells here. Along with other factors formed during the destruction phase and the existing and newly-migrated cells, the basal membranes are responsible for creating an environment that stimulates division of satellite cells, the prerequisite for successful muscle repair (Chargé and Rudnicki 2004, Shi and Garry 2006). The extent of damage to the basal membranes resulting from the injury—whether they have been completely destroyed or are still intact—is therefore extremely important. If they are still intact, they can serve as a template for new muscle fiber (**Fig. 4.5**).

Note

Satellite cells are activated by factors in the local environment—for example, components of the basal membrane.

Satellite cell division reaches a maximum after 2–3 days (Chargé and Rudnicki 2004, Shi and Garry 2006). However, the stimulus for this process starts just 2 hours after the muscle injury, via trophic factors released by incoming neutrophils. Macrophages migrating to the site of the damage are also involved in regulating the process. Research has shown that after macrophages are depleted, their absence leads to a complete failure of muscle healing (Tidball 2005). The macrophages are involved both in the regulation of cell division and also in the differentiation of satellite cells and their survival. The differentiation phase begins following the cell division phase. This reaches a

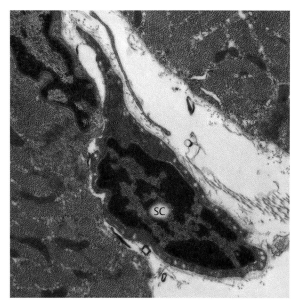

Fig. 4.3   An activated satellite cell (SC) in regenerating muscle.

major intermediate stage after ~ 2 weeks with the reconstruction of the regular cellular architecture, and it also represents a transition to the remodeling phase (Shi and Garry 2006).

Regulation of Satellite Cells

The process of muscle fiber repair, parts of which are very similar to the development of fetal muscle fiber, is subject to complex regulation. In addition to the influence of growth factors and cytokines, it is also controlled by the extracellular matrix and its components, as well as mechanical and metabolic factors. This also explains why differences can arise in muscle fiber repair and in the course of healing, depending on the type of damage involved and on subsequent treatment.

Activation of the satellite cells is induced by the growth factors and signal proteins released in the vicinity of the injury; these mainly include the following groups (Grefte et al. 2007, Le Grand et al. 2009):

- Fibroblast growth factors (FGF)
- Transforming growth factors (TGF-β)
- Insulin-like growth factors (IGF-1 and -2)
- Hepatocyte growth factor (HGF)
- The interleukin-6 (IL-6) family (leukocyte inhibitory factor, LIF)
- Wnt signal protein (Wnt7a)

As muscle regeneration through satellite cells involves a precisely regulated sequential process, the temporal sequence and the relation of the growth factors to one another have to be meticulously coordinated (**Fig. 4.6**). A more detailed description of the sequential release of all the growth factors involved and the regulatory signifi-

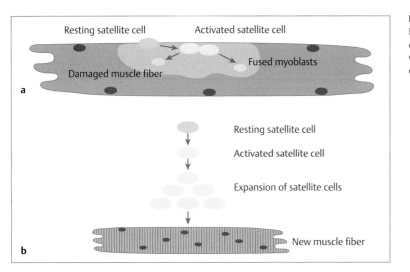

Fig. 4.4a, b   Muscle fiber regeneration. Following initial expansion of the satellite cell pool, satellite cells fuse in some cases with the remaining muscle fiber (**a**), or with each other to form a new muscle fiber (**b**).

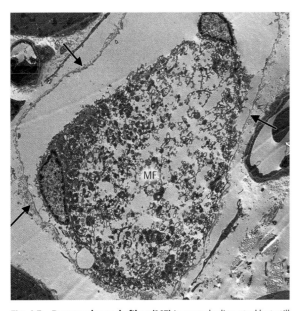

Fig. 4.5   Damaged muscle fiber (MF) is severely disrupted but still has an intact basement membrane (arrows).

cance of each of them is beyond the scope of this chapter. Only a few key functions of the most important growth factors are presented below.

- *FGF and HGF*. These are responsible for early activation of the satellite cells in particular and may play a significant role in increasing proliferation and thus the expansion of the satellite cell pool.
- *IGF-1*. Increased proliferation of satellite cells is also attributed to this factor; in addition, it has a direct effect on protein synthesis and thus on muscle-fiber hypertrophy. It may also support the survival of myogenic cells, and it has a positive effect on myogenic differentiation.

- *IGF-2*. This factor is up-regulated during the later phase of muscle regeneration and may play a role in differentiation in this context.
- *TGF-β*. The significance of the transforming growth factors is more complex, as different members not only regulate myoblast fusion, but also inhibit myoblast activity and satellite cell proliferation. Myostatin appears to play quite an interesting role here; this substance inhibits satellite cell proliferation, which in principle might counteract the process of regeneration. Its timing is, however, very finely tuned, with the result that it is up-regulated particularly during the destruction phase. It is thought that, at this point, myostatin has the task of preventing satellite cell proliferation from occurring too early, when the cell detritus has not yet been completely removed.
- *LIF*. By contrast, this factor, while stimulating satellite cell proliferation, does not affect further differentiation processes.

During satellite cell expansion and differentiation, a series of transcription factors are produced sequentially that are responsible for regulating muscle cell regeneration. The program is based on embryonic regulatory mechanisms. During the early regenerative phase, when the satellite cells or myoblasts are proliferating and subsequently maturing, Pax7, MyoD, and later Myf5 are produced. When differentiation begins, the factors Mrf4 and myogenin are synthesized; these are thought to be responsible for regulating differentiation and myoblast fusion. If there is well-ordered and well-coordinated sequential production of these factors, structural restoration of skeletal muscle fibers is complete after 14 days (**Fig. 4.6;** Chargé and Rudnicki 2004, Shi and Garry 2006, Gayraud-Morel et al. 2009). The fibers have not apparently reached their original size at this point, but they already have the structure of a mature muscle fiber, with peripheral nuclei. Following this phase, both an increase in size and remodeling of the

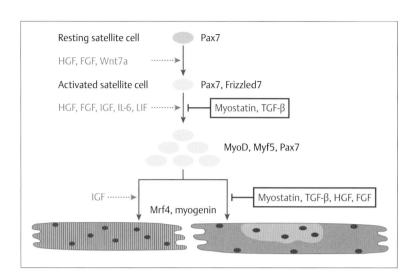

muscle fiber take place—processes which under optimal conditions lead to complete restoration of muscle function.

> *Note*
>
> **When healing progresses smoothly, the muscle fibers are already restored after 14 days. However, they have not yet reached their maximum size, and the muscle-fiber phenotype has yet to be adapted (Shi and Garry 2006).**

Particularly during the late phase of regeneration and remodeling, exercise stress appears to have positive effects on muscle healing, as discussed below (see p. 122).

> *Practical Tip*
>
> **Controlled exercise can accelerate healing, particularly during the late phase of regeneration, when the muscle fibers have achieved their original structure, and during further restructuring in the remodeling phase.**

Formation of Extracellular Matrix

In parallel with muscle fiber repair, extracellular matrix forms in the vicinity of the wound. This is important for regeneration, and it is also a process that affects the structural outcome of muscle repair and its functional outcome in particular. Formation of the extracellular matrix is important for restoring the mechanical capabilities of muscle tissue, on the one hand, as tensile strength and power transmission both depend on the extracellular matrix. On the other hand, muscle fibers also require extracellular matrix for regeneration and maintenance processes (**Fig. 4.7**).

Collagen Formation

The excessive formation of extracellular matrix that usually occurs represents a problem. It mainly involves excess generation of fiber collagen, which leads to defective healing, as it forms a stable collagen matrix that prevents muscle fibers from filling the defect and later, during the remodeling phase, is only broken down with difficulty.

The four collagen types mainly found in muscle tissue are types I, III, IV, and V. Collagen types I and III are distributed in the epimysium, perimysium, and endomysium. Whereas intact muscle contains collagen I chiefly in the epimysium and perimysium, collagen III is located primarily in the endomysium, which is also the main location of collagen types IV and V.

It is mainly collagen III that is produced during the initial muscle healing process, even before migration of fibroblasts occurs and myotubes are synthesized, but collagen IV and V can also be detected. It is only at a later stage that larger amounts of collagen I are produced in the wound. During the repair phase, therefore, the wound mainly contains collagen III, and the ratio of type I to type III collagen shifts in favor of collagen III. Normalization of the collagen ratios in muscle is thus part of the remodeling phase.

The migration of fibroblasts, which are responsible for the majority of extracellular matrix production starts during the first 48 hours after the injury and precedes actual myotube synthesis. In the first 5 days following injury, collagen production exceeds myosin production—implying that rapid production of extracellular matrix is the top priority, taking precedence even over muscle regeneration. This is especially the case when rupture of muscle fibers and fascicles (bundles) has occurred, with damage to blood vessels, as seen in particular with injuries starting at the level of minor partial muscle tears. This leads to bleeding, with subsequent hematoma formation. Due to

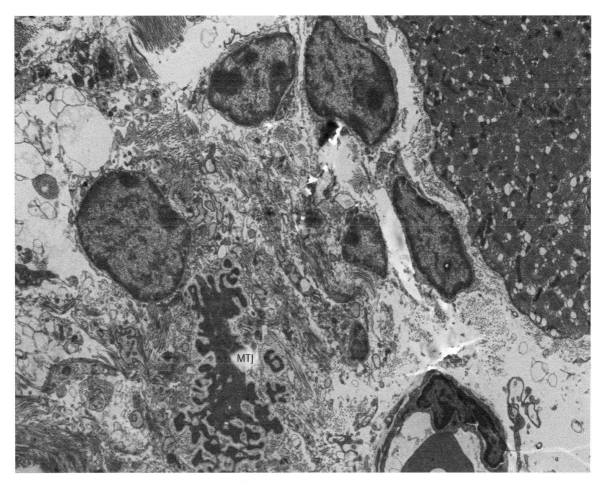

Fig. 4.7 **An area of fibrosis, with macrophages and fibroblasts in the region of a myotendinous junction (MTJ) in regenerating skeletal muscle**.

its high fibrin and fibronectin content, the hematoma is in practice structured into early granulation tissue, representing a skeleton for the subsequent fibroblast influx. The fibroblasts form the extracellular matrix, which in turn gives the granulation tissue fibrous stability. This stabilization of the granulation tissue helps to produce some mechanical stability in the wound.

The first extracellular matrix molecules that are produced, even before collagen III, are tenascin C (a proteoglycan) and fibronectin (a glycoprotein). The peculiarities of these early extracellular matrix molecules include their extreme tensile plasticity and their elastic properties, which contribute to the granulation tissue's high retraction capacity and thus help reduce the size of the scar region. The early extracellular matrix molecules are replaced by collagen III within a matter of days and by collagen I over the course of the following weeks. During these events, the size of the scar decreases substantially; mechanical load appears to play an essential role in the process, as the extracellular matrix component in the

damaged area remains increased only in muscle that has been immobilized over a long period of time.

With regard to the stability of damaged muscle, it may be noted that the fibrous scar area limits the overall stability of the damaged muscle only for the first 10 days (Järvinen et al. 2005).

Note

In the first 10 days following more severe muscle injury, it is newly-formed connective tissue that determines its stability; after that, it is the actual muscle tissue.

After this, the weak spot is the muscle in the region of the musculotendinous junctions, and renewed damage occurs in this area. As a rule, complete stability of the scar is only achieved after a matter of weeks. The extent to which this process can be influenced is discussed below (see p. 122).

Problem: Excessive Scar Formation

Although most muscle injuries are associated with temporary, morphologically detectable fibrous scar formation, which later heals without any structural or functional deficits in the muscle, there are cases in which excessive fibrous scarring develops, permanently impairing muscle fiber regeneration (**Fig. 4.8**). The causes of overwhelming scar formation may include inflammation, bleeding, or poor revascularization of the muscle. There are indications that inhibitors of TGF-β, important for activating fibroblasts and the production of extracellular matrix, may reduce the amount of fibrous scar formation. TGF-β inhibitors include decorin, suramin, and interferon-γ (IFN-γ). Decorin also influences collagen fibril formation and the associated aggregation of collagen I fibrils (Järvinen et al. 2005). A better understanding of the complex regulatory mechanisms involved in muscle fiber regeneration and the formation of the extracellular matrix in injured muscle is central to developing new approaches and optimizing treatment strategies in the future.

Note

Fibrous scar formation is dependent on the extent of muscle injury and on local factors at the site of the wound, which regulate the development of the extracellular matrix.

Neovascularization

Both muscle fiber regeneration and fibrous scar formation can take place only when the tissue is well supplied with nutrients. This requires an adequate vascular supply, so that blood vessel formation is a limiting factor, as in nearly every type of tissue regeneration (Smith et al. 2008). It is therefore surprising that relatively little research into blood vessel development in damaged muscle has been carried out. Neovascularization appears to start on the third day after the injury; this is comparable with the temporal sequence during revascularization of skin wounds.

Note

Muscle tissue can regenerate only when blood vessels are formed early enough and in sufficient quantities.

The structural changes that take place during the first few days at the site of the wound lead to the development of an environment that promotes vessel growth, characterized by a specific extracellular matrix. This contains large amounts of fibronectin, for example—a substance that promotes the migration of endothelial cells and the new growth of endothelial cells associated with it. The endothelial cells then aggregate to form a substrate for new blood vessels. In addition to the specific extracellular matrix, there are numerous growth factors and cytokines that promote the growth of new vessels when they are released into the wound. The newly-formed capillaries orient themselves toward the center of the wound, thus ensuring both revascularization of the wound region, originating in the wound periphery, and an adequate supply of oxygen and nutrients (Järvinen et al. 2005).

Note

Vascularization requires a growth-promoting environment; the composition of the connective tissue plays a central role in this context.

The supply of oxygen leads to an increasingly aerobic metabolic state in the wound region. The improved oxy-

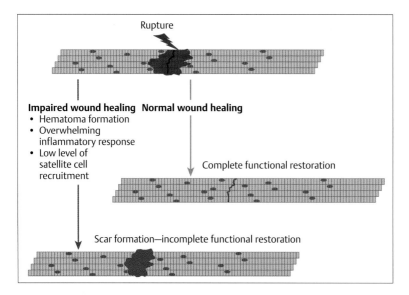

Fig. 4.8 Normal/impaired wound healing. Normal wound healing processes result in complete functional restoration, with formation of a stable myotendinous junction in the area of the scar. In cases of impaired wound healing, substitution of muscle by scar tissue takes place, resulting in incomplete functional restoration of the muscle.

gen supply is particularly important during the later phases of muscle fiber regeneration. At the onset of muscle fiber regeneration, the fibers still have a low aerobic capacity and a primarily anaerobic metabolism, as they have only very few mature mitochondria. Their metabolism switches to become aerobic as they continue to mature. An adequate capillary supply is necessary in order for this to take place (Järvinen et al 2005, Tee et al. 2007).

Evidence of the chronological sequence of blood vessel development has been provided by histological studies, and above all by data on the chronological sequence of the expression of angiogenic factors in damaged muscle tissue. The growth factors basic fibroblast growth factor (bFGF) and TGF-β, initially found in the wound, promote the migration of endothelial cells into the wound area. Vascular endothelial growth factor (VEGF) is synthesized starting on the third day after the injury and reaches a maximum level after 5 days. It regulates various cell-biological processes via VEGF receptor 1 and VEGF receptor 2, which are produced in the endothelial cells depending on the extent of endothelial differentiation. VEGF receptor 2 is primarily responsible for the division and migration of endothelial cells, while VEGF receptor 1 initiates the stabilization process in newly-formed blood vessels. In general, a range of vascular growth factors and their receptors are markedly increased from the third day until approximately the fifth day after injury (Järvinen et al. 2005, Smith et al. 2008).

Reinnervation

As with vascular development, disturbances in the structural and functional restoration of muscle can also be caused by unsuccessful regeneration of intramuscular nerves. Although muscle regeneration also takes place in denervated muscle, subsequent atrophy of the muscle fibers will ensue during the remodeling phase, at the very latest, in the absence of innervation processes. Reinnervation of muscle fibers requires the outgrowth of new axons originating from the proximal nerve stump. The new axons only have a relatively short distance to grow, as this involves peripheral intramuscular nerve injuries, and the process thus takes place quite quickly and does not usually limit regeneration (Järvinen et al. 2005). Local factors in the extracellular matrix (e.g., agrin, laminin, tenascin C) and factors released by the muscle fibers (e.g., IGF-1, FGF-5, nitrogen monoxide) induce and regulate the new formation of motor end plates in the muscle fibers (Sanes et al. 1998; Järvinen et al. 2005).

Laboratory Markers for Diagnosis and Healing

Serum markers such as creatine kinase, slow and heavy myosin chains, and myoglobin are of limited use, as they are already elevated due to the stress caused by exercise and competitive forms of physical exertion, making it almost impossible to distinguish between injury-related and stress-related increases. It is still unclear whether any additional serum factors could be used that would also specifically reflect the healing process in muscle injuries.

During the first two phases of muscle regeneration, a range of cytokines and growth factors are released that can be assigned, at least in part, to the individual phases of muscle healing (Guerrero et al. 2008, Smith et al. 2008; see **Table 4.2**)—for example:

- *Destruction phase:*
  TNF-α, IL-1α and IL-1β, IL-6, and bFGF
- *Inflammation:*
  Macrophage inflammatory protein-1α (MIP-1α), monocyte chemoattractant protein-1 (MCP-1), granulocyte colony-stimulating factor (GCSF), macrophage colony-stimulating factor (MCSF), VEGF, IL-8, and IFN-γ
- *Regeneration:*
  IGF-1, HGF, platelet-derived growth factor (PDGF), VEGF, TGF-β, macrophage migration inhibitory factor (MIF), and LIF

It remains to be determined whether these markers can be used to monitor the healing process. Another aspect that has so far been almost completely overlooked is whether it might be possible to detect degradation products from the extracellular matrix in the blood in cases of muscle injury. Since the degradation and later reconstruction of the extracellular matrix are important processes in muscle injury and regeneration, the question arises of whether the detection of degradation products stemming from the extracellular matrix in the blood might provide information about the severity of the muscle injury and might also reflect the healing process. Our own research has shown that degradation products from the extracellular matrix, as well as proteases originating in muscle that are responsible for breaking down the extracellular matrix, can be detected in the blood even after a single exercise unit. In general, there is considerable scope for further development of laboratory testing in connection with muscle injuries and the subsequent healing processes.

Factors Influencing Healing

Nutrition

The extent to which nutrition may have prophylactic effects against muscle injuries, or may be able to limit them and promote muscle repair, has been a topic of debate for some time.

Antioxidants

In particular, administration of antioxidants has been discussed in connection with limiting the secondary muscle damage caused by the early inflammatory response. Inflammatory cells migrating during the destruction phase, particularly neutrophils, produce large amounts of free oxygen radicals, which in turn lead to further cell damage in the already damaged muscle. However, a precise explanation of the mechanism of effect of free oxygen radicals has not yet been provided.

The main antioxidants used are vitamins C and E. However, results have been inconsistent. One series of studies described positive effects on pain and muscle damage markers such as creatine kinase, but a lack of effectiveness and even negative effects have also been reported. From the point of view of the mechanisms involved, preventing excessive load due to free oxygen radicals is important for inhibiting lipid-related, protein-related, and DNA-related damage, which can lead to the destruction of additional muscle fibers. Early treatment with antioxidants thus does appear to make sense. However, free radicals also act as signal molecules, which promote the production and release of growth factors, for example, and thus have wound-healing effects. This would also explain why delayed muscle regeneration has been observed in studies in which antioxidants have been administered. A detailed assessment of the effects of antioxidants in cases of muscle injury is not possible at present. However, administering them during the destruction phase, when there is excess production of free oxygen radicals that can intensify secondary muscle damage, would seem to be the most likely use. Administering antioxidants later than that appears at least to be problematic (Goldfarb 1999, Howatson and van Someren 2008).

> **Note**
> Antioxidants should be administered above all during the early phase of the muscle healing process.

Carbohydrates and Proteins

Supplying carbohydrates and protein is another supportive treatment option in cases of muscle injury. However, it has also not yet been fully clarified whether carbohydrate and protein supplementation has positive effects. A series of studies have been conducted on the issue of the significance of carbohydrates and proteins; either carbohydrates *or* proteins, or carbohydrates *and* proteins, were administered for different periods in the investigations. The supplemented amounts ranged from a single dose administered after the injury to treatments lasting several days.

Carbohydrates

In general, despite the reduced storage and resynthesis of glycogen in injured muscle, the results yielded in connection with the administration of carbohydrates alone have not been particularly promising, and a positive influence on the regeneration of damaged muscle has not been conclusively demonstrated. One possible explanation for the absence of any effects of carbohydrate application is the insulin resistance that develops in injured muscle. This may additionally, although not necessarily, be associated with a reduction in glucose transporters (such as GLUT-4) in the new muscle fibers. There is also evidence that the muscle fibers are unable to transform glucose into its storage form, glycogen, due to reduced enzyme activity (hexokinase and glycogen synthase). It might therefore be speculated that the carbohydrates administered are not able to increase the muscle's glycogen reserves sufficiently.

Protein

The situation looks somewhat more favorable with regard to protein or amino acid supplements. It has been shown that administering protein, particularly over a period of several days, leads to a reduction in signs of injury. The extent to which this effect might be further enhanced by combining carbohydrates and proteins has not yet been adequately clarified, although some speculations have been made (Howatson and van Someren 2008).

Age

Age is a factor that not only affects the physiological functioning of skeletal muscle, leading to sarcopenia, but also has a negative impact on muscle regeneration. It was previously thought that the decline in muscle regeneration observed during the aging process was an effect of an age-related reduction in the number of satellite cells, or at least a result of functional limitations in the satellite cells in aging muscle tissue. However, there has been no proof that any reduction in the number of satellite cells actually occurs, and studies have in fact confirmed in individual cases that there is actually an *increase* in the relative and absolute numbers of satellite cells in skeletal muscle. Regardless of the current unclear state of knowledge on this topic, however, it may be noted that aging skeletal muscle still has sufficient amounts of satellite cells for muscle regeneration (Carosio et al. 2011).

This may suggest that it is the functioning of satellite cells in skeletal muscle that declines with increasing age, rather than their numbers. Experimental studies involving cross-transplantation of satellite cells from skeletal muscle in young animals into skeletal muscle in older animals, and vice versa, have provided further information on the underlying mechanisms. It is not the satellite cells themselves that are responsible for impaired regeneration—leading to an impaired muscle regeneration process as a result of an intrinsic loss of functionality. Instead, there appears to be a change in the environment, with differences between older and younger muscle tissue that impair satellite cell–dependent regeneration. While successful muscle regeneration can be achieved in young mice using satellite cells from older mice, satellite cells in old mice stemming from young mice lose their capacity for regeneration. These results suggest that systemic factors responsible for successful activation, and therefore necessary for satellite-cell function, are altered in older mice. These changes in the environment might be due to local changes in muscle, but might also be caused by changes in the organism as a whole. For new treatment approaches in the future, it will be vital to identify the systemic changes that occur in muscle tissue during the aging process and to investigate how they arise.

Influence on Phagocytosis

One approach here involves the reduced ability of aging skeletal muscle to resolve hematomas and cell detritus through phagocytosis via inflammatory cells.

This also underlines the major physiological importance of the inflammatory process during the initial phase after muscle injury.

Influence on Signaling Pathways

In addition to phagocytosis, other changes at the level of signaling pathways due to the altered environment have also been described. For example, two signaling pathways that are important for satellite cell mobilization and differentiation and are therefore also important for muscle fiber regeneration are altered in skeletal muscle tissue in older animals. These are the Notch protein and Wnt signaling pathways, which already serve to regulate the early process of embryonic and fetal myogenesis and play a part in the activation and regulation of satellite cells during muscle regeneration.

Initially, the Notch signal pathway leads to activation and expansion of existing satellite cells in damaged muscle. Following a transition to regulation dominated by the Wnt signal pathway, satellite cell differentiation into myoblasts and myotubes is initiated. Advancing age is associated with a decrease in Notch activity in skeletal muscle, with the result that the satellite cell pool cannot be sufficiently expanded. The two signaling pathways have to be meticulously coordinated in order to ensure a successful and adequate muscle regeneration process. Thus, the prevalence of certain Wnt signals may well lead to satellite cell differentiation, but without the previous expansion of the satellite pool, the number of satellite cells is not sufficient to stimulate adequate muscle regeneration. In addition, production of the extracellular matrix in the damaged muscle is also regulated via the Wnt signal pathway, so that increased activity of certain Wnt signals may lead to fibrosis in the injured muscle, and in turn to scar fibrosis (**Fig. 4.9**). The activity of certain Wnt signals in aging skeletal muscle is increased, giving rise to a scenario in which muscle fiber regeneration is negatively influenced and fibrosis is positively influenced. For therapeutic purposes, an experimentally tested approach involving inhi-

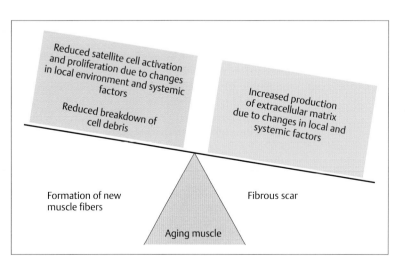

Fig. 4.9 Influence of age on muscle regeneration. In aging skeletal muscle, changes in the structure of the muscle tissue (influenced by local growth factors, extracellular matrix, and oxidative stress) and a concentration of systemic factors (hormones, growth factors) take place. These alterations lead to a reduction in satellite cell expansion and increased formation of extracellular matrix. The lower activity level of phagocytic cells has a direct effect on the clearance of cell debris.

Reduced satellite cell activation and proliferation due to changes in local environment and systemic factors

Reduced breakdown of cell debris

Increased production of extracellular matrix due to changes in local and systemic factors

Formation of new muscle fibers

Fibrous scar

Aging muscle

bition of the Wnt signal pathway might lead to a reduction in fibrosis and improved muscle fiber regeneration.

Influence on Growth Factors

In addition to the signaling pathways described above, there are also growth factors that are altered in aging skeletal muscle. Impaired skeletal muscle regeneration following injury is attributed to these factors. IGF-1 may play a special role here, as it intervenes sequentially in the regulation of expansion and differentiation of the satellite cell pool. IGF-1 production declines with advancing age, supporting the assumption that there is a causal relationship linking it to deteriorating muscle regeneration following injury. This has been confirmed in the context of animal experiments.

Myostatin, another growth factor in the TGF-β family, does not appear to show any altered expression in aging skeletal muscle, but it should still be mentioned here, as it may represent a possible approach in the treatment of muscle injuries, since inhibition of myostatin also leads to improved muscle regeneration in aging skeletal muscle.

Overall, the changes in growth factors that take place in skeletal muscle in older individuals are considerably more complicated even than this. However, the significance of these changes for impaired skeletal muscle regeneration in aging skeletal muscle has not yet been demonstrated for many of these growth factors.

Influence on the Extracellular Matrix and Antioxidative Capacity

In aging skeletal muscle, the extracellular matrix and antioxidative capacity are also altered. Both of these factors impair regeneration processes in skeletal muscle; however, there is as yet insufficient information about the significance of these alterations in relation to muscle healing processes in older individuals. There is a clear need for further research in this area, as it may be speculated that these are key factors that may play a major role in the changes observed during the aging process.

Exercise

The effects of specific exercise approaches in the treatment of muscle injuries have to be considered from various points of view. The severity of the injury and the temporal components of the exercise therapy need to be taken into account.

Approaches in Various Degrees of Muscle Injury

Early Mobilization in Cases of Muscle Firmness

In case of minor injuries (particularly muscle firmness) an initial effort must be made to achieve moderate early mobilization of the injured muscle in order to limit damage and reduce pain. It has been postulated that tissue-dam-

aging substances can be flushed out by means of light exercise during the first hours or days through improved circulation and that this may result in an increased release of endorphins, with analgesic effects (Howatson and van Someren 2008).

> *Practical Tip*
>
> **Early mobilization following muscle injury is useful, but it should only take place with strict monitoring of the stress placed on the muscle relative to the degree of injury.**

However, the results with this approach are unclear, and further research is needed to obtain better evidence on the value of early mobilization and the methods used to provide early exercise.

Initial Immobilization after Minor Partial Muscle Tears

In cases of more extensive injury, starting at the level of minor partial muscle tears (in which more obvious structural damage has taken place), initial immobilization lasting 3–5 days (or longer for more severe injuries) is recommended. This corresponds to a time frame encompassing the destruction phase (2–3 days) and the start of the regeneration phase and coincides with the period during which the maximum inflammatory reaction takes place.

> *Practical Tip*
>
> **Muscle injuries starting at the level of minor partial tears should not be subjected to stress until ~ 3–5 days after the event, and the exercise should then involve endurance-focused walking exercises. At this point, the ruptured ends of the muscle fibers, mainly in the region of the myotendinous junctions in the muscle, ought to have been reconnected and stabilized by temporary scar tissue.**

> *Note*
>
> **A muscle's loading capacity has been reached when a temporary scar has formed.**

This may be important when it comes to preventing secondary damage and the associated expansion of the muscle injury. There is also evidence that early mobilization during the first few days after injury leads to the development of a dense extracellular matrix, which in turn obstructs the growth of muscle tissue. In contrast, mobilization after 3–5 days has the effect of optimizing the formation of new muscle fibers in the still-immature extracellular matrix, as this can still be easily broken down and displaced (Järvinen et al. 2005).

Effects of Exercise

Influence on the Extracellular Matrix

In addition, components and catabolic products of the extracellular matrix are involved in regulating growth processes in many different tissues. This suggests that one of the effects of mobilization is to modulate the extracellular matrix in such a way as to promote its growth. Very little is currently known about the precise exercise-induced changes that take place in the extracellular matrix in damaged muscle. However, our own experimental studies in humans have shown that individual exercise interventions lead to extracellular matrix processing that is associated with the release of matrix-splitting proteases.

Influence on Muscle Growth

As exercise leads to activation of hypertrophic and hyperplastic muscle growth, the question arises as to the extent to which it also influences functional and structural regeneration through direct stimulation of muscle growth. In experimental animal models, Richard-Bulteau and colleagues showed that when exercise is performed initially for 1–2 hours, and later with increasing intensity directly after the destruction phase, it reduces the time needed for complete regeneration of muscle mass from 8 to 3 weeks, following total damage to the soleus muscle induced by a muscle toxin (Richard-Bulteau et al. 2008).

Although this was an animal experiment that may not necessarily correspond fully to muscle toxin–induced damage, with mechanical damage and tearing of muscle fibers and the muscle fascicle (bundle) and additional bleeding into the tissue, it may provide information capable of explaining why early functional loading through exercise interventions can promote regeneration of muscle tissue. The study shows that increased cell division takes place in the damaged muscle, which may derive at least in part from satellite cells. This type of expansion of the satellite cell pool available for further differentiation and for producing muscle fiber can increase the numbers of nuclei coding for protein synthesis in muscle. This effect can mainly be achieved during the early regeneration phase, as it is at this time that initial expansion of the satellite pool takes place (see p. 114). This suggests that it is important to start exercise as early as possible.

Activation of satellite cells and the corresponding alteration and up-regulation of satellite cell–activating factors also lead to a longer-lasting increase in cell division in the damaged muscle.

Activation of the mammalian target of rapamycin (mTOR) signaling pathway is also observed in addition to satellite cell activation. This pathway plays an important part in the regulation of protein synthesis and degradation. It can generally be assumed that activation of satellite cells, which leads to an increase in their numbers, also increases the number of muscle fiber nuclei. This in turn enhances transcription capacity in the new or regenerated muscle fibers, and in connection with subsequent intensified activation of protein synthesis mechanisms, accelerates the increase in muscle mass. In addition, mTOR activation through inhibition of transcription factor FoxO leads to a reduction in protein breakdown and apoptosis in the skeletal muscle fibers, shifting the balance between protein and fiber synthesis, on the one hand, and protein and fiber breakdown on the other, in favor of synthesis (Gayraud-Morel et al. 2009; **Fig. 4.10**).

Although the research findings are highly promising, the question of whether they can be transferred to humans remains to be answered, as the damage model used produces a slightly different type of tissue change. For example, it does not lead to hematoma formation in the muscle—a process that has a major influence on the course of muscle regeneration. In addition, a central issue is how much load the damaged muscle can tolerate at what stage during the process of muscle healing without suffering further tearing. In general, early exercise loading is an extremely interesting treatment option even in cases of higher-grade muscle injury, but it still requires more detailed investigation.

Drug-Based Therapy

Nonsteroidal anti-inflammatory drugs or glucocorticoids are often used to treat muscle injuries. Although these agents are frequently used, their therapeutic value is extremely questionable (Järvinen et al. 2005, Howatson and van Someren 2008).

Nonsteroidal Anti-Inflammatory Drugs

There are almost no studies supporting the value of nonsteroidal anti-inflammatory drugs (NSAIDs) in the treatment of human muscle injuries. Animal experiments suggest that an effect on the muscle injury can be achieved during the destruction phase. This takes place through a reduction in the early inflammatory response in the damaged muscle area, preventing the associated secondary damaging reaction. However, as the early inflammatory reaction also plays an essential role in the ordered sequence of wound healing and muscle regeneration, the

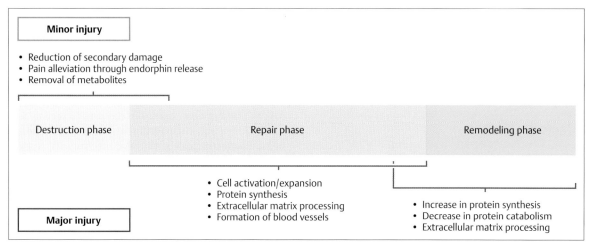

Fig. 4.10   Early exercise intervention can lead to better and faster muscle healing of both minor and major injuries.

question arises of whether drug-based therapy using non-steroidal anti-inflammatory drugs has a positive or negative influence on the healing process. The mainly experimental studies that have been conducted on the use of nonsteroidal anti-inflammatory drugs have also not produced a clear picture. It is therefore currently recommended that the use of NSAIDs should be limited to the early phase (destruction phase) (Järvinen et al. 2007).

Practical Tip

According to the current state of knowledge on the subject, administration of NSAIDs should be limited to the first few days following injury (destruction phase).

No negative effects on the later course of healing or tensile strength, or on the contractile activity of the injured muscle, have been described when NSAIDs are limited to the early phase following injury.

Glucocorticoids

Glucocorticoid administration appears to be considerably more problematic. Glucocorticoids are generally regarded as catabolic hormones that slow the healing process. This leads to delayed elimination of hematoma and necrotic tissue, as well as delayed regeneration of muscle tissue. It has also been reported that the mechanical properties of the regenerated muscle are poorer (Järvinen et al. 2007).

Caution

Glucocorticoids can markedly slow down the healing process and can cause muscle necrosis when they are injected.

New Treatment Approaches

Increasing knowledge about the mechanisms responsible for delayed or inadequate muscle repair following injury is leading to new therapeutic approaches. For example, treatments involving growth factors such as IGF-1 or using myostatin inhibitors are certainly promising options for promoting the regeneration of muscle fiber. On the other hand, excessive scar tissue formation can be prevented by TGF-β inhibitors such as decorin, for example (Järvinen et al. 2005).

Although these treatment strategies are at present suitable for practical application only with certain reservations, they may open up new therapeutic options. However, controlled and time-limited administration of specific drugs in defined phases of the muscle healing process is essential. Additional data pertaining to the mechanisms of the effects involved are still required.

Physical Measures

Various physical measures form part of the standard program following muscle injury. It has to be decided whether the specific case requires measures for reducing secondary damage after muscle injury or measures intended to have a positive effect on the healing process.

Cryotherapy

Cryotherapy, preferably using iced water, is one of the initial measures after acute muscle injuries. It is usually carried out immediately after the injury and is intended to reduce the inflammatory reaction in particular, as well as any bleeding occurring in the tissue. The aim is generally to help reduce swelling, edema, and hematoma formation, as well as pain.

Immediate cryotherapy reduces swelling, edema, and hematoma formation, as well as pain, and is the first step in treatment for better and faster healing.

However, the objective results obtained in research studies are not nearly as positive as subjective impressions of successful ice treatment. It has not yet been clearly established how long and how often cryotherapy has to be administered to be effective. It has been suggested that intermittent treatment over several hours is needed in order to achieve the effects on the local inflammatory reaction and hematoma formation mentioned above.

In terms of its mechanism of effect, cryotherapy leads to reduced local enzyme reactions, cell metabolism, neurotransmission, and blood supply. The effectiveness of longer phases of intermittent cryotreatment has yet to be investigated in greater detail in clinical and experimental studies.

Compression

Cryotherapy represents only one part of an initial treatment strategy involving rest, ice, compression, and elevation—RICE. Compression is the second step in this procedure. It is a matter of controversy whether compression is effective, but in consideration of the mechanism of its effects, immediate compression in muscle injuries involving vascular rupture should prevent severe bleeding into the tissues and thus potential secondary damage, as well as delaying the onset of the regeneration phase (Howatson and van Someren 2008).

Practical Tip
Direct compression of the muscle following injury prevents more extensive bleeding and consequently secondary damage as well.

Massage

Massage is an extremely nuanced and valuable treatment measure for all types of muscle injury. It is important to apply the correct technique at the right moment (for more details, see Chapter 14).

The effectiveness of massage results from a reduction in the inflammatory reaction due to a decrease in neutrophil infiltration and a reduction in vascular permeability brought about by increased prostaglandin release in the damaged muscle (Howatson and van Someren 2008).

Caution
Massaging an injured area too soon after a partial muscle tear, with hemorrhage or a contusion hematoma, is contraindicated as the mechanical stimulus can easily give rise to foci of calcification, leading to myositis ossificans (see also Chapter 6).

Ultrasound and Electrotherapy

Additional physical therapy methods that are used include therapeutic ultrasound and electrotherapy. Electrotherapy is often used to treat musculoskeletal injuries. One electrical therapy approach is known as transcutaneous electrical nerve stimulation (TENS). This is mainly used to alleviate pain and inhibit the inflammatory response. It has been speculated that pain relief with TENS is achieved by inhibiting presynaptic pain-conducting fibers in the damaged muscle (Järvinen et al. 2005, Howatson and van Someren 2008).

In general, there appears to have been insufficient research to date into the physical measures administered for muscle injuries. In addition to further clinical research, more studies are needed particularly to clarify the mechanisms responsible for the effects of individual forms of physical therapy. This would make it possible to define target dosages, application times, and time points for initiating each form of treatment—since dose–effect relationships are also relevant in physical therapy. However, systematic studies of these relationships are still largely lacking.

References

Best TM, Hunter KD. Muscle injury and repair. Phys Med Rehabil Clin N Am 2000; 11(2): 251–266

Byrne C, Twist C, Eston R. Neuromuscular function after exercise-induced muscle damage: theoretical and applied implications. Sports Med 2004; 34(1): 49–69

Carosio S, Berardinelli MG, Aucello M, Musaró A. Impact of ageing on muscle cell regeneration. Ageing Res Rev 2011; 10(1): 35–42

Chargé SB, Rudnicki MA. Cellular and molecular regulation of muscle regeneration. Physiol Rev 2004; 84(1): 209–238

Clarkson PM, Hubal MJ. Exercise-induced muscle damage in humans. Am J Phys Med Rehabil 2002; 81(11, Suppl): S52–S69

Gayraud-Morel B, Chrétien F, Tajbakhsh S. Skeletal muscle as a paradigm for regenerative biology and medicine. Regen Med 2009; 4(2): 293–319

Goldfarb AH. Nutritional antioxidants as therapeutic and preventive modalities in exercise-induced muscle damage. Can J Appl Physiol 1999; 24(3): 249–266

Grefte S, Kuijpers-Jagtman AM, Torensma R, Von den Hoff JW. Skeletal muscle development and regeneration. Stem Cells Dev 2007; 16(5): 857–868

Guerrero M, Guiu-Comadevall M, Cadefau JA, et al. Fast and slow myosins as markers of muscle injury. Br J Sports Med 2008; 42(7): 581–584, discussion 584

Howatson G, van Someren KA. The prevention and treatment of exercise-induced muscle damage. Sports Med 2008; 38(6): 483–503

Hurme T, Kalimo H, Lehto M, Järvinen M. Healing of skeletal muscle injury: an ultrastructural and immunohistochemical study. Med Sci Sports Exerc 1991; 23(7): 801–810

Järvinen TAH, Järvinen TLN, Kääriäinen M, et al. Muscle injuries: biology and treatment. Am J Sports Med 2005; 33(5): 745–764

Järvinen TAH, Järvinen TLN, Kääriäinen M, et al. Muscle injuries: optimising recovery. Best Pract Res Clin Rheumatol 2007; 21 (2): 317–331

Le Grand F, Jones AE, Seale V, Scimè A, Rudnicki MA. Wnt7a activates the planar cell polarity pathway to drive the symmetric expansion of satellite stem cells. Cell Stem Cell 2009; 4(6): 535–547

Richard-Bulteau H, Serrurier B, Crassous B, et al. Recovery of skeletal muscle mass after extensive injury: positive effects of increased contractile activity. Am J Physiol Cell Physiol 2008; 294(2): C467–C476

Sanes JR, Apel ED, Burgess RW, et al. Development of the neuromuscular junction: genetic analysis in mice. J Physiol Paris 1998; 92(3–4): 167–172

Shi X, Garry DJ. Muscle stem cells in development, regeneration, and disease. Genes Dev 2006; 20(13): 1692–1708

Smith C, Kruger MJ, Smith RM, Myburgh KH. The inflammatory response to skeletal muscle injury: illuminating complexities. Sports Med 2008; 38(11): 947–969

Tee JC, Bosch AN, Lambert MI. Metabolic consequences of exercise-induced muscle damage. Sports Med 2007; 37(10): 827–836

Tidball JG. Inflammatory processes in muscle injury and repair. Am J Physiol Regul Integr Comp Physiol 2005; 288(2): R345 R353

Further Reading

Proske U, Morgan DL. Muscle damage from eccentric exercise: mechanism, mechanical signs, adaptation and clinical applications. J Physiol 2001; 537(Pt 2): 333–345

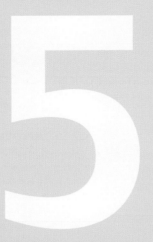

5

Epidemiology of Muscle Injuries in Soccer

J. Ekstrand

Consensus of Study Design   *128*

Material   *129*

Method   *129*

Results   *129*

Localization of Muscle Injuries
in Soccer Players   *129*

Injury Incidence   *130*

Injury Risk   *131*

Injury Severity   *132*

Recurrent Injuries   *132*

Examination Procedures:
MRI and Ultrasound   *132*

Evaluation of Data   *134*

Notes

Muscle Injuries in Soccer Players
- Muscle injuries constitute 35% of all soccer injuries.
- Of these, 55% affect the thighs (17% quadriceps, 37% hamstrings, of which 86% affect the biceps femoris), 30% affect the hip/groin area, and 13% affect the calf muscles.
- The most common single type of injury is hamstring injury (12%).
- A male elite-level team can expect ~ 18 muscle injuries each season (seven in hamstrings, three in quadriceps, five or six in the groin/hip, and two or three calf lesions).
- The risk of injury is six times higher during match play.
- The risk of injury increases with age only in the case of calf injuries.
- The risk of injury with thigh and hip/groin lesions increases over time in match play.
- Muscle injuries are more common from August to April (when many league matches are played).
- Of these, 96% occur in noncontact situations, and only 2% due to fouls.
- Thigh and calf injuries cause more moderate to severe injuries in comparison with hip/groin injuries.

Repeat Injuries
- Sixteen per cent of injuries are repeat injuries (more common in the hip/groin area in comparison with other areas).
- Repeat injuries cause a 30% longer period of absence (sometimes even more).

Hamstrings
- Of these injuries, 86% affect the biceps femoris muscle.
- The risk is 11 times higher during matches.
- Related to high velocity (running/sprinting).
- Evenly distributed between the two halves of matches.
- Mean absence time: 16 days.

Quadriceps
- Of these injuries, 88% affect the rectus femoris.
- The risk is four times higher in matches.
- They are related to shots at goal.
- More common in the first half of matches.
- Mean absence time: 18 days.

The high prevalence of muscle injuries in soccer is well documented (Ekstrand and Gillquist 1983, Hawkins et al. 2001, Askling et al. 2003, Ekstrand et al. 2003, 2006, and 2011a, Andersen et al. 2004, Hägglund et al. 2005b, 2009a, and 2009b, Waldén et al. 2005a, 2005b, and 2007, Árnason et al. 2008, Ekstrand et al. 2011a). The ultimate goal is therefore to prevent or reduce these injuries.

Practical Tip

Identifying and describing the injury problem is an important first step toward preventing injuries.

According to the van Mechelen model (van Mechelen et al. 1992), prevention of sports injury can be seen as a four-step sequence:
1. The extent of the injury problem is evaluated through injury surveillance.
2. Injury risk factors and injury mechanisms are established.
3. On the basis of this information, preventive strategies are introduced.
4. These strategies are evaluated by repeating step one.

This means that when one is aiming to prevent injuries, it is essential to conduct injury surveillance studies in order to evaluate the epidemiology of the injuries that take place.

Consensus of Study Design

A fundamental problem associated with the epidemiological assessment of data concerned with soccer injuries is the inconsistent manner in which injury is defined and the way in which data are collected and recorded (Inklaar 1994, Dvorak and Junge 2000, Junge and Dvorak 2000). Commonly, researchers compare the results from their own study with results from other published studies. However, the methodological differences between studies may be greater than any statistically significant differences between the studies concerned (Ekstrand and Karlsson 2003, Hägglund et al. 2005a).

Meaningful comparisons of the epidemiology of exposure and injury can only be made between studies that use similar study designs, definitions, and methods. A methodological consensus for soccer injury studies was recently established by the International Federation of Association Football (FIFA) and Union of European Football Associations (UEFA) in cooperation with representatives from major soccer research groups throughout the world (Fuller et al. 2006). The aim of this chapter is to present some results from in-depth studies on male professional soccer in Europe that were conducted using the methodology set out in the consensus agreement.

Material

The study population consisted of three cohorts:
- The UEFA Champions League (UCL) cohort
- The Swedish Super-League cohort
- The Danish Super-League cohort

The UCL cohort was followed over seven consecutive seasons (2001–2008). Twenty-three teams from 10 countries that had been playing regularly in the UEFA Champions League in the previous decade were chosen by UEFA to participate in the study.

The Swedish Super-League, with 16 teams, was followed during the 2001, 2002, and 2005 seasons, and eight teams from the Danish Super-League were followed during the 2001–2002 season. All players in the first team squads were included in the study. The total cohort includes 134 team seasons and ~850 000 hours of exposure.

Method

The methodology used has been described elsewhere in detail (Hägglund et al. 2005a, Fuller et al. 2006). Each team doctor was provided with attendance record forms and was responsible for completing these forms with data about the players' attendances at training sessions and matches. The attendance records included all training sessions and matches. Only coach-directed sessions that included physical activity were recorded.

Definition: Injury

A recordable injury was defined as an injury resulting in a player being unable to take full part in training or match play at any time following the injury. All injuries were recorded on a special card. The injury card consisted of a single page on which all injuries were listed in tabular form. Each injury was followed until the final rehabilitation date. A player was considered injured until the medical staff allowed full participation in all types of training or match play.

Structural injuries such as total and partial muscle tears, as well as functional disorders such as fatigue-induced, spine-related or neuromuscular muscle disorders, were included, while contusions, hematomas, tendon ruptures, and chronic tendinopathies were not.

Definition: Injury Severity

Injury severity was defined as the number of days elapsing from the date of injury to the date of return to full participation in team training and availability for match selection:
- Minimal (1–3 days)
- Mild (4–7 days)
- Moderate (8–28 days)
- Severe (> 28 days)

Definition: Recurrent Injury

A recurrent injury was defined as the same type of injury to the same side and location within 2 months after the final rehabilitation day following the previous injury.

Results

A total of 2365 muscle injuries were recorded in 900 players (mean age 26 ± 4 years, range 17–40 years). According to the consensus grouping (Fuller et al. 2006), muscle injuries constituted 35% of all injuries (in comparison with sprain/ligament injuries and hematoma/contusion/bruise injuries, which constituted 18% and 16% of all injuries, respectively).

Localization of Muscle Injuries in Soccer Players

As **Fig. 5.1** shows, 98% of all muscle injuries in soccer affect the thighs (55%), the hip/groin area (30%), or the calf muscles (13%). At the elite level, hamstring muscle injury is the most common single type of injury, representing 12% of all injuries.

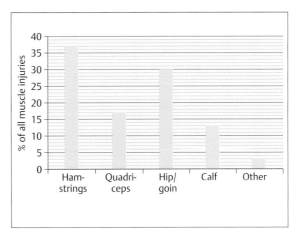

Fig. 5.1 Localizations of muscle injuries in soccer players.

Injury Incidence

The overall injury incidence (injuries/1000 hours) was 2.8 for all muscle injuries. On average, a male elite-level team with a squad of 25 players can expect ~ 18 muscle injuries each season. Ten of these will be thigh muscle injuries (seven hamstrings and three quadriceps), five or six will be groin injuries, and two or three will be calf injuries.

Figure 5.2 shows the distribution of muscle injuries during a season for teams that have a fall–spring season. Muscle injuries are more common during the August to April period, when many league matches are played. During January, when many leagues have a winter break and fewer matches are played, the risk of thigh and hip/groin injury (but not calf injury) is reduced.

Figure 5.3 shows the injury incidence over seven seasons for the UCL cohort. The injury risks for all muscle injuries, as well as for the most common subtypes, were fairly stable over the period, with only minor differences between seasons.

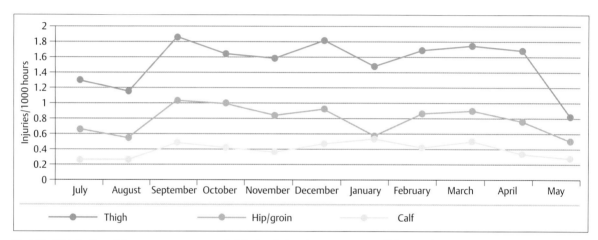

Fig. 5.2 Distribution of the most common muscle injuries during the soccer season (fall–spring).

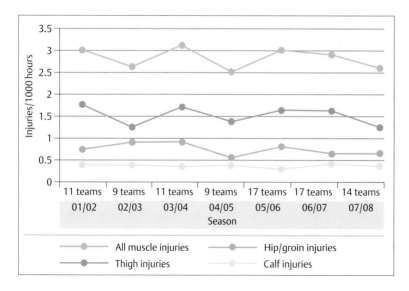

Fig. 5.3 Incidence of muscle injuries in Champions League teams over 7 years.

Injury Risk

Note

The risk of injury is six times higher at matches.

In total, the risk of sustaining a muscle injury is six times higher during match play in comparison with training (9.6/1000 match-hours vs. 1.6/1000 training hours). Two-thirds of all hamstring injuries occur during matches, in comparison with 52% of calf injuries, 48% of hip/groin injuries, and 42% of quadriceps injuries.

Muscle Injuries and Age

As seen in **Fig. 5.4**, the risk of sustaining a muscle injury generally increases with age.

During match play, however, the injury risk increases with age for sustaining a calf injury but for quadriceps injuries, hamstring injuries, and muscle injuries in the hip/groin region, no such effect was noticed (**Fig. 5.5**).

Variation in Injury Risk during Matches

The risk of thigh muscle injuries increases over time in both the first and second halves of matches (**Fig. 5.6**). A similar tendency is seen for hip/groin injuries in the first half, while the risk of calf injuries is fairly constant until the last 15 minutes of the match, when the risk increases substantially.

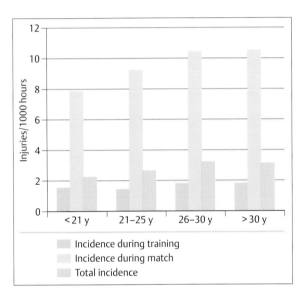

Fig. 5.4 The risk of sustaining a muscle injury in different age groups.

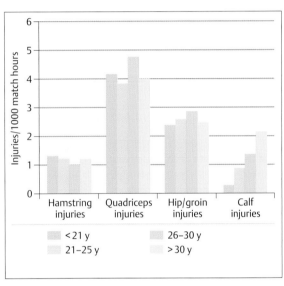

Fig. 5.5 The risk of sustaining a muscle injury during match play in different age groups.

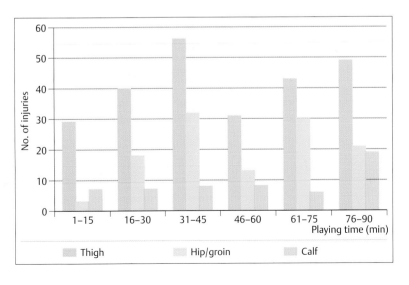

Fig. 5.6 Distribution of muscle injuries during a match.

Injuries Due to Contact Situations and Foul Play

Note

Almost all injuries occur in noncontact situations.

As many as 96% of all muscle injuries occur in noncontact situations, only 4% being sustained during contact. Furthermore only 2% of match-play muscle injuries are due to foul play specified by the referee.

Injury Severity

As seen in **Fig. 5.7**, 39–62% of all muscle injuries are moderate, causing absences from training and matches lasting between 8 and 28 days. Some 9–13% of muscle injuries are severe, causing absences lasting more than 28 days. In general, thigh and calf injuries cause more moderate to severe injuries in comparison with hip/groin injuries.

Recurrent Injuries

About 16% of muscle injuries in elite soccer are recurrent injuries.

Note

A recurrent injury is an injury of the same type and at the same site as an index injury and occurs no more than 2 months after a player's return to full participation following the index injury.

The risk of recurrent injury is higher for hip/groin injuries in comparison with thigh and calf injuries (**Fig. 5.8**). On average, repeat injuries caused a 30% longer period of absence than the initial injury (17 versus 13 days; $P < 0.001$).

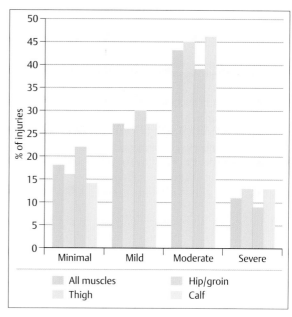

Fig. 5.7   Severity of muscle injuries.

Examination Procedures: MRI and Ultrasound

The diagnostic procedures used for thigh muscle injuries were investigated in the UCL cohort during the 2007–08 season. Of the 159 thigh muscle injuries, 72 (45%) were examined with magnetic resonance imaging (MRI; some with ultrasound as well). Seventy (44%) were examined with ultrasound, and 11% were diagnosed only clinically.

Of the 14 clubs that participated during that season, two clubs examined almost all thigh muscle injuries (> 90%) with MRI, while two clubs did not perform any MRI examinations at all during the period. Seven clubs used mainly MRI for diagnosis, and seven used mainly ultrasound.

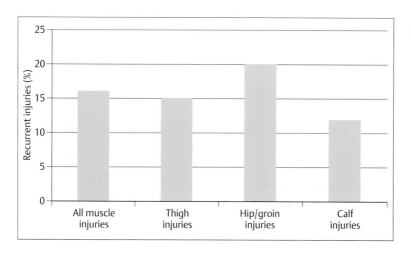

Fig. 5.8   Percentage of recurrent injuries for all muscle injuries and the most common muscle injury subtypes.

Hamstring Injuries

According to the MRI findings, the majority of hamstring injuries are to the biceps femoris muscle (86%).

Two out of three hamstring injuries occurred at matches, and the risk of sustaining a hamstring injury during a match was 11 times higher than during training. As hamstring injuries are known to be related to high-velocity loading (sprinter's injury), this finding may be related to the high intensity of top-level matches (Askling et al. 2007). The hamstring injuries were evenly distributed between the two halves of the matches (51% vs. 49%).

The majority of hamstring injuries (52%) were due to running or sprinting, while 17% were due to overuse. Almost all hamstring injuries were noncontact injuries, with 97% sustained without contact with other players. According to the referees, only 1.5% of the match play injuries were due to foul play. Thirteen per cent of the injuries were recurrent injuries.

Figure 5.9 shows the distribution of thigh muscle injuries over the season for the Champions League teams. Hamstring injuries were more common during the competitive season (September to May). It seems reasonable to assume that the finding of a higher risk of hamstring injury during the competitive season is due to the fact that more, and more intensive, matches are played during that period.

In general, a soccer team with 25 players can expect approximately seven hamstring injuries per season, with a total absence of ~110 days. On average, a hamstring injury causes 16 days of absence (range 1–128 days), with a mean of 10 missed training sessions (range 0–90) and three missed matches (range 0–27). Fourteen per cent of the injuries will be severe, causing absences lasting more than 4 weeks. Injuries sustained during matches cause significantly longer periods of absence in comparison with injuries sustained during training (18.3 vs. 11.9 days; $P < 0.001$).

Quadriceps Injuries

According to the MRI findings, the majority of quadriceps injuries occur to the rectus femoris muscle (88%). The majority of the quadriceps injuries occur during training, and the risk of sustaining a quadriceps injury during a match is four times greater than during training (1.1 vs. 0.3/ 1000 hours).

The majority of quadriceps injuries (62%) occur in the first half of the matches, and the peak risk was noted between minutes 16 and 45 of the first half, when 40% of all quadriceps injuries occur.

As many as 28% of all quadriceps injuries occur during shots at goal, in contrast to hamstring injuries, in which only 1.5% of injuries occur during goal shots ($P < 0.001$). The finding that the risk of quadriceps injuries peaks at the end of the pre-season preparation period might be explained by more intensive practice of shooting during training in this period. As with hamstring injuries, the majority of quadriceps injuries were noncontact injuries, 96% being sustained without contact with other players. None of the match-play injuries were due to foul play. As with hamstring injuries, 13% of the injuries were recurrent injuries.

Figure 5.9 shows the distribution of injuries over the season. The highest risk of sustaining a quadriceps injury was seen in August, during the end of the pre-season preparation period. In contrast to hamstring injuries, no increase in risk was seen during the competitive season.

A team with 25 players can expect approximately three quadriceps injuries each season, with a total absence period of ~50 days. On average, a quadriceps injury causes 18 days of absence, with a mean of 12 missed training sessions and three missed matches. Nineteen per cent of the injuries will be severe, causing absences lasting more than 4 weeks. In contrast to hamstring injuries, there were no significant differences in the number of absence days between injuries sustained at matches and injuries sustained during training (20 versus 17 days; not significant).

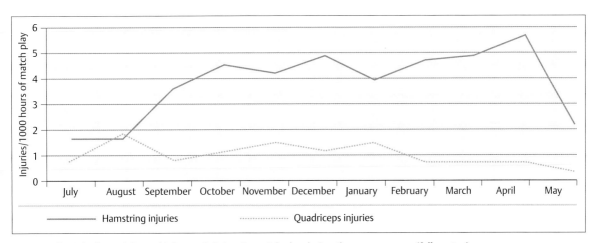

Fig. 5.9 The risk of sustaining a thigh muscle injury in match play during the soccer season (fall–spring).

Evaluation of Data

In view of the difficulty of generalizing findings about muscle injuries, this chapter concentrates on muscle injuries in a homogeneous group of male elite soccer players in Europe. Each sport has its own injury profile, and even within one sport there may be differences relative to gender, age, competitive level, etc. There is an example of this in the discussion of age and risk for muscle injuries in this chapter. When one looks at all muscle injuries occurring in elite soccer, a general increase with age is observed (**Fig. 5.4**). Similar findings are often referred to in the literature (Lindenfeld et al. 1994, Dvorak and Junge 2000, Árnason et el. 2004, Junge and Dvorak 2004). However, when a subanalysis of the risk for different types of muscle injuries in different age groups is carried out (see **Fig. 5.5**), which is possible if the material is large enough, it is found that the increase with age only applies to calf injuries and not to hamstring injuries, quadriceps injuries, or hip/groin injuries.

In addition, meaningful comparisons of the epidemiology of injury can only be made between studies that essentially use the same study design, definitions, and methods. Until now, however, methodological differences between studies may have been greater than the reported differences in their results (Waldén 2007).

Another problem with comparisons of muscle injuries is that a wide range of pathological findings are normally included—total and partial muscle tears, as well as muscle firmness and cramps, in the consensus definition. In addition, possible differences in the locations, grade, and type of muscle injuries in different sports have so far hardly been evaluated at all (Askling et al. 2007).

References

Andersen TE, Engebretsen L, Bahr R. Rule violations as a cause of injuries in male Norwegian professional football: are the referees doing their job? Am J Sports Med 2004; 32(1, Suppl): 62S–68S

Árnason Á, Sigurdsson SB, Gudmundsson Á, Holme I, Engebretsen L, Bahr R. Risk factors for injuries in football. Am J Sports Med 2004; 32(1, Suppl): 5S–16S

Árnason Á, Andersen TE, Holme I, Engebretsen L, Bahr R. Prevention of hamstring strains in elite soccer: an intervention study. Scand J Med Sci Sports 2008; 18(1): 40–48

Askling C, Karlsson J, Thorstensson A. Hamstring injury occurrence in elite soccer players after preseason strength training with eccentric overload. Scand J Med Sci Sports 2003; 13(4): 244–250

Askling CM, Tengvar M, Saartok T, Thorstensson A. Acute first-time hamstring strains during high-speed running: a longitudinal study including clinical and magnetic resonance imaging findings. Am J Sports Med 2007; 35(2): 197–206

Dvorak J, Junge A. Football injuries and physical symptoms. A review of the literature. Am J Sports Med 2000; 28(5, Suppl): S3–S9

Ekstrand J, Gillquist J. Soccer injuries and their mechanisms: a prospective study. Med Sci Sports Exerc 1983; 15(3): 267–270

Ekstrand J, Karlsson J. Editorial. The risk for injury in football. Scand J Med Sci Sports 2003; 13: 147–149

Ekstrand J, Karlsson J, Hodson A, eds. Football Medicine. London: Martin Dunitz (Taylor & Francis Group); 2003

Ekstrand J, Timpka T, Hägglund M. Risk of injury in elite football played on artificial turf versus natural grass: a prospective two-cohort study. Br J Sports Med 2006; 40(12): 975–980

Ekstrand J, Hägglund M, Waldén M. Injury incidence and injury patterns in professional football: the UEFA injury study. Br J Sports Med 2011a; 45(7): 553–558

Ekstrand J, Hägglund M, Waldén M. Epidemiology of muscle injuries in professional football (soccer). Am J Sports Med 2011b; 39(6): 1226–1232

Fuller CW, Ekstrand J, Junge A, et al. Consensus statement on injury definitions and data collection procedures in studies of football (soccer) injuries. Br J Sports Med 2006; 40(3): 193–201

Hägglund M, Waldén M, Bahr R, Ekstrand J. Methods for epidemiological study of injuries to professional football players: developing the UEFA model. Br J Sports Med 2005a; 39(6): 340–346

Hägglund M, Waldén M, Ekstrand J. Injury incidence and distribution in elite football—a prospective study of the Danish and the Swedish top divisions. Scand J Med Sci Sports 2005b; 15(1): 21–28

Hägglund M, Waldén M, Ekstrand J. Injuries among male and female elite football players. Scand J Med Sci Sports 2009a; 19 (6): 819–827

Hägglund M, Waldén M, Ekstrand J. UEFA injury study—an injury audit of European Championships 2006 to 2008. Br J Sports Med 2009b; 43(7): 483–489

Hawkins RD, Hulse MA, Wilkinson C, Hodson A, Gibson M. The association football medical research programme: an audit of injuries in professional football. Br J Sports Med 2001; 35(1): 43–47

Inklaar H. Soccer injuries. I: Incidence and severity. Sports Med 1994; 18(1): 55–73

Junge A, Dvorak J. Influence of definition and data collection on the incidence of injuries in football. Am J Sports Med 2000; 28 (5, Suppl): S40–S46

Junge A, Dvorak J. Soccer injuries: a review on incidence and prevention. Sports Med 2004; 34(13): 929–938

Lindenfeld TN, Schmitt DJ, Hendy MP, Mangine RE, Noyes FR. Incidence of injury in indoor soccer. Am J Sports Med 1994; 22 (3): 364–371

van Mechelen W, Hlobil H, Kemper HC. Incidence, severity, aetiology and prevention of sports injuries. A review of concepts. Sports Med 1992; 14(2): 82–99

Waldén M, Hägglund M, Ekstrand J. Injuries in Swedish elite football—a prospective study on injury definitions, risk for injury and injury pattern during 2001. Scand J Med Sci Sports 2005a; 15(2): 118–125

Waldén M, Hägglund M, Ekstrand J. UEFA Champions League study: a prospective study of injuries in professional football during the 2001–2002 season. Br J Sports Med 2005b; 39(8): 542–546

Waldén M. Epidemiology of injuries in elite football [dissertation]. Dept. of Health and Society, University of Linköping, Sweden; 2007

Waldén M, Hägglund M, Ekstrand J. Football injuries during European Championships 2004–2005. Knee Surg Sports Traumatol Arthrosc 2007; 15(9): 1155–1162

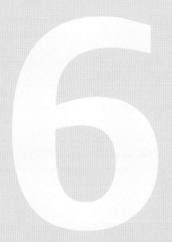

Terminology, Classification, Patient History, and Clinical Examination

H.-W. Müller-Wohlfahrt
P. Ueblacker
A. Binder
L. Hänsel

Translated by Gertrud G. Champe

Why a New Classification?   *136*
Short Review of the Current Literature   *137*

Terminology of Muscle Injuries   *137*
Classification of Muscle Injuries   *137*
Consensus Conference on Muscle
Terminology and Development of
a New Comprehensive Classification
System   *139*
Type 1 and 2:
Functional Muscle Disorders   *145*
Types 3 and 4:
Structural Muscle Injuries   *149*
Contusion Injuries   *153*

Patient History   *155*

Examination of Muscle Injuries   *156*
Examination Techniques   *156*
Typical Findings on Examination   *160*
Other Muscle Injuries and Causes
of Muscle Symptoms   *162*

Complications   *163*
Post-Stress Muscle Imbalance   *163*
Recurrence   *163*
Seroma and Cyst   *163*
Fibrosis/Scarring   *165*
Traumatic Compartment Syndrome   *165*
Myositis Ossificans and
Heterotopic Ossification   *165*
Muscle Hernia   *165*

Why a New Classification?

The paper "Terminology and classification of muscle injuries in sport: The Munich consensus statement" by Müller-Wohlfahrt et al., published in the *British Journal of Sports Medicine* in 2012, is freely available via www.bjsm.com and www.pubmed.org.

Due to a lack of adequate information, muscle injuries are often regarded as harmless. People often say, "It'll heal up again, whether it takes 3 weeks or 6 weeks or longer." Competitive athletes such as professional soccer players see it differently, however. For them, a great deal depends on how long the injury is going to keep them off the field. An injury can undo the effects of long weeks of training, cost a player his regular place on the team, involve serious financial losses, and can have a significant effect on performance morale. Even for recreational athletes, however, correct assessment of the injury, comprehensive advice, and therapy are extremely important.

An athlete has to comply with the schedules and time frames that the physician treating the injury gives him, which provide him with both guidance and a goal. If the healing process does not progress as expected, the situation can become increasingly difficult, since issues of whether the diagnosis is correct and whether the treatment is suitable arise.

Although muscle injuries are the most frequent type of sports injury and represent more than 30% of all injuries in soccer, for instance (Järvinen et al. 2005; Waldén et al. 2005, Ekstrand et al. 2011a), it can be seen almost every day that the injuries are poorly evaluated and given inadequate therapy, even in elite athletes. For instance, 6 weeks are estimated for the treatment of a minor partial muscle tear, but only 10 days for therapy of a moderate partial muscle tear. In the past, even plaster casts were ap-

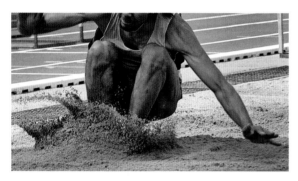
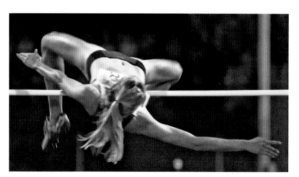
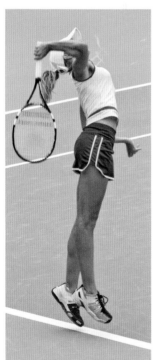
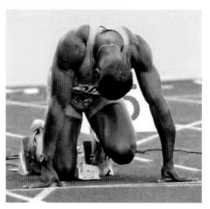
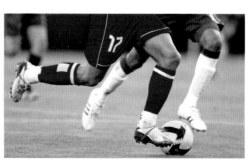

Fig. 6.1

plied. Some athletes are dismissed from training with instructions to return when they think the injury has healed, while others are prescribed absolute rest after a functional muscle disorder.

These contradictory measures are a sign of uncertainty and ignorance, and also of the inconsistency of clinical and imaging diagnoses and the fact that a practical classification system has so far not yet been available. Moreover, the terminology used in the field of muscle injuries lacks clear definitions and is therefore used extremely inconsistently.

Unfortunately, the topic of muscle injury still receives little attention at conferences on orthopedic medicine, sports medicine, and traumatology—in contrast to the techniques of bone and joint surgery. There is also an unfortunate lack of information on the diagnosis and treatment of muscle injuries. This is often attributed to the fact that adequate numbers of representative injuries can only be observed in specialized centers. The same argument can also be applied to other types of injury, however.

In our view, it is high time for the musculature to be raised to the level of a major medical topic and for a differentiated, informative, and practice-oriented classification of injuries to be established on the basis of the physiological course of each of the injuries (**Fig. 6.1**). Guidelines need to be developed so that differentiated treatment programs can be offered.

This book is specifically intended to stimulate discussion of frequently occurring muscle injuries so that diagnostic, therapeutic, and preventive measures can be further improved in the future.

Short Review of the Current Literature

While the literature currently available on the topic includes numerous books about sports orthopedics, often with overlapping content, there is a lack of standard works on potential muscle injuries and methods of examining and treating them. More extensive overviews of sports orthopedics, orthopedics, traumatology, and sports medicine usually only have a few pages on the muscles, and the information they provide is often not consistent. There are consequently only a few points on which it is possible to provide citations from the literature, so that in terms of evidence we can only fall back on the numerous muscle injuries that we have examined and treated in the past. The authors contributing to the present volume, and in particular the senior author, Hans-Wilhelm Müller-Wohlfahrt, have evaluated and treated thousands of athletic muscle injuries since 1976.

To date there have only been very few studies on the differential diagnosis, treatment, and evaluation of muscle injuries, despite the considerable clinical significance of this type of injury (Järvinen et al. 2005, Orchard et al. 2005 and 2008). This is not only due to the wide variation in the severity of the injuries, but also to the fact that the injuries can occur in different muscles and at different points in the muscles, making it very difficult to design research studies (Järvinen et al. 2005 and 2007). Up to now, studies have been concerned almost exclusively with the genesis of a "strain" or the genesis of lesions that are considered to represent "strain."

The best and most consistent data are available in the literature on the epidemiology of muscle injuries, especially in soccer. Muscle injuries constitute 31% of all injuries in elite soccer (Ekstrand et al. 2011b). The high prevalence of these injuries in soccer and other sports is well documented (Alonso et al. 2009, Andersen et al. 2004, Árnason et al. 2004, Borowski et al. 2008, Brophy et al. 2010, Feeley et al. 2008, Hägglund et al. 2009, Hawkins et al. 2001, Lopez et al. 2012, Malliaropoulos et al. 2010, Malliaropoulos et al. 2011, Waldén et al. 2005). However, very little information is available in the international literature on the definitions of muscle injuries or on systems for classifying them.

Terminology of Muscle Injuries

A review of the current literature on the topic in English showed that there is no standardization of the terminology used in the field of muscle injuries; terms are used indiscriminately by researchers and clinicians.

"Muscle strain," for example, is one of the terms most frequently used to describe athletic muscle injury. However, it is used in extremely variable ways in the literature and everyday practice and without any clear definition. While some authors use "muscle strain" synonymously with structural muscle tears, others also use the word "strain" to refer to nonstructural muscle injuries.

Hägglund et al. define "muscle strain" as "acute distraction injury of muscles and tendons" (Hägglund et al. 2005). But this definition is rarely used, either in the literature or colloquially among medical staff treating muscle injuries or caring for top-level athletes with muscle injuries.

> ### Note
> Terms used in the field of muscle injuries, such as "strain," are not clearly defined and are used inconsistently.

Classification of Muscle Injuries

Fundamentals

As muscles are heterogeneous and have a complex functional and anatomic organization, developing a universally applicable classification is a challenge. Unambiguous differentiation and classification is much more difficult with muscle injuries than it is for fractures or ligament and tendon injuries, for example. The muscles have many different sizes and shapes; some are long, like the biceps femoris, with tendon insertions on bone at both ends, and cross two joints. Others are short, some have long muscle bellies, and others again have long tendons. Muscle fibers may be aligned with tendons in a colinear fashion (unipennate), or fibers can insert at an angle on an intramuscular tendon (bipennate) (Armfield et al. 2006).

The fact that 16% of muscle injuries in elite soccer (see Chapter 5) and 30% of those in Australian football (Orchard et al. 1997) are recurrent injuries, which are associated with a 30% longer period of absence from competition than the original injury (Ekstrand et al. 2011b), emphasizes the critical importance of correct evaluation, diagnosis, and treatment of the index muscle disorder.

Current Classification Systems

Athletic muscle injuries are a heterogeneous group of muscle disorders that have traditionally been difficult to define and categorize. Earlier attempts to establish classification systems for muscle have simply used categories such as delayed-onset muscle soreness (DOMS), strains (distraction injuries), and contusions (compression injuries) (Ekstrand et al. 2011b). Various classification systems have been published in the literature, but there is little consistency within studies (Bryan Dixon 2009) or in everyday practice.

A grading system for muscle injuries that has been more widely used was devised by O'Donoghue. This system uses a classification based on the severity of injury relative to the amount of tissue damage and associated *functional* loss. It categorizes muscle injuries into three grades, ranging from grade 1 (no appreciable tissue disruption) and grade 2 (tissue damage and reduced strength in the musculotendinous unit) to grade 3 (complete disruption of the musculotendinous unit and complete loss of function) (O'Donoghue 1962).

Ryan published a classification for quadriceps injuries that has also been applied to other muscles. In this classification, grade 1 represents tearing of a few muscle fibers with intact fascia. Grade 2 is tearing of a moderate number of fibers, with the fascia remaining intact. Grade 3 injury involves tearing of many fibers with partial tearing of the fascia, and grade 4 injury is a complete tear of the muscle and fascia (Ryan 1969).

In 1995, Takebayashi et al. published an ultrasound-based three-grade classification system, ranging from grade 1 injury (less than 5% of the muscle involved) to grade 2 (partial tear, with more than 5% of the muscle involved) to grade 3 (complete tear) (Takebayashi et al. 1995). Peetrons has recommended a similar grading system (Peetrons 2002).

The classification currently most widely used is based on magnetic resonance imaging (MRI) and has four grades: grade 0, no pathological findings; grade 1, muscle edema only, but without tissue damage; grade 2, partial muscle tear; and grade 3, complete muscle tear (Stoller 2006).

The International Federation of Association Football (FIFA) F-MARC *Football Medicine Manual,* considered to be one of the most practical and comprehensive references in the field of sports injuries, classifies thigh muscle injuries into "direct" and "indirect" types, differentiating only "strains" from "contusions" and intramuscular from intermuscular hematomas. Unfortunately, no further subclassification is provided or discussed (Dvorak et al. 2009).

The most recently published classification system, by Chan et al., is imaging-based (Chan et al. 2012), although many authors have stated that the diagnosis and prognosis of muscular injuries should normally be mainly based on clinical findings, with radiological methods such as MRI or ultrasound being used for additional information in order to confirm a diagnosis (Ekstrand et al. 2012, Kerkhoffs et al. 2012).

In our opinion, the current classification systems are inadequate. None of the classifications are subclassified, so that the grading is only rough and injuries of differing sizes, and therefore with different prognoses, fall into the same grading.

The classification by Takebayashi et al. can be criticized on the grounds that it is difficult to measure whether a volume of muscle fiber is greater or less than 5%. Since we are dealing with an amount expressed in terms of percentage—that is, a relative size—the size of an injury of equal grade may differ depending on the volume of the muscle (e.g., it would be smaller in the sartorius in comparison with the biceps femoris). However, the anatomic configuration—that is, the size of the muscle fibrils, fibers, and bundles (fascicles) in each of an individual's muscles—is approximately the same, so that minor or moderate partial muscle tears, independently of the size of the muscle, will always have about the same dimensions. It is only in more extensive injuries such as subtotal muscle tears that the size of the affected muscle is relevant, since a subtotal tear in a small muscle has different dimensions than in a large muscle.

Note

Most of the classifications established so far are not comprehensive enough to be capable of reliably describing all of the muscle injuries that occur in sports.

Until recently there has been no classification that has described and subclassified disorders for which there is no macroscopic evidence of structural damage in professional athletes. However, a Union of European Football Associations (UEFA) muscle injury study (Ekstrand et al. 2012) has emphasized the high clinical relevance of these nonstructural muscle disorders. Ekstrand's study included data from a 4-year observation period of MRI findings obtained within 24–48 hours after injury and demonstrated that the majority of injuries (70%) were less than MRI grade 2 and thus did not involve any macroscopic structural injury to the muscle. However, these injuries were responsible for more than 50% of the periods of absence for club players (Ekstrand et al. 2012). In addition to the fact that muscle disorders of this type are very frequent, they can lead to structural injuries such as partial tears if they remain unrecognized and untreated. A comprehensive system for defining and classifying athletic muscle injury therefore needs to include these nonstructural or "functional" muscle disorders as well.

The diversity of diagnoses resulting from the lack of a consistent classification system covering all forms of athletic muscle disorders and the lack of an agreed terminology limit communication between the members of the medical team involved in caring for the athlete. In view of this, and on the basis of the findings of the UEFA study, it is clear that a more efficient grading and classification system needs to be developed that better reflects the differentiated range of muscle injuries seen in athletes.

Consensus Conference on Muscle Terminology and Development of a New Comprehensive Classification System

Terminology

In early 2011, the authors conducted a survey based on the hypothesis that the use of terms for muscle lesions in English is highly inconsistent. Thirty scientists and team doctors, all native English speakers, were asked to complete a questionnaire on the terminology of muscle injuries. The recipients of the questionnaires were invited on the basis of their international scientific reputation and extensive expertise as team doctors for national or first-division sports teams from the United Kingdom, Australia, the United States, FIFA, UEFA, and the International Olympic Committee. The experts included were responsible for covering a variety of different sports with high rates of muscle injury, including soccer, rugby, Australian football, and cricket.

Their responses to the survey confirmed our belief that there is marked variability in the use of the medical terminology relating to muscle injury—for example, for terms such as "strain," "tear," "pulled muscle," and "muscle hypertonia." The survey demonstrated among other things that the term "strain" is not well defined and is used categorically to cover a wide range of muscle injuries, including "functional" and "structural" disorders. The survey also clearly showed that even among sports experts, there is considerable inconsistency in the use of the terminology for muscle injuries and that there is no clear definition, differentiation, or use of the distinction between "functional" and "structural" muscle disorders. There is therefore limited comparability in the complex field of athletic muscle injuries, and this directly influences the day-to-day management of these injuries and also affects physicians' ability to develop novel therapies and to carry out systematic research and present publications on this extremely important topic.

On the basis of these findings, we organized a consensus meeting of international sports medicine experts, held on March 3, 2011 in Munich, to review the results of the survey and to discuss terminology and classification systems for athletic muscle injuries. The following members took part in the meeting (in alphabetical order):
- Prof. Dieter Blottner (author of Chapter 1)
- Prof. Jan Ekstrand (author of Chapter 5)
- Dr. Bryan English (team physician of Chelsea Football Club)
- Prof. William E. Garrett, Jr. (one of the editors of the present volume and author of Chapter 13)
- Dr. Lutz Hänsel (one of the editors of the present volume and co-author of Chapters 6, 7, 11, 12, and 16)
- Dr. Gino M.M.J. Kerkhoffs (Department of Orthopedic Surgery, Orthopedic Research Center, Academic Medical Center, University of Amsterdam)
- Dr. Steve McNally (team physician of Manchester United)
- Dr. Kai Mithoefer (Harvard Medical School; Director of Research for Major League Soccer; team physician for the United States Soccer Federation)
- Dr. Hans-Wilhelm Müller-Wohlfahrt (editor of the present volume and co-author of Chapters 6, 11, 12, and 16)
- Dr. John Orchard, MD, PhD (Associate Professor, University of Sydney; team physician for the Australian cricket team and for Sydney Roosters rugby league team)
- Dr. Patrick Schamasch (Medical and Scientific Director of the International Olympic Committee, Lausanne, Switzerland)
- Dr. Leif Swärd (Associate Professor, University of Göteborg, Sweden; team physician for Sweden's national soccer team and previously for England)
- PD Dr. Peter Ueblacker (one of the editors of the present volume and co-author of Chapters 6, 7, 11, 12, and 16)
- Prof. C. Niek van Dijk (Department of Orthopedic Surgery, Academic Medical Center, University of Amsterdam)

Practical and systematic terms for athletic muscle injuries were established at the conference (**Table 6.1**).

The survey clearly showed that the term "strain" is given different meanings and lacks differentiation. It is also a biomechanical term, and we therefore do not recommend its use. Instead, we propose using the term "tear" for structural injuries to muscle fibers/bundles that lead to a loss of continuity and contractile properties. The term "tear" better reflects structural characteristics, as opposed to the mechanism of injury, and this clearly differentiates it from *functional* injuries and allows more accurate and consistent description of injuries in order to improve communication.

Table 6.1   Terminology for muscle injuries in accordance with the 2011 Munich Consensus Conference (Müller-Wohlfahrt et al. 2012)

Category of disorder/injury	Type of disorder/injury	Definition
A Indirect muscle disorder/injury		
Functional muscle disorder		Acute indirect muscle disorder *without macroscopic evidence* of muscular injury. Often associated with a circumscribed increase in muscle tone to varying extents and predisposing to tears. Based on the etiology, there are several subcategories of functional muscle disorder
	Muscle firmness (tightness)	Increase in muscle tone to varying extents, predisposing to tears
	Fatigue-induced muscle disorder	Circumscribed longitudinal increase in muscle tone (firmness) due to overexertion, change of playing surface, or change in training patterns
	Delayed-onset muscle soreness (DOMS)	More generalized muscle pain following unaccustomed, eccentric deceleration movements
	Spine-related neuromuscular muscle disorder	Circumscribed longitudinal increase in muscle tone (firmness) due to functional or structural *spinal/lumbopelvic* disorder
	Muscle-related neuromuscular muscle disorder	Circumscribed (spindle-shaped) area of increased muscle tone (firmness). May result from dysfunctional neuromuscular control, such as reciprocal inhibition
Structural muscle injury		Any acute indirect muscle disorder *with macroscopic evidence* of muscle injury
	Minor partial muscle tear	Structural muscle injury, tear with a maximum diameter of less than a muscle fascicle/bundle (anatomically *intra*fascicular/bundle tear)
	Moderate partial muscle tear	Structural muscle injury, tear with a diameter of more than a muscle fascicle/bundle (anatomically *inter*fascicular/bundle tear)
	Subtotal/complete muscle injury	Structural muscle injury involving the subtotal/complete muscle diameter
	Tendinous avulsion	Structural tendinous injury involving the bone–tendon junction
B Direct muscle injury		
	Laceration	*Direct* muscle trauma. External injury including muscular, subcutaneous, and cutaneous tissue
	Muscle contusion	*Direct* muscle trauma, caused by blunt external force. Leading to diffuse or circumscribed hematoma. Not necessarily accompanied by structural damage to muscle tissue
Terminology lacking specific recommendation		
Strain	Not well defined and used indiscriminately for anatomically and functionally different muscle injuries (see text)	
Pulled muscle	A lay term for various undefined types/grades of muscle injury	
Hardening	Highly inconsistent use	
Hypertonia	Highly inconsistent use	
Induration	Highly inconsistent use	

Note

Undifferentiated use of the term "strain" is no longer recommended, as it is a biomechanical term that is not well defined and is used indiscriminately for anatomically and functionally different muscle injuries. Instead of this, we propose that the term "tear" should be used for structural injuries (Müller-Wohlfahrt et al. 2012).

In addition to defining the terminology, those attending the conference also carried out a detailed review of the structural and functional anatomy and physiology of muscle tissue, the epidemiology of injuries, and currently existing classification systems for athletic muscle injuries during the one-day meeting. A classification system was discussed, compared with existing classifications, reclassified, and approved. This grading system was basically developed during the last 30 years in everyday practice at the Müller-Wohlfahrt Center for Orthopedics and Sports Medicine in Munich. A preliminary version of it was published in the German edition of this book in 2010.

New Classification System

The muscle injury classification presented here is based on extensive, long-term experience and has been used successfully in the everyday management of athletic muscle injuries. The classification is empirically based and includes some new aspects of athletic muscle injuries that have not yet been described in the literature, specifically the highly relevant *functional muscle injuries*. An advanced muscle injury classification that distinguishes these injuries as separate clinical entities is extremely important for successful management of athletes with muscle injury and provides a basis for future comparative studies, as there are generally only limited scientific data for muscle injuries (Müller-Wohlfahrt et al. 2012).

The comprehensive new classification system (**Fig. 6.2**) distinguishes between indirect and direct muscle injuries. Indirect muscle injuries are subclassified into those *without* macroscopic evidence of structural damage (functional muscle disorders) and muscle injuries *with* macroscopic evidence of structural damage (structural muscle injuries).

Functional muscle injuries are subclassified into those that are overexertion-related (types 1a and 1b) and neu-

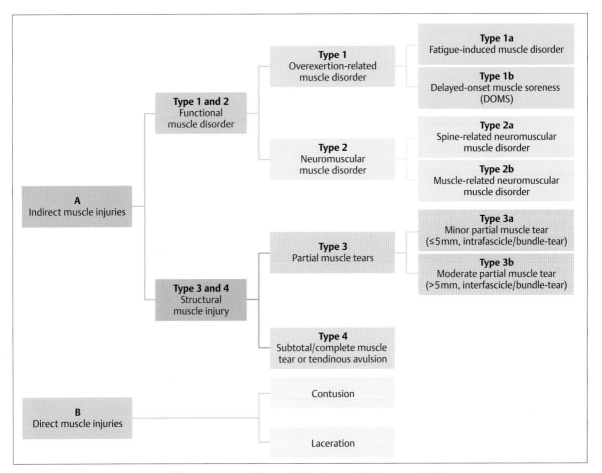

Fig. 6.2 Classification of acute muscle injuries in accordance with the 2011 Munich Consensus Conference.

Table 6.2   Comprehensive muscle injury classification: type-specific definitions and clinical presentations (adapted from Mueller-Wohlfahrt et al. 201

A   Indirect muscle injuries

Functional muscle disorders

Painful muscle disorder *without* **macroscopic evidence of muscle fiber damage**

Type	1a	1b	2a
Classification	Fatigue-induced painful muscle disorder	Delayed-onset muscle soreness (DOMS)	Spine-related* neuromuscular muscle disorder
Definition	Functional, indirect; overexertion-related	Functional, indirect; overexertion-related	Functional, indirect; neuromuscular
Description	Circumscribed longitudinal increase in muscle tone (firmness) due to overexertion, change of playing surface or change of training patterns	More generalized muscle pain after unaccustomed deceleration movements (eccentric contractions) or after long-lasting metabolic overload.	Circumscribed longitudinal increase in muscle tone due to functional or structural spinal disorder. (*Note: includes lumbopelvic region and sacroiliac joint)
Symptoms	Aching, increasing firmness. Dull ache to stabbing pain, increasing with continued activity. Can provoke pain at rest	Acute inflammatory pain, stiff, weak muscles. Pain at rest	Aching firmness. Dull ache to stabbing pain, increasing with continued activity (e.g., sprinting). No pain at rest
Onset/history	During or after activity within 24 h	Some hours after activity	During activity
Location	Focal involvement up to entire length of muscle	Mostly entire muscle or muscle group	Muscle bundle or larger muscle group along entire length of muscle
Frequently affected muscles	Dependent on sport-specific muscle recruitment and demands	Mostly untrained muscles or muscle groups	Rectus femoris, adductors, hamstrings, gastrocnemius–soleus
Palpation, clinical findings	On bilateral comparison, firm muscle band, no edema. Dull, diffuse, tolerable pain. Athlete reports "muscle tightness". Defensive reaction on muscle stretching. Pressure pain	Edematous swelling, stiff muscles. Limited range of motion in adjacent joints. Pain on isometric contraction. Therapeutic stretching leads to relief. Pressure pain	Circumscribed longitudinal increase in muscle tone. Discrete edema between muscle and fascia. Occasional skin sensitivity, defensive reaction on muscle stretching. Pressure pain
Ultrasound/MRI	Negative	Negative or edema only	Negative or edema only
MRI classification	0	0/1	0/1
Treatment	Conservative. Physical modalities and physical therapy, massage	Conservative. Physical modalities and physical therapy. Stretching, anti-inflammatory medication, rest or light exercises	Conservative. Physical modalities and physical therapy, *no* massage. Combined lumbosacral and local muscle infil
Duration (with optimal treatment)	< 1 week. Early aerobic running mostly possible on day 1 after onset	< 1 week	< 1 week. Early aerobic running mostly possible on day 1 after onset
Possible complications	Post-stress muscle imbalance—i.e., overcompensation of adjacent uninjured muscle groups. Functional compartment syndrome with severe increasing exercise-induced pain up to resting pain. Progression to structural injury	Usually harmless process. Progression to structural injury theoretically possible if symptoms are ignored	Post-stress muscle imbalance—i.e., over-compensation of adjacent uninjured muscle. Functional compartment syndrome with seve increasing exercise-induced pain up to restin. Progression to structural injury

B   Direct muscle injuries

Muscle contusion and laceration

b	3a	3b	4
Structural muscle injuries			
Any acute distraction injury of a muscle *with* macroscopic evidence of muscle fiber damage			
Muscle-related neuromuscular muscle disorder	Minor partial muscle tear	Moderate partial muscle tear	Subtotal/complete muscle tear/ tendinous avulsion
Functional, indirect; neuromuscular	Structural, indirect; partial tear	Structural, indirect; partial tear	Structural, indirect
Circumscribed spindle-shaped area of increased muscle tone. May result from dysfunctional neuromuscular control such as reciprocal inhibition	Acute distraction injury. Tear with a maximum diameter of less than a muscle fascicle/bundle	Acute distraction injury. Tear with a diameter of greater than a fascicle/ bundle	*Complete muscle rupture:* Acute distraction injury. Tear involving the subtotal/ complete muscle diameter. *Tendinous avulsion:* Involving the bone–tendon junction
Aching, gradually increasing muscle firmness and tension. Cramplike pain	Sharp, needlelike or stabbing pain. Athlete often experiences a "snap" followed by a sudden onset of localized pain	Stabbing, sharp pain, often noticeable tearing at time of injury. Athlete often experiences a "snap" followed by a sudden onset of local-ized pain	Impactlike, dull pain at time of injury. Athlete experiences a "snap"
Rapid onset during activity. Player tries to relieve symptoms by stretching	During activity, sudden onset	During activity, sudden onset. Possibly followed by fall	During activity, sudden onset. Often followed by fall
Mostly along the entire length of the muscle belly	Primarily muscle–tendon junction	Primarily muscle–tendon junction	Muscle–tendon junction/ bone–tendon junction
Hamstrings, gastrocnemius–soleus	Rectus femoris, hamstrings, adductors, gastrocnemius–soleus	Rectus femoris, adductors, hamstrings, gastrocnemius–soleus	Rectus femoris proximal, hamstrings, adductor longus; proximal
Circumscribed (spindle-shaped) area of increased muscle firmness, edematous swelling	Well-defined localized pain. Probably palpable defect in fiber structure up to 5 mm within a firm muscle band	Well-defined localized pain. Palpable defect in muscle structure	Larger (several cm) defect in muscle. Tendinous avulsion: palpable gap, hematoma. Probable muscle retraction
Therapeutic stretching leads to relief. Pressure pain without central painful point	Stretch-induced pain aggravation. Possible hematoma (usually invisible on skin surface). Pressure pain	Pain with movement. Stretch-induced pain aggravation. Often pronounced hematoma. Pressure pain	Severe pain with movement, loss of function. Massive hematoma
Negative or edema only	Positive for fiber disruption (< 5 mm) on high-resolution MRI. Intramuscular hematoma	Positive for significant fiber disruption (> 5 mm) possibly includ-ing some retraction. Often with fascial injury and intramuscular hematoma	Subtotal/complete discontinuity of entire muscle/tendon. Possible wavy tendon morphology, depending on retraction. With fascial injury and intramuscular hematoma
0/1	2	2	3
Conservative	Conservative	Conservative	Surgery recommended for tendinous avulsion with significant muscle retraction
Physical modalities and physical therapy	Physical modalities and physical therapy	Physical modalities and physical therapy	
Local infiltration. (Lumbosacral infiltra-tion in treatment-resistant cases)	Local infiltration	Local infiltration	In conservative cases: local infiltration
< 1 week	~ 10–14 days	~ 6 weeks	~ 12 weeks plus
Early aerobic running mostly possible on day 1–2 after onset	Early aerobic running mostly possible on day 5 after injury	Aerobic running mostly possible 2–3 weeks after injury	
Progression to structural injury	Recurrence, progression of tear, hematoma, myositis ossificans	Recurrence, progression of tear, hematoma, myositis ossificans, cyst formation, scarring	Recurrence, progression of tear, hematoma, myositis ossificans, cyst formation, scarring. Tendinous avulsion: recurrence, progression of tear, hematoma, myositis ossificans, cyst formation, scarring. Muscle retraction, loss of function

143

romuscular muscle disorders (types 2a and 2b). On the basis of the anatomy, *structural muscle injuries* are subclassified into partial tears (types 3a and 3b) and complete tears/tendinous avulsions (type 4).

A classification is only useful if it provides direction for therapy. With this basic idea in mind, we established divisions with increasing relevance for the athlete, for the severity of the injury, and for the duration of therapy (increasing from left to right in **Table 6.2**). **Table 6.2** shows the classification, the type-specific clinical characteristics, and details of the patient's history, as well as the treatment for each type (see also Chapter 11).

Scientific data supporting the classification system presented here, which is based on clinical experience, are still lacking. We hope that our work will stimulate research—based on the suggested terminology and classification—to prospectively evaluate the prognostic and therapeutic implications of the new classification and to specify each subclassification. A validation study by the UEFA Champions League Injury Study, involving several UEFA Champions League teams and teams in the English Premier League, is currently in progress in order to prospectively evaluate the prognostic and therapeutic implications of the new classification.

Location of the Injury

It is important to mention the location of the injury. Muscles that are frequently involved in disorders and injuries often cross two joints or have a more complex architecture, such as the adductor longus, undergoing eccentric contraction and primarily containing fast-twitch type II muscle fibers (Anderson et al. 2001, Noonan and Garrett 1999). Ninety-two percent of injuries affect the four major muscle groups in the lower limbs: hamstrings 37%, adductors 23%, quadriceps 19%, and calf muscles 13% (Ekstrand et al. 2011b). As many as 96% of all muscle injuries occur in noncontact situations, and the risk of sustaining a muscle injury is six times higher during match play than during training sessions (Ekstrand et al. 2011b). Some studies have suggested that muscles with a high proportion of fast-twitch muscle fibers are more vulnerable to injury (Noonan and Garrett 1999; see also the comments on the pennation angle in Chapter 1).

Increased susceptibility to injury is also seen in muscles that only run over a single joint, especially the adductor longus (Garrett 1996). Injuries to this muscle, as well as the other muscles in the adductor group, occur in hurdle races due to the abduction movement of the trailing leg with subsequent adduction movement over the hurdle, for instance, or in soccer in final kicks with the inner arch of the foot.

In view of the frequency of various injuries in soccer, in tennis or handball, in track and field, and in other sports, this classification is particularly directed at muscle injuries in the lower extremities. However, the classification can also be applied to the upper limb. A javelin thrower or tennis player is also more likely to suffer a muscle injury

in the legs rather than in the arms. Muscle injuries to the upper extremities are rare; the biceps and triceps brachii, as well as the pectoralis major, are the ones most likely to be injured. Tears in the pectoralis major occur in sports disciplines involving throwing and pushing, among others. The tendon tears of the rotator cuff that occur in sports, particularly in the older population, which are repeatedly described as sports injuries, are thoroughly described in the relevant specialist works and are therefore not included in this book. Injuries to the abdominal muscles occur in tennis, for instance, as a result of explosive striking movements.

Note

In sports, muscle injuries in the lower extremities are many times more frequent than those in the upper extremities.

Age

Age is also an important factor. In the many years of our observations, our impression is that muscle injuries increase markedly after the age of ~25 years, and at least for calf injuries there is evidence of this (see Chapter 5).

Changes of Surface

Practical Tip

Changes of surface—for example, from grass to a hard and unyielding gym floor or hard court—lead via input from the joints to different ranges of challenge to the musculoskeletal system. In other words, they lead to a receptor-mediated change in muscle tone:

- Action potentials are conducted from the joint receptors to the spinal cord via γ-afferents and from there via $γ_2$-efferents to the muscle spindle. Whereas the afferents react γ-dynamically with rapid adaptation, the efferents adapt slowly and create an elevated muscle tone (γ-static reflex response).
- Via type II afferents (flower-spray endings), action potentials are conducted to the spinal cord and from there via α-motor neurons to the striated muscle.

The reflex is triggered via:

- Mechanoreceptors type I and II:
  - Type I: slowly adapting receptors; these measure the joint position and affect type I muscle fibers (slow twitch fibers)—that is, the postural and/or tonic muscles.
  - Type II: rapidly adapting receptors; acceleration detectors; these are connected in a reflex arc directly via the spinal cord with type II muscle fibers (fast-twitch fibers)
- Golgi mechanoreceptors, type III

Alternatively, the reflex can result from overfacilitated spinal column segments.

The increased proprioception in the internal structures of the joints provoked by a change of surface inevitably leads to an increase in muscle tone and to premature muscle fatigue; this reaction would inhibit the healing process after a muscle injury. It must therefore be absolutely avoided during regenerative training (buildup phase).

Classic examples of an unfavorable and unnecessary change of surface in the case of soccer players are warm-up training on artificial turf, as well as stress tests (sprinting) on a Tartan Track synthetic surface instead of natural grass.

Type 1 and 2: Functional Muscle Disorders

According to Fuller et al., a sports injury is defined as "any physical complaint sustained by an athlete that results from a match/competition or training, irrespective of the need for medical attention or time loss from sportive activities" (Fuller et al. 2006). This also means irrespective of any structural damage. According to this definition, functional muscle disorders, irrespective of any structural muscle damage, also represent injuries. However, the term "disorder" may be able to differentiate functional disorders from structural injuries better. The term "functional muscle disorder" was therefore specifically chosen by the consensus conference.

As mentioned above, a UEFA study on muscle injury (Ekstrand et al. 2012) emphasizes the high clinical relevance of nonstructural muscle disorders. The study by Ekstrand et al. included data from a 4-year observation period of MRI examinations obtained within 24–48 hours after injury and demonstrated that the majority of injuries (70%) were less than MRI grade 2 and were therefore without macroscopic structural injury to the muscle. However, these injuries caused more than 50% of the periods of absence for club players (Ekstrand et al. 2012). In addition to the fact that these muscle disorders are very frequent, they can lead to structural injuries such as partial tears if they remain unrecognized and untreated. A comprehensive system for defining and classifying athletic muscle injury therefore needs to include these nonstructural or functional muscle disorders.

Note

Functional disorders are more frequent than structural injuries in professional sports.

Why should functional muscle disorders be graded? It is important to define a distinct category of functional muscle injury not only because of the different pathogenesis involved, but more importantly because it has different implications for treatment. Functional muscle injuries are always indirect disorders—i.e., not caused by external forces—and they show no macroscopic evidence of muscular injury. In animal studies, muscle fatigue has been shown to predispose to this type of injury. One study showed that in the hind leg of the rabbit, fatigued muscles absorb less energy in the early stages of stretching in comparison with nonfatigued muscle (Garrett 1996). Fatigued muscle also shows increased stiffness, which has been shown to predispose to subsequent injury. It is thought that this is partly due to altered biomechanics, which may be protective to the injured muscle but detrimental to adjacent uninjured muscle. Studies have demonstrated that reduced flexibility is significantly associated with muscle injuries. Many authors have emphasized the importance of warming up before activity and of maintaining flexibility, since a decrease in muscle stiffness is seen with warming up (Garrett 1996). A study by Witvrouw et al. (Witvrouw et al. 2003) found a strong correlation between preseason hamstring firmness (tightness) and subsequent hamstring injury in athletes. Laboratory studies have shown the detrimental effect of muscle stiffness and the critical importance of stretching and warm-up. Muscles such as the hamstrings are viscoelastic and therefore have the property of stress relaxation. Increasing the length of the musculotendinous unit causes a reduction in strain. Garrett (1996) showed in a rabbit model that simulating warm-up by stretching a muscle isometrically and then stimulating the muscle increases the longitudinal stretch required for failure.

Note

The integrity of the muscle structure remains intact in functional muscle disorders.

It should be added that a functional muscle disorder or a minor muscle injury that heals within days or a few weeks is of little significance for recreational athletes, as they are usually fully capable of continuing play or training during the treatment period. However, such disorders or injuries prevent an elite athlete from achieving full sports performance and require adequate treatment. Since decisions regarding return to play and player availability have significant financial or strategic consequences for the player and the team, functional muscle disorders are extremely important in professional athletics. This was another reason why functional muscle disorders, which might be considered minor and irrelevant at first glance, were included in this comprehensive classification.

Functional muscle disorders are multifactorial and can be classified into subgroups that reflect their clinical origin, including "overexertional" and "neuromuscular" muscle disorders. This is important, as the origin of a muscle disorder influences the treatment pathway (Müller-Wohlfahrt et al. 2012).

Figure 6.3 illustrates the anatomic location and extent of *functional* and structural muscle disorders/injuries.

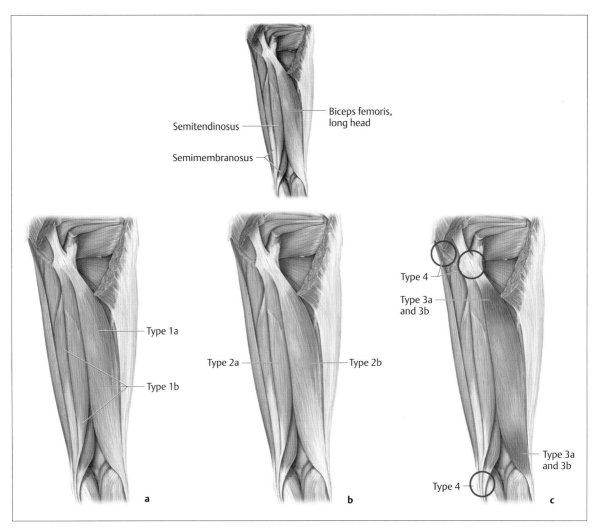

Fig. 6.3   Anatomy of the location and extent of *functional* and *structural* muscle disorders/injuries.

Type 1: Overexertion-Related Muscle Disorder

Type 1a: Fatigue-Induced Muscle Disorder

Muscle fatigue has been shown to predispose to injury (Opar et al. 2012). Fatigued muscle also demonstrates increased stiffness, which has been shown to predispose to subsequent injury (Wilson AJ and Myers PT, unpublished data, 2005).

Fatigue-induced muscle disorders are not always easily differentiated from muscle-related neuromuscular muscle disorders (type 2a). One characteristic is that the increased muscle tone extends over the entire length of a muscle and sometimes even of a muscle group. Depending on the cause, there is an onset of pulling, an increasing sense of tension, and finally pain.

Mair et al. investigated the role of fatigue in muscle injuries using the extensor digitorum longus muscles of rab-

bits. The rabbit muscles were fatigued and then stretched to failure and compared with the contralateral controls. The force to muscle failure was reduced in the fatigued leg in all groups. The authors concluded that fatigued muscles need to absorb less energy before reaching the degree of stretch that causes injuries (Mair et al. 1996).

On examination, the muscle is rigid, inelastic, and shortened. The athlete no longer feels secure and therefore—in soccer, for example—changes his positional play to avoid long sprints in rapid succession; he holds back in his style of playing. The danger of a structural injury during a sprint is particularly high in this phase, and the player suspects this. This can lead to a willingness to be substituted. The explanation is given in a statement such as "The muscle shut down," which expresses the essence of the problem very well.

Fatigue-induced muscle disorder, caused by fatigue or overload, can develop for instance during or after high-intensity training or a change of surface in the first 24 hours after overload. Depending on the cause, there is a slight pull, as well as an increased feeling of tension with persistent stress and finally a strong pull that can become piercing pain. Most often, there is no focal pain and usually no pain at rest. The athlete feels limited in his physiological range of motion. Clinically, there is no edema in the periphery of the muscle, and the hardening can be called "dry." Stretching causes a defense reaction. Fatigue-induced muscle disorder can be well treated with physical therapies such as electrotherapy, combined with massage.

Type 1b: Delayed-Onset Muscle Soreness (DOMS)

Delayed-onset muscle soreness has to be differentiated from fatigue-induced muscle injury (Böning 2002). DOMS occurs several hours after unaccustomed deceleration movements while the muscle is stretched by external forces (eccentric contractions), whereas fatigue-induced muscle disorder can also occur during athletic activity.

DOMS develops primarily in untrained individuals as a result of dynamically negative eccentric contractions with unfamiliar braking movements, which is why delayed-onset muscle soreness occurs more frequently in sports that require frequent stopping and starting (such as squash, tennis, soccer, strength sports, and hill running) than in running disciplines. It only develops in trained athletes when there is particularly strong or new exertion; recreational athletes are affected by unaccustomed training after a long interval or in altered training conditions.

Until the beginning of the 1980s, it was thought that DOMS was caused by lactate deposition in the affected muscles. This theory was contradicted by the fact that in sports associated with high lactate values, such as middle-distance running, symptoms involving delayed-onset muscle pain are rare. Technical improvements in diagnostic options made it possible to obtain visual evidence that delayed-onset muscle pain is caused by tears in the sarcomeres of individual muscle fibrils, especially around the Z disks. This was first demonstrated using electron microscopy in 1983 (Fridén et al. 1983). Numerous studies in recent decades have supported the view that microtrauma is the cause of delayed-onset muscle pain (Böning 2002).

The symptoms of DOMS occur at the earliest a few hours after exertion (in contrast to fatigue-induced muscle disorder, which can also occur during athletic activity), presumably as the result of secondary reactions, autolysis, and catabolism of the disrupted fiber structures as well as secondary edema. The primary damage to the muscle fibrils is not noticed as painful, since the pain sensors lie extracellularly in the surrounding connective tissue.

There has been discussion of a rare form of DOMS that develops after long-lasting intensive metabolism—for example, after marathons—in which inflammatory reactions with infiltration of leukocytes can be demonstrated (Böning 2002).

DOMS is not triggered by the same exertion over a period of several weeks (Mair et al. 1995); it does not cause any lasting residual damage (Böning 2002).

Type 2: Neuromuscular Muscle Disorder

Type 2a: Spine-Related Neuromuscular Muscle Disorder

The term "neuromuscular" was specifically chosen by the consensus panel to describe muscle problems involving neurogenic dysregulation. These disorders have to be clearly differentiated from neurological/neuromuscular diseases.

Two different types of neuromuscular disorder can be distinguished: a spinal or spinal nerve–related (central) type and a neuromuscular end plate–related (peripheral) type. Since muscles act as a target organ, their state of tension is modulated by electrical information from the motor component of the corresponding spinal nerve. Thus, irritation of a spinal nerve root can cause an increase in the muscle tone (see also Chapter 12).

As early as the 1980s, the senior author of this chapter (Hans-Wilhelm Müller-Wohlfahrt) began to regard the spine as being the cause of many muscle injuries and started to take this into account in treatment. This led among other things to the observation that there is a spontaneous decrease in tone after lumbar infiltration therapy (as discussed in Chapter 11) and the publication of research on the connection between lumbar spine pathology and muscle injuries (Müller-Wohlfahrt and Montag 1985, Müller-Wohlfahrt et al. 1992, Müller-Wohlfahrt 2006).

In recent years, this approach has increasingly been taken up by other authors as well. It is known that back injuries are very common in elite athletes, particularly at the L4/L5 and the L5/S1 level (Ong et al. 2003); lumbar pathology such as disk prolapse at the L5/S1 level may present with hamstring and/or calf pain and limitations in flexibility, which may result in or mimic a muscle injury (Orchard et al. 2004). However, Orchard et al. state that theoretically, any pathology relating to the lumbar spine, lumbosacral nerve roots or plexus, or sciatic nerve could result in hamstring or calf pain (Orchard et al. 2004). This could range from transient and fully reversible *functional* disturbances to permanent *structural* changes, which may be congenital or acquired. Other clinicians have also supported the concept of "back-related" (or more specifically, lumbar spine–related) hamstring injury (Orchard 2001, Verrall et al. 2001, Woods et al. 2004), although this is a controversial paradigm for researchers, as no specific mechanism has ever been identified for such injuries (Orchard et al. 2004). It might be argued that this mainly represents a back problem, with a secondary muscle disorder, not an actual muscle injury. However, the secondary muscular disorder prevents the athlete from taking part in sports and requires comprehensive treatment that includes the primary problem as well, in order to facilitate a return to sport.

However, this type of injury would logically require different forms of treatment from muscle–tendon injuries alone (Hoskins and Pollard 2005). It is therefore important that assessment of hamstring injuries should include a biomechanical evaluation, especially of the lumbar spine, pelvis, and sacrum (Woods et al. 2004).

Lumbar manifestations are not present in all cases, but the examiner and therapist have to carry out a specific search for them. Negative structural findings in the lumbar spine do not exclude nerve root irritation, due to the absence of the dynamic component that occurs in athletes' highly dynamic movements. In the absence of structural findings, functional lumbar disturbances such as lumbar or iliosacral blocking can also cause spine-related muscle disorders (Müller-Wohlfahrt 2001). The diagnosis is then established through a precise clinical and functional examination. Back-related muscle injuries are usually MRI-negative or only show edema (Orchard et al. 2004). Many clinicians also believe that athletes with lumbar spine pathology are more strongly predisposed to develop hamstring strains, although this has not been confirmed in prospective studies. Verrall et al. showed that soccer players with a history of lumbar spine injury had a higher rate of MRI-negative posterior thigh injury, but not of actual structural hamstring injury (Verrall et al. 2001).

The peripheral band of muscle fibers affected is firm (tight) along its whole length, and not only in a spindle-shaped area in a limited section, as in muscle-related neuromuscular muscle disorders (**Fig. 6.3**). As in fatigue-induced muscle disorder, the athlete feels a pulling to piercing pain that increases with persisting stress. Usually there is no resting pain. On palpation, the affected muscle is painful on pressure; sometimes there is pain just on touch.

Injection therapy is a possible treatment for the cause of the neurogenic disorder in the area of the corresponding spinal segment or iliosacral joint (see Chapter 11).

Caution

The cause of spine-related neuromuscular muscle disorders lies in structural and/or functional lumbar or iliosacral disorders.

However, dysfunctional causes are also treated, such as lumbar joint blockage or blocking of the iliosacral joints, which can lead to firmness in the functionally corresponding muscles. The athlete often does not report lumbar or iliosacral problems, but will consider them possible when specifically questioned. Spontaneous relief follows after mobilization of the affected joints.

Note

Lumbar or iliosacral joint blocking can lead to firmness in the functionally corresponding muscles. It is usually spontaneously reversible after joint mobilization.

Type 2b: Muscle-Related Neuromuscular Muscle Disorder

Disturbances of reciprocal inhibition or Renshaw inhibition can compromise the functional units that coordinate the agonists and antagonists (Müller-Wohlfahrt and Montag 1985). The results may include increased resistance to voluntary movements, making it necessary to increase the tone of the agonist muscles through increased activity of their individual motor units and the recruitment of additional motor units. Muscle tone is mainly under the control of the gamma loop, and activation of the α-motor neurons remains mainly under the control of motor descending pathways. Sensory information from the muscle is carried by ascending pathways to the brain. Ia afferent signals enter the spinal cord on the α-motor neurons of the associated muscle, but branches also stimulate interneurons in the spinal cord that act via inhibitory synapses on the α-motor neurons of antagonistic muscles. In this process, simultaneous inhibition of the α-motor neurons to antagonistic muscles (reciprocal inhibition) occurs to support muscle contraction of agonistic muscle (see Chapter 2) (Müller-Wohlfahrt et al. 2012). Dysfunction of these neuromuscular control mechanisms can result in significant impairment of normal muscle tone and can cause neuromuscular muscle disorders, when inhibition of antagonistic muscles is disturbed and agonistic muscles over-contract to compensate this (see Chapter 2) (Müller-Wohlfahrt et al. 2012). Increasing fatigue with a decline in muscle force will increase the activity of the α-motor neurons of the agonists through Ib disinhibition. The rising activity of the α-motor neurons can lead to an over-contraction of the individual motor units in the target muscle resulting in a painful muscle firmness which can prevent an athlete from sportive activities (see Chapter 2) (Müller-Wohlfahrt et al. 2012). The increase in muscle tone takes place within a few moments, a few steps or a few minutes, so that involvement of the synaptic stimulus-conducting system in the development of the condition must be assumed. The clinical evidence available to support this became the basis for further consideration. The muscle becomes inelastic, and typically there is cramping pain, which is usually not acute at first (Müller-Wohlfahrt 2001 and 2006). There is as yet no scientific proof of these concepts, but they appear to be correct from clinical observations and the success of specific therapy.

Although these ideas about the cause of the cramping pain that athletes experience and identify as "pulling" have not yet been generally accepted, due to a lack of description and publications, many athletes and trainers have already become aware of them, as seen in the increasing use of the concept of "neuromuscular injury."

The athlete often tries to resolve increased muscle tension on his own, by shaking the affected leg. But loosening—that is, releasing the tension and the pain—can usually not be achieved in that way. At first, the athlete thinks that he can still go on running. This may be possible at a slow pace, but at higher speeds, the pain quickly increases, the muscle tone becomes unphysiologically elevated, and the athlete is stopped in his tracks by what is probably hypoxemic pain. This pain only affects a limited, usually spindle-shaped, section of muscle. The athlete feels a need to stretch the muscle, but soon realizes that this will not solve the problem.

Note

Muscle-related neuromuscular muscle disorders usually occur in the muscle belly, whereas structural muscle injuries are more frequent in the area of the muscle–tendon junction.

The longer the muscle continues to be exposed to stress, the more marked the problem of strain becomes; ignoring the symptoms—for instance, in an attempt to sprint—can lead to structural injury. This is why it is so important to diagnose these lesions correctly and distinguish them from harmless muscle symptoms (for the fundamental physiological factors, see also Chapter 2).

Note

The integrity of the muscle structure remains intact in these forms of muscle disorder. It is the neuromuscular function that is disordered.

Clinically, there is neither interruption of the muscle contour, nor bleeding, nor a focal pain center as in structural injuries. Instead, there is a spindle-shaped, swollen zone as a result of the dysregulation of tone that only affects a specific section of the muscle. The symptoms are initially hard to detect by palpation. It is often only in the hours following the start of symptoms, due to the further increase in tone, that the diagnosis can be confirmed by a follow-up examination.

Practical Tip

If adequate therapeutic measures are not taken immediately, a further increase in muscle tone is observed in the hours after injury.

Muscle-related neuromuscular muscle disorders can be caused by insufficient warm-up or an abrupt change in stress—for example, switching abruptly from running backward to running forward. They can also be triggered by uncoordinated rapid movement patterns—for example, after a fall. An extreme shift in rhythm can also be causative—for example, when an athlete catches on a hurdle and the use of agonists and antagonists is insufficiently trained (when earlier training units or the warm-up program before a competition have not included sufficiently qualified and quantified sport-specific movement patterns).

In this context, it is worth noting that the frequency of these lesions has decreased significantly since stretching—with targeted dynamic mobility exercises without long static pauses, but with short intermittent stretching phases—became an established component of preparation for competitions. This ensures that sport-specific muscles in particular are well warmed up and that the best possible elasticity is achieved (see also Chapter 15).

In conclusion, it is important to recognize *functional* muscle disorders, as they can affect the athlete's ability to perform and can act as prodromal injuries, which if they are not recognized and treated can progress to *structural* muscle injuries, leading to a prolonged absence from competition. Importantly, these are also the most common muscle disorders in high-level athletes (Ekstrand et al. 2011b).

Types 3 and 4: Structural Muscle Injuries

The most important *structural* athletic muscle injuries (injuries in which there is macroscopic evidence of muscle damage) are *indirect* injuries—that is, stretch-induced injuries caused by a sudden forced lengthening beyond the elastic limits of muscles that occurs during a powerful contraction (internal force). It is the weakest point that tears: In mature patients—i.e., in most athletes—the musculotendinous junction, in adolescents the apophysis, and in elderly patients with tendon degeneration it is the diseased tendon that fails, rather than the musculotendinous junction (Taylor et al. 1993). Theoretically, a tear can occur anywhere along the muscle–tendon–bone chain. Structural injuries are usually located at the muscle–tendon junction (Clanton and Coupe 1998, Garrett 1996), since this area presents anatomic weak points. The quadriceps muscle and hamstrings are frequently affected, as they have large intramuscular or central tendons and can be injured along this interface (Garrett et al. 1989, Hughes et al. 1995).

Note

A structural muscle injury is usually located at the muscle–tendon junction, but can also occur anywhere in the muscle along the muscle–tendon–bone chain.

Type 3: Partial Muscle Tears

Most *indirect structural* injuries are partial muscle tears. Clinical experience shows that they have different prognostic relevance according to their size. *Indirect structural* injuries therefore need to be subclassified as well. Previous classification systems categorized them into injuries with focal fiber rupture of less than 5% of the muscle and focal fiber rupture of more than 5% of the muscle (Takebayashi et al. 1995, Peetrons 2002). Since this grading refers to the complete muscle size, it is relative and not consistently measurable. In this classification, different grades of muscle injuries have different sizes in various muscles—for example, they are smaller in the biceps femoris in comparison with the gracilis muscle. In addition, there is no differentiation within grade 2 or 3 injuries, so that many

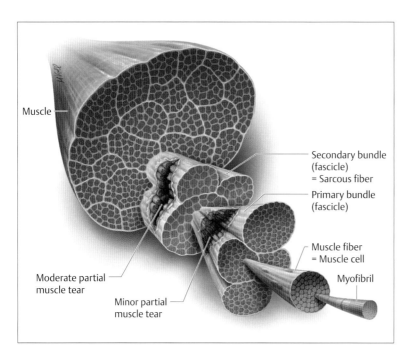

Fig. 6.4   Anatomy of the location and extent of partial muscle tears.

Muscle

Secondary bundle
(fascicle)
= Sarcous fiber

Primary bundle
(fascicle)

Muscle fiber
= Muscle cell

Moderate partial
muscle tear

Myofibril

Minor partial
muscle tear

structural injuries that have different prognostic implications are subsumed into grade 3.

A grading of *structural* injuries based on anatomic findings is better and more consistent. It may seem difficult to draw clear distinctions between partial muscle tears, due to the heterogeneity of the muscles, which may be structured very differently. However, clinical experience shows that most partial injuries can be assigned to one of two types, either a minor or a moderate partial muscle tear, which ultimately has implications for treatment and for periods of absence from sports. Preliminary data from the UEFA Champions League Study support this clinical observation.

Anatomic Background

Detailed familiarity with the muscular macroanatomy and microanatomy is important for understanding and correctly defining and classifying *indirect structural* injuries. To begin with, it must be pointed out that a symptomatic minor partial muscle tear always affects a large number of muscle fibers.

Anatomically, an individual skeletal muscle fiber represents a multinuclear cell with a diameter of 10–100 μm. An isolated tear of a single muscle fiber is therefore usually not clinically relevant (see **Fig. 1.22**; also compare the structural principles of skeletal muscle, discussed in Chapter 1).

> *Note*
>
> **Isolated tears of an individual muscle fiber are not clinically apparent.**

Muscle fibers are anatomically organized into primary and secondary muscle fascicles (bundles). About 200–250 muscle fibers constitute a primary bundle, with an average cross-sectional area of 1 mm² (Schünke et al. 2005), and are surrounded by a layer of connective tissue, the internal perimysium.

Secondary muscle bundles ("sarcous" or "flesh" fibers), with a diameter of 2–5 mm (depending on the athlete's training status) consist of several primary bundles and are surrounded by the external perimysium. They are visible to the human eye. Secondary muscle bundles have structures that can be palpated by an experienced examiner during clinical examination of healthy and injured athletes. Multiple secondary bundles constitute the muscle (**Fig. 6.4**).

> *Note*
>
> **Secondary muscle bundles (fascicles) are macroscopically visible.**

Type 3a: Minor Partial Muscle Tear (Intrafascicular/Bundle Tear)

Due to the heterogeneity of the muscles, which can be structured very differently as a result of hypertrophy or atrophy, it seems difficult to distinguish clearly between minor and moderate partial muscle tears. However, taking the anatomic factors mentioned above into account, and reflecting experience in everyday clinical work with muscle injuries, upper limits for a minor partial muscle tear in comparison with a moderate partial muscle tear can be assumed at a cross-sectional area of ~5 mm (based on the size of a secondary fascicle [bundle] or sarcous fiber).

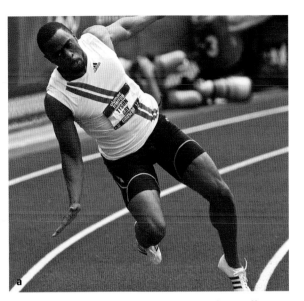

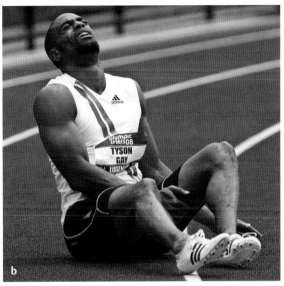

Fig. 6.5a, b Top sprinter Tyson Gay, then aged 26, suffering a moderate partial muscle tear in the left semimembranous muscle during the 100-m sprint at the US trials in July 2008. As a result of the extensive injury, the athlete is unable to prevent a fall. The fall can be interpreted as a sudden functional deficit in the muscles, but also as a defense reflex of the organism trying to prevent even more extensive damage (Photo: Rob Finch/The Oregonian).

Involvement of the adjacent connective tissue, especially the perimysium, epimysium, and fascia, also distinguishes a minor from a moderate partial muscle tear, in addition to size. Concomitant injury of the external perimysium appears to play a special role. This connective-tissue structure has an intramuscular barrier function of some sort when bleeding occurs. It may be injury to this structure (with optional involvement of the muscle fascia) that differentiates a moderate from a minor partial muscle tear.

Note

Minor partial muscle tears appear to correspond anatomically to injuries to a "sarcous/flesh fiber"— a secondary bundle (fascicle).

Figure 6.4 illustrates the anatomy of the location and extent of partial muscle tears.

Muscle healing—that is, fiber regeneration—always originates in satellite cells in the basal membrane, which are resting myofibroblasts or stem cells that are activated after an injury and serve as a source of new myoblasts (Best and Hunter 2000, Shi and Garry 2006; see also Chapter 4). The expression of collagen, especially types I and III, can in some conditions lead to the development of scarring or fibrosis. Minor partial muscle tears usually heal completely, while moderate partial tears usually result in defective healing with scar formation.

Depending on the severity of the injury, the athlete usually experiences a sharp piercing to cutting pain in a partial muscle tear. More rarely, the injury is felt as a sharp burning sensation. The athlete immediately adopts a protective posture or gait, knowing that he cannot continue playing and usually realizing at once that this would exacerbate the injury.

There is often intramuscular bleeding, which requires special therapeutic attention, as large hematomas disturb the healing of the muscle fibers and obstruct treatment. Externally visible hematomas are not expected in minor partial muscle tears, but due to the significantly increased rate of muscle perfusion during increased muscle activity, hematomas can be considerable. Especially in structural injuries, immediate first aid with cooling and compression is essential.

Type 3b: Moderate Partial Muscle Tear (Interfascicular/Bundle Tear)

As mentioned above, it is difficult to distinguish clearly between a minor partial muscle tear and a moderate one. Anatomically, the structural damage in a moderate partial muscle tear affects several secondary bundles (see **Fig. 6.4**). Falls may occur in serious partial muscle tears; this is caused by a functional deficit and a protective reflex to prevent even worse damage (**Fig. 6.5**). Clinically, a defect of 10 mm or more can often be found (for illustrations, see Chapters 7 and 8).

The external perimysium, the connective-tissue structure that forms the scaffolding for the muscle fibers and stabilizes them, is significantly involved in the injury; moreover, the muscle fascia is often involved, so that an intermuscular hematoma results. The extent of the bleeding can vary considerably, depending on whether first aid with cooling and compression is administered, and can often be seen externally, usually distal to the tear (due to gravity). But it can also be proximal, depending on the location.

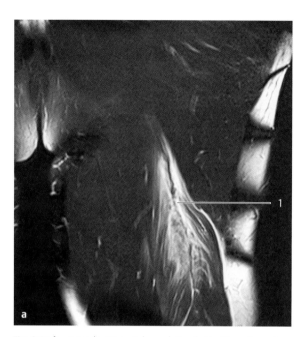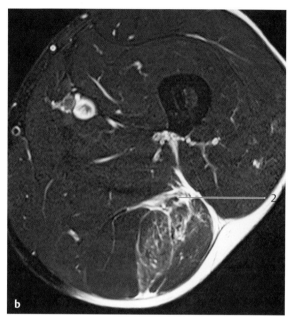

Fig. 6.6a, b   A moderate partial muscle tear in the biceps femoris muscle (1) in a 33-year-old professional soccer player in the Italian Series A, with intermuscular hematoma surrounding the sciatic nerve (2).

> **Caution**
>
> The real size of the actual structural defect is significant for classification, not the extent of a hematoma or edema.

The injury is usually located at the musculotendinous junction, but can also occur anywhere in the muscle along the muscle–tendon chain.

A special form is (partial) tearing of the intramuscular tendon (see the anatomic description in Chapter 1)—for example, (partial) tearing of the central tendon of the rectus femoris muscle. (Another special case is an isolated tear of the fascia, which usually has different biomechanical characteristics.)

> **Caution**
>
> A large muscle injury to the hamstrings, especially if it is close to the ischial nerve, can lead to special symptoms. As a result of mechanical irritation of the ischial nerve, the injured athlete experiences, among other things, a sudden, shooting, cramping pain in the hamstrings that can extend as far as the calf muscles. Because of the intense pain, it is possible for the real extent of the muscle lesion to be overestimated (see **Fig. 6.6**).

A (partial) tear of the distal gastrocnemius muscle is called "tennis leg," as the eccentric load on landing after jumps—for example, when serving, or after sideways and backward stepping—can lead to a tear (Lohrer 2007). The main area of involvement is the medial portion distal to the musculotendinous junction. This type of injury has to be distinguished from a tear of the Achilles tendon.

As mentioned above, it appears difficult to differentiate clearly between partial muscle tears due to the heterogeneity of the muscles, which can be structured very differently. Technical capabilities today (MRI and ultrasound) are not precise enough to conclusively determine and prove the effective muscular defect within the injury zone of the hematoma and/or fluid seen on MRI, which is slightly oversensitive at times (Jarvinen et al. 2005) and usually leads to overestimation of the actual damage (Müller-Wohlfahrt et al. 2012). The challenge for future research will be to find a way of precisely defining the size that describes the cut-off level between a minor and a moderate partial muscle tear.

Type 4: Subtotal/Complete Muscle Tear or Tendinous Avulsion

An extensive muscle injury can be further differentiated as a subtotal muscle tear. The distinction depends on the relative size of the muscle, even in the present classification. This appears useful, as a subtotal tear of the sartorius muscle, for example, differs in extent from a subtotal tear of the biceps femoris muscle.

Complete muscle tears with discontinuity of the entire muscle are very rare. Subtotal muscle ruptures and tendinous avulsions are more frequent (**Fig. 6.7**; for further illustrations, see also Chapters 7 and 8). Clinical experience shows that injuries involving more than 50% of the

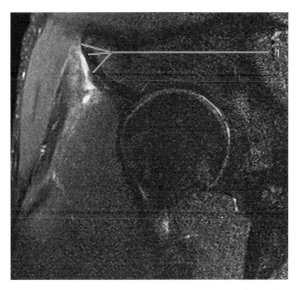

Fig. 6.7 Complete avulsion of the rectus femoris tendon at the anterior inferior iliac spine in a professional soccer player. The injury was surgically treated. 1, point of tear.

muscle diameter (subtotal tears) usually have a similar healing time to that of complete tears.

Tendinous avulsions are included in the classification system, since biomechanically they represent a total tear of the origin or insertion of the muscle. The most frequently involved locations are the proximal rectus femoris, the proximal hamstrings, the proximal adductor longus, and the distal semitendinosus.

Intratendinous lesions in the free or intramuscular tendon also occur. Pure intratendinous lesions are rare. The most frequent type is a tear near the muscle–tendon junction (e.g., in the intramuscular tendon of the rectus femoris muscle). Tendinous injuries are consistent either with the partial tear (type 3) or (sub-)total tear (type 4) in our classification system and can be included in that aspect of the classification (Müller-Wohlfahrt et al. 2012).

Clinically, there is also intermuscular bleeding, which can become quite large and can often be detected externally very early.

In professional sports, a tendinous avulsion can occur at the tendinous attachment after local (e.g., intratendinous) injection of corticoids, but also after taking substances that promote increased strength such as anabolics, since these substances lead to an imbalance between muscle strength and resistance to tendon tearing.

In our experience, the lumbar spine is very often involved as a cause of structural injuries associated with functional or structural disorders (**Fig. 6.8**). Unfortunately, there have been no informative research studies on this topic in professional sports, and empirical medicine is therefore the only source of information. However, the causal relationship between functional disorders and injuries to the spine and peripheral muscles is increasingly being taken into account in the literature (Müller-Wohlfahrt 2001, Best 2004, Orchard et al. 2004; see also Chapter 12).

A possible vicious circle involved in the pathogenesis of a structural muscle injury can be pictured as follows. Initially there is a nerve root irritation caused by disk protrusion or prolapse, spondylolisthesis, degenerative changes, joint blockages, or incorrect joint position. Even without perceptible lumbar symptoms, this leads to increased impulse emission from the motor neuron fibers to the muscles, which elevates the muscle tone in the corresponding supply area both paravertebrally and peripherally. As a result of muscle firmness, the musculature is more susceptible to tearing (see also Chapter 12).

Contusion Injuries

In contrast to *indirect* injuries (caused by internal forces), lacerations or contusions are caused by *external* forces. Thus, muscle contusions are classified as acute direct muscle injuries.

Contusion injuries are most frequently encountered in contact sports such as soccer, handball, ice hockey, etc., and differ widely in their extent (Beiner and Jokl 2001). The severity of the injury depends on the contact force, the contraction state of the affected muscle at the moment of injury, and other factors. Contusions can be graded into mild, moderate, and severe (Ryan et al. 1991).

The most frequently injured muscles are the exposed rectus femoris and the intermediate vastus, lying next to the bone, with limited room for movement when exposed to a direct blunt blow. Contusion injury can lead to either diffuse or circumscribed bleeding, which displaces or compresses muscle structures but typically does not tear the muscle fibers by longitudinal distraction. Contusions are therefore not necessarily accompanied by structural damage to muscle tissue.

Note

Bleeding caused by a contusion displaces or compresses muscle fibers, but they are usually not torn in a longitudinal way.

In muscle contusion, as for the other injuries, palpation is the simplest, fastest, and most accurate diagnostic tool. Although imaging methods such as ultrasonography or more rarely MRI are now being used more, especially to determine the extent of the injury, the clinical examination is still definitive for assessment (Beiner and Jokl 2001).

The whole area is usually painful on pressure; a large hematoma can be extremely painful. The hematoma can often even be seen on the skin, as the subcutaneous vessels are also traumatized. A distinction is made between a subfascial and an epifascial hematoma. A circumscribed hematoma may be punctured; massive hematomas that result in muscle death have to be surgically cleared.

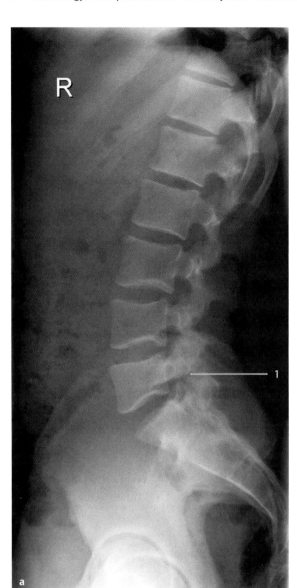

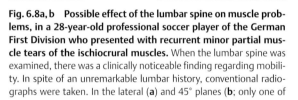

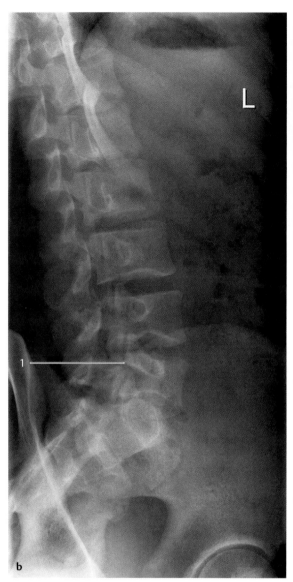

Fig. 6.8a, b   Possible effect of the lumbar spine on muscle problems, in a 28-year-old professional soccer player of the German First Division who presented with recurrent minor partial muscle tears of the ischiocrural muscles. When the lumbar spine was examined, there was a clinically noticeable finding regarding mobility. In spite of an unremarkable lumbar history, conventional radiographs were taken. In the lateral (**a**) and 45° planes (**b**; only one of the oblique views is shown here), these showed bilateral spondylolysis of the lumbar vertebra without spondylolisthesis (see also Chapter 12). After appropriate therapy with lumbar injection and stabilization exercises for the lumbar spine (core exercises), the muscular problems resolved. The player has since been playing for over 3 years without any further symptoms or recurrences.

The prognostic relevance is different from that in indirect distraction injuries. In most cases of muscle contusion, rapid resolution of symptoms can be expected with adequate therapy and hemoabsorption. Even athletes with more severe contusions can often continue playing for a longer time, whereas even a smaller indirect structural injury forces the player to stop at once (see Case 7 in Chapter 16).

A possible complication after muscle contusion, especially after a premature attempt at massage therapy or training, is the development of myositis ossificans (**Fig. 6.9**). An additional complication is the development of compartment syndrome in the compartment in which the contusion bleeding is located. If surgical fascial section is delayed, muscle necrosis can set in rapidly.

Muscle contusions were defined at the consensus conference as: "Direct muscle trauma, caused by blunt external force. Leading to diffuse or circumscribed hematoma. Not necessarily accompanied by structural damage to muscle tissue."

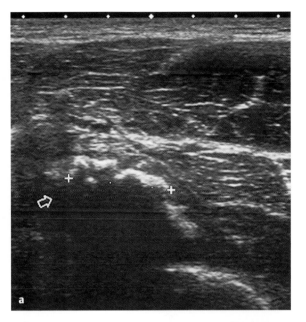

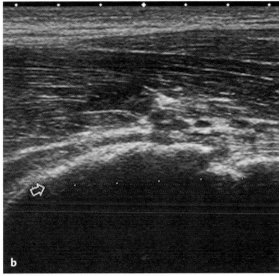

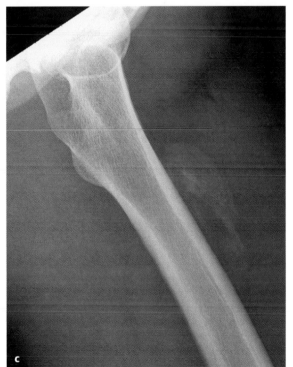

Fig. 6.9a–e X-ray, ultrasonography, and MRI of an extensive myositis ossificans in the proximal medial vastus muscle. This 33-year-old defender of the first Italian soccer league "Series A" sustained a contusion trauma to the left anterior thigh 4 weeks earlier. After inappropriate treatment with massage, the player complained of muscle firmness. Therapy after correct diagnosis consisted of lymphatic drainage and water gymnastics. Massage was avoided and indometacin was prescribed.

a, b Ultrasonography: Transversal and longitudinal sections demonstrating the large calcification (echo-rich formation with acoustic shadowing) within the muscle in an extension of 80 × 25 mm.

c Lateral X-ray confirming the diagnosis of a heterotopic ossification.

Patient History

As so often happens in medicine, an accurate diagnosis can often be reached by taking a patient history that concentrates on the injury (see also **Table 6.2**). Numerous questions are essential here:

- When did the injury occur?
- What did the athlete perceive at the moment of injury?
- Was there an external factor, a collision?
- Did he feel a stitch, or a "snap"; did the stitch feel like a needle or like a knife?
- Was the pain cramplike, developing over several steps or did it strike suddenly?
- Or did he notice a painful pull?

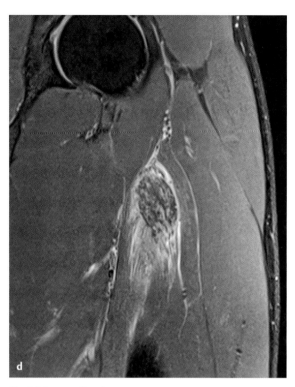 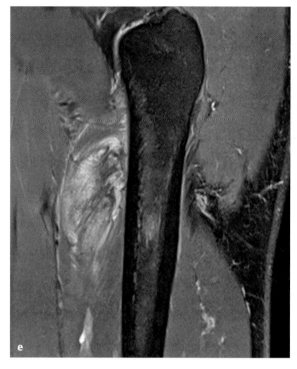

Fig. 6.9d, e *continued*

d, e MRI: Coronal and sagittal sections showing the myositis ossificans within an old intramuscular hematoma with signs of inflammatory muscular activity. Note: The calcification can be much better revealed in ultrasonography and X-ray and could be missed in MRI.

- Was the pain focal, or did it run along the whole muscle?
- Was there a fall after the muscle injury, or was the athlete able to go on running or try to continue playing?
- Did he feel signs of muscle fatigue?
- Did the muscle stretch well during warm-up, or did it take longer than usual?
- Did the legs feel heavy before the injury?
- Did the athlete train on unaccustomed new surfaces (e.g., a hard court or frozen ground)?
- Was there a change of shoes or orthotics?
- Were there new training exercises (to which a trained and highly sensitive muscle frequently reacts)?
- Was there a new trainer?
- How intense was the training stress during the previous few days?
- How many games took place during what period of time?
- Were the intervals between training sessions sufficient?
- Was there an earlier muscle or tendon injury or pain in the area of the neighboring joints or the motor chain?
- Did the spine cause problems?
- Was there an infection?

As can be seen from **Table 6.2** classifying muscle injuries, many of these questions are essential in order to arrive at an initial identification of the category. The patient history, in combination with the clinical and imaging examination, usually leads to a firm diagnosis followed by appropriate therapy.

Examination of Muscle Injuries

Examination Techniques

As always in medicine, treatment for muscle injuries has to start with a precise diagnosis, on the basis of which appropriate and targeted therapy can be initiated immediately. Our approach for diagnosis is to include a combination of the best diagnostic tools currently available, in order to address the current lack of clinical and scientific information and the lack of sensitivity and specificity of existing diagnostic modalities. A careful combination of diagnostic modalities, including medical history, inspection, clinical examination, and imaging will most likely lead to an accurate diagnosis—which should certainly be mainly based on the clinical findings and medical history and not on imaging alone, as the technology and sensitivity of imaging methods for detecting *structural muscle injury* are still undergoing development (Müller-Wohlfahrt et al. 2012).

Note

Note

For diagnosis, information should always be combined from:
1. Medical history/symptoms
2. Inspection, clinical examination, functional testing, and injury location
3. Imaging (ultrasound, MRI)

We start by inspecting the injured leg. Is there any swelling, or a visible hematoma? Inspection of the muscle contour after the athlete has tensed the muscles and pulled up the legs reveals whether there is any muscle retraction suggesting a more severe muscle injury.

Functional examination of the adjacent joints, as well as dynamic checking of the tensed muscles, should be performed as the next diagnostic steps. In case of a hamstring injury, the range of motion of the hip and knee in the injured leg may be decreased in comparison with the healthy leg (Kerkhoffs et al. 2012). Careful passive prestretching of the affected muscles can help differentiate a tear (which is painful on stretching) from a *functional* problem (which may be relieved with stretching).

Palpation

On of the most important aspects of the clinical examination is precise palpation of the injured muscle. This is indispensable for correct assessment and for initiating of appropriate measures at the right spot. A diagnosis relying on imaging alone can never take the place of a good clinical examination (Noonan and Garrett 1999, Bryan Dixon 2009). Only palpation is able to identify the tone, the condition of the musculature, possible scarring or adhesions, etc., which imaging diagnosis misses. Ultrasound and MRI can supplement these impressions, which are so important for evaluating the patient's readiness to play again, but they cannot replace them.

Palpation has to be practiced intensively to make it possible to grasp and evaluate the variety of the skeletal musculature. The smaller the muscle injury, the more difficult it is to reach an accurate diagnosis.

Note

Palpation by an experienced examiner is superior to imaging.

Deciding when full sport-specific activity is possible again is just as important as reaching the correct diagnosis. Significant experience in palpation, which allows correct assessment at the first examination and at repeated clinical check-ups, is a prerequisite for this.

A brief account of how the first author gained his initial experience in the importance of palpation may be of interest here. He became responsible for medical care for the Bayern Munich soccer team in the 1976/1977 season. Shortly before this, the club had won the European Champion Clubs' Cup for the third time. At that level, it was expected that a correct diagnosis would be reached immediately when accidents and injuries occurred—even without equipment, which was in short supply in those days and in any case was not available in the stadium—and that the best possible therapy would be initiated at once. So the expected standards were very high from the start. Just like today, the trainer or manager would always ask immediately after an injury, "What's wrong with the player?" and "When will he be able to play again?" For understandable reasons, incorrect assessments were not an option. Then as now, there was no alternative to training and perfecting one's skills in the palpation and clinical examination of injuries.

Admittedly, the examination of the skeletal muscles requires a certain amount of experience, good empathy, and intuitive talent. A physical therapist or team physician who is in daily contact with the muscles of elite athletes for examination and massage is of course able to train more rapidly and intensively in evaluating muscular problems.

Learning to palpate muscle injuries can be compared with learning cardiac auscultation. To begin with, a medical student understands little about the heart; later, he becomes able to hear the sounds, and after a great deal of practice even the very soft ⅙ heart sounds. It is the same with muscle injuries: initially, you can feel the noticeable interruptions of the structure in a larger partial tear; later on, differences in muscle tone, small structural defects, and finally the tiniest fluid deposits can also be identified. Another way of picturing training in tactile skills is to compare it with learning Braille. Here again, structures have to be felt which to the inexperienced seem too small and too complex to be able to provide any information.

Before the examination, the patient is positioned in such a way that the muscles being examined are slightly stretched; a second step in the examination takes place with the muscles relaxed—for example, with a bent knee joint (**Fig. 6.10**). It is important here to ensure that knee flexion during an examination of the rectus femoris muscle causes a slight stretching of the muscle, and relaxation of the muscle(s) during an examination of the hamstrings.

What information can be obtained from detailed palpation? Firstly, the examiner should obtain a differentiated impression of the muscle tone of the uninjured, contralateral side. This makes it possible to assess the individual physiological tension, which can vary widely.

Note

The physiological muscle tone of athletes is highly individualized and depends on training stress, type of sport (e.g., sprinting, hurdles, soccer), and other factors. It can also be different on the two sides.

The examining hand then slides broadly several times over the region of the injury that has been indicated by the patient. Impressions of the tissue—skin, subcutaneous tissue, fascia, and even the musculature already—are obtained. Next, the temperature is felt; and then a search is

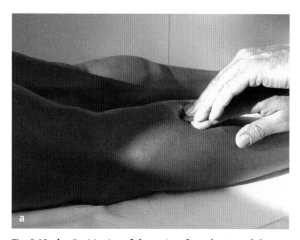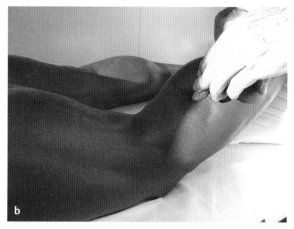

Fig. 6.10a, b Positioning of the patient for palpation of the musculature. It should be noted that knee flexion causes muscle stretching during examination of the rectus femoris muscle, but causes muscle relaxation during examination of the ischiocrural muscle.

a The examination is first performed with slightly passively tensed muscles.

b In a second stage of the examination, the relaxed muscles are palpated.

made by palpation for a band of contracted muscle that has a higher tone than the surrounding muscles. Usually, the injury is in this muscle. Where there is normal tone, a muscle injury is fairly unlikely.

Practical Tip

A muscle injury is usually located in a muscle that has a band of contraction with increased tone.

Note

A well-trained muscle can compensate better for a small partial tear.

Palpation is performed with moderate pressure and moves the skin, so that the fingertip slides on the muscle (**Fig. 6.11**). In the affected muscle bundle that has a higher tone than the surrounding muscles, the examiner tries to feel the injury by repeatedly sliding the fingers from proximal to distal and back again, and also across the grain of the fibers. The examiner should identify with the injured area as he palpates and thinks himself into the anatomic shapes and conditions; at the same time, he should observe the injured person, paying attention to visual and acoustic responses to sensation.

Practical Tip

The examination proceeds by comparing the two sides, first with relaxed and then with slightly tensed muscle, palpating from proximal to distal and then back, and also across the grain of the fibers.

Simply pressing the muscle is not enough. The examination should be performed quietly and without time pressure, so that the examiner can find his way into the anatomic situation.

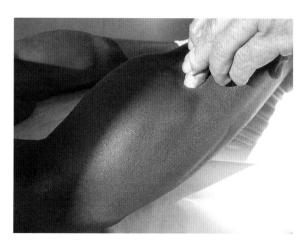

Fig. 6.11 Palpation technique. Palpation is carried out with moderate pressure and with inclusion of the skin in such a way that the fingertip slides back on the muscle from proximal to distal and also across the direction of the fibers.

For an experienced examiner, it is easier to reach a diagnosis, as the current findings are mentally compared with the mnemic imprint (engram) of typical findings observed in the past for similar injuries.

The clinical examination should include passive and active functional diagnosis over the full physiological range of motion. The examiner should ask the injured athlete to contract the muscles with the same force on both sides so that differences in the muscle outlines can be noted (**Fig. 6.12**). Careful passive prestretching of the affected muscles can help differentiate a partial tear from a muscle-related neuromuscular muscle disorder, as prestretching hurts in the former but is tolerated in the latter and tends to relieve the pain.

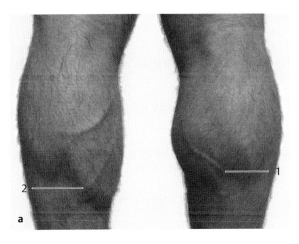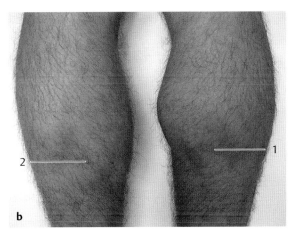

Fig. 6.12a, b   A change in the muscle outline is already visible on inspection in large muscle injuries. This is a professional soccer player who has suffered a complete avulsion of the medial head of the gastrocnemius muscle. 1, retracted medial head of the gastrocnemius; 2, normal insertion on the other side.

a In the relaxed state.

b On contraction of the calf.

> *Note*
>
> **Passive stretching is tolerated in muscle-related neuromuscular muscle disorders but not in (partial) muscle tears.**

Ultrasound Diagnosis

Ultrasound examination is useful in addition to palpation (see also Chapter 7). The quality of the instruments and the examiner's level of experience are definitely the limiting factors here. Although ultrasound can never replace a clinical examination, it does provide valuable imaging documentation of the injury, can show the difference between a functional and a structural injury, and can identify and localize a hematoma. The course of the injury can also be documented in images.

Magnetic Resonance Imaging (MRI)

MRI (see also Chapter 8) is now being used more and more frequently. In our opinion, it is not yet optimally suited to providing an exact image of a small structural injury. All too often, especially where the image quality is inadequate, it exaggerates the extent of the actual injury by the way it visualizes the extent of edema or bleeding. However, the technology and its sensitivity for detecting *structural muscle injury* are continuing to evolve. We recommend MRI for every injury that is suspicious for *structural muscle injury*. MRI is helpful in determining whether edema is present, in what pattern, and if there is a structural lesion, including its approximate size (Müller-Wohlfahrt et al. 2012). MRI is also helpful for confirming the site of an injury and any tendon involvement (Askling et al. 2007). However, it must be pointed out that MRI alone is not sufficiently sensitive to measure the extent of

muscle tissue damage accurately. For example, it is not possible to judge from the scans where edema or hemorrhage (displayed as a strong signal) are obscuring muscle tissue that has not been structurally damaged (Müller-Wohlfahrt et al. 2012).

Ekstrand et al. reported that there is a significantly and clinically relevant more rapid return to sports in MRI-negative cases (without edema) in comparison with MRI grade I injuries (with edema, but without fiber tearing) (Ekstrand et al. 2001b). Similar findings have also been described by others (Verrall et al. 2001). However, muscle edema is a very complex issue, and in our opinion too little is known about it so far. We therefore mention in the classification system that there are several *functional disorders* that may present *with or without* edema (see **Table 6.2**). This is in our view the best way of handling the currently insufficient data (Müller-Wohlfahrt et al. 2012). We believe that discussion of the phenomenon of edema is premature at present, but will become a focus of advanced research in the future, with more precise imaging and with studies based on a common terminology and classification.

Laboratory Diagnosis

The information provided by laboratory values is marginal for evaluating muscle injuries. After training stress, athletes almost always have elevated creatine kinase and myoglobin levels. The creatine kinase can rise to several thousand units per liter (see Chapters 3 and 9).

> *Note*
>
> **Laboratory values are not informative for interpreting muscle injuries. Creatine kinase and myoglobin are usually elevated after training stress.**

Typical Findings on Examination

The findings for the individual muscle disorders and injuries, so far as this is descriptively possible, are presented below (see also **Table 6.2**).

Type 1a: Fatigue-Induced Muscle Disorder

Clinically, there is a muscle band that is firm in comparison with the contralateral side. This is usually detectable along the entire length of the muscle. There is dull pain over a wide area; on stretching, there is a defensive reaction. In contrast to spine-related neuromuscular muscle disorder, this lesion usually does not present with edema.

Type 1b: Delayed-Onset Muscle Soreness (DOMS)

Whereas fatigue-induced muscle disorders lead to aching and increasing, circumscribed firmness, with a dull ache to stabbing pain that increases with continued activity, and with no pain at rest, DOMS causes a characteristic acute inflammatory pain with stiff and weak muscles and pain at rest and on movement. The range of motion of adjacent joints is secondarily limited; pain is at a maximum after 1–3 days. Isometric contractions are particularly painful.

DOMS pain resolves spontaneously within a few days, usually a week, in contrast to fatigue-induced muscle disorder, which can persist for several weeks if it remains unrecognized and untreated and can cause structural injuries such as partial tears. These two types of functional muscle disorder therefore have to be distinguished.

Recommended measures for pain reduction in DOMS are mild activities that promote circulation, and relaxed training with avoidance of any force exertion (e.g., relaxed cycling, water exercises), careful passive stretching and heat treatment (sauna) and, if necessary, nonsteroidal anti-inflammatory drugs.

Thorough warm-up, stretching and massage, and antioxidants, enzymes, magnesium, zinc and alkaline minerals are administered to improve muscle function. Information about effects is only available for the first of these measures (McHugh 1999).

Type 2a: Spine-Related Neuromuscular Muscle Disorder

The affected muscle band is firm along its entire length (the contralateral side should be compared) and shows a small edema between muscle and fascia. This edema can sometimes also be visualized sonographically or on MRI. The muscle is painful on palpation; when it is stretched, the pulling sensation increases, and the athlete shows a defensive reaction. Sometimes even the skin is sensitive to touch.

It is essential to examine the lumbar spine, the iliosacral spine, and possibly the hip joints. The cause of the disorder can be identified here in the form of a functional segmental problem, blockage, another type of dysfunction, or a structural problem—for example, a prolapsed disk or spondylolisthesis.

Type 2b: Muscle-Related Neuromuscular Muscle Disorder

A spindle-shaped, thickened zone can be palpated which is swollen with edema and extends over 10–20 cm, usually in the area of the muscle belly. The integrity of the tissue is maintained; no interrupted fibers, hematoma, or focal pain can be detected. Therapeutic stretching does not elicit a defensive reaction and can even help relieve the symptoms.

Clinical Case

A specific example of incorrect evaluation of a muscle-related neuromuscular muscle disorder: Detailed diagnostic work, including palpation and functional tests, during the half-time interval in an international soccer game confirmed the diagnosis of a type 2a lesion in a midfield player. Initial therapeutic measures such as muscle release, strain–counterstrain, and spray and stretch were carried out. These measures already led to improvement in the symptoms. This was followed by injection therapy. A liniment bandage was applied, and the player was given medications (without nonsteroidal anti-inflammatory drugs or other pain medication).

The player's club was informed of these measures in writing. The next day, the team physician requested an MRI, which led to diagnosis of a moderate partial muscle tear. A rest period of several weeks was ordered. The reason for this was the fluid that had been injected the day before, which was incorrectly overinterpreted on the MRI as representing hematoma or edema. Due to insufficient resolution of the muscle structures on the MRI, the fluid expansion had been evaluated as the only criterion for a partial muscle tear.

However, the healing process progressed rapidly; the player was able to train again after a few days and competed in a league game after 9 days. This course unequivocally contradicted the diagnosis suggested on the basis of the MRI.

Type 3a: Minor Partial Muscle Tear (Intrafascicular/Bundle Tear)

This type of injury usually occurs in the area of the musculotendinous junction. Fairly large interruptions of muscle tissue on a scale of millimeters are detected within a firm muscle.

During the first minutes of a partial muscle tear, the structural defect is filled with only a little blood; as time goes on, there is usually increased bleeding into the muscle gap, which makes the latter harder to find on palpation. A structural injury is therefore best diagnosed immediately after the injury. First aid plays an important role in later evaluation of the severity of the injury; when first-aid treatment has been optimal (with compression and ice water), a minor partial muscle tear appears less severe (not only on imaging) than if there has been no treatment or only delayed treatment.

A minor partial muscle tear is focally painful on pressure; however, the pain focus indicated by the patient is not necessarily the same as the point of the tear. In contrast to a muscle-related neuromuscular muscle disorder, the athlete cannot tolerate stretching of the muscle.

In the hours after injury, an inflammation lasting for several days develops and the injured area becomes swollen. The portions of the muscle bundle lying immediately distal and proximal to the injury develop a tone that is often considerably elevated. The muscle is attempting through this mechanism to protect the torn area (defensive spasm). Palpation has to locate this type of ribbonlike shortened band of muscle fibers, which has a higher tone than the surrounding musculature. The injury can usually be found in this muscle band.

Type 3b: Moderate Partial Muscle Tear (Interfascicular/Bundle Tear) and Type 4: Subtotal/Complete Muscle Tear or Tendinous Avulsion

A moderate partial muscle tear is also usually found at the musculotendinous junction and this is also the case, although much less frequently, with a complete muscle tear. A tendinous avulsion of the muscle is often called a "complete muscle tear," although in this case the muscle is intact.

In a moderate partial muscle tear, examination reveals a pressure-sensitive center; the interruption of the muscle structure is clearly palpable and can often extend for more than 10 mm. If the fascia is also injured, a rapidly growing, extensive intermuscular hematoma develops; if the fascia is not injured, the hematoma can only expand within the muscle. Here again, later evaluation largely depends on the initial treatment and the extent of bleeding into the structural defect.

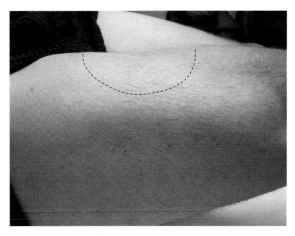

Fig. 6.13 A subtotal tear of the rectus femoris in a recreational soccer player. Inspection from the side shows a distinct depression of the muscle outline (dotted line).

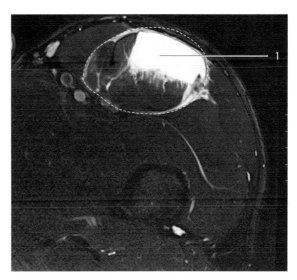

Fig. 6.14 An extensive old seroma in the rectus femoris muscle in a professional soccer player who was released for full training with this lesion by his team's medical division. 1, seroma; dotted line, boundary of the rectus femoris muscle.

There is also pain on movement, and even attempted slight stretching can intensify the symptoms. Moreover, there is a significant functional deficit and pronounced hematoma in the area of the injury. In a partial muscle tear, it can be seen that the muscle outline is changed in comparison with the contralateral side (**Fig. 6.13**).

In overlooked more severe muscle injuries, there is often significant hardening proximal and distal to the tear; the stump ends can be felt until consolidation. A seroma can sometimes be palpated. Overlooked large injuries of this type can even be observed in elite athletes who are supposedly receiving first-class medical care (**Fig. 6.14**).

In tendinous avulsion of the muscle, there is circumscribed pain on pressure at the point of the tear—for ex-

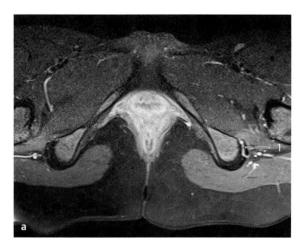 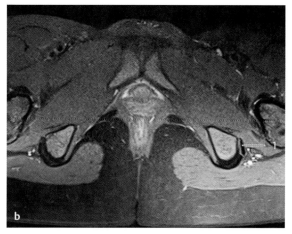

Fig. 6.15a, b Partial deinsertion of the semimembranosus tendon at the ischial tuberosity (1) with associated peritendinitis in a 22-year-old professional dancer. The origins of the tendons from the semitendinosus and biceps femoris muscles are intact.

a Initial MRI at the first visit, after 12 weeks of unsuccessful therapy at another institution.

b MRI during the subsequent course, after 8 weeks of adequate therapy with injections at the ischial tuberosity and along the course of the muscle to decrease tone, along with physical thera-

py and instructions not to stretch the ischiocrural muscle. The images during the subsequent course show distinct closing of the distance from the tendon to the tuberosity, from a previous dehiscence of 3.6 mm to 1.6 mm (1), although the situation is not yet normal.

ample, at the ischial tuberosity in avulsion of the proximal hamstrings. The tendon stump can often be palpated, and the tendon and muscle show a loss of tension. In functional testing, the muscle contracts but cannot deploy its force via the torn tendon, so that joint movement is either absent or distinctly reduced.

Practical Tip

Proximal hamstring avulsions at the origin (ischial tuberosity) can be treated conservatively if no significant retraction is found (**Fig. 6.15**).

Other Muscle Injuries and Causes of Muscle Symptoms

Functional Compartment Syndrome

Functional compartment syndrome rarely occurs in sports, but it must not be omitted from the differential diagnosis. The syndrome, which results from prolonged intensive training or competition, mediated primarily through the fatigue mechanism, involves muscle firmness and ischemia, with inflammatory tissue reactions and finally intramuscular edema formation with a painful increase in pressure in the affected muscle bed.

Clinical Case

In advance of the soccer World Cup in 2006, there was an event that attracted considerable public attention: during training in the days before the match, one of the players developed muscle symptoms in the calf

that resolved with treatment, so that he thought he would still be able to play in the opening match. However, with treatment still incomplete and with positive, conspicuous findings on palpation, he was advised for medical reasons against playing, due to the risk of further damage and a potential need for early substitution during the match, with all the possible consequences for the team.

After 2 more days of rest and intensive treatment with oral enzymes, lumbar infiltration to relieve muscle tone, and sympathetic down-regulation (see Chapter 11), as well as physical and physical-therapy measures, he was able to return to complete participation in the subsequent matches.

Apophyseal Avulsion

In young people, apophyseal avulsions occur most frequently in the area of the pelvis. The cause is an incorrect relationship between growing muscle power and the tensile strength of the cartilaginous portions of the apophyses (Best 1995, Wolff 2007).

Here again, a clinical examination with detailed palpation is informative. Additional diagnostic measures include conventional radiological imaging, sonography, and, if necessary, MRI.

The most frequently seen locations are in the anterior superior iliac spine, with the origins of the sartorius and the tensor fasciae latae muscles, and in the anterior inferior iliac spine, with the origin of the rectus femoris muscle (**Fig. 6.16**).

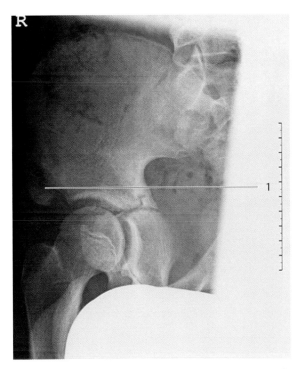

Fig. 6.16 An apophyseal avulsion of the rectus femoris muscle at the anterior inferior iliac spine (1) in a 14-year-old junior soccer player.

Apophyseal avulsions can usually be treated conservatively. A sufficiently long period of rest from sports, lasting up to 12 weeks, is essential.

Other Conditions

Symptoms in the skeletal muscles are among the most frequent in medicine. They have a wide variety of causes, and the differential diagnosis is often difficult. Among many other things, muscle pain that develops in individuals with a significant vitamin D deficiency has to be considered. A comprehensive overview of nontraumatic differential diagnoses is given in Chapter 9.

Complications

Post-Stress Muscle Imbalance

Post-stress muscle imbalance involves overcompensation of adjacent uninjured muscle groups. Continual stress results in an increase in the muscle tone in an adjacent muscle in the same muscle group, which can also be injured by continuing stress.

Recurrence

Of all the common sports injuries, muscle injuries have one of the highest recurrence rates after return to play (Orchard and Best 2002). The recurrence rate for hamstring injuries is about 14% in track and field athletes (Malliaropolous et al. 2011), about 16% in professional soccer (Ekstrand et al. 2011b), 23% in rugby (Brooks et al. 2006), and around 30% in professional Australian football (Orchard and Best 2002, Orchard et al. 2005).

One plausible cause of recurrent muscle injures, which are significantly more severe than the first injury (Ekstrand et al. 2011b, Best 1995), is a premature return to full activity due to the injury being underestimated. Healing of muscle and other soft tissue is a gradual process. The connective (immature) tissue scar produced at the injury site is the weakest point in the injured skeletal muscle (Jarvinen et al. 2005), with full strength in the injured tissue taking time to return, depending on the size and location of the injury. Previous injury without total healing of muscle tissue and without total recovery of tensile strength thus predisposes to a more severe recurrent injury. Only mature scar is as stiff as or even stronger than healthy muscle. It appears plausible that athletes often return to sport before muscle healing is complete. As Malliaropolous et al. have stated, "it is therefore crucial to establish valid criteria to recognize severity and avoid premature return to full activity and the risk of reinjury" (Malliaropolous et al. 2010). However, there are at present no consensus guidelines or agreed criteria for a safe return to sport following muscle injury.

> *Note*
> **If a muscle injury is misdiagnosed, there is a very high risk of reinjury.**

In our opinion, recurrences can be significantly reduced if precise evaluation and diagnosis are carried out. These are critical for adequate assessment and treatment of a muscle injury. Since the pain caused by a *structural* muscle injury often subsides shortly after the injury, this may tempt the patient to use the injured muscle at a preinjury level. Regular follow-ups with up-to-date assessment of healing progress are critically important for making any adjustments that may be needed in the timing and nature of proposed therapies.

> *Note*
> **Pain is not a good indicator for safe return to sport, as it often subsides shortly after the injury.**

Seroma and Cyst

Particularly in the case of more severe tears, a seroma can form that remains clinically inapparent for a time. It is also possible for intramuscular cysts to develop after an exten-

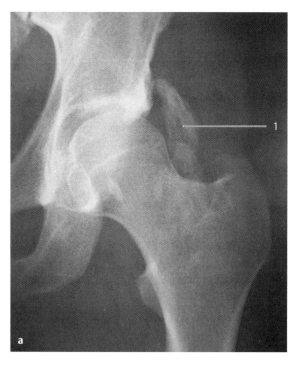

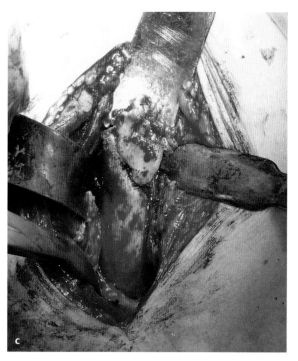

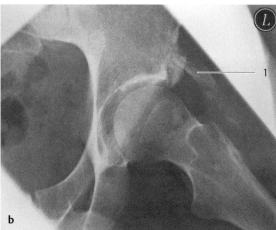

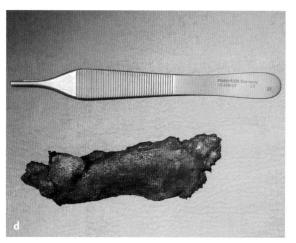

Fig. 6.17a–d   Heterotopic ossification after an old, overlooked avulsion injury of the reflected head of the rectus femoris muscle in a 40-year-old amateur athlete. The ossification bridge had reduced hip flexion to 95° and internal rotation to 0°. (Images **c** and **d** kindly provided by Prof. M. Dienst.)

a, b Anteroposterior (**a**) and axial conventional (**b**) radiographs.
1, ossification bridge.
c Exploration via the anterior approach used in the Smith-Petersen operation in the fascia of the tensor fasciae latae muscle to protect the lateral femoral cutaneous nerve. Resection of the

ossification bridge, which extended laterally as far as the pars reflecta and arched to the lateral capsule, without further injury to the muscle.
d Size of the main resection specimen: 10 × 4 × 3 cm. The consistency resembled cortical bone.

sive injury. A cyst differs from a seroma in that it is encapsulated (for images, see Chapters 7 and 8).

Fibrosis/Scarring

Both a circumscribed and a diffuse hematoma can become fibrotic as a result of ingrowth of connective tissue. A larger or smaller fibrotic scar can form and may lie inside or outside of the muscle. If the scar has not yet become stable during the course of healing, it will tear if there is premature exertion. If a scar heals in a stable state, it is practically impossible to stretch it and it can be palpated as a gross hardening. If the scar is intramuscular, therefore, tears in the normal proximal and distal adjacent muscle bundles, which have to take over the elasticity function, are not uncommon (see Chapters 7 and 8).

Traumatic Compartment Syndrome

Traumatic compartment syndrome can occur particularly in cases of muscle contusion with massive bleeding and without injury to the fascia. It is caused by an increase in pressure resulting from bleeding in the corresponding muscle bed surrounded by fascia. The lower leg is primarily affected; involvement of the thigh is not as frequent, and involvement of the arms is rare. The increase in pressure disrupts the (micro-)circulation, causing a transitory to permanent loss of nervous and muscular function and even possible tissue death, in the form of necrosis. The first and most important symptom is unbearable pain, and less frequently a neurovascular deficit. Surgical splitting of the affected compartment is usually indispensable in a traumatic compartment and must be carried out at an early stage.

In an extensive structural injury, in which there may also be profuse bleeding, the blood may escape from the compartment as a result of the often concomitant injury to the fascia, so that compression of structures is very rare.

Myositis Ossificans and Heterotopic Ossification

Extraosseous calcification or heterotopic ossification can occur at almost any location of a former injury. Myositis ossificans is the intramuscular form and occurs, for instance, after contusion injuries with extensive bleeding, especially if massage was administered early to the injured area (see **Fig. 6.9**).

The first dense, calcified shadows can be seen 7–10 days after the trauma on conventional radiographs (Wolff 2007), and earlier on ultrasound. These are hyperechoic structures (see Chapters 7 and 8), which with further progression can develop into heterotopic bone material with spongy and cortical portions. The calcifications are frequently missed on MRI, as they are often indistinguishable from other tissue such as tendons, etc.

Treatment depends on the symptoms. Surgical resection is indicated when there is extensive ossification, with limitation of muscular function or joint movement (**Fig. 6.17**).

Prophylactic administration of nonsteroidal anti-inflammatory agents (e.g., indometacin) or anti-inflammatory radiation can be considered.

Muscle Hernia

Muscles can protrude through a defect in the fascia after an extensive muscle injury, causing an externally visible "swelling." During training, this can cause pain, increased protrusion, and a loss of function. If the symptoms are pronounced, surgical closure of the fascia or widening of the fascial defect by fasciotomy is necessary. The latter becomes necessary if closure of the fascia would cause increased pressure in the compartment.

References

Alonso JM, Junge A, Renström P, Engebretsen L, Mountjoy M, Dvorak J. Sports injuries surveillance during the 2007 IAAF World Athletics Championships. Clin J Sport Med 2009; 19 (1): 26–32

Anderson K, Strickland SM, Warren R. Hip and groin injuries in athletes. Am J Sports Med 2001; 29(4): 521–533

Andersen TE, Engebretsen L, Bahr R. Rule violations as a cause of injuries in male Norwegian professional football: are the referees doing their job? Am J Sports Med 2004; 32(1 Suppl): 62S–68S

Armfield DR, Kim DH, Towers JD, Bradley JP, Robertson DD. Sports-related muscle injury in the lower extremity. Clin Sports Med 2006; 25(4): 803–842

Árnason Á, Sigurdsson SB, Gudmundsson Á, Holme I, Engebretsen L, Bahr R. Risk factors for injuries in football. Am J Sports Med 2004; 32(1, Suppl): 5S–16S

Askling CM, Tengvar M, Saartok T, Thorstensson A. Acute first-time hamstring strains during high-speed running: a longitudinal study including clinical and magnetic resonance imaging findings. Am J Sports Med 2007; 35(2): 197–206

Beiner JM, Jokl P. Muscle contusion injuries: current treatment options. J Am Acad Orthop Surg 2001; 9(4): 227–237

Best TM. Muscle–tendon injuries in young athletes. Clin Sports Med 1995; 14(3): 669–686

Best TM. Soft-tissue injuries and muscle tears. Clin Sports Med 1997; 16(3): 419–434

Best TM, Hunter KD. Muscle injury and repair. Phys Med Rehabil Clin N Am 2000; 11(2): 251–266

Best TM. Commentary to: Lumbar spine region pathology and hamstring and calf injuries in athletes: Is there a connection? Br J Sports Med 2004; 38(4): 504

Böning D. Delayed-Onset Muscle Soreness (DOMS). Dtsch Arztebl 2002; 99(6): 372–377

Borowski LA, Yard EE, Fields SK, Comstock RD. The epidemiology of US high school basketball injuries, 2005–2007. Am J Sports Med 2008; 36(12): 2328–2335

Brooks JH, Fuller CW. The influence of methodological issues on the results and conclusions from epidemiological studies of sports injuries: illustrative examples. Sports Med 2006; 36 (6): 459–472

Brophy RH, Wright RW, Powell JW, Matava MJ. Injuries to kickers in American football: the National Football League experience. Am J Sports Med 2010; 38(6): 1166–1173

Bryan Dixon J. Gastrocnemius vs. soleus strain: how to differentiate and deal with calf muscle injuries. Curr Rev Musculoskelet Med 2009; 2(2): 74–77

Chan O, Del Buono A, Best TM, Maffulli N. Acute muscle strain injuries: a proposed new classification system. Knee Surg Sports Traumatol Arthrosc 2012; 20(11): 2356–2362

Clanton TO, Coupe KJ. Hamstring strains in athletes: diagnosis and treatment. J Am Acad Orthop Surg 1998; 6(4): 237–248

Dvorak J, Junge A, Grimm K. Thigh injuries. In: FIFA, eds. FIFA F-Marc football medicine manual. 2nd ed. Zurich: FIFA; 2009: 176–181

Ekstrand J, Karlsson J. The risk for injury in football. There is a need for consensus about definition of the injury and the design of studies. Scand J Med Sci Sports 2003;13:147–149

Ekstrand J, Hägglund M, Waldén M. Injury incidence and injury patterns in professional football: the UEFA injury study. Br J Sports Med 2011a; 45(7): 553–558

Ekstrand J, Hägglund M, Waldén M. Epidemiology of muscle injuries in professional football (soccer). Am J Sports Med 2011b; 39(6): 1226–1232

Ekstrand J, Healy J, Waldén M, Lee J, English B, Hägglund M. Hamstring muscle injuries in professional football: the correlation of MRI findings with return to play. Br J Sports Med 2012; 46(2): 112–117

Feeley BT, Kennelly S, Barnes RP, et al. Epidemiology of National Football League training camp injuries from 1998 to 2007. Am J Sports Med 2008; 36(8): 1597–1603

Fridén J, Sjöström M, Ekblom B. Myofibrillar damage following intense eccentric exercise in man. Int J Sports Med 1983; 4 (3): 170–176

Fuller CW, Ekstrand J, Junge A, et al. Consensus statement on injury definitions and data collection procedures in studies of football (soccer) injuries. Clin J Sport Med 2006; 16(2): 97–106

Garrett WE Jr, Rich FR, Nikolaou PK, Vogler JB III. Computed tomography of hamstring muscle strains. Med Sci Sports Exerc 1989; 21(5): 506–514

Garrett WE Jr. Muscle strain injuries. Am J Sports Med 1996; 24 (6, Suppl): S2–S8

Hägglund M, Waldén M, Bahr R, Ekstrand J. Methods for epidemiological study of injuries to professional football players: developing the UEFA model. Br J Sports Med 2005; 39(6): 340–346

Hägglund M, Waldén M, Ekstrand J. Injuries among male and female elite football players. Scand J Med Sci Sports 2009; 19 (6): 819–827

Hawkins RD, Hulse MA, Wilkinson C, Hodson A, Gibson M. The Association Football medical research programme: an audit of injuries in professional football. Br J Sports Med 2001;35 (1): 43–47

Hoskins WT, Pollard HP. Successful management of hamstring injuries in Australian Rules footballers: two case reports. Chiropr Osteopat 2005; 13(1): 4–8

Hughes C IV, Hasselman CT, Best TM, Martinez S, Garrett WE Jr. Incomplete, intrasubstance strain injuries of the rectus femoris muscle. Am J Sports Med 1995; 23(4): 500–506

Järvinen TA, Järvinen TL, Kääriäinen M, Kalimo H, Järvinen M. Muscle injuries: biology and treatment. Am J Sports Med 2005; 33(5): 745–764

Järvinen TA, Järvinen TL, Kääriäinen M, et al. Muscle injuries: optimising recovery. Best Pract Res Clin Rheumatol 2007; 21(2): 317–331

Kerkhoffs GM, van Es N, Wieldraaijer T, Sierevelt IN, Ekstrand J, van Dijk CN. Diagnosis and prognosis of acute hamstring injuries in athletes. Knee Surg Sports Traumatol Arthrosc 2013; 21(2): 500–509

Lohrer H. Muskelverletzungen. In: Dickhuth HH, Mayer F, Röcker K, Berg A, eds. Sportmedizin für Ärzte. Cologne: Deutscher Ärzte-Verlag; 2007: 397–398

Lopez V Jr, Galano GJ, Black CM, et al. Profile of an American amateur rugby union sevens series. Am J Sports Med 2012; 40(1): 179–184

McHugh M. Can exercise-induced muscle damage be avoided? Br J Sports Med 1999; 33(6): 377

Mair J, Mayr M, Müller E, et al. Rapid adaptation to eccentric exercise-induced muscle damage. Int J Sports Med 1995; 16(6): 352–356

Mair SD, Seaber AV, Glisson RR, Garrett WE Jr. The role of fatigue in susceptibility to acute muscle strain injury. Am J Sports Med 1996; 24(2): 137–143

Malliaropoulos N, Papacostas E, Kiritsi O, Papalada A, Gougoulias N, Maffulli N. Posterior thigh muscle injuries in elite track and field athletes. Am J Sports Med 2010; 38(9): 1813–1819

Malliaropoulos N, Isinkaye T, Tsitas K, Maffulli N. Reinjury after acute posterior thigh muscle injuries in elite track and field athletes. Am J Sports Med 2011; 39(2): 304–310

Müller-Wohlfahrt HW, Montag HJ. Diagnostik und Therapie der sogenannten Muskelzerrung, Diagnosis and therapy of "pulled muscle." Dtsch Z Sportmed 1985; 11: 246–248

Müller-Wohlfahrt HW, Montag HJ, Kübler U. Diagnostik und Therapie von Muskelzerrungen und Muskelfaserrissen. Dtsch Z Sportmed 1992; 3: 120–125

Müller-Wohlfahrt HW. Diagnostik und Therapie von Muskelzerrungen und Muskelfaserrissen. Sportorthopädie – Sporttraumatologie 2001; 17: 17–20

Müller-Wohlfahrt HW. Diagnostik und Therapie von Zerrungen und Muskelfaserrissen im Hochleistungssport. Frankfurt am Main: Deutscher Fussball-Bund; 2006

Mueller-Wohlfahrt HW, Haensel L, Mithoefer K, et al. Terminology and classification of muscle injuries in sport: The Munich consensus statement. Br J Sports Med 2012; Epub ahead of print. Open access on: www.bjsm.com or www.pubmed.org

Noonan TJ, Garrett WE Jr. Muscle strain injury: diagnosis and treatment. J Am Acad Orthop Surg 1999; 7(4): 262–269

O'Donoghue DH. Treatment of injuries to athletes. Philadelphia: Saunders; 1962: 51–56

Ong A, Anderson J, Roche J. A pilot study of the prevalence of lumbar disc degeneration in elite athletes with lower back pain at the Sydney 2000 Olympic Games. Br J Sports Med 2003; 37(3): 263–266

Opar DA, Williams MD, Shield AJ. Hamstring strain injuries: factors that lead to injury and re-injury. Sports Med 2012; 42 (3): 209–226

Orchard JW, Marsden J, Lord S, Garlick D. Preseason hamstring muscle weakness associated with hamstring muscle injury in Australian footballers. Am J Sports Med 1997; 25(1): 81–85

Orchard JW. Intrinsic and extrinsic risk factors for muscle strains in Australian football. Am J Sports Med 2001; 29(3): 300–303

Orchard J, Best TM. The management of muscle strain injuries: an early return versus the risk of recurrence. Clin J Sport Med 2002; 12(1): 3–5

Orchard JW, Farhart P, Leopold C. Lumbar spine region pathology and hamstring and calf injuries in athletes: is there a connection? Br J Sports Med 2004; 38(4): 502–504, discussion 502–504

Orchard JW, Best TM, Verrall GM. Return to play following muscle strains. Clin J Sport Med 2005; 15(6): 436–441

Orchard JW, Best TM, Mueller-Wohlfahrt HW, et al. The early management of muscle strains in the elite athlete: best practice in a world with a limited evidence basis. Br J Sports Med 2008; 42(3): 158–159

Peetrons P. Ultrasound of muscles. Eur Radiol 2002; 12(1): 35–43

Ryan AJ. Quadriceps strain, rupture and charlie horse. Med Sci Sports 1969; 1: 106–111

Ryan JB, Wheeler JH, Hopkinson WJ, Arciero RA, Kolakowski KR. Quadriceps contusions. West Point update. Am J Sports Med 1991; 19(3): 299–304

Schünke M, Schulte E, Schumacher U, et al. Thieme atlas of anatomy. Stuttgart–New York: Thieme; 2005

Shi X, Garry DJ. Muscle stem cells in development, regeneration, and disease. Genes Dev 2006; 20(13): 1692–1708

Stoller DW. Magnetic resonance imaging in orthopaedics and sports medicine. 3rd ed. Philadelphia: Lippincott Williams & Wilkins, 2006

Takebayashi S, Takasawa H, Banzai Y, et al. Sonographic findings in muscle strain injury: clinical and MR imaging correlation. J Ultrasound Med 1995; 14(12): 899–905

Taylor DC, Dalton JD Jr, Seaber AV, Garrett WE Jr. Experimental muscle strain injury. Early functional and structural deficits and the increased risk for reinjury. Am J Sports Med 1993; 21(2): 190–194

Verrall GM, Slavotinek JP, Barnes PG, Fon GT, Spriggins AJ. Clinical risk factors for hamstring muscle strain injury: a prospective study with correlation of injury by magnetic resonance imaging. Br J Sports Med 2001; 35(6): 435–439, discussion 440

Waldén M, Hägglund M, Ekstrand J. UEFA Champions League study: a prospective study of injuries in professional football during the 2001–2002 season. Br J Sports Med 2005; 39(8): 542–546

Witvrouw E, Danneels L, Asselman P, D'Have T, Cambier D. Muscle flexibility as a risk factor for developing muscle injuries in male professional soccer players. A prospective study. Am J Sports Med 2003; 31(1): 41–46

Wolff R. Spezielle Krankheitsbilder im Hüftbereich. In: Dickhuth HH, Mayer F, Röcker K, Berg A, eds. Sportmedizin für Ärzte. Cologne: Deutscher Ärzte-Verlag; 2007: 373–375

Woods C, Hawkins RD, Maltby S, Hulse M, Thomas A, Hodson A; Football Association Medical Research Programme. The Football Association Medical Research Programme: an audit of injuries in professional football—analysis of hamstring injuries. Br J Sports Med 2004; 38(1): 36–41

Ultrasonography

L. Hänsel
P. Ueblacker
A. Betthäuser

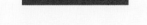

Translated by Terry Telger

Introduction *170*

**Relevant Physical Phenomena
and Artifacts** *170*
Absorption and Attenuation *171*
Reflection and Reflection Artifact *171*
Scatter *171*
Acoustic Shadow *171*
Acoustic Enhancement *171*
Reverberations *172*
Mirror-Image Artifact *172*

**Ultrasonographic Examination
of Skeletal Muscle** *172*
Ultrasonography of Normal Muscle
Tissue/Sonoanatomy *174*
Ultrasonography of
Pathological Conditions *185*

Ultrasonography of Complications *195*
Seroma, Cyst *195*
Fibrosis, Scar *195*
Myositis Ossificans *197*
Heterotopic Ossification *198*
Compartment Syndrome *198*

Introduction

While the importance of musculoskeletal ultrasonography has increased tremendously in recent years, the technical literature is still fragmentary as far as skeletal muscle imaging is concerned. In most textbooks on musculoskeletal ultrasound, the sections dealing with skeletal muscle usually illustrate only contusion-related hematomas or large structural defects in muscle. This very limited differentiation is likely to disappoint interested readers and practitioners who regularly examine skeletal muscles with ultrasound.

The fact is that ultrasonography can do much more. Among the soft tissues, muscles are one of the best adapted to ultrasound examination (Peetrons 2002). Although ultrasound does not have sufficient resolution to define structures on the scale of muscle fibers, even small muscular lesions can be visualized. When interpreted in the context of a detailed history and clinical examination, this cost-effective imaging modality will usually be able to furnish a diagnosis. It should be added, however, that the ultrasound examination of skeletal muscle takes time. It involves more than just holding a transducer briefly over the muscle of interest. Instead, the examiner must proceed slowly and deliberately, scanning the muscles in two planes while searching for abnormalities and making side-to-side comparisons.

This procedure is time-consuming. It requires a calm setting and an experienced examiner. This may help explain why ultrasonography, despite its improved technical capabilities, has been increasingly overshadowed by magnetic resonance imaging (MRI).

Ultrasound can be highly rewarding in orthopedic diagnosis and is commonly used for musculoskeletal imaging (Krappel and Harland 1997, Woodhouse an McNally 2011, Lee et al. 2012). The main advantages of ultrasonography are its easy availability and low cost. This makes ultrasound superior to MRI, especially for follow-up examinations. With a little practice, the examiner can quickly distinguish a functional muscle disorder without evidence of structural damage from a structural injury such as a moderate partial muscle tear (type 3b lesion) with associated hematoma, which is the key sign of a muscle tear. This means that the first and main goal of ultrasound is to assess whether or not a muscle tear is present (Peetrons 2002). With some experience, ultrasound can assess the need for further investigation by MRI and determine whether a hematoma is present that can or should be percutaneously aspirated to promote the healing of injured structures.

> **Note**
>
> The ideal time for the examination is between 2 and 48 hours after the muscle trauma. Before 2 hours, the hematoma is still forming. After 48 hours, the hematoma may have spread outside of the muscle (Peetrons 2002).

Moreover, as ultrasound does not expose patients to ionizing radiation, it can be repeated as often as desired. Dynamic imaging is also possible. Disadvantages are the relatively long examination time, the long learning curve, and the marked examiner-dependence of findings. The latter can be reduced, however, by following a standard protocol when acquiring and documenting findings (see **Table 7.1**).

Familiarity with normal findings is essential for effective use of ultrasound.

For physicians who see and treat competitive athletes, ultrasonography is an indispensable link in the diagnostic chain. Whereas doctors formerly had to rely on the clinical impression and manual examination, we now have access to portable, high-performance ultrasound scanners that can even be used in the locker room.

There have already been initial realistic reports on ultrasound probes that can be connected to smartphones. This may become a standard tool for future generations of sports medicine practitioners.

Relevant Physical Phenomena and Artifacts

The resolution of diagnostic ultrasound is significantly higher than that of other modalities (Woodhouse and McNally 2011). The maximum lateral resolution is slightly less than the axial resolution. The following formula is used to calculate resolution:

$$\frac{\text{Sound velocity}}{\text{Frequency}} = \frac{1540\ ^{\text{m}}/\text{s}}{\text{MHz}}$$

This means that an ultrasound transducer operating at a frequency of 7.5 MHz would have an axial resolution of 0.2 mm.

> **Note**
>
> A 7.5-MHz transducer has an axial resolution of 0.2 mm and a lateral resolution of 0.4 mm. A 12-MHz transducer halves these values, but the higher-frequency sound does not penetrate as deeply into the tissue.

Conversely, the soft-tissue contrast of ultrasound is not as good as MRI (Woodhouse and McNally 2011).

A variety of physical phenomena affect the ultrasound image:

- Absorption
- Reflection
- Scatter
- Refraction
- Diffraction

The first three of these are the ones most relevant to everyday ultrasonography. It is also important to be aware

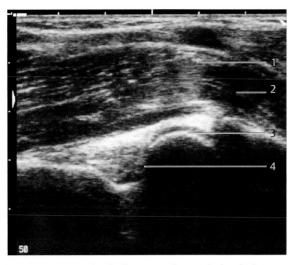

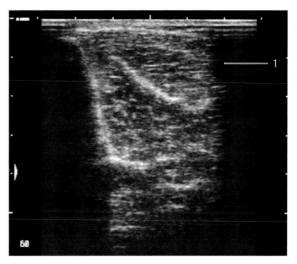

Fig. 7.1   An example of reflection artifact, in the brachialis muscle. Any obliquity of the ultrasound beam relative to a scanned interface may affect echogenicity.

1 Brachialis muscle scanned at a 90° angle
2 Brachialis muscle scanned at an oblique angle
3 Bone surface scanned at a 90° angle
4 Bone surface scanned at an oblique angle

Fig. 7.2   Coupling artifact at the edges of the image, caused by air trapped between the transducer and skin.

1 Air between the transducer and the skin surface

of the principal artifacts that occur in ultrasound imaging of muscle. Some artifacts can add useful information to the examination. (Examples of this include acoustic shadowing behind an ossifying area and acoustic enhancement behind structures with increased fluid content.)

Absorption and Attenuation

As sound waves pass through tissue, they are absorbed and converted into heat. When this occurs, the echo amplitudes returned to the transducer are also diminished. Time gain compensation (TGC) can correct for this effect by amplifying echoes as a function of their distance from the transducer.

Reflection and Reflection Artifact

An ultrasound image is generated by echo signals reflected from the interfaces of tissues that have different acoustic impedances. When the acoustic impedance is high, a high degree of sound reflection occurs. For example, all of the incident sound waves are reflected from bone, causing an acoustic shadow to appear behind the bony surface. But if the ultrasound beam strikes an interface at an oblique angle, that structure will appear less echogenic than in the case of an "orthograde" or 90° beam angle ("reflection artifact," **Fig. 7.1**).

Scatter

The smoother the surface of a structure, the greater the effect of beam angle on echogenicity, or the apparent brightness of the structure in the ultrasound image. But a rough surface will always reflect some of the sound waves back to the transducer. Because of this scattering effect, the surface may still appear echogenic (bright) even though the beam angle deviates significantly from the optimum 90° value. Without scatter, it would be extremely difficult to image a rounded surface contour with ultrasound.

Acoustic Shadow

"Acoustic shadow" is the term applied to the hypoechoic or echo-free zone that forms behind a strong reflector (e.g., calcium, bone, foreign body) or absorber (e.g., air) of sound. If the acoustic coupling between the transducer and skin is faulty, any trapped air will produce a "coupling artifact"—a vertical black streak passing down the entire image (**Fig. 7.2**). Also, an overlying structure of increased density (e.g., degenerated muscle or an area of incipient myositis ossificans) may locally decrease the echogenicity of a strong reflector such as bone (**Fig. 7.3**).

Acoustic Enhancement

Structures located behind tissue with a high fluid content appear more echogenic than neighboring structures, as fluid is a better conductor and the sound waves therefore undergo less attenuation. For example, if a segment of bone suddenly appears more echogenic that the adjacent bone, the cause may be edema or hematoma overlying that portion of the bone. The examiner therefore needs to give particular attention to structures that show an apparent local increase in echogenicity.

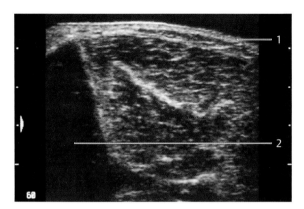

Fig. 7.3   Acoustic shadow behind the tibia and fibula.

1   The skin layer appears along the full length of the transducer
2   Acoustic shadow cast by the tibial bone

Reverberations

Ultrasound waves are often reflected back and forth at highly reflective interfaces. This gives rise to reverberations, which appear as parallel linear echoes behind the structure (e.g., standoff pad or patellar tendon). The echoes are equally spaced on the image, but diminish in intensity with increasing distance from the transducer (**Fig. 7.4**).

Mirror-Image Artifact

"Ghost images" can form deep to strong reflectors, appearing as a mirror-image duplication of the near-field image. The artifact is displayed at a greater depth because the transit time of the reflected sound waves is doubled (**Fig. 7.5**).

Ultrasonographic Examination of Skeletal Muscle

The ultrasound imaging of skeletal muscle is certainly more difficult than imaging other skeletal structures such as the shoulder joint, for which valid standards with reproducible scan planes have been developed. Skeletal muscle is so heterogeneous that it is difficult to establish uniform rules, at least as far as the fiber structure is concerned. It is usually helpful to compare the right and left sides. There are cases in which a finding that appears abnormal initially is suddenly found to be completely normal. An example of this is the proximal tendon of the rectus femoris muscle, which consistently casts a posterior acoustic shadow because of its density, so that underlying structures cannot be evaluated and may appear abnormal at first sight.

As in all ultrasound examinations, lesions that are detected in skeletal muscle should be scanned in two mutually perpendicular planes. But even with two muscles that are directly adjacent to each other, such as the rectus femoris and sartorius, scans in the longitudinal and transverse planes may differ considerably due to the variable anatomic course of the muscles (**Fig. 7.6**).

It is important to note the following basic technical criteria for ultrasound scanning:

- Appropriate transducer
- Correct settings
- Correct focal depth
- Correct beam angle
- Above all: correct orientation

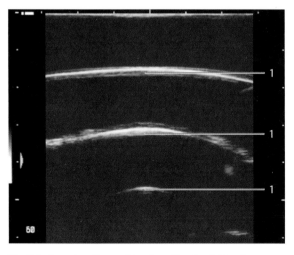

Fig. 7.4   Reverberations arising from the standoff pad.

1   Equally spaced reverberation artifacts

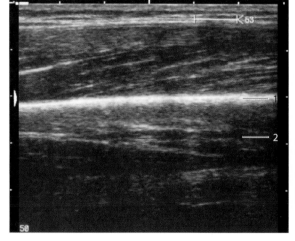

Fig. 7.5   Mirror-image artifact mimics muscle tissue "inside" the humerus. This artifact is easily identified by pressing the transducer more firmly against the skin, causing a mirror image of the compressed triceps muscle to appear "behind" the humeral cortex.

1   Bone surface
2   Mirror-image artifact

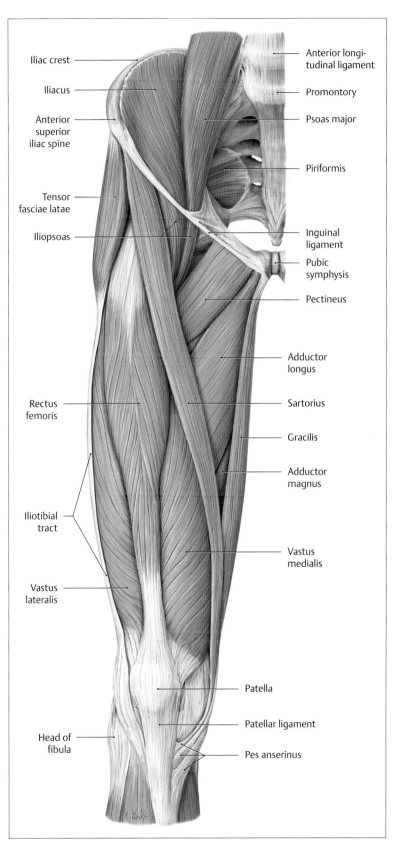

Iliac crest

Iliacus

Anterior superior iliac spine

Tensor fasciae latae

Iliopsoas

Rectus femoris

Iliotibial tract

Vastus lateralis

Head of fibula

Anterior longitudinal ligament

Promontory

Psoas major

Piriformis

Inguinal ligament

Pubic symphysis

Pectineus

Adductor longus

Sartorius

Gracilis

Adductor magnus

Vastus medialis

Patella

Patellar ligament

Pes anserinus

Fig. 7.6 Anatomy of the right thigh muscles, anterior view. The fascia has been removed as far as the iliotibial tract on the lateral side. The nonparallel orientation of the rectus femoris and sartorius muscles should be noted. This makes it necessary to rotate the transducer when scanning these two muscles, in order to obtain true longitudinal and transverse scans relative to the course of the muscles (from Thieme Atlas of Anatomy, General Anatomy and Musculoskeletal System, © Thieme 2005, Illustration by Karl Wesker).

Table 7.1   Standard protocol recommended for the ultrasound examination of skeletal muscles

Standard protocol
• Use side-by-side display so that the sides can be compared
• Use bone as a reference structure (landmark) whenever possible
• Obtain dynamic scans whenever possible:
• Make the patient tense the muscle
• Move the joint
• Optional: vary the transducer pressure (compressibility of target structure?)
• Optional: distal manual muscle compression (to distinguish vein from hematoma in a Doppler scan)

Table 7.2   Criteria for interpreting ultrasound findings

Location	
Margins	Shape
	Size
Structure	Echogenicity
	Internal echo pattern
Consistency	Solid
	Liquid
	Compressible
Blood flow	Increased
	Decreased

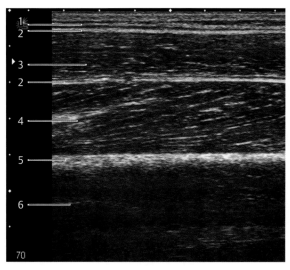

Fig. 7.7   Typical appearance of normal skeletal muscle in longitudinal section, seen here in the quadriceps femoris. The line near the top of the image is the subcutaneous tissue (1). Beneath that is the muscle fascia (2), which appears as a highly echogenic linear band. Next comes the typical striate pattern of the skeletal muscle (here the rectus femoris, 3), followed by another myofascial band (2). Beneath that is the striate structure of the vastus intermedius (4), followed by the highly echogenic band of the femoral cortex (5). Structures deep to the femoral cortex are obscured by acoustic shadowing (6).

Detailed knowledge of anatomy is essential in differentiating the muscles, especially in their proximal and distal portions.

Table 7.1 shows a recommended standard protocol for the ultrasound examination of muscles.

When a finding is evaluated (**Table 7.2**), first its relationship to known structures (landmarks) is described, and then its margins are scrutinized to determine shape and size. Next, its structure is evaluated in terms of echogenicity and internal echo pattern. The echo pattern may be described as typical, atypical, mottled, homogeneous, or inhomogeneous. Consistency is then evaluated, followed by an assessment of blood flow if a Doppler instrument is being used.

Ultrasonography of Normal Muscle Tissue/Sonoanatomy

Note

Familiarity with normal findings is essential for effective use of ultrasonography.

There is disagreement regarding the smallest cross-sectional size of a muscle injury that is detectable by ultrasound. Most authors believe that the smallest definable structural unit is the "primary bundle (= fascicle)," which consists of numerous muscle fibers surrounded by perimysium (Dock et al. 1990, Gerber et al. 2000). Single muscle fibers have a diameter of ~ 10–100 µm. Multiple fibers are grouped together to form the primary bundle, also called a fascicle, which is surrounded in turn by a connective-tissue sheath or septum, the perimysium (Schünke et al. 2004) (see Chapter 1).

When viewed in longitudinal section, the primary muscle bundle appears as a parallel array of hypoechoic, homogeneous bands 1–2 mm thick. The connective-tissue septa appear echogenic because of their collagen content (Yeh and Rabinowitz 1982) and are responsible for the typical pennate pattern. Viewed in cross-section, the intramuscular septa appear as echogenic stipples distributed over a hypoechoic background. The fascia surrounding the muscle, also called the epimysium, appears as a prominent echogenic structure (**Fig. 7.7**).

Note

The primary bundle (fascicle) has a pennate echo pattern when viewed in longitudinal section and a stippled pattern when viewed in cross-section.

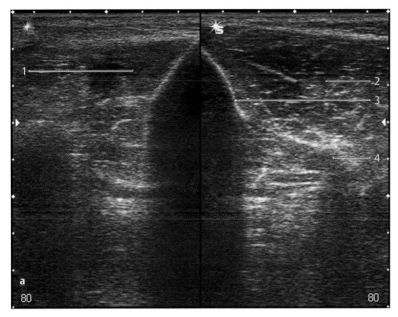

Fig. 7.8a, b   Effect of age and level of conditioning on the ultrasound appearance of skeletal muscle.

a Side-to-side comparison of the tibialis anterior muscle. The anterior tibial compartment appears normal on the right image. The image on the left side of the body shows partial loss of the normal muscular structure due to compression-related atrophy (following a compartment syndrome).

1   Atrophy of the tibialis anterior muscle
2   Normal tibialis anterior muscle of contralateral side
3   Tibial cortex (lateral)
4   Fibula

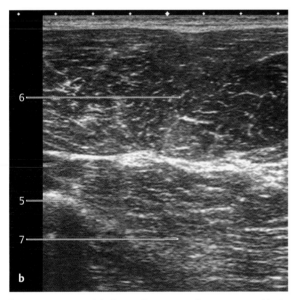

b Transverse scan of the biceps femoris muscle in a 24-year-old athlete (a decathlon competitor). Notable features are the large muscle volume and the small proportion of connective-tissue elements (especially in the long head).

5   Posterior femur
6   Biceps femoris muscle, long head
7   Biceps femoris muscle, short head

Factors that Affect Imaging

In addition to the level of physical conditioning, ultrasound imaging of skeletal muscles also depends on the muscle tone, age, and gender of the individual being examined. The skeletal muscle appears less echogenic in ath-

letically trained individuals (**Fig. 7.8b**) and male adolescents (Reimers et al. 2004), while in older persons it is more echogenic due to a relative increase in the proportion of collagen.

Hypertrophy or atrophy of muscle represents a long-term adaptation to functional demands on the muscle and its innervation. An increase in the volume of the muscle cells, leading to hypertrophy, decreases the relative amount of connective tissue in the muscle, giving the hypertrophic muscle a generally less echogenic appearance. Atrophy, on the other hand, is marked by a relative increase in the volume of septa and fascia, reducing the overall volume of the muscle (relative to the opposite side) and causing it to appear more echogenic (**Fig. 7.8**).

However, echogenicity is also dependent on the beam angle and instrument settings. Muscle that is scanned at an orthograde angle appears more echogenic (reflection artifact), while structures scanned at a tangential angle appear more hypoechoic (**Fig. 7.9**). A high transducer pressure will also increase the echogenicity of all structures and should therefore be avoided.

Note

The sonographic appearance of skeletal muscle is very heterogeneous on both an intramuscular and intermuscular scale. A muscle may contain a mixture of hypoechoic and hyperechoic features, and this pattern also depends on the transducer angle. If there is any doubt, it is usually helpful to compare the right and left sides. The transducer pressure should be as light as possible. In all cases, the most echogenic view should be selected for a side-to-side comparison. This view is found by gently angling the transducer back and forth.

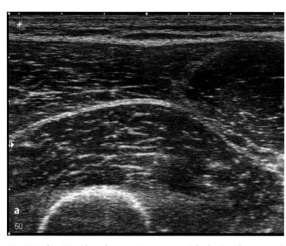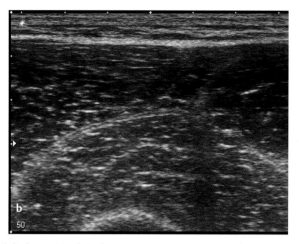

Fig. 7.9a, b Muscle echogenicity varies with the incidence angle of the beam. Muscle in the same anatomic region scanned at an orthograde angle (**a**) and at a tangential angle (**b**).

Examination Technique

The target structures in an ultrasonographic examination of skeletal muscle are located no more than a few centimeters beneath the skin. In a large thigh, for example, the femur is surrounded by a muscular envelope ≈ 6 cm thick. A transducer frequency of 7.5 MHz is recommended, owing to its high resolution. Modern scanners allow the operating frequency to be adjusted over a certain range. For example, a transducer can be operated at 6.0 MHz for scanning deep muscles and at 10.0 MHz for scanning the tendons of the hand.

> ### Note
>
> Not all muscles are equally accessible to ultrasound imaging. Visibility may even vary between the proximal and distal ends of the same muscle. For example, while the distal portion of the gastrocnemius muscle may be very clearly defined, a trained eye is needed to evaluate the proximal gastrocnemius. The soleus muscle is also difficult to evaluate, as it consistently has a faint and heterogeneous internal echo pattern.

In all cases, a detailed past and current medical history should be taken to obtain information about the probable findings. This is followed by a clinical examination with careful palpation of the affected area that has been indicated by the patient (for technique, see Chapter 6). The surrounding muscles should also be palpated and compared with the opposite side to detect any reactive hypertonicity in the adjacent muscles. The rest of the work-up can be facilitated by marking the area of interest identified by the history and palpation with a skin marker.

> ### Practical Tip
>
> Marking the area of interest during the clinical examination will facilitate ultrasound imaging. Remarkable findings are verified, measured, marked, and evaluated in transverse and longitudinal scans.

We recommend starting the ultrasonographic examination with a transverse scan to provide initial orientation. The muscle is then systematically surveyed by moving the scanning plane slowly down the muscle and back up again. Any apparent abnormalities should be compared with the opposite side. The transducer pressure should be as light as possible, since compressing the muscle may obscure small lesions. This is aided by using enough ultrasound gel to ensure optimum acoustic coupling. To improve coupling on a convex surface such as the anterior lower leg, it may be helpful to use a standoff pad. The transducer should be angled back and forth until the most echogenic view of the muscle is obtained; then the image can be compared with the uninjured contralateral side as a reference.

Power Doppler, if available, is useful for evaluating the neovascularization of an injured area or inflammatory reactions, and it can grade the activity of ossification in injured muscle (Campbell et al. 2005, Koulouris and Connell 2005). Doppler technique is also helpful in distinguishing a vein from a hematoma. This differentiation may be aided by brief manual compression of the distal portion of the muscle. In the case of a vein, this maneuver will evoke a typical color flow signal.

Practical Tip

- Work calmly and deliberately.
- Hold the transducer as lightly as possible against the skin.
- Use enough gel for good acoustic contact.
- Start with transverse scans for better anatomic orientation.
- Scan completely through the muscle in longitudinal and transverse planes.
- Make the patient tense the muscle being imaged.

Note

Transverse scans are best for anatomic orientation. Longitudinal scans are better for detecting small lesions, as they display the fiber architecture of the muscle.

Practical Tip

By definition and convention, the transducer should be positioned so that the left side of the image is superior in longitudinal scans and medial in transverse scans. Thus, for example, when the left leg is scanned from the posterior side and the patient is viewed from the distal or inferior aspect, the transducer should be reversed to preserve the conventional orientation.

Ultrasonographic Examination of the Lower Limbs

Anterior Thigh

A detailed knowledge of anatomy is an essential prerequisite for every ultrasound examination of muscle. **Figure 7.10** shows an anatomic cross-section of the thigh, displaying the muscles on the anterior and posterior sides.

The anatomy of the proximal anterior thigh is relatively complex, mainly due to the arrangement of the muscles (sartorius, rectus femoris, tensor fasciae latae) and to the large caliber and obliquity of the rectus tendon (**Fig. 7.11**). It is easier to define and identify the individual muscles of the quadriceps group, which can be clearly visualized in most patients (**Fig. 7.12**).

Caution

Dense acoustic shadowing behind thick tendons such as the proximal rectus tendon may be mistaken for a structural discontinuity in the muscle.

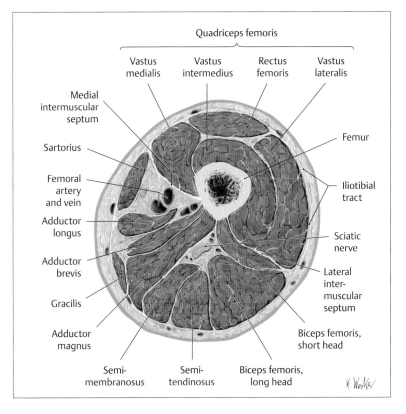

Fig. 7.10 Anatomic cross-section of a thigh, proximal view (from Thieme Atlas of Anatomy, General Anatomy and Musculoskeletal System, © Thieme 2005, Illustration by Karl Wesker).

Quadriceps femoris

Vastus medialis — Vastus intermedius — Rectus femoris — Vastus lateralis

Medial intermuscular septum

Sartorius

Femoral artery and vein

Adductor longus

Adductor brevis

Gracilis

Adductor magnus

Semimembranosus — Semitendinosus — Biceps femoris, long head

Femur

Iliotibial tract

Sciatic nerve

Lateral intermuscular septum

Biceps femoris, short head

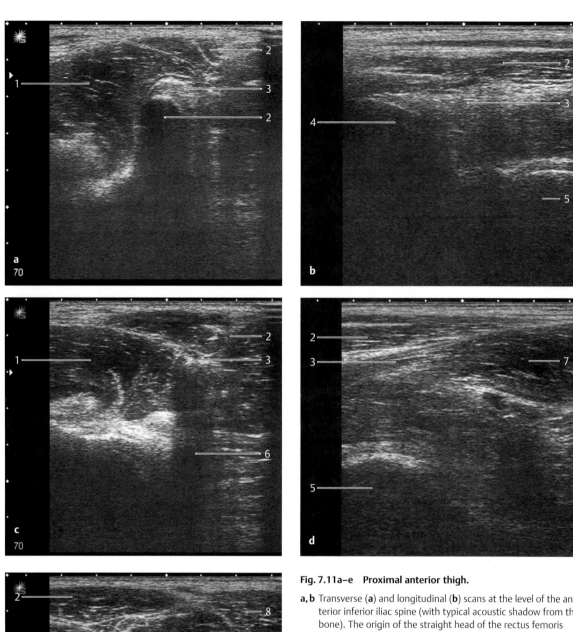

Fig. 7.11a–e   Proximal anterior thigh.

a, b Transverse (**a**) and longitudinal (**b**) scans at the level of the anterior inferior iliac spine (with typical acoustic shadow from the bone). The origin of the straight head of the rectus femoris tendon is clearly visible anteriorly.

c, d Transverse (**c**) and longitudinal (**d**) scans at the level of the hip joint. The powerful rectus femoris tendon casts a distinct shadow, especially in the transverse scan, which is typical at this site and should not be mistaken for a structural injury. The iliopsoas muscle crosses the hip joint anteriorly.

e Transverse scan of the upper thigh. All the muscles can be clearly identified as described.

1 Iliopsoas
2 Sartorius
3 Rectus femoris tendon (straight head)
4 Anterior inferior iliac spine
5 Femoral head
6 Acoustic shadow
7 Rectus femoris
8 Tensor fasciae latae

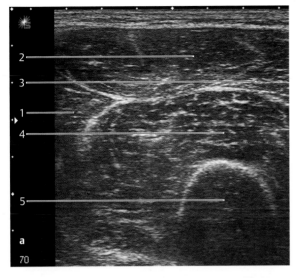

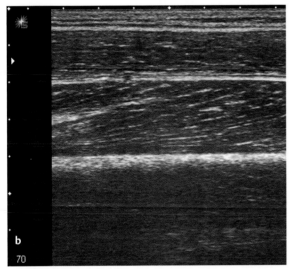

Posterior Thigh (Hamstrings)

The proximal and middle thirds of the posterior thigh (hamstrings) are dominated by the large muscle bellies of the biceps femoris, semitendinosus, and semimembranosus.

The anatomy of the posterior thigh muscles (hamstrings) is illustrated in **Fig. 7.13**.

The interfascial tissue planes are difficult to evaluate with ultrasound, especially the areas between the semimembranosus and semitendinosus muscles and between the semitendinosus and biceps femoris. A shadow is often found at these sites. The transducer has to be angled to detect lesions, which are not uncommon in this region (**Fig. 7.14**). In the distal part, the semitendinosus tendon appears as a long, thin, medial structure that directly overlies the semimembranosus muscle and tapers distally (**Fig. 7.15**). The course of the biceps femoris muscle and tendon is clearly visible on the lateral side (**Fig. 7.16**).

Adductors

Some experience and anatomic knowledge are needed to consistently define the adductors with ultrasound, distinguish them from one another, and detect lesions. This is due to the course of the muscles and their relatively complex anatomy near their origin on the pubic ramus (**Fig. 7.17**).

Figure 7.18 illustrates the complex anatomy of the adductor muscles.

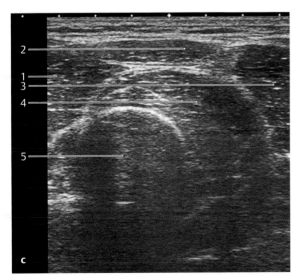

Fig. 7.12a–c Normal ultrasound findings at the mid-thigh level.

a Transverse scan.
b Longitudinal scan.
c Distal thigh level. All muscles in the quadriceps femoris group are visualized. The relative sizes of the individual muscles change distally.

1 Vastus medialis
2 Rectus femoris
3 Vastus lateralis
4 Vastus intermedius
5 Femur

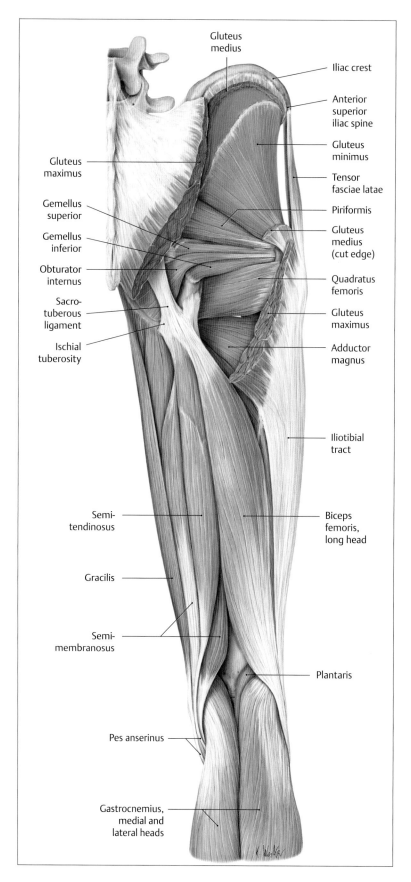

Fig. 7.13 Anatomy of the right thigh muscles, posterior view. The gluteus maximus and medius have been partially removed (from Thieme Atlas of Anatomy, General Anatomy and Musculoskeletal System, © Thieme 2005, Illustration by Karl Wesker).

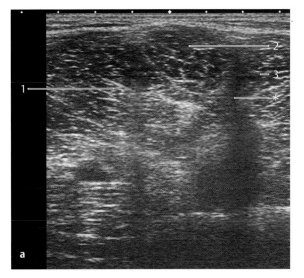

Fig. 7.14a, b   Posterior upper thigh.

a The transverse scan through the posterior upper thigh simultaneously displays the semitendinosus, semimembranosus, and biceps femoris muscles. Special attention should be given to the sonographic "gap" (*) at the interface of the three muscles (see text).

b The medial transverse scan simultaneously displays the semitendinosus, semimembranosus, and adductor magnus muscles. Longitudinal scans should always be accurately correlated with the transverse scans to determine which muscle belly is being imaged.

1 Semimembranosus
2 Semitendinosus
3 Biceps femoris
4 Adductor magnus

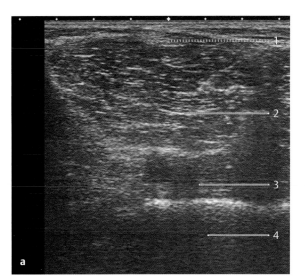
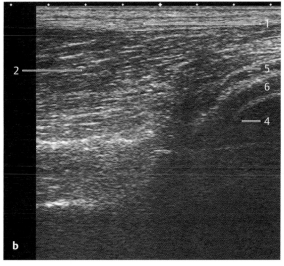

Fig. 7.15a, b   The semitendinosus tendon is clearly defined in the medial portion of the lower thigh. The tendon directly overlies the semimembranosus muscle belly.

a Transverse scan.
b Longitudinal scan.

1 Semitendinosus tendon
2 Semimembranosus
3 Medial head of gastrocnemius
4 Medial femoral condyle
5 Cartilage of medial femoral condyle

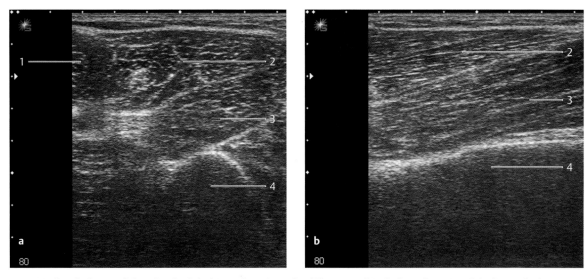

Fig. 7.16a, b The long and short heads of the biceps femoris can be differentiated in the lateral portion of the lower thigh.

a Transverse scan.
b Longitudinal scan.

1 Semitendinosus
2 Long head of biceps femoris
3 Short head of biceps femoris
4 Femur

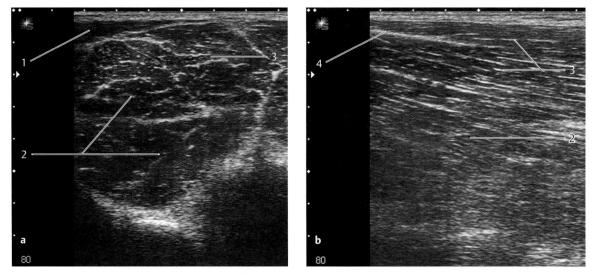

Fig. 7.17a, b The ultrasonographic anatomy of the adductor muscles is difficult to interpret and requires some experience.

a The transverse scan (here through the medial portion of the upper thigh) does not always display the individual muscles as clearly as in this example.
b Even in the longitudinal scan, it is often difficult to identify the individual adductor muscles in comparison with other muscle groups.

1 Gracilis
2 Adductor magnus
3 Adductor longus
4 Adductor longus tendon

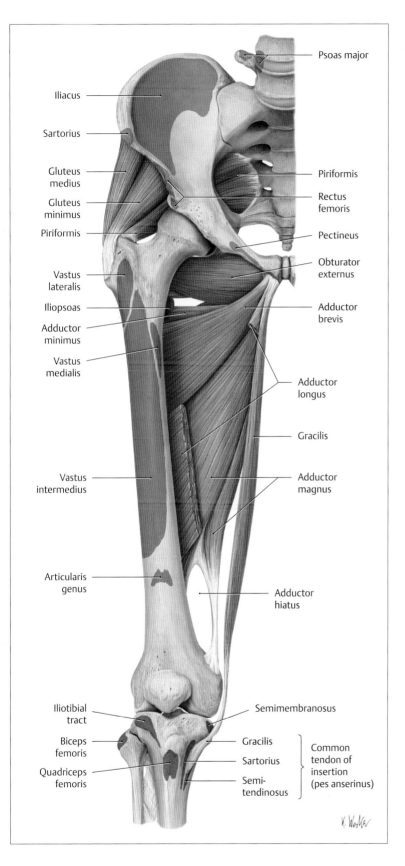

Iliacus

Sartorius

Gluteus
medius

Gluteus
minimus

Piriformis

Vastus
lateralis

Iliopsoas

Adductor
minimus

Vastus
medialis

Vastus
intermedius

Articularis
genus

Iliotibial
tract

Biceps
femoris

Quadriceps
femoris

Psoas major

Piriformis

Rectus
femoris

Pectineus

Obturator
externus

Adductor
brevis

Adductor
longus

Gracilis

Adductor
magnus

Adductor
hiatus

Semimembranosus

Gracilis

Sartorius

Semi-
tendinosus

Common
tendon of
insertion
(pes anserinus)

Fig. 7.18   Muscular anatomy of the medial right thigh, displaying the adductors. The quadriceps femoris, iliopsoas, tensor fasciae latae, and pectineus muscles are intact. The adductor longus muscle has been partially removed (from Thieme Atlas of Anatomy, General Anatomy and Musculoskeletal System, © Thieme 2005, Illustration by Karl Wesker).

Calf

Ultrasound examination of the calf does not usually present any major difficulties. The gastrocnemius muscle bellies are consistently well defined and can be tracked distally as they taper into the Achilles tendon (**Fig. 7.19**). It may be difficult to define the origins of the gastrocnemius muscles at the back of the knee and to evaluate the soleus muscle. The soleus has an atypical pennate structure on ultrasound and often appears faint, making it difficult to evaluate for possible lesions. Often it is helpful to compare the right and left sides.

The anatomic cross-section in **Fig. 7.20** shows the anterior and posterior muscles of the lower leg. As the posterior muscles are more commonly injured, they are of greater interest in ultrasound examinations.

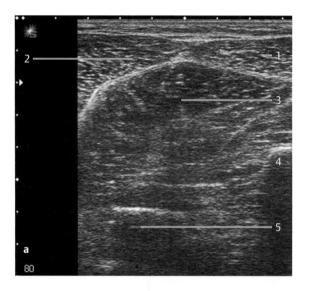

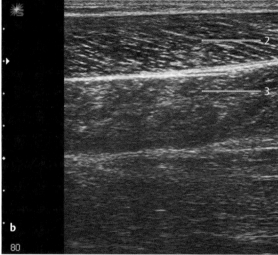

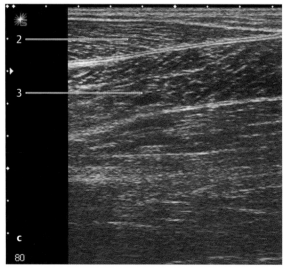

Fig. 7.19a–c   The calf muscles. The gastrocnemius and soleus muscles can always be positively identified in transverse and longitudinal scans (**a, b**) through the proximal and middle thirds of the calf. The soleus muscle is somewhat more difficult to interpret. The sharply tapered muscle bellies of the medial and lateral heads of the gastrocnemius should be noted in particular (**c**). The muscles of the deep flexor compartment are more difficult to identify.

1   Lateral head of gastrocnemius
2   Medial head of gastrocnemius
3   Soleus
4   Fibula
5   Tibia

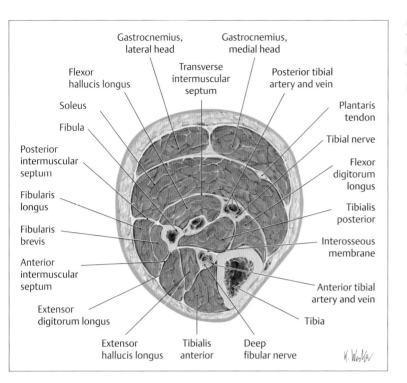

Fig. 7.20 Anatomic cross-section through a right lower leg in the prone position, proximal view (from Thieme Atlas of Anatomy, General Anatomy and Musculoskeletal System, © Thieme 2005, Illustration by Karl Wesker).

Ultrasonography of Pathological Conditions

Fatigue-Induced Painful Muscle Disorder (Type 1a Lesion)

As a functional disorder, fatigue-induced painful muscle disorder is not associated with any conspicuous ultrasound abnormalities. There are no consistently reproducible changes that are seen on ultrasound. Occasionally, the affected muscle area may appear more or less echogenic (brighter) than the surrounding muscle (**Fig. 7.21**). Again, a side-to-side comparison is often helpful. The main role of ultrasonography with a type 1a lesion is to exclude structural damage and support the clinical diagnosis based on palpation findings.

Delayed-Onset Muscle Soreness (Type 1b Lesion)

The situation is similar in patients with delayed-onset muscle soreness (DOMS), which does not cause any macroscopic structural alterations that are detectable on ultrasonography (although ultrastructural changes may be present). The muscle may appear less echogenic than normal, due to inflammatory edema.

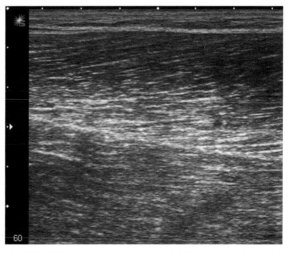

Fig. 7.21 Ultrasound appearance of fatigue-induced painful muscle disorder. The affected area may appear more or less echogenic than the surrounding muscle (longitudinal scan). Usually, there are no pathological findings seen on ultrasound.

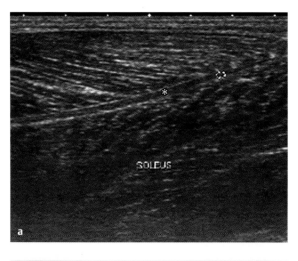
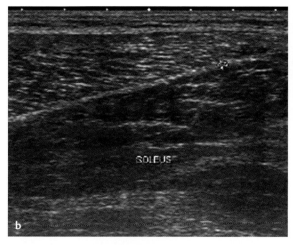
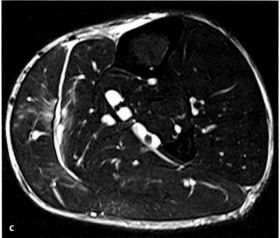

Fig. 7.22a–d Longitudinal scan of the calf.

a Thin intermuscular edema is visible between the medial gastrocnemius and soleus (∗).

b Absence of edema on the contralateral side.

c,d Representative transverse (**c**) and longitudinal (**d**) Magnetic resonance images of the same lesion on the same day.

Spine-Related Neuromuscular Muscle Disorder (Type 2a Lesion)

Ultrasonographic exclusion of any macroscopic damage alone allows an experienced examiner to classify this muscle problem as belonging to the class of functional muscle disorders. This type of disorder may induce autonomic effects (see Chapter 6) leading to the development of intermuscular edema. The edema band can be detected sonographically (**Fig. 7.22**) and lends further support to the clinical diagnosis.

Muscle-Related Neuromuscular Muscle Disorder (Type 2b Lesion)

A fourth type of nonstructural muscle lesion is the common entity of a type 2b lesion. Again, the main role of ultrasound is to exclude structural injury and thus confirm the diagnosis based on the history and palpable findings. The circumscribed, spindle-shaped area of edematous swelling in the muscle belly is palpable by an experienced examiner, but it is difficult to visualize with ultrasound and cannot be reproducibly detected with current instruments.

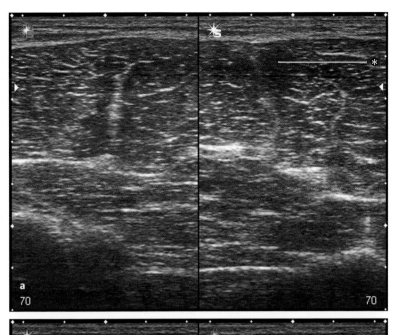

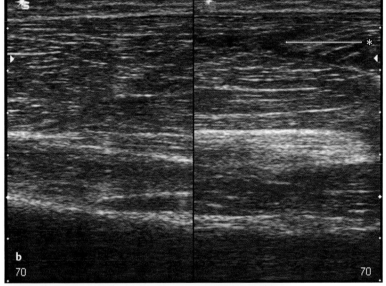

Fig. 7.23a–c   Ultrasound appearance of minor partial muscle tears.

a, b Transverse (**a**) and longitudinal (**b**) scans of the biceps femoris muscle in a 27-year-old top international sprinter (400 m). While sprinting on the previous day, the athlete had felt a sudden stabbing pain in the back of his thigh (left image in each set with normal findings).

c Transverse scan of a minor partial muscle tear (Type 3a injury) in the proximal semitendinosus muscle of a 23-year-old professional soccer player.

* Structural discontinuity

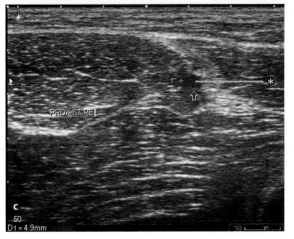

Minor Partial Muscle Tear (Type 3a Lesion)

The muscle fiber (in anatomic nomenclature, a single muscle cell measuring 10–100 μm in diameter) is well below the resolution limit of current ultrasound scanners, so a single torn muscle fiber cannot be visualized with this technique (Fornage 2000). In addition, tearing of a single muscle fiber (i.e., a single muscle cell) does not have any functional or therapeutic relevance.

However, ultrasonography can certainly detect tearing of multiple primary and secondary bundles (fascicles) that are more than several millimeters in size (**Fig. 7.23**), as well as secondary changes such as hematoma (Bily and Kern 1998, Konermann and Gruber 2007) and edema. Again, the associated hematoma is the key sign of a muscle tear (Peetrons 2002). The prominence of these secondary changes is highly variable, depending on whether first aid has been rendered with a cold pack and compression.

Note

The heterogeneous echo pattern caused by the varying fiber structure of muscle can mimic the appearance of a small muscular lesion. Interpretation can be assisted by comparing the sides and perhaps by dynamic imaging while the muscle is contracted and relaxed.

Moderate Partial Muscle Tear (Type 3b Lesion)

The injury appears as a larger structural discontinuity with an associated hematoma. Often the hematoma is visible as a diffuse intramuscular hemorrhage both proximal and distal to the rupture site, as well as a localized hematoma filling the muscle gap (if present). An intermuscular hematoma is present in some cases due to fascial disruption. It should be noted that the extent of the hematoma does not necessarily match the size of the tear.

Ultrasound reveals discontinuity in the muscle fibers and septa in the rupture or hematoma (**Fig. 7.24**). The muscle fibers may appear broadened by the mass effect of the hemorrhage, and the fascia may be raised into a convex bulge (**Fig. 7.24b**). A standoff pad will help reduce the contact pressure, especially on the anterior lower leg, making it easier to detect subtle bulges in the muscle fascia without causing a coupling artifact.

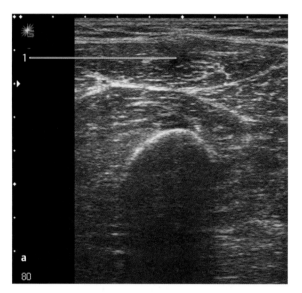

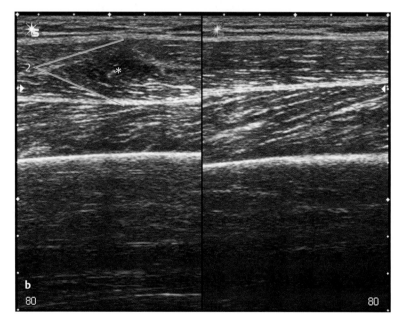

Fig. 7.24a–g Ultrasound appearance of moderate partial muscle tears.

a, b Transverse (**a**) and longitudinal (**b**) scans of a moderate partial muscle tear in the rectus femoris of a 22-year-old professional soccer player who had felt a sudden shooting pain in his anterior thigh during a match, forcing him to leave the field. The convex bulge on the muscle fascia, caused by the mass effect of the hematoma, should be noted (**b**, left image; the right image shows the normal contralateral side).

1 Muscle tear
2 Bulging muscle fascia

* Structural defect with hematoma

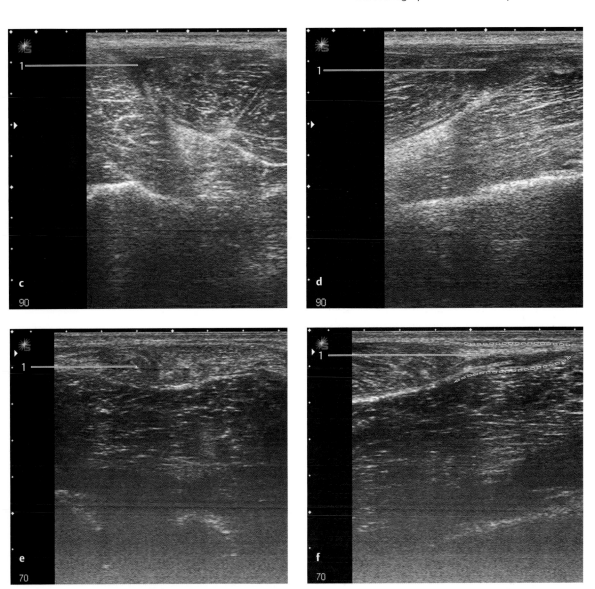

Fig. 7.24c–g Ultrasound appearance of moderate partial muscle tears.

c, d Transverse (**c**) and longitudinal (**d**) scans of a moderate partial muscle tear in the distal biceps femoris of a 30-year-old professional soccer player. The longitudinal scan clearly demonstrates the rupture site at the musculotendinous junction.

e–g Transverse (**e**) and longitudinal (**f**) scans of a moderate partial muscle tear in the distal portion of the gastrocnemius medial head. The patient is a 30-year-old professional soccer player who, while training 2 days earlier, had felt a sudden, stabbing calf pain with an immediate functional deficit. The longitudinal scan in particular (**f**) clearly shows a rupture at the distal musculotendinous junction.

A longitudinal scan of the medial head of the uninjured gastrocnemius muscle is shown for comparison (**g**).

1 Moderate partial muscle tear

The timing of the ultrasound examination after the injury is another important consideration that influences the interpretation of findings. As a large injured area heals, it appears increasingly echogenic due to progressive scar formation. Follow-ups are important for early detection of complications such as seroma formation or ossification.

Subtotal or Complete Muscle Tear/ Tendinous Avulsion

A full-thickness tear of a muscle through its belly or at the muscle–tendon junction is rare. It is more common for a tendon to be avulsed from its origin or insertion. The following tendons are most commonly affected by this type of injury:

- The rectus femoris tendon at the anterior inferior iliac spine (**Fig. 7.25**)
- The proximal hamstring tendons
- The distal semitendinosus tendon (**Fig. 7.26**)
- The proximal adductor longus tendon
- The junction of the gastrocnemius muscles with the Achilles tendon
- The distal biceps femoris

Sonographic diagnosis of these lesions may be difficult and requires experience, time, a knowledge of anatomy, and in most cases comparison with the opposite side. The examiner evaluates the retraction of the tendon, the degree of associated hemorrhage, and possible concomitant injuries to surrounding structures.

A bony avulsion of the apophysis from the pelvis may occur in patients in their growth years and can be classified into various grades (Betthäuser and Bartschat 2003).

Contusion

A contusion may result from external blunt trauma to the muscle causing vascular injury and internal bleeding. Muscle fiber disruption is rare, as the traumatizing force tends to displace and compress. Bleeding occurs due to shear and crush forces on the muscle tissue (see also Chapter 6).

The injury may cause diffuse intramuscular bleeding, circumscribed hematoma, or only edema. The ultrasound appearance of a hematoma is highly variable and depends on the age of the lesion (**Fig. 7.27**). A fresh hematoma under pressure is somewhat more echogenic, due to its high cellular content (**Fig. 7.27 g**), so it may be difficult to distinguish from muscle. The surrounding fascia appears more convex than its counterpart on the opposite side (**Fig. 7.27 h**). The same is true of diffuse intramuscular bleeding, which increases the muscle volume. A side-to-side comparison is helpful and sometimes essential for appreciating a size change (assuming the absence of some other cause, such as atrophy). As the hematoma liquefies over a period of days, it can be identified as an echo-poor structure, often presenting a round or oval shape.

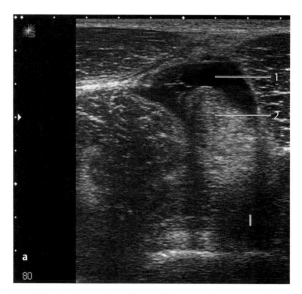 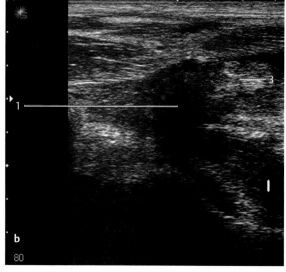

Fig. 7.25a, b Proximal avulsion of the rectus femoris tendon in a 24-year-old top international sprinter (100 m) who had felt a definite tearing in the proximal anterior thigh while competing 4 days earlier. The injury forced him to drop out of the race. The retracted rectus femoris tendon and surrounding hematoma are clearly visualized.

a Transverse scan.
b Longitudinal scan.

1 Structural defect with hematoma
2 Rectus femoris tendon
3 Retracted rectus femoris tendon

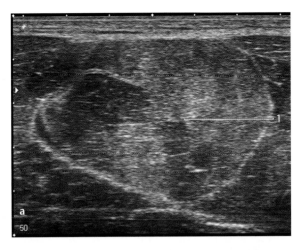

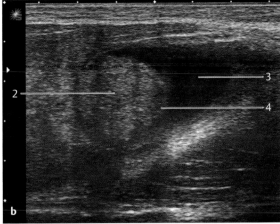

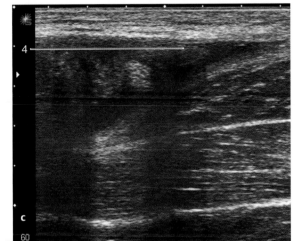

Fig. 7.26a–e   Distal avulsion of the semitendinosus tendon in a 23-year-old top international sprinter (100 m) who had felt a sudden, painful tearing on the medial side of the distal thigh while running. He was unable to train after the injury.

a   Transverse scan. The semitendinosus muscle appears hyperechoic and inhomogeneous due to tendon retraction.

b, c   The longitudinal scan demonstrates the avulsed tendon stump and conspicuous surrounding hematoma/seroma.

d, e   Magnetic resonance images for comparison and orientation.

1   Semitendinosus muscle
2   Retracted semitendinosus
3   Seroma
4   Stump of semitendinosus tendon

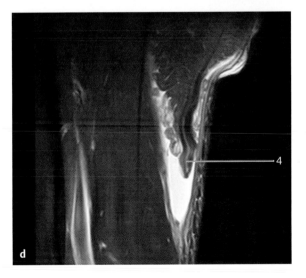

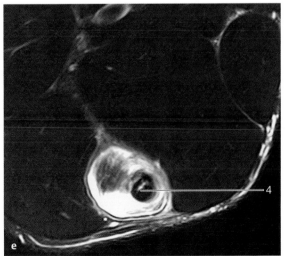

Fresh blood has a high corpuscular content and is more echogenic immediately after the trauma than 1–2 days later. It is therefore often difficult to distinguish from surrounding muscle in the acute stage. A side-to-side comparison is helpful for recognizing volume differences that may suggest intramuscular bleeding. It is also helpful to compare the structure of the muscle on the right and left sides.

Fresh hematomas should be measured for documentation and follow-up. The transverse and longitudinal scans can be used to calculate volumes, particularly in circumscribed hematomas.

Practical Tip

This simple formula can be used to estimate the approximate volume of a hematoma:
Length × width × depth × 0.5

Once a circumscribed hematoma has been localized on ultrasonography, it can easily be aspirated with a percutaneous needle using a sterile technique.

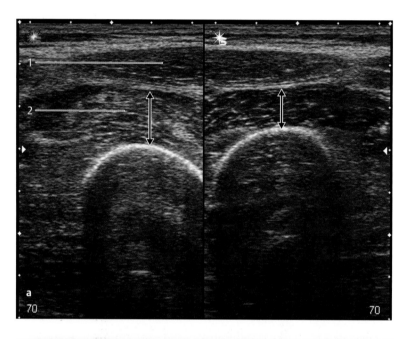

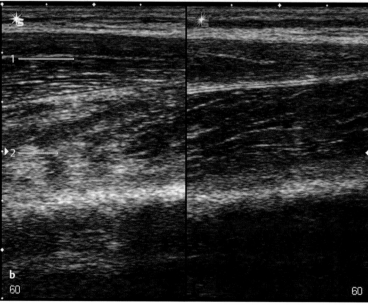

Fig. 7.27a–h Ultrasound and magnetic resonance imaging (MRI) appearance of muscle contusions.

a, b Transverse (**a**) and longitudinal (**b**) scans of diffuse intramuscular bleeding in the vastus intermedius of a 21-year-old professional soccer goalkeeper whose knee had been injured the previous day in a violent collision with an opposing player. The increased volume (↕) of the contused muscle is evident when compared with the normal opposite side (right-hand image in each set).

1 Rectus femoris
2 Increased echogenicity in the vastus intermedius, caused by diffuse intramuscular bleeding

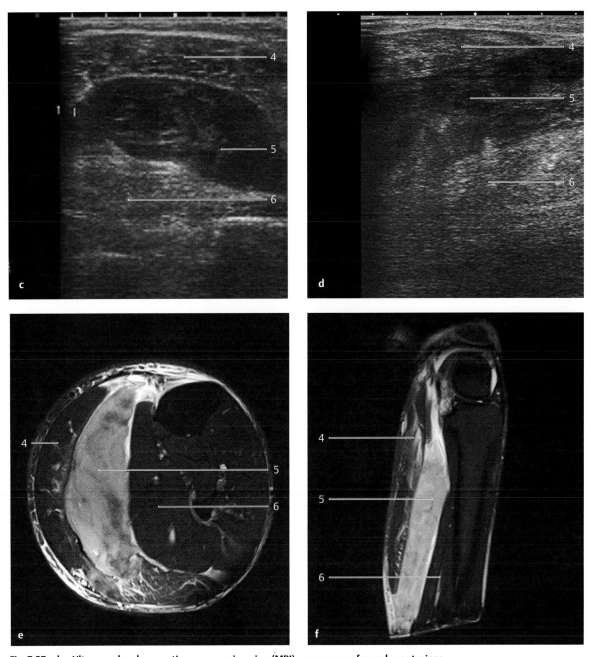

Fig. 7.27a–h   Ultrasound and magnetic resonance imaging (MRI) appearance of muscle contusions.

c, d Transverse (**c**) and longitudinal (**d**) scans of a massive hematoma between the gastrocnemius and soleus muscles following
an extensive contusion injury at the musculotendinous junction
of the medial and lateral heads of the gastrocnemius. Measuring 18 × 9 × 3.5 cm, the hematoma required immediate evacuation to prevent an impending compartment syndrome.

e, f MRIs for comparison and orientation.

4 Medial head of the gastrocnemius
5 Hematoma
6 Soleus muscle

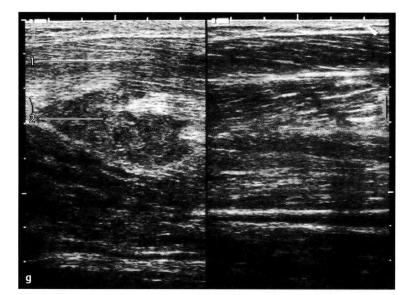

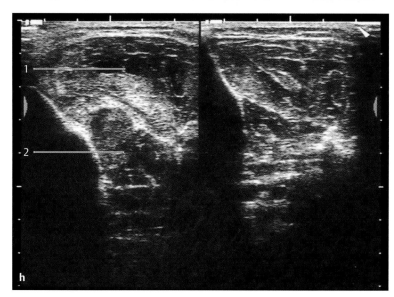

Fig. 7.27a–h   Muscle contusions. Contusion injury of the lower leg (g, h).

g   Longitudinal scan of the tibialis anterior muscle. The image on the left shows a hematoma under pressure (110 mmHg). The normal opposite side is seen on the right.

h   Transverse scan of the tibialis anterior, which is under pressure (110 mmHg here). The fascia in the left image shows a convex bulge (normal findings at right). Often a hematoma is absent, however, and the pressure is caused simply by an edematous increase in muscle volume at the expense of the adjacent muscle. The subcutaneous fat layer is often thickened.

1   Tibialis anterior
2   Hematoma

Ultrasonography of Complications

Seroma, Cyst

Seromas are circumscribed fluid collections at the site of a former injury. They always have more or less rounded margins. A cyst is distinguished by its capsular boundary. A seroma, unlike a fresh hematoma or fibrosis, is always echo-free (**Fig. 7.28**), although it may contain internal septa. It is difficult to distinguish a liquefied hematoma from a seroma using ultrasound.

Fibrosis, Scar

A circumscribed or diffuse hematoma, with or without structural injury, may undergo fibrous transformation over time due to connective-tissue ingrowth, forming a scar of variable size. This scar tissue is considerably more echogenic than the surrounding tissue. It is located at the former injury site and is generally easy to detect on ultrasound, especially in a side-to-side comparison (**Fig. 7.29**).

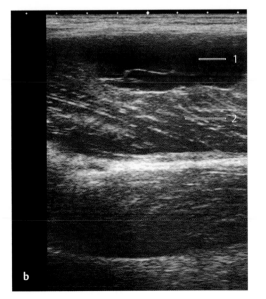

Fig. 7.28a, b   A large seroma with an internal septum in a 21-year-old professional soccer player who had been medically released for full training after a prior injury. The lesion resolved with percutaneous aspiration, infiltration, and physical therapy. The patient was able to resume a full training schedule 3 months later.

a   Transverse scan. The image on the left shows normal contralateral findings.
b   Longitudinal scan.

1   Seroma with septation
2   Rectus femoris
3   Vastus intermedius

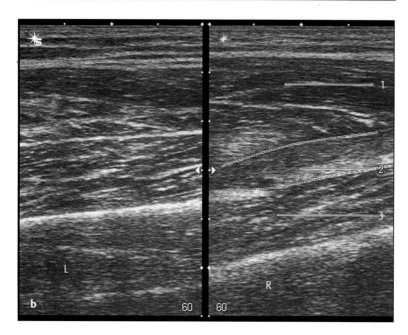

Fig. 7.29a, b Pronounced fibrotic changes following a partial muscle tear in the rectus femoris of a 31-year-old professional soccer player. The transverse (**a**) and longitudinal (**b**) scans clearly demonstrate the fibrosis, which is located beneath the rectus femoris and is partially compressing the muscle. The normal left side is shown for comparison.

1 Rectus femoris
2 Fibrosis
3 Vastus intermedius

Myositis Ossificans

The intramuscular foci of calcification that form in myositis ossificans can always be recognized by their high-amplitude surface echoes, accompanied by some degree of posterior shadowing (**Fig. 7.30a, b**). On the other hand, foci of calcification, especially when small, may be missed within a large muscular volume. As with other abnormalities, ultrasound detection requires a calm, time-consuming, and detailed survey of the muscle. In later follow-ups, the examiner will generally have no difficulty in locating a comparable scan plane. When foci of calcification are detected on ultrasonography, conventional radiography using a soft-tissue technique can be performed to complete the documentation (**Fig. 7.30c, d**).

Foci of myositis ossificans should be precisely measured in two planes so that accurate assessments can be made over time. If the surrounding tissue appears very hypoechoic and edematous, it is likely that active ossification is still present. This can be verified with laboratory tests detecting an elevation of bone-specific alkaline phosphatase.

Practical Tip

MRI is inferior to ultrasound for determining whether early, circumscribed myositis ossificans (calcified foci) is present. Smaller foci in muscle tissue are easily missed on MR images.

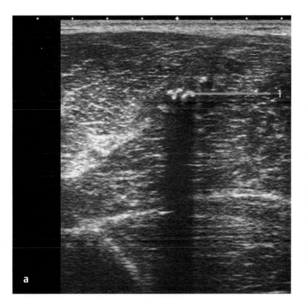

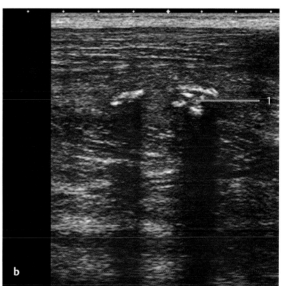

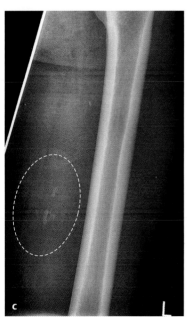

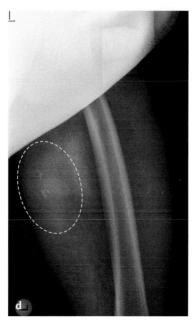

Fig. 7.30a–d   Myositis ossificans in a 23-year-old professional soccer player who had sustained an extensive semi-membranosus muscle injury 3 weeks earlier. He returned to play prematurely, leading to the formation of calcified foci (1) that are detectable sonographically by their high echogenicity and acoustic shadows.

a   Transverse scan.
b   Longitudinal scan.
c, d   Conventional radiographs can be helpful for accurate localization of calcified foci.

Heterotopic Ossification

Heterotopic ossification has to be distinguished from myositis ossificans, which is always an intramuscular process. In principle, foci of ossification may occur at old injury sites anywhere in the body. Tendon avulsions are most relevant in evaluating the injuries discussed in this chapter. Examples include avulsion of the proximal rectus femoris tendon (**Fig. 7.31**) or a proximal hamstring tendon. Avulsion of the rectus apophysis from the pelvis in adolescents may lead to the formation of a very large ossification with the appearance of a "pseudotumor."

Compartment Syndrome

The intramuscular pressure may rise following a muscular injury (especially a contusion) that does not disrupt the fascia, leading to a compartment syndrome affecting a single muscle. Ultrasound shows an increased muscle volume, rounding of the fascia, increased echogenicity, and a "ground-glass appearance" with a reduction in the normal pennate markings (**Fig. 7.32**; Löffler 1989 and 2005).

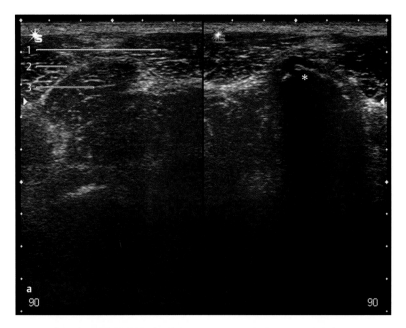

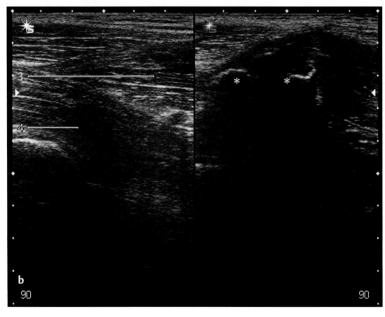

Fig. 7.31a, b Marked extraosseous calcifications (heterotopic ossification) in a 40-year-old recreational athlete. Five months earlier, the patient had suffered an avulsion of the reflected head of the rectus femoris that was not recognized as such, and inadequate treatment was provided. Subsequent plaquelike ossifications were clearly detectable on ultrasound by their posterior acoustic shadows. The images on the left show normal contralateral findings. The ossifications caused severe limitation of hip rotation. They were surgically removed, and the rectus tendon was repaired.

a Transverse scan.
b Longitudinal scan.

1 Sartorius
2 Tensor fasciae latae
3 Rectus femoris
4 Iliopsoas
* Heterotopic ossification

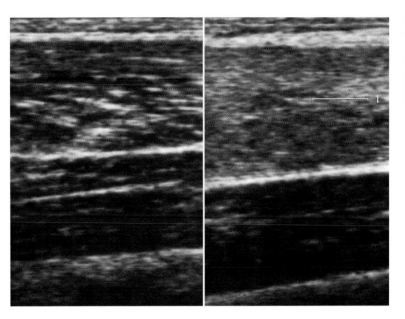

Fig. 7.32 Compartment syndrome following a rectus femoris contusion, marked by increased echogenicity and a typical loss of the normal pennate pattern. The image on the left shows normal contralateral findings (Photo courtesy: L. Loeffler).

1 Ground-glass appearance

Clinical Case

A 51-year-old man presented the day after experiencing a sudden shooting pain on the medial side of the left calf while playing tennis. The patient left the tennis court and self-treated the injury with cold compresses. When examined the next day, the calf appeared clinically normal, with no visible signs of hematoma formation and with normal-appearing contours. Despite marked regional tenderness over the distal portion of the medial gastrocnemius, plantar flexion was possible with almost no pain. The painful area felt spongy on palpation, but there was no definite, circumscribed, palpable defect in the muscle.

Ultrasound scans showed loss of the sharp distal taper of the medial gastrocnemius muscle fibers into the Achilles tendon, with a small associated fluid collection (**Fig. 7.33**). This led the examiner to diagnose a "partial distal avulsion of the medial gastrocnemius on the left side." Subsequent MRI yielded the images shown in **Fig. 7.34**, and the interpreting radiologist summarized (and underestimated) the injury as a "pulled muscle in the left calf (distal medial gastrocnemius) with fluid streaks along the muscle fibers extending distally to the musculotendinous junction. The proximal Achilles tendon appears normal. Mild effusion is noted along the fascial planes of the gastrocnemius, especially between the gastrocnemius and soleus muscles."

The patient was informed of the ultrasound diagnosis and given an estimated recovery time of at least 6 weeks. The treatment regimen was as follows:

- Three local infiltrations , injected through eight needles placed along the muscle
- Supportive zinc paste bandages
- Heel wedge
- Oral enzyme therapy
- Immediate institution of manual lymph drainage
- Complete abstinence from sports for 1 week, followed by ergometric exercises

The pain quickly subsided, and initial healing was uneventful. At the end of 3 weeks, the patient carelessly (as he was not feeling any new pain in the leg) jumped over a mound of snow at the edge of a sidewalk. He again experienced a sudden, shooting pain at the previous injury site. Ultrasound revealed marked proximal displacement of the medial gastrocnemius muscle, accompanied by a fresh hematoma (**Fig. 7.35**).

The hematoma had to be aspirated on several occasions. Despite these measures and repeated compression bandaging, the hematoma did not resolve completely, however, and an extensive fibrous scar formed at the injury site (**Fig. 7.36**). This did not cause functional disability. Twelve weeks after the original injury, the patient was able to resume tennis and jogging. Six months later, he was still free of complaints and had not experienced a recurrence.

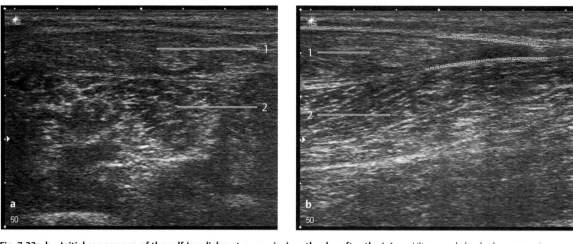

Fig. 7.33a, b Initial appearance of the calf (medial gastrocnemius) on the day after the injury. Ultrasound clearly shows a post-traumatic fluid collection (hematoma) and loss of the sharp distal taper of the gastrocnemius.

a Transverse scan.
b Longitudinal scan.

1 Medial gastrocnemius
2 Soleus

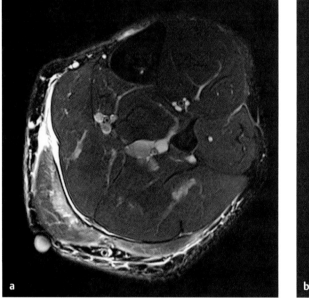
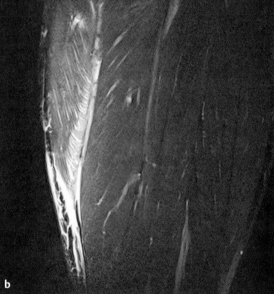

Fig. 7.34a, b MRI on the day after the injury (see text). Representative transverse (**a**) and longitudinal (**b**) images are shown.

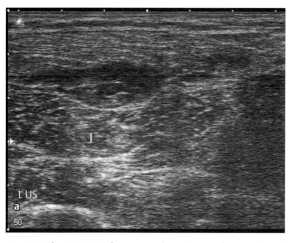 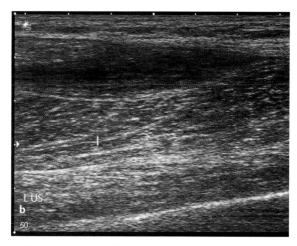

Fig. 7.35a, b Extensive hematoma formation and retraction of the medial gastrocnemius after the patient jumped over an obstacle during the healing period.

a Transverse scan.　　　　　　　　　　　**b** Longitudinal scan.

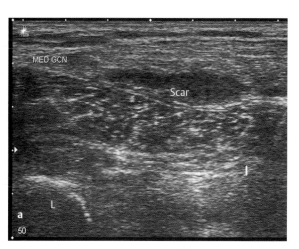 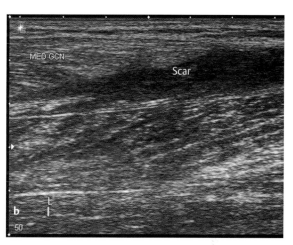

Fig. 7.36a, b Despite multiple aspirations and compression therapy, the hematoma persisted in this case and underwent fibrous transformation.

a Transverse scan.　　　　　　　　　　　**b** Longitudinal scan.

Note from the authors. The comprehensive selection of ultrasound images shown in this chapter were collected over a 6-month period (from the start of the planning phase for the German edition of this book until the manuscript was submitted)—showing the large number and variety of muscle injuries the authors see in their everyday practice, along with the course of the injuries and the associated complications.

References

Betthäuser A, Bartschat T. Wertigkeit bildgebender Verfahren am Hüftgelenk des Sportlers. Sport-Orthopädie Sport-Traumatologie 2003; 19: 322–327

Bily W, Kern H. Diagnosis, first aid and classification of muscle injuries in sports medicine. [Article in German] Sportverletz Sportschaden 1998; 12(3): 87–93

Campbell SE, Adler R, Sofka CM. Ultrasound of muscle abnormalities. Ultrasound Q 2005; 21(2): 87–94, quiz 150, 153–154

Dock W, Grabenwöger F, Happak W, et al. Sonography of the skeletal muscles using high-frequency ultrasound probes. [Article in German] Rofo 1990; 152(1): 47–50

Fornage BD. The case for ultrasound of muscles and tendons. Semin Musculoskelet Radiol 2000; 4(4): 375–391

Gerber TA, Prim J, Michel BA. Sonographie des Bewegungsapparats. Stuttgart: Thieme; 2000: 19–20

Konermann W, Gruber G. Sonographie am Stütz- und Bewegungsapparat. 2nd ed. Stuttgart: Thieme; 2007: 27

Koulouris G, Connell D. Hamstring muscle complex: an imaging review. Radiographics 2005; 25(3): 571–586

Krappel F, Harland U. Current role of ultrasonography in orthopedics. Results of a nationwide survey. [Article in German] Z Orthop Ihre Grenzgeb 1997; 135(2): 106–111

Lee JC, Mitchell AW, Healy JC. Imaging of muscle injury in the elite athlete. Br J Radiol 2012; 85(1016): 1173–1185

Löffler L. Ultraschalldiagnostik am Bewegungsapparat. Stuttgart: Thieme; 1989

Löffler L. Sonographie in Sportverletzungen und Sportschäden. In: Engelhardt M, Krüger-Franke M, Pieper H-G, Siebert CH, eds. Praxiswissen Halte- und Bewegungsorgane. 1st ed. Stuttgart: Thieme; 2005: 7–15

Peetrons P. Ultrasound of muscles. Eur Radiol 2002; 12(1): 35–43

Reimers CD, Gaulrapp H, Kehle H. Sonographie der Muskeln, Sehnen und Nerven. 2nd ed. Cologne: Deutscher Ärzteverlag; 2004

Schünke M, Schulte E, Schumacher U. Prometheus – Allgemeine Anatomie und Bewegungssystem. Stuttgart: Thieme; 2004

Woodhouse JB, McNally EG. Ultrasound of skeletal muscle injury: an update. Semin Ultrasound CTMR 2011; 32(2): 91–100

Yeh HC, Rabinowitz JG. Ultrasonography and computed tomography of inflammatory abdominal wall lesions. Radiology 1982; 144(4): 859–863

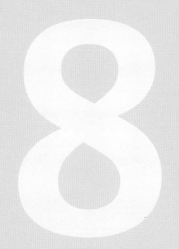

8

Magnetic Resonance Imaging

J. Böck
P. Mundinger
G. Luttke

Relevant Anatomic Microstructure   *204*

**MRI Examination Technique
and Normal Findings**   *204*
Examination Technique   *204*
MRI of Normal Muscle   *205*

**MRI of Functional Muscle
Disorders and Structural Injuries**   *208*
Fatigue-Induced Functional Muscle
Disorder (Type 1a) and Delayed-Onset
Muscle Soreness (Type 1b)   *208*
Spine-Related Neuromuscular
Muscle Disorder (Type 2a)   *208*
Muscle-Related Neuromuscular
Muscle Disorder (Type 2b)   *208*
Minor Partial Muscle Tear (Type 3a)   *209*
Moderate Partial Muscle Tear (Type 3b)   *209*
Subtotal or Complete Muscle Tear
and Tendinous Avulsion (Type 4)   *211*
Muscle Contusion, Laceration   *211*
Muscle Herniation   *213*
Muscle Denervation   *213*
Chronic Tendinosis, Tendon Rupture   *213*

Complications   *215*
Seroma/Cyst   *215*
Fibrosis/Scar   *215*
Myositis Ossificans   *215*
Heterotopic Ossification   *215*
Compartment Syndrome   *216*

Differential Diagnosis   *216*
Muscle Edema Pattern   *216*
Fatty Atrophy Pattern   *216*
Tumor, Hematoma, Bony Avulsion Pattern   *216*

Prognostic Criteria   *217*

Risk Factors for Recurrent Muscle Injury   *217*

Specific Muscle Injuries   *217*
Quadriceps Muscle   *217*
Hamstring Muscles   *220*
Adductor Longus Muscle   *220*
Gastrocnemius Muscle   *220*
Less Frequently Involved Muscles   *220*

Summary   *220*

In comparison with all of the other imaging modalities available, magnetic resonance imaging (MRI) has excellent intrinsic contrast. The spatial resolution of MRI has been improving with each new generation of the system. Along with ultrasonography, MRI is therefore now the imaging modality of choice for evaluating musculotendinous injuries (Boutin et al. 2002). Associated injuries in bone, joints, and soft tissues such as tendons, ligaments, cartilage and meniscus can be documented or excluded in a single MRI examination. It can be justifiably claimed that MRI is the most robust and versatile imaging tool for evaluating muscle injuries.

MRI, ultrasonographic, and clinical findings provide the basis for classification, treatment, and prognosis in muscle injuries. Functional disorders have to be differentiated from structural injuries; rehabilitating structural injuries too rapidly may interfere with the healing process and can even lead to complications. By contrast, early mobilization after functional muscle disorders is usually unproblematic. This chapter follows the consensus on terminology and classification established by Müller-Wohlfahrt et al. and presented in this book (see Chapter 6).

Relevant Anatomic Microstructure

Histologically, the structural unit is the muscle fiber, a polynuclear cell with a diameter of ~ 10–100 µm. Groups of 200–250 muscle fibers are contained in a layer of connective tissue and thus form the primary muscle bundles (fascicles). Up to 12 primary muscle bundles are surrounded by the epimysium and form the macroscopically appreciable secondary muscle bundles (sarcous fibers). Their diameter is in the range of 1–2 mm, or up to 5 mm in athletes, depending on their training status. Groups of secondary muscle bundles, not specifically addressed in the literature, may be termed tertiary muscle bundles. These are associated with type 3b lesions (moderate partial muscle tear) in the Müller-Wohlfahrt et al. classification (see Chapter 6). All of the tertiary muscle bundles together form the entire muscle belly.

The junction between muscle and tendon—the musculotendinous interface—is the weakest segment in the load transmission chain in adults. In children and adolescents, avulsion of the apophysis is the most frequent injury type. Older adults with preexisting degenerative changes typically suffer from ruptures of the tendons.

> *Note*
>
> **The musculotendinous interface is the weakest segment in the load transmission chain in adults.**

Musculotendinous injuries frequently occur during contraction and simultaneous (usually sudden) eccentric load on the tensed muscle. Typically, muscles that course over two joints and that contain fast-twitch fibers are affected. The rectus femoris, hamstring, and gastrocnemius muscles are therefore the muscles that are most frequently involved. Eccentric contractions also occur in muscles that course over only one joint, such as the adductor muscles, and particularly the adductor longus muscle.

MRI Examination Technique and Normal Findings

Examination Technique

MRI is now an integral part of medical imaging, particularly in the fields of orthopedics and traumatology. Due to its excellent spatial and contrast resolution, MRI can provide good visualization of both the location and the extent of musculotendinous injuries. Unlike radiography and computed tomography, MRI examination is not associated with exposure to ionizing radiation. Musculoskeletal injuries in younger patients and children can therefore be safely imaged with MRI.

The physical principle of MRI is based on the magnetic properties of atomic nuclei with uneven numbers of protons and neutrons. Hydrogen nuclei are abundant in the human body and therefore play a major role in imaging. Due to their magnetic moment, the spin axes describe a motion similar to that of a spinning top. Depending on the strength of the MRI system's static magnetic field (15 000–30 000 times stronger than the Earth's magnetic field), a proportion of the spins are oriented in the direction of the magnetic field. The direction of the spins is altered when they are exposed to a high-frequency impulse. This process is associated with energy uptake and is termed resonance—hence magnetic *resonance* imaging. The spinning motion and the magnetic relationship between neighboring spins are thus altered. The release of this energy is called relaxation and can be detected with appropriate antennas ("coils"). Additional smaller magnetic fields, spatially and temporally varying magnetic gradients, are used to modulate the large static magnetic field strength and thus help localize the source of the signal in the body. Using magnetic gradients, it is possible to selectively excite a thin two-dimensional slice or a larger three-dimensional volume of tissue in the body and reconstruct a two-dimensional or three-dimensional matrix.

Depending on whether the longitudinal change in spin orientation or the transverse spin–spin interaction is studied, T1-weighted, T2-weighted, or proton density–weighted images can be produced, which differ in the tissue contrast provided.

- On *T1-weighted images,* for example, fat is bright ("hyperintense"), while water is dark.
- On *T2-weighted images,* fluid is hyperintense and fat is just slightly less hyperintense than fluid.
- On *proton density–weighted images,* fluid is darker than on T2-weighted images, but the spatial resolution is better.

The sensitivity of MRI for detecting musculotendinous injuries can be significantly improved using fat-suppression techniques. Specifically designed high-frequency pulses are able to suppress the otherwise high signal from fat. Fluids, blood, and edema are consequently displayed with high signal intensity. Since the signal intensity of normal muscle is low to intermediate on most pulse sequences, the best contrast between normal and injured muscle is obtained with T2-weighted fat-saturated images. If a higher spatial resolution is desired, proton density–weighted fat-suppressed images may be chosen.

Improved detection of pathological findings is also possible with intravenous administration of specific contrast media containing chelated gadolinium, a rare earth metal. On T1-weighted or T1-weighted fat-saturated images, the presence of gadolinium increases the signal intensity and thus contrast with surrounding tissue. Gadolinium is primarily enriched in the blood vessels and may accumulate in areas of hypervascularity and hyperperfusion. From the blood vessels, it may exit into the extracellular fluid compartment, where it accumulates locally depending on vascular permeability and the size of the extravascular compartment.

A state-of-the-art 1.5-tesla MRI system, with dedicated high-resolution surface coils, was used for the examinations presented in this chapter (Espree, Siemens, Erlangen, Germany). All of the images shown in this chapter were acquired using T1-weighted images and proton density–weighted or T2-weighted fat-saturated images.

Practical Tips

- High field strength (1.5/3.0 T) should be used.
- High spatial resolution (dedicated surface coils (**Fig. 8.1**).
- T2-weighted fat-saturated images generate more contrast (**Fig. 8.2**), while proton density–weighted fat-saturated images generate better spatial resolution.
- Multiplanar slice orientation: always axial, in addition coronal and/or sagittal image orientation (**Fig. 8.3**).
- T1-weighted images in one image orientation are usually sufficient.
- Strict limitation of the field of view according to the clinical symptoms and ultrasound provides better spatial resolution.

Note

MRI systems with a lower magnetic field strength, and/or an inappropriate examination technique—particularly with insufficient spatial resolution and contrast resolution—may result in erroneous interpretation. This typically involves overestimation of the degree of injury, as adequate differentiation between the muscle injury itself, edema, and hematoma is not possible.

MRI of Normal Muscle

Normal muscle tissue is characterized by uniform signal intensity; individual secondary muscle bundles cannot be differentiated (**Fig. 8.4**). After a therapeutic intramuscular injection, the injected fluid is distributed in the connective-tissue layers, such as the epimysium, creating sufficient contrast for visualizing the secondary muscle bundles (**Fig. 8.4**). A physiologic increase in signal intensity can be observed in muscle tissue approximately 30 minutes after intense exercise. This results from extravasation of fluid, resulting in an increased extravascular fluid volume.

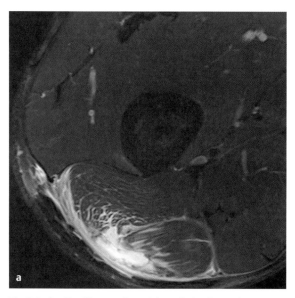
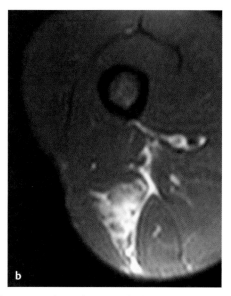

Fig. 8.1a, b Significance of spatial resolution for evaluating a moderate partial muscle tear in the biceps femoris muscle. (See also **Fig. 8.8a, b**: axial images of the same muscle lesion).

a Differentiation between the lesion, hematoma, and secondary muscle fascicles (bundles) is significantly improved with the higher spatial resolution provided by a surface coil and an optimized field of view.

b Diffuse signal alteration at lower spatial resolution.

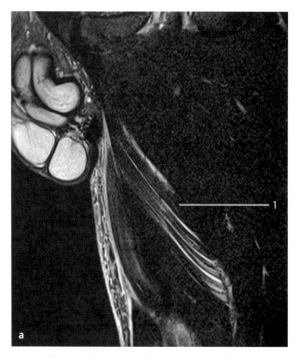
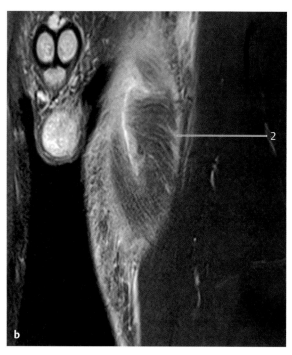

Fig. 8.2a, b Significance of pulse sequence selection for visualizing secondary muscle fascicles (bundles) in a minor partial muscle tear of the adductor longus muscle. There is excellent contrast of secondary muscle bundles due to edema.

a Improved evaluation of fiber continuity (1) in the T2-weighted fat-saturated image. Coronal oblique section.

b In proton density–weighted fat-saturated images, the definition of the secondary muscle bundles (2) is less clear. Coronal section.

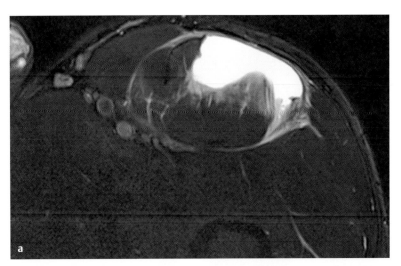

Fig. 8.3a–c   Subtotal muscle tear of the rectus femoris muscle. Large defect (over one-third of the cross-sectional area of the muscle), hematoma, musculofascial separation. See also **Fig. 8.15**.

a Axial section.
b Coronal section.
c Sagittal section.

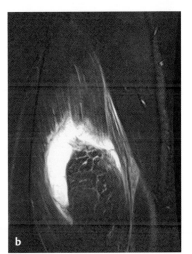
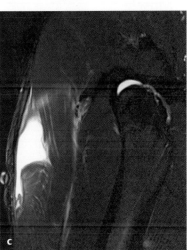

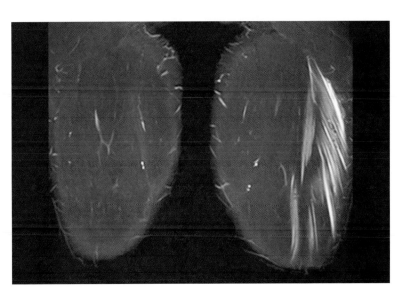

Fig. 8.4   Status following an intramuscular injection into the left rectus femoris muscle in a patient with fatigue-induced muscle disorder. Secondary muscle bundles are visualized through the infiltrated fluid. On the normal contralateral side, the muscle tissue is homogeneous, without visualization of secondary muscle bundles. Coronal section.

MRI of Functional Muscle Disorders and Structural Injuries

Fatigue-Induced Functional Muscle Disorder (Type 1a) and Delayed-Onset Muscle Soreness (Type 1b)

Patients with fatigue-induced functional muscle disorder (type 1a) or delayed-onset muscle soreness (DOMS; type 1b) are not typically referred for MRI. A feathery appearance in the muscle tissue, caused by transient edema, may develop in some functional lesions. There is no discontinuity in the secondary muscle bundles (fascicles).

Spine-Related Neuromuscular Muscle Disorder (Type 2a)

Patients with spine-related neuromuscular muscle disorder (type 2a) are more likely referred for MRI for imaging of the lumbar spine. If MRI of the involved muscle is performed, some discrete accumulations of epifascial or subfascial fluid may be observed. There is no discontinuity in the secondary muscle bundles.

Muscle-Related Neuromuscular Muscle Disorder (Type 2b)

Some fluid/edema is evident between the secondary muscle fascicles (bundles) and is predominantly located in the epimysium. The fluid's high signal intensity creates contrast, revealing the secondary muscle bundles (with a feathery appearance). All of the secondary muscle bundles visualized can be followed without discontinuity (**Fig. 8.5**). The image after intramuscular injection (in the absence of a musculotendinous injury) is quite similar (see **Fig. 8.4**). The integrity of the secondary muscle bundles and the absence of architectural distortion can be evaluated on this basis. In this type of injury, no confluent intramuscular hematoma is seen. Frequently, perifascial edema with high signal intensity around the muscle belly is apparent (De Smet and Best 2000).

If there is insufficient spatial resolution (e.g., with obsolete MRI systems, inadequate imaging technique, or inappropriate coils with insufficient spatial resolution), a diffuse signal alteration is seen in the area of the injury (see **Fig. 8.2a**); differentiation between type 1, type 2, and type 3 injury may be difficult or even impossible, and there is a tendency to overestimate the type of injury.

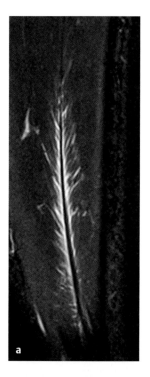

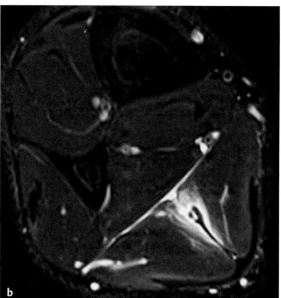

Fig. 8.5a, b   Muscle-related neuromuscular muscle disorder of the soleus muscle. All of the secondary muscle bundles are intact, but are visualized through edema in the musculotendinous junction, typically involving only a well-defined region of the muscle.

a Sagittal section.
b Axial section.

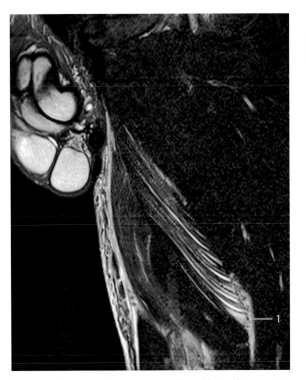

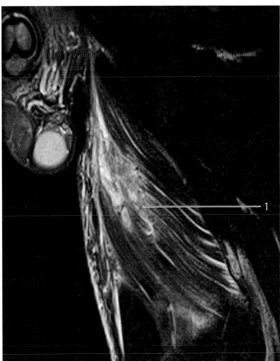

Fig. 8.6 Minor partial muscle tear in the adductor longus muscle. Both edema and hematoma help display the secondary muscle bundles, most of which are intact. Only a few secondary muscle bundles at the inferior aspect of the lesions are ruptured (1). Oblique coronal section.

Fig. 8.7 Moderate partial muscle tear in the adductor longus muscle. Secondary muscle bundles are depicted with high contrast; discontinuity can be seen in numerous secondary muscle bundles (1). There is hematoma in the muscle defect. Oblique coronal section.

Minor Partial Muscle Tear (Type 3a)

The secondary muscle bundles are visualized with the presence of blood and edema. Discontinuity in one or just a few secondary muscle fascicles (bundles) is noted. Retraction may cause a wavy course in the secondary muscle bundles. Type 3a injury is characterized by a group of torn primary, and possibly secondary, muscle bundles with a maximum cross-sectional area of up to 5 mm (**Fig. 8.6**). A small or larger intramuscular hematoma is frequently seen. Optimal primary care (ice, compression) can considerably reduce the extent of hematoma formation.

Caution

There is a tendency to overestimate the type of lesion due to insufficient discrimination of actually ruptured secondary muscle bundles, blood, and edema, particularly when there is insufficient spatial resolution and/or contrast resolution.

Moderate Partial Muscle Tear (Type 3b)

A larger group of secondary muscle bundles with a cross-sectional diameter of more than 5 mm is ruptured. This type of injury can be further classified according to whether less than one-third (**Figs. 8.7** and **8.8**), one-third to two-thirds (see **Fig. 8.3**), or more than two-thirds of the cross-sectional area of the muscle is torn (Boutin et al. 2002). Typically, an intramuscular hematoma is seen between the retracted parts of the muscle. A larger interfascial hematoma may also be present, with considerable —usually distal—extension.

A special form of type 3b injury is a partial tear of the intramuscular tendon, frequently without relevant tearing of secondary muscle bundles. The discontinuity in the hypointense intramuscular tendon is clearly seen on MRI images. The tendon may be partially retracted in the longitudinal direction. The unruptured secondary muscle bundles are visualized due to the presence of edema and blood, and have a wavy course toward the retracted parts of the tendon (**Fig. 8.9**).

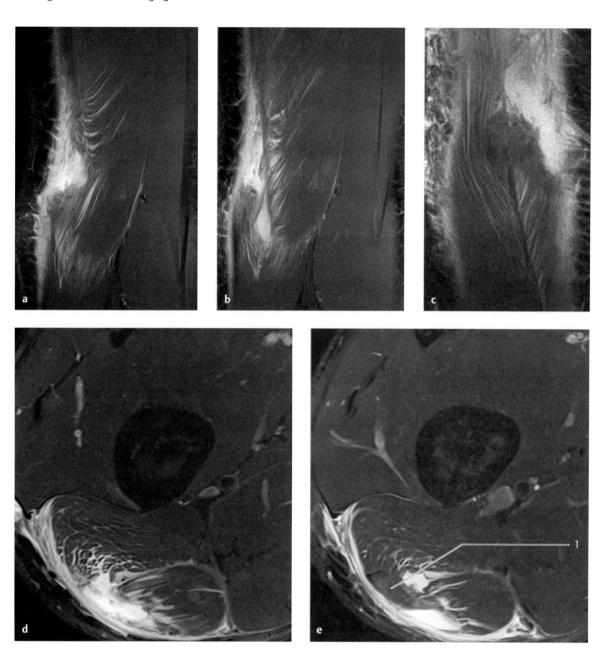

Fig. 8.8a–e   Moderate partial muscle tear at the musculotendinous interface of the biceps femoris. For the follow-up examination, see **Fig. 8.16**.

a, b Retraction, muscle gap, bundle deviation, hematoma.
   Sagittal section.
c   Visualization of the musculotendinous stump. Coronal section.

d   Gap with hematoma. Axial section.
e   Distal musculotendinous stump (1). Axial section.

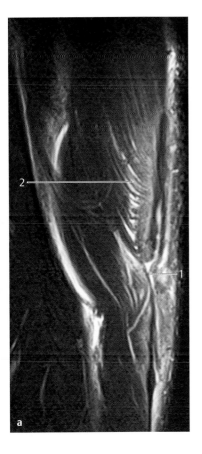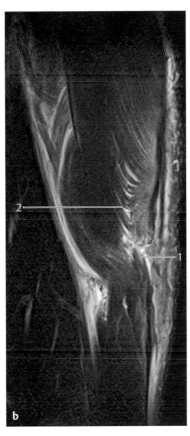

Fig. 8.9a, b   An intramuscular tendinous rupture in the biceps femoris muscle (a variant of moderate partial muscle tear). There is a tendinous gap, with slight retraction of the tendon ends (1). The undulating course of the secondary muscle bundles is caused by retraction (2). Most of the secondary muscle bundles are intact. Sagittal sections.

Subtotal or Complete Muscle Tear and Tendinous Avulsion (Type 4)

This injury is characterized by the interruption of (almost) all secondary muscle bundles, which typically show a wavy course due to retraction. There is extensive hematoma between the retracted muscle stumps. Functionally equivalent special forms of the type 4 lesion are:

- Avulsion of the apophysis
- (Bony) tendon avulsion
- Purely tendinous rupture at the level of the tendon or the musculotendinous interface

Traumatic apophyseolysis (functionally a type 4 lesion) is typically seen in children or adolescents and can often be diagnosed on the basis of conventional radiography alone. Special forms include undisplaced and displaced avulsions of a nonunited infantile apophysis. In some cases, the diagnosis is based on MRI, and follow-up examinations demonstrate the course of the healing process (**Fig. 8.10**). Partial (**Fig. 8.11**) and complete (**Fig. 8.12**) tendinous avulsions, without (**Figs. 8.11** and **8.12**) or with (**Fig. 8.13**) a bony fragment, can be differentiated on the basis of MRI.

Complete, purely tendinous tears of the musculotendinous interface are also classified as type 4 injuries. The morphologic criteria correspond to those described for purely tendinous partial tears of the musculotendinous interface.

Muscle Contusion, Laceration

Contusion is caused by direct blunt trauma. Different degrees of injury with edema, diffuse bleeding, circumscribed hematoma, and, rarely, crushing injury are seen. MRI shows an increased cross-sectional area of the muscle, with geographic signal-intensity changes (edema, hematoma). The volume of a hematoma can be assessed to facilitate follow-up. Edema and diffuse hemorrhage cause a feathery pattern of secondary muscle bundles in the periphery of the lesion. Complications of contusion are seromas, myositis ossificans, and (less frequently) compartment syndrome (see p. 215).

Laceration is caused by direct penetrating trauma, including penetration of the skin. In the MRI image, however, direct muscle injuries like contusions and lacerations cannot be differentiated from indirect injuries, like (partial) tears. Consequently, referral to the medical history of the patient is recommended. MRI shows a circumscribed area with discontinuous secondary muscle bundles, edema, and hematoma. Due to associated injuries in the muscle fascia, muscle herniation may develop (see p. 213).

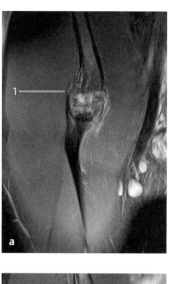 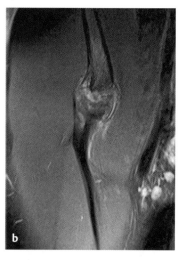 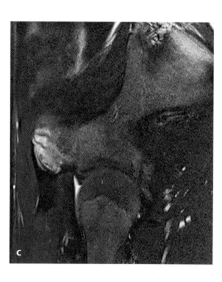

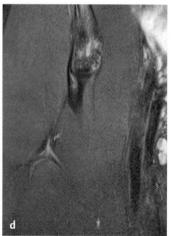 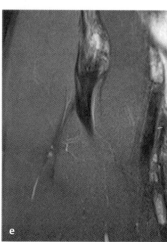

Fig. 8.10a–e Traumatic apophyseolysis of the rectus femoris muscle (caput rectum), with follow-up assessment.

a Edema, hemorrhage, moderate dehiscence, angulation, and lateral dislocation (1). Coronal section.

b–e The follow-up examination 6 weeks later, after adequate therapy, showing remodeling. Lateral periosteum can be distinguished again. Coronal sections (**b, d,** and **e**), and sagittal section (**c**).

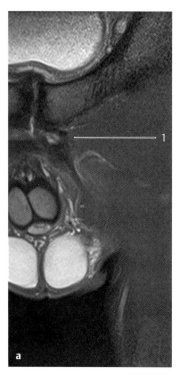 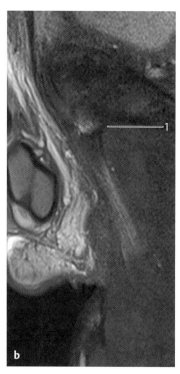

Fig. 8.11a, b Partial avulsion of the adductor longus tendon. The lateral fascicle and fascicle to the arcuate ligament are visible (1).

a Coronal section.

b Sagittal section.

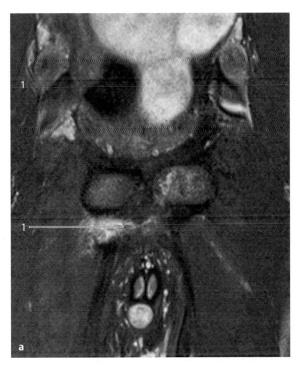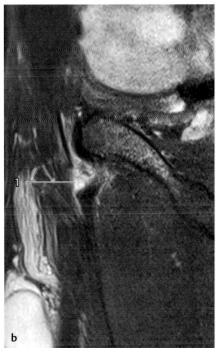

Fig. 8.12a, b   Complete avulsion of the adductor longus tendon. Retraction of the tendon (1), intact bony origin.

a Coronal section.   **b** Sagittal section.

Muscle Herniation

By definition, herniation refers to muscle tissue protruding through a gap in a fascia. The etiology is either (penetrating) trauma or increased intramuscular pressure, such as seen in muscle hypertrophy or compartment syndrome. In the latter cases, herniation occurs through the weakest areas of the fascia (typically through preformed gaps at the level of penetrating blood vessels and nerves). The middle or distal tibialis anterior muscle or other muscles of the lower leg are frequently affected, and the muscles of the thigh or forearm much less frequently. MRI shows the muscle's atypical protrusion, as well as its cause, the gap in the fascia. In uncomplicated cases, the herniated muscle has a regular signal intensity, similar to that of the unherniated portions of the muscle. Rarely, there may be associated muscle ischemia and/or entrapment neuropathy, with a pathologic signal intensity.

Muscle Denervation

In athletes, nerve compression syndromes may be caused by (atypical) muscle hypertrophy, ganglia, hematomas, or spinal disk disease. MRI can frequently identify the site of entrapment and can also visualize the typical effects on the affected muscle(s). Occasionally, pathologic signal intensity and contrast enhancement can be seen in the nerve. Initially, after 2–3 weeks, muscle edema may be present. The distribution corresponds to the innervation pattern of the spinal or peripheral nerve. Chronic denervation is characterized by atrophy and fatty degeneration of the muscle. Atrophy results in a decreased cross-sectional area of the muscle. Fatty infiltration is best demonstrated as a feathery pattern on T1-weighted images, on which fat is bright and the secondary muscle bundles are dark. Rarely, pseudoatrophy develops as a consequence of excessive accumulation of intramuscular fat, with a pathognomonic MRI image (increased cross-sectional area and feathery image on T1-weighted images, with a high proportion of fat).

Chronic Tendinosis, Tendon Rupture

Purely tendinous injuries are usually seen in elderly patients with preexisting chronic tendinosis. Minor trauma can cause a partial or complete tear in the tendon. Partial tears are characterized by partial interruption of the tendon fibers, without retraction. Complete tears show retracted tendon stumps.

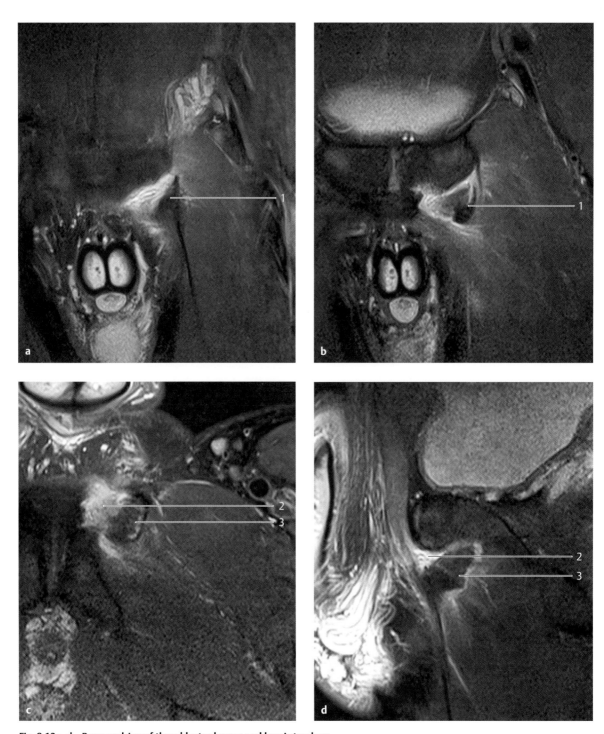

Fig. 8.13a–d   Bony avulsion of the adductor longus and brevis tendons.

a, b Retraction of the tendon (1). Coronal section.

c, d Gap (2) and tendon with avulsed bony fragment (3). Axial (**c**) and sagittal (**d**) sections.

Complications

Seroma/Cyst

Incomplete resorption of fluid accumulations or hematomas results in seromas or cystoid lesions. MRI shows well-demarcated, homogeneous structures with a high signal intensity on T2-weighted images. In a seroma, blood degradation products (mainly hemosiderin in the chronic phase) may be seen, causing more heterogeneous signal characteristics.

Fibrosis/Scar

Healed musculotendinous lesions may be accompanied by irregular fibrotic thickening or scar formation at the level of the musculotendinous interface (**Fig. 8.14**).

Myositis Ossificans

Different phases can be distinguished, both clinically and on the basis of imaging. The acute or pseudoinflammatory phase and the subacute phase show uncharacteristic findings on MRI images (early: swelling, edema, geographic area with altered signal intensity and pathologic contrast uptake; later: fat in central cancellous areas). In the chronic phase, intramuscular calcification occurs and has a tendency to decrease in size. Mature ossification is composed of both cortical and cancellous bone. The cortical bone is characterized by low signal intensity, while in the cancellous center dark trabeculae and bright fat are seen on T1-weighted images. The differential diagnosis includes inflammatory and neoplastic processes. A biopsy is usually not required, particularly when MRI is complemented with conventional radiography, ultrasound, and computed tomography. Initial calcium deposits can be detected with these imaging modalities only a few weeks after the development of symptoms. The end stage shows a heterotopic intramuscular ossification, which is pathognomonic for the disease (see also Chapters 6 and 7).

Heterotopic Ossification

The chronic stage of myositis ossificans corresponds to an intramuscular heterotopic ossification. Heterotopic ossifications also occur in other locations—for example, after tendon avulsion or in hematomas in different locations.

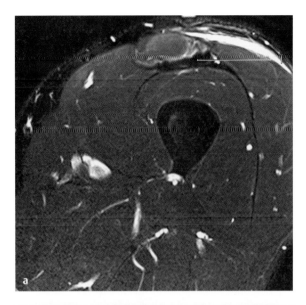

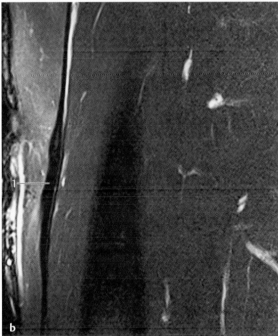

Fig. 8.14a, b An older muscle injury in the rectus femoris muscle. Fibrosis (scar plate) with irregular thickening of the intramuscular tendon (1).

a Axial section.
b Sagittal section.

Compartment Syndrome

Two types of compartment syndrome can be differentiated, on the basis of both clinical and MRI findings: traumatic, frequently caused by major hemorrhage; and functional, due to overuse. Typically, the affected muscle compartment is enlarged due to hemorrhage, edema, and/or hypertrophy (May et al. 2000). The increased pressure in the compartment—for example, due to hemorrhage in the presence of intact fascia—may cause vessel and nerve compression, muscle necrosis, and herniation through fascial gaps.

Characteristic MRI findings include a pathologic signal intensity due to edema and hemorrhage, and in the later stage due to fatty degeneration, fibrosis, dystrophic calcifications, loss of volume caused by atrophy, and thickening of the fascia. The differential diagnosis includes uncomplicated muscle injuries, thrombosis, and lymphedema. Venous thrombosis can be detected with MRI, particularly if intravenous contrast is used. Lymphedema primarily affects the subcutaneous tissue. The topographic distribution of lymphedema is not limited by the borders of muscle compartments.

Differential Diagnosis

Muscle Edema Pattern

A feathery appearance of muscle tissue, caused by edema, fluid, or blood, is seen not only after muscle injuries, but also characterizes delayed-onset muscle soreness (DOMS) (Evans et al. 1998, Marqueste et al. 2008). Muscle edema is observed hours to days after intense exercise; the edema can last considerably longer than the symptoms, up to 3 weeks (Fleckenstein et al. 1989).

The same pattern may be present in ischemic, necrotic, inflammatory, infectious, and neoplastic diseases (May et al. 2000). The early phases of myositis ossificans and compartment syndrome, subacute denervation, and infectious or autoimmune myositis may also present with the pattern of muscle edema. A feathery appearance in the muscle can also be seen after surgery, radiotherapy, and intramuscular infiltration (see **Fig. 8.4**). The distribution of the findings may be helpful (May et al. 2000); for example, dermatomyositis and polymyositis are symmetrically distributed in the muscles of the pelvis and thighs. After radiotherapy, the distribution of muscle edema is limited to the radiation field.

Note

The pattern of muscle edema has a nonspecific MRI appearance and a wide range of differential diagnoses. Despite its morphologic similarity, the pattern of fatty atrophy (see below) has distinct imaging characteristics if the appropriate examination technique is used.

Fatty Atrophy Pattern

Fatty atrophy of the muscle—for example, after untreated tendon avulsion, denervation, or corticosteroids—also shows a feathery pattern of typically atrophied secondary muscle bundles.

- The pattern of muscle edema can be differentiated using both T2-weighted or proton density–weighted fat-suppressed images and T1-weighted images.
- The latter should be acquired at least in one imaging plane in every MRI examination of the musculoskeletal system.
- Muscle atrophy starts to develop during the second week after trauma and may become irreversible after only 4 months.

Practical Tip

T1-weighted images make it easier to distinguish between the pattern of muscle edema and the pattern of fatty atrophy (see above).

Tumor, Hematoma, Bony Avulsion Pattern

This pattern is seen with muscle lesions, particularly if a larger hematoma is present, with myositis ossificans, neoplasm, abscess, parasitosis, and sarcoidosis (May et al. 2000, Bonvin et al. 2008). Intramuscular or intermuscular hematoma undergoes absorption within 6–8 weeks. Older hematomas may appear as pseudocysts or, with peripheral contrast enhancement, mimicking an abscess. Occasionally, they have to be differentiated from tumors such as rhabdomyosarcoma (see below). The pattern of intramuscular injections occasionally also resembles hematomas.

Fat can be found in benign or malignant lipomatous tumors, myositis ossificans, or hemangiomas. Tissue characterization is possible by simultaneously using T2-weighted or proton density–weighted fat-suppressed and T1-weighted imaging (Palmer et al. 1999). Fluid–fluid layers in a process indicate hematoma, abscess, or necrosis.

Malignant tumors are unlikely in the absence of contrast uptake, but on the other hand an abscess or old hematoma may demonstrate predominantly peripheral contrast uptake. A nodule with contrast uptake in an inhomogeneous hemorrhagic node may be neoplasm, granulation tissue, or myositis ossificans (May et al. 2000). However, contrast can diffuse into a fluid retention and thus appear as a node with contrast uptake. To minimize the time available for diffusion, fast pulse sequences should be used after contrast administration (Boutin et al. 2002).

An avulsion, particularly in the subacute to chronic phase, may occasionally resemble a neoplastic process (osteosarcoma, chondrosarcoma) or infectious process (abscess). The MRI findings may be ambiguous even if intravenous contrast is used. Clinical and laboratory findings may be helpful in difficult cases (Bonvin et al. 2008). If there is any doubt, comparison with previous imaging examinations, follow-up imaging, or additional modalities such as conventional radiography and/or computed tomography can be used to avoid biopsy in most cases.

Prognostic Criteria

If MRI confirms a clinically suspected muscle injury, this fact alone is associated with a less favorable prognosis (in comparison with a patient with normal MRI findings, independently of the type of injury) (Verrall et al. 2003, Gibbs et al. 2004). The cross-sectional area of the injured muscle correlates with the time required for rehabilitation (Slavotinek et al. 2002, Gibbs et al. 2004). These circumstances are taken into consideration in the classification of muscle injuries by Müller-Wohlfahrt et al. through a distinction between minor (type 3a) and moderate partial muscle tears (type 3b) (see Chapter 6).

In general, the rehabilitation time is particularly longer after injuries to the quadriceps muscle with involvement of the central tendon (Cross et al. 2004). Nevertheless, with optimal treatment, even extended injuries (**Fig. 8.15**, see also **Fig. 8.3**) can show rapid and favorable healing progress (**Figs. 8.16** and **8.17**). The healing process in a case of traumatic apophyseolysis is shown in **Fig. 8.10**.

Risk Factors for Recurrent Muscle Injury

Depending on its extent (as documented by MRI), a previous injury is a risk factor for future muscle injuries in the same muscle group. This is well documented for injuries to the hamstring muscles (Verrall et al. 2001). The longitudinal extent of the primary injury correlates with the risk of a repeat injury. The recurrent injury is frequently more extended than the primary tear (Koulouris et al. 2007a). Old injuries frequently leave scar tissue, which can be documented by MRI (see also p. 215 and **Fig. 8.14**).

> *Note*
> **A recurrent tear is frequently more extended than the original tear.**

Specific Muscle Injuries

Quadriceps Muscle

The rectus femoris muscle is most frequently involved in quadriceps injuries (Cross et al. 2004, Ouellette et al. 2006, Gyftopoulos et al. 2008). A special feature of this muscle is its double tendinous origin, with one cordlike tendon originating from the anterior inferior iliac spine (caput rectum, direct head) and the other consisting of the more variable tendinous plate (caput reflexum, indirect head), which originates from the superior aspect of the anterolateral acetabular rim and from the capsule of the hip joint. The indirect head is particularly prone to injury (Ouellette et al. 2006).

The direct head fuses into the anterior muscle fascia, while the indirect head dips into the muscle belly (Gyftopoulos et al. 2008). Excellent MRI differentiation of the two heads and their injuries is shown in **Fig. 8.18**. For further injuries of the rectus femoris muscle, see **Figs. 8.10, 8.14, 8.15**, and **8.17** (see also Chapter 13).

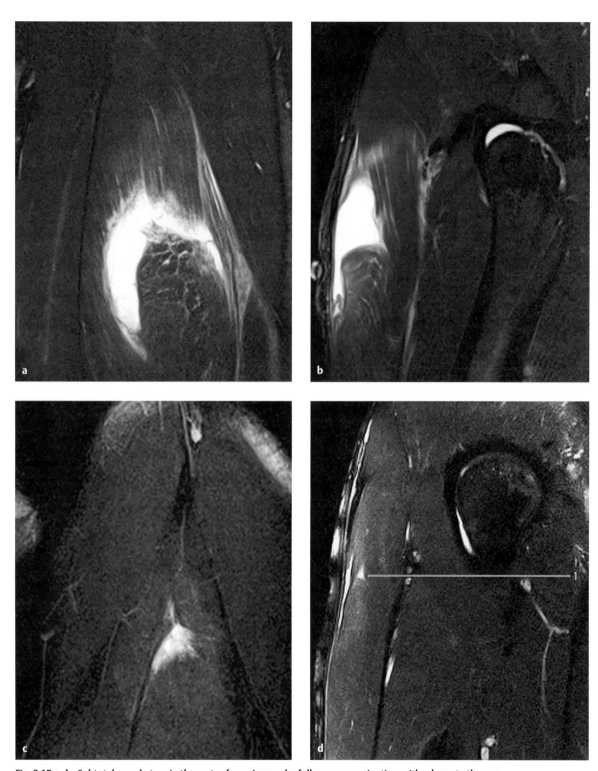

Fig. 8.15a–d   Subtotal muscle tear in the rectus femoris muscle: follow-up examination with adequate therapy.
(For further imaging levels, see **Fig. 8.3**).

a, b A large defect at the musculotendinous interface, hematoma, and musculofascial dehiscence.
Coronal (**a**) and sagittal (**b**) sections.

c, d The follow-up examination after 7 weeks shows significant improvement, with a small residual seroma (1).
Coronal (**c**) and sagittal (**d**) sections.

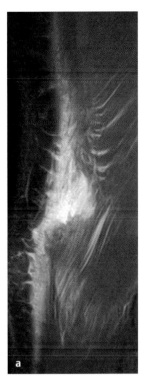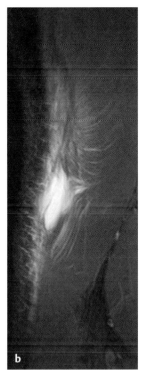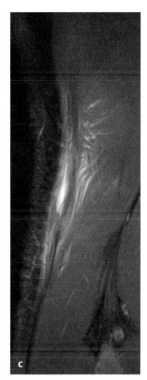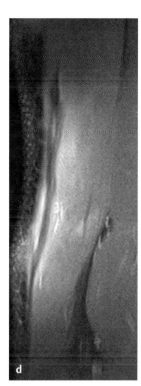

Fig. 8.16a–d   A moderate partial muscle tear in the biceps femoris muscle at the musculotendinous interface, with follow-up examination after adequate therapy showing resolving hematoma and fibrous bridging of the gap.

a The acute situation on the day after the trauma, with retraction, a muscle gap, and bundle deviation. For further imaging levels, see **Fig. 8.8**. Coronal sections.

b Follow-up image 10 days after the trauma.

c Follow-up image 31 days after the trauma.

d Follow-up image 6 weeks after the trauma. The defect has been bridged with a hypointense fibrotic strand.

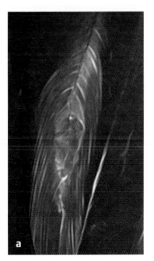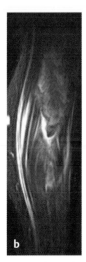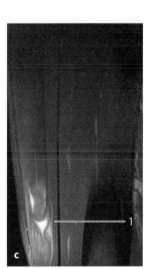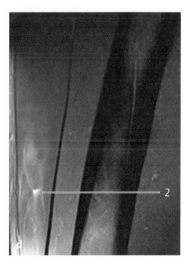

Fig. 8.17a–d   An extensive moderate partial muscle tear in the rectus femoris muscle with follow-up assessment during adequate therapy.

a, b On the first day, there is discontinuity of the central musculo-tendinous interface with hematoma. The retracted proximal tendon has an undulating course. Intact secondary muscle bundles with a curvilinear orientation toward the retracted tendon can be seen. Coronal (**a**) and sagittal (**b**) sections.

c Follow-up image after 3 weeks (1). Sagittal section.

d Follow-up image after 6 weeks (2). Sagittal section.

Hamstring Muscles

This muscle group—the biceps femoris (see **Figs. 8.1, 8.8, 8.9, 8.16**), semitendinosus, and semimembranosus muscles (**Fig. 8.19**)—is most often affected in runners (Askling et al. 2007b), dancers (Askling et al. 2007a), jumpers, and football players—in whom the long head of the biceps femoris is particularly prone to injury (De Smet and Best 2000, Slavotinek et al. 2002). These muscles extend the hip and flex the knee. Their course over two joints partly explains their frequent involvement in injuries. The high proportion of fast-twitch muscle fibers in these muscles further increases their vulnerability.

Partial, often quite extended, tears of the musculotendinous interface are frequent. The tears may occur both at the origin and insertion of the affected muscle. Partial or complete avulsions from the ischial tuberosity frequently involve the common origin of the biceps femoris and semitendinosus muscles (Koulouris and Connell 2005). Bony avulsion of the apophysis is frequent in children. Slow stretching to do the splits can lead to a quite characteristic injury (Askling et al. 2007a).

Adductor Longus Muscle

Typical injuries to the adductor longus muscle include proximal tendon avulsions (see **Figs. 8.11, 8.12, 8.13**), but minor (see **Fig. 8.6**) and moderate partial muscle tears (see **Fig. 8.7**) are also observed.

Gastrocnemius Muscle

The gastrocnemius muscle (see **Figs. 8.20** and **8.21**) and other muscles of the posterior lower leg can be affected, particularly the soleus (see **Fig. 8.5**), plantaris, and popliteus muscles. The medial head of the gastrocnemius muscle is most frequently involved among tennis players, skiers, and runners (Koulouris et al. 2007b). A partial tear of the musculotendinous unit is almost always present (Bencardino et al. 2000, Verrall et al. 2003, Koulouris et al. 2007b).

Less Frequently Involved Muscles

These include the pectoralis major muscle in the upper part of the body (Zvijac et al. 2006), the iliopsoas muscle (Bui et al. 2008), and the quadratus femoris muscles in the pelvic region (O'Brien and Bui-Mansfield 2007). The evaluation and classification of these injuries also follow the criteria and classification presented in this chapter and Chapter 6.

Summary

MRI is one of the cornerstones of musculoskeletal imaging, specifically in the diagnosis of muscle injuries. Injuries to the muscular or musculotendinous unit can be characterized and classified on the basis of MRI. A complete evaluation of all accompanying lesions, including those in bones and joints, can also be carried out during the same examination.

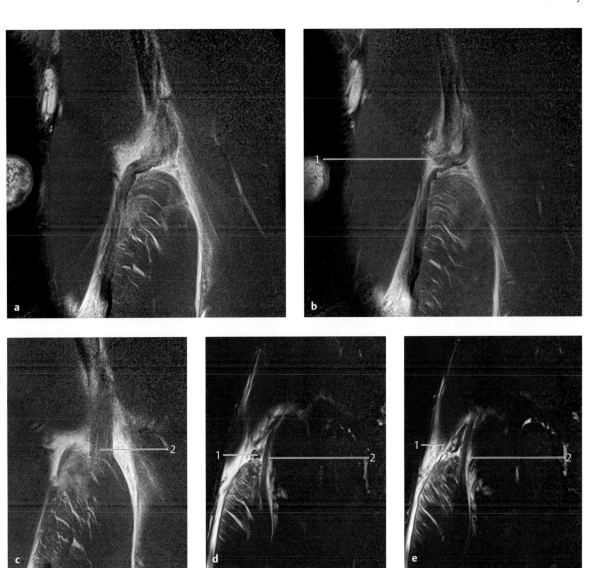

Fig. 8.18a–i   Rupture of the proximal tendon of the caput rectum of the rectus femoris muscle.

a, b Subtotal rupture of the caput rectum (direct head) tendon (1).
c   The caput reflexum (indirect head). Coronal section.
d, e Sagittal sections.

1   Caput rectum tendon
2   Caput reflexum tendon (largely intact)

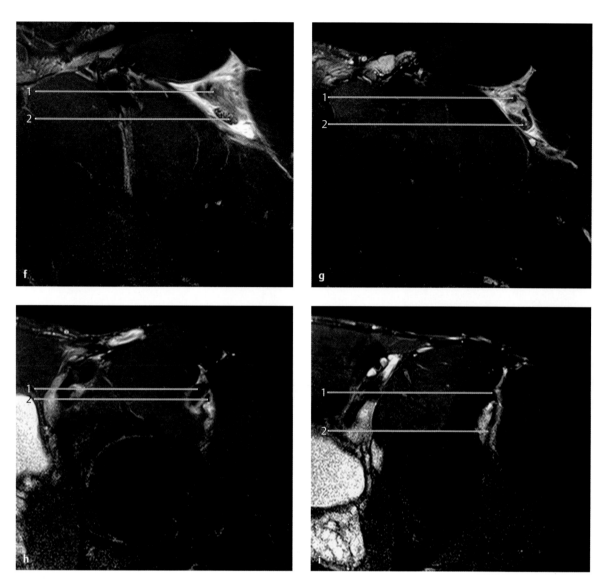

Fig. 8.18a–i   Rupture of the proximal tendon of the caput rectum of the rectus femoris muscle.

f–i   The axial images (from distal to proximal) show the distal stump of the caput rectum (**f**), the gap in the course of the caput rectum (**g**), and the proximal stump of the caput rectum (**h**). There is partial periosteal avulsion of the caput reflexum from the anterolateral acetabular rim (**i**).

1   Caput rectum tendon
2   Caput reflexum tendon

(See also Chapter 13)

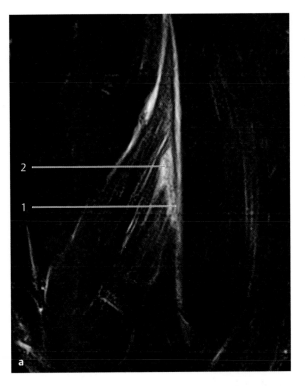

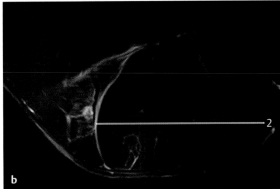

Fig. 8.19a, b **Partial rupture of the intramuscular tendon and moderate partial muscle tear of the semimembranosus muscle.**

a Coronal section.
b Axial section.

1 Partial rupture of the intramuscular tendon
2 Focal musculotendinous separation

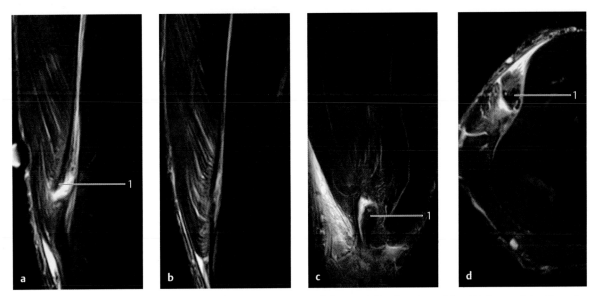

Fig. 8.20a–d **Moderate partial muscle tear in the gastrocnemius medialis muscle/focal rupture of the distal musculotendinous interface.** Partial tearing of a musculotendinous plug (1).

a, b Gap, retraction and hematoma. Sagittal sections.
c   Coronal section.

d Axial section.

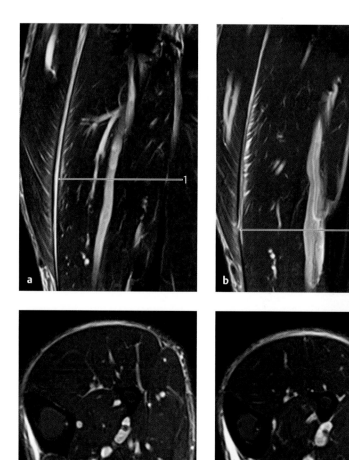

Fig. 8.21a–d   Moderate partial muscle tear/focal rupture of the distal intramuscular tendon of the gastrocnemius medialis muscle. All of the secondary muscle bundles are intact.

a, b Coronal sections.
c, d Focal musculotendinous separation. Axial sections.

1 Largely intact intramuscular tendon
2 Focal rupture

References

Askling CM, Tengvar M, Saartok T, Thorstensson A. Acute first-time hamstring strains during high-speed running: a longitudinal study including clinical and magnetic resonance imaging findings. Am J Sports Med 2007a;35(2): 197–206

Askling CM, Tengvar M, Saartok T, Thorstensson A. Acute first-time hamstring strains during slow-speed stretching: clinical, magnetic resonance imaging, and recovery characteristics. Am J Sports Med 2007b;35(10): 1716–1724

Bencardino JT, Rosenberg ZS, Brown RR, Hassankhani A, Lustrin ES, Beltran J. Traumatic musculotendinous injuries of the knee: diagnosis with MR imaging. Radiographics 2000; 20 (Spec No): S103–S120

Bonvin A, Racloz G, Hoffmeyer P. Musculoskeletal tumours misdiagnosed as sports injuries. [Article in French] Rev Med Suisse 2008; 4(184): 2750–2753

Boutin RD, Fritz RC, Steinbach LS. Imaging of sports-related muscle injuries. Radiol Clin North Am 2002; 40(2): 333–362, vii

Bui KL, Ilaslan H, Recht M, Sundaram M. Iliopsoas injury: an MRI study of patterns and prevalence correlated with clinical findings. Skeletal Radiol 2008; 37(3): 245–249

Cross TM, Gibbs N, Houang MT, Cameron M. Acute quadriceps muscle strains: magnetic resonance imaging features and prognosis. Am J Sports Med 2004; 32(3): 710–719

De Smet AA, Best TM. MR imaging of the distribution and location of acute hamstring injuries in athletes. AJR Am J Roentgenol 2000; 174(2): 393–399

Evans GFF, Haller RG, Wyrick PS, Parkey RW, Fleckenstein JL. Submaximal delayed-onset muscle soreness: correlations between MR imaging findings and clinical measures. Radiology 1998; 208(3): 815–820

Fleckenstein JL, Weatherall PT, Parkey RW, Payne JA, Peshock RM. Sports-related muscle injuries: evaluation with MR imaging. Radiology 1989; 172(3): 793–798

Gibbs NJ, Cross TM, Cameron M, Houang MT. The accuracy of MRI in predicting recovery and recurrence of acute grade one hamstring muscle strains within the same season in Australian Rules football players. J Sci Med Sport 2004; 7(2): 248–258

Gyftopoulos S, Rosenberg ZS, Schweitzer ME, Bordalo-Rodrigues M. Normal anatomy and strains of the deep musculotendinous junction of the proximal rectus femoris: MRI features. AJR Am J Roentgenol 2008; 190(3): W182–W186

Koulouris G, Connell D. Hamstring muscle complex: an imaging review. Radiographics 2005; 25(3): 571–586

Koulouris G, Connell DA, Brukner P, Schneider-Kolsky M. Magnetic resonance imaging parameters for assessing risk of recurrent hamstring injuries in elite athletes. Am J Sports Med 2007a;35(9): 1500–1506

Koulouris G, Ting AYI, Jhamb A, Connell D, Kavanagh EC. Magnetic resonance imaging findings of injuries to the calf muscle complex. Skeletal Radiol 2007b;36(10): 921–927

Marqueste T, Giannesini B, Fur YL, Cozzone PJ, Bendahan D. Comparative MRI analysis of T2 changes associated with single and repeated bouts of downhill running leading to eccentric-induced muscle damage. J Appl Physiol 2008; 105(1): 299–307

May DA, Disler DG, Jones EA, Balkissoon AA, Manaster BJ. Abnormal signal intensity in skeletal muscle at MR imaging: patterns, pearls, and pitfalls. Radiographics 2000; 20: S295–S315

O'Brien SD, Bui-Mansfield LT. MRI of quadratus femoris muscle tear: another cause of hip pain. AJR Am J Roentgenol 2007; 189(5): 1185–1189

Ouellette H, Thomas BJ, Nelson E, Torriani M. MR imaging of rectus femoris origin injuries. Skeletal Radiol 2006; 35(9): 665–672

Palmer WE, Kuong SJ, Elmadbouh HM. MR imaging of myotendinous strain. AJR Am J Roentgenol 1999; 173(3): 703–709

Slavotinek JP, Verrall GM, Fon GT. Hamstring injury in athletes: using MR imaging measurements to compare extent of muscle injury with amount of time lost from competition. AJR Am J Roentgenol 2002; 179(6): 1621–1628

Verrall GM, Slavotinek JP, Barnes PG, Fon GT, Spriggins AJ. Clinical risk factors for hamstring muscle strain injury: a prospective study with correlation of injury by magnetic resonance imaging. Br J Sports Med 2001; 35(6): 435–439, discussion 440

Verrall GM, Slavotinek JP, Barnes PG, Fon GT. Diagnostic and prognostic value of clinical findings in 83 athletes with posterior thigh injury: comparison of clinical findings with magnetic resonance imaging documentation of hamstring muscle strain. Am J Sports Med 2003; 31(6): 969–973

Zvijac JE, Schurhoff MR, Hechtman KS, Uribe JW. Pectoralis major tears: correlation of magnetic resonance imaging and treatment strategies. Am J Sports Med 2006; 34(2): 289–294

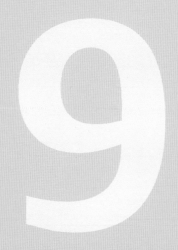

9

Differential Diagnosis of Muscle Pain

B. Schoser

Translated by Terry Telger

Special Diagnostic Issues 228
Pain History in Myalgia 228
Creatine Kinase 228
Indications for Muscle Biopsy 229

Neurologic Disorders 230
Clinical Symptoms and Lesion Location 230
Lesions of the First or Second
Motor Neuron 232
Peripheral Nerve Lesions 232
Muscle Cramps 232

**Hereditary Muscle Diseases
with Myalgia** 233
Degenerative Myopathies 233
Hereditary Metabolic Myopathies 234
Nondystrophic and Dystrophic
Myotonias 235

Acquired Muscle Diseases with Myalgia 235
Inflammatory Muscle Diseases
with Myalgia 235
Endocrine Myopathies 237
Toxic Myopathies with Myalgia 237
Rheumatologic Diseases 238
Myofascial Pain Syndrome 239

**Relationship of Myalgia to the Classification
of Muscle Injuries** 242
Fatigue-Induced Muscle Disorder
(Type 1a) Differentiated from Myalgia 242
Spine-Related Neuromuscular Muscle
Disorder (Type 2a) Differentiated from
a Myofascial Trigger Point 242
Muscle-Related Neuromuscular Muscle
Disorder (Type 2b) Differentiated from
a Myofascial Trigger Point 242
Partial Muscle Tears (Type 3) Differentiated
from a Myofascial Trigger Point 242

Besides sports-related injuries, even competitive athletes may suffer from various acute and chronic forms of muscle pain and congenital muscle diseases that can significantly limit their performance. This chapter deals with congenital and acquired muscle disorders that are associated with muscle pain. The chapter concludes by relating muscle pain to the classification of muscle injuries presented in this book.

> **Caution**
>
> Inspection and palpation are still the cornerstones of neuromuscular diagnosis. All subsequent tests, no matter how sophisticated, serve only to substantiate the primary clinical working diagnosis, which is usually syndromic. It makes no sense to reverse this sequence.

Special Diagnostic Issues

Besides the clinical examination techniques described earlier in this book, it is necessary to consider some special issues involved in the neuromuscular evaluation and classification of muscle pain:

- *Cramps* are transient, involuntary, usually very painful and visible contractions of individual muscles.
- *Fasciculations* are short, involuntary contractions of muscle fibers in a motor unit, based on spontaneous discharges of the innervating axons. Fasciculations are ubiquitous, visible, repetitive, and arrhythmic. They can be induced by mechanical manipulations such as tapping or pinching a muscle.
- *Myokymia* is a visible, involuntary "quivering" of muscle bundles that is not strong enough to move adjacent joints.
- *Myotonia* refers to the delayed relaxation of a muscle, which takes longer than normal to relax after voluntary contraction or mechanical stimulation.
- *Contracture* generally refers to the fixed, clinically visible shortening of a muscle, caused by fibrous tissue proliferation in damaged muscle parenchyma. This differs from a "physiologic" contracture, which is a permanent, electrically silent state of muscle shortening that is in principle reversible. The activation of actin and myosin filaments leads to local muscle shortening, which compresses the associated longitudinal and horizontal capillaries, resulting in local ischemia and hypoxia—like that occurring at a trigger point in myofascial pain syndrome.
- *Spasm* refers to the more sustained involuntary contraction of a muscle or muscle group.
- *Tetany* is a state of neuromuscular hyperexcitability. The permanent form of tetany is tetanus, which is also associated with permanent muscle contractions.

Pain History in Myalgia

A standard pain history should be elicited in patients whose primary complaint is muscle pain. First, it should be determined whether the pain follows a constant, intermittent, or remitting pattern. Other key concerns are the frequency and duration of the pain and whether it is increasing over time. The examiner should ask specifically about location and distribution (e.g., focal, segmental, lateralized, or generalized), referral pattern, and whether the pain sensation is superficial or deep. Whole-body diagrams are very helpful in documenting this information. The character of the pain should be described in the patient's own words. We also use a standard pain questionnaire to characterize and quantify the pain more precisely and identify affective components. A depression inventory may be added for further differentiation. The differentiation between rest pain and exercise-induced pain can supply useful etiologic information. In addition to emotional distress, there may be other precipitating factors such as fatty foods, a carbohydrate-rich diet, cold, stress, lack of sleep, infections, or drugs that should also be identified. The examiner should also ask about and test for concomitant neuromuscular and neurologic symptoms such as muscle weakness, muscular atrophy, or muscle cramps, as well as any motor difficulties associated with walking, running, stair-climbing, or other activities.

> *Practical Tip*
>
> Whole-body diagrams are helpful in documenting the location and distribution of pain.

Creatine Kinase

Despite its known limitations, serum creatine kinase is still the most important laboratory marker for neuromuscular diseases.

The skeletal muscles normally contain 96% of all creatine kinase in the body. Creatine kinase is the enzyme responsible for the reversible conversion of adenosine triphosphate (ATP) and creatine into adenosine diphosphate (ADP) and phosphocreatine during intracellular energy transfer between the mitochondria and cytosol. Creatine kinase is synthesized in the form of creatine kinase M (CK-M), creatine kinase B (CK-B), and creatine kinase Mi (CK-Mi). Usually measured in the serum, creatine kinase activity includes isoenzymes in the form of the dimers CK-MM, CK-MB, CK-BB, and two macro-creatine kinases.

A marked elevation of serum creatine kinase can be measured in patients with acute myositis, muscular dystrophy, and rare metabolic myopathies (which cause up to a 20-fold increase). Nonmuscular diseases such as polyneuropathies and motor neuron disease may also raise creatine kinase levels to as much as 1000 U/L. Ten studies including a total of 371 patients with "idiopathic" high creatine kinase levels showed evidence of a possible causal neuromuscular disorder in 51% of the patients, on the basis of their family history and personal history of occupational and recreational physical activity. In 27% of the patients, a relationship was found between physical activity and elevated creatine kinase levels. Neurologic examination showed evidence of neuromuscular disease in 11% of the patients. A cause could not be established in 42% of the patients, despite clinical examination, electromyography, and muscle biopsy. Myalgia referable to an electrolyte imbalance (low potassium, calcium, magnesium, and sodium, or elevated sodium) may be apparent even at rest, presenting clinically with muscle cramps and elevated creatine kinase. Hyperuricemia is another potentially important cause.

Macro-Creatine Kinase

Macro-creatine kinase is present when the CK-MB fraction is 15% higher than the total creatine kinase activity. Its presence can be confirmed by performing creatine kinase electrophoresis. Differential diagnosis is aided by noting that the concomitant detection of a high serum myoglobin level suggests primary damage to muscle fibers as the cause.

> *Practical Tip*
>
> **A myoglobin assay is helpful only in the differential diagnosis of macro-creatine kinase and should not be considered a routine test.**

Types of macro-creatine kinase:
- *Macro-creatine kinase type 1* is a postsynthetic isoenzyme of CK-BB, bound to specific immunoglobulins and having a total molecular weight > 200 kDa. Macro-creatine kinase type 1 is unlikely to have any pathogenic significance. It is most prevalent in older individuals, especially women, and is present in 0.3% of all patients with elevated creatine kinase.
- *Macro-creatine kinase type 2* is an oligomer of mitochondrial creatine kinase (CK-Mi). To date, it has been detected only in the setting of severe diseases, including neoplasias and cirrhosis of the liver.

Creatine Kinase in Healthy Individuals and Athletes

A marked elevation of serum creatine kinase levels (up to > 1000 U/L; 180 U/L or less is normal) may also be measured in healthy individuals following increased physical activity, unaccustomed occupational or recreational exertion, after alcohol consumption, and especially in recreational or competitive athletes after training or game exposure.

> *Practical Tip*
>
> **Intramuscular injections and athletic activity should be avoided for at least 72 hours before the creatine kinase level is determined. Repeated creatine kinase tests are strongly advised before any conclusions are drawn on the presence or absence of disease.**

The recommended work-up for the differential diagnosis of elevated serum creatine kinase levels is outlined in **Fig. 9.1**.

Rhabdomyolysis

A variety of acquired (toxic or inflammatory) and hereditary (degenerative or metabolic) myopathies can lead to rhabdomyolysis, which denotes an acute, massive rise in creatine kinase levels to far above 1500 U/L. The rise tends to progress in subsequent hours and may be associated with urinary excretion of myoglobin (**Fig. 9.2**).

> *Note*
>
> **Very massive and peracute forms of rhabdomyolysis (with creatine kinase levels rising above 20 000 U/L within 2 h) may lead to acute renal failure—a medical emergency that requires immediate treatment and further investigation.**

Indications for Muscle Biopsy

Molecular-genetic test methods have reduced the need for muscle biopsy. Accurate phenotype characterization by clinical examination, electromyography, and special laboratory tests can establish a primary DNA diagnosis for fascioscapulohumeral muscular dystrophy, the myotonic dystrophies (DM1 and DM2), oculopharyngeal muscular dystrophy, as well as Emery–Dreifuss and lamin A/C muscular dystrophy. As for the limb-girdle syndromes, a direct gene mutation analysis is justified only in patients with suspected Duchenne muscular dystrophy. Otherwise a muscle biopsy is indicated, due to the great number and variety of the different genetic forms. Congenital structural myopathies, hereditary metabolic myopathies, and acquired myopathies are still the domain of diagnostic muscle biopsy (**Table 9.1**).

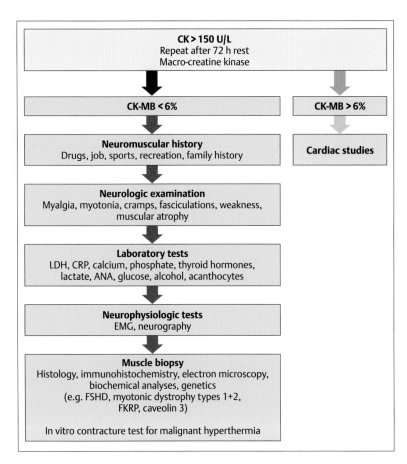

Fig. 9.1 Flow chart for the differential diagnosis of elevated serum creatine kinase levels.

ANA antinuclear antibodies
CK creatine kinase
CRP C-reactive protein
EMG electromyography
FKRP gene encoding for fukutin-related protein
FSHD fascioscapulohumeral muscular dystrophy
LDH lactate dehydrogenase

Table 9.1 Indications for muscle biopsy

Mandatory

In patients with suspected:

- Muscular dystrophies, myofibrillar myopathies
- Congenital structural myopathies
- Myositis
- Metabolic and mitochondrial myopathies
- Rhabdomyolysis (but only after 4 weeks!)

Optional

In patients with:

- Muscular involvement by a systemic disease (e.g., vasculitis, sarcoidosis, systemic lupus erythematosus, amyloidosis, or paraneoplasia)
- Unexplained disorders characterized by muscle weakness, myalgia, or elevated serum creatine kinase
- Suspected malignant hyperthermia

Neurologic Disorders

Clinical Symptoms and Lesion Location

A syndromic phenotypic classification is an important aid in the localization of nerve lesions (**Fig. 9.3**). Systemic diseases are more likely to cause symmetrical deficits, whereas focal lesions more often produce unilateral manifestations. Systemic diseases of muscle, such as congenital or acquired inflammatory myopathies, usually present with proximal limb-girdle weakness and atrophy consistent with a proximal myopathic syndrome. By contrast, systemic lesions affecting a peripheral nerve tend to produce distal manifestations such as a distal symmetrical polyneuropathy syndrome. Lesions of a peripheral neuron cause early hyporeflexia or areflexia by interrupting the reflex arc. By contrast, a muscle disease will cause lost or diminished reflexes only after the muscle parenchyma has become severely atrophied or a fixed contracture has developed. Trophic and sensory disturbances almost always result from lesions of the nerve roots, plexus, or peripheral nerve. Fasciculations, defined as spontaneous visible contractions of motor units in hypotrophic or atrophic muscle, are an important diagnostic indicator of

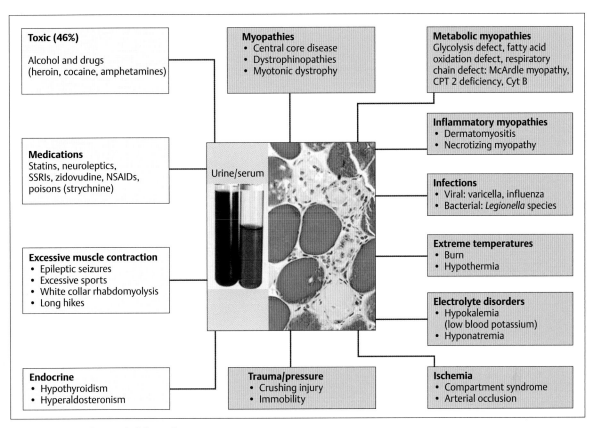

Fig. 9.2 Causes of acute rhabdomyolysis.

CPT   carnitine palmitoyltransferase
Cyt B   cytochrome B
NSAIDs nonsteroidal anti-inflammatory drugs
SSRIs   serotonin reuptake inhibitors

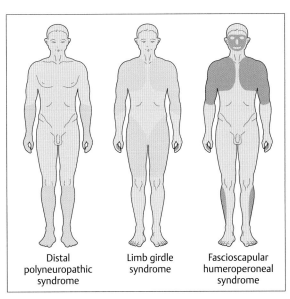

Fig. 9.3 Clinical syndromes in neuromuscular diseases.

anterior horn or ventral root lesions (**Fig. 9.4**). Mild fasciculations may also occur in peripheral neuropathies and in the absence of disease ("benign fasciculations" in normal muscle tissue).

Practical Tip

"Benign fasciculations" may occur in healthy individuals and athletes. They always involve a nonatrophic, nonparetic muscle. A common example is the periorbital muscle twitch that may occur after ingesting caffeine, smoking, or after sleep deprivation.

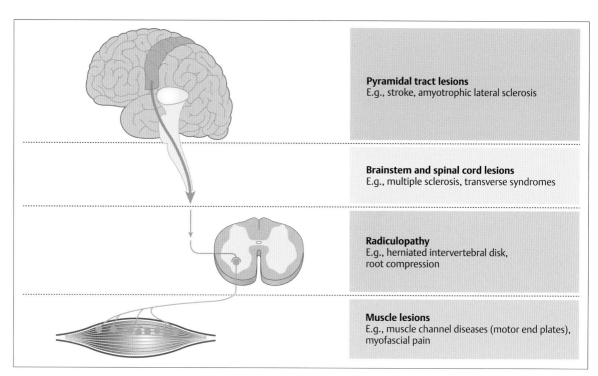

Fig. 9.4   Differential diagnosis of increased muscle tone.

Lesions of the First or Second Motor Neuron

A lesion of the first motor neuron will cause a spastic or dystonic increase in muscle tone and may lead to painful firmness of the affected limb muscle. Muscle pain in the shoulder girdle, especially on initiating movement, is typical of extrapyramidal motor disease such as Parkinson syndrome (rigor, akinesia). Spinal cord lesions lead to projected muscle pain and are associated with complex neurologic symptoms.

Congenital (spinal muscular atrophy) or idiopathic lesions of the second motor neuron (amyotrophic lateral sclerosis) may also be associated with myalgia. As in spasticity and dystonia, they are usually caused by secondary myofascial pain or musculoskeletal pain syndromes resulting from the unphysiologic loading of joints and tendons based on muscular atrophy or a central dysregulation of muscle tone. Muscle cramps are a common associated finding. Inflammatory, traumatic and congenital spinal cord disorders such as syringomyelia may also be associated with muscle pain. Patients with "stiff-person syndrome" experience episodes of severe, shooting, asymmetrical stiffness accompanied by cramping of the truncal and proximal limb muscles, along with myoclonic spasms of abdominal and paraspinal muscles. Muscle cramps and spasms may be provoked by emotional stress, muscular stretching, or tactile stimulation.

Peripheral Nerve Lesions

Peripheral nerve lesions cause a neuropathic pain that is distinct from the "nociceptor pain" occurring after tissue trauma. However, neuropathic pain may also be accompanied by nociceptor pain in myalgia, resulting in a mixed pain pattern. One example is acute polyradiculitis (Guillain–Barré syndrome), which features mixed pain and autonomic disturbances. Another example is neuromyotonia, which is characterized by continuous muscle fiber activity. Patients complain of increased muscle tension that starts in the distal extremities. The diagnosis is suggested clinically by myokymia, painful muscle cramps, and muscle stiffness.

Muscle Cramps

Muscle cramps usually occur without a detectable cause. They often occur at rest and at night and most commonly affect the calf muscles, especially the soleus muscle. The soleus is an almost purely tonic muscle composed of slow-twitch type I fibers. Given its fiber composition and its possible endowment with nociceptors, the soleus muscle is extremely susceptible to cramping. Cramps appear to be significantly more common in muscles with a high proportion of type I fibers. A cramp is usually initiated neurogenically in the terminal intramuscular portions of the efferent axons. Before a patient is diagnosed with

Table 9.2 Studies necessary in the differential diagnosis of muscle cramps

History
• Mechanisms that provoke muscle cramps
• Family history, drug history
Assessment of neurologic and neuromuscular status
Electrophysiologic testing where appropriate
• Electromyography
• Nerve conduction velocities
Laboratory tests
• Electrolytes, including magnesium
• Kidney and liver values
• Blood glucose
• Thyroid hormones
• Uric acid
• Creatine kinase

Table 9.3 Differential diagnosis of muscle cramps

Acquired myopathies	Alcohol
Hereditary myopathies	
• Metabolic myopathies	Glycogenosis, type 5 (McArdle disease); MAD deficiency, etc.
• Myotonias	Myotonic dystrophy, types 1 and 2
• Degenerative myopathies	Becker dystrophinopathy
	Central core disease
	Brody myopathy
	Rippling muscle disease
Neurogenic cause	Polyneuropathy
	Motor neuron diseases (ALS, SMA, Kennedy)
	Neuromyotonia
	Root irritation syndromes (herniated disk)
Central nervous cause	Stiff-person syndrome (spinal cord)
	Tetanus, strychnine (spinal cord)
	Brainstem seizures
Metabolic cause	Uremia
	Hyperthyroidism, hypothyroidism
	Electrolyte disorders (diarrhea, vomiting)
Drug side effects	Beta blockers, scopolamine, theophylline, terbutaline, salbutamol, neuroleptics, isoniazid, oral contraceptives, morphine preparations, steroids, etc.

ALS, amyotrophic lateral sclerosis; MAD, myoadenylate deaminase; SMA, spinal muscular atrophy

"idiopathic muscle cramps," the following frequent symptomatic causes should be investigated:
• Hypovolemia
• Hyponatremia
• Uremia
• Pregnancy
• Hypothyroidism
• Hyperuricemia
• Pharmacologic effects
• Systemic neurologic diseases associated with a spastic increase in muscle tone
• Rare central motor disorders, such as stiff-person syndrome
• Rare muscle diseases such as myotonias and metabolic myopathies

Table 9.2 lists the studies that are necessary in the differential diagnosis of muscle cramps, and **Table 9.3** lists the possible diagnoses that should be considered.

Selected cases may require additional function studies (e.g., exercise testing) and possibly a Doppler ultrasound examination of the arteries and veins.

Hereditary Muscle Diseases with Myalgia

Degenerative Myopathies

Degenerative myopathies are genetically based abnormalities affecting the structure of the muscle membrane or intracellular structural components. The cardinal symptoms of these diseases are muscular weakness and atrophy, and elevated serum creatine kinase levels are usually present. Myalgia is a feature of numerous degenerative myopathies. It is believed to be caused by muscle fiber necrosis, with an associated clearance of necrotic cells and activation of muscular nociceptors.

More detailed information on muscular dystrophies can be found at http://neuromuscular.wustl.edu (Neuromuscular Disease Center, Washington University, St. Louis, Missouri, USA) and http://www.baur-institut.de (Friedrich Baur Institute, Munich, Germany).

Hereditary Metabolic Myopathies

The metabolic myopathies include glycogen and lipid storage diseases and mitochondrial myopathies. This group is characterized by disturbances of carbohydrate metabolism, fatty acid metabolism, oxidative phosphorylation, and energy production or purine metabolism.

The main symptoms of metabolic myopathies are:
- Exercise intolerance
- Exercise-induced muscle cramps
- Weakness or rhabdomyolysis

Glycogen Storage Diseases

Static glycogen storage diseases such as Pompe disease present clinically with progressive muscle weakness and atrophy, while "dynamic" glycogen storage diseases such as McArdle myopathy are marked by exercise intolerance, early loss of stamina, painful muscle contractures, cramps, and myoglobinuria. Skeletal muscle with a primary defect of cytosolic glycogenolytic metabolism lacks the ability to produce lactic acid during exercise, resulting in a rise of intracellular pH.

Inherited as an autosomal-recessive trait, McArdle myopathy (phosphorylase deficiency, glycogen storage disease type 5) is the most common glycogen storage disease in the adult population. Its prevalence is estimated at one in 100 000 births. Histopathology shows a vacuolar myopathy with negative phosphorylase histochemistry. McArdle myopathy is characterized by a significant depletion of high-energy ATP and phosphocreatine during aerobic and ischemic low-level exercise, accompanied by a rise in intracellular pH. Reduction of the adenine nucleotide pool appears to cause muscle membrane excitation, leading to a disturbance of muscle contractility. These energy deficits may contribute to typical clinical symptoms such as muscle stiffness and painful contractures, early fatigue, and muscle cramps. Myalgias are most frequently reported in the thighs and upper arms. The quality of the pain is usually likened to that of a muscle cramp or "charley horse" soreness.

Fatty Acid Oxidation Disorders (β-Oxidation)

This group of metabolic myopathies present clinically with progressive muscle weakness (e.g., primary or secondary carnitine deficiency), exercise intolerance with muscle cramps (e.g., carnitine palmitoyltransferase deficiency), or recurrent episodes of rhabdomyolysis.

Fatty acid oxidation disorders, like glycogen storage diseases, are multisystemic, involving not just the skeletal muscle and myocardium but also the liver and other organs. Fatty acid oxidation disorders are generally manifested in childhood by symptoms such as hypoketotic hypoglycemia, which may be triggered by fasting, exercise, or infection and may have a fatal course.

Fatty acids are an important energy source for the heart, skeletal muscle, liver, and kidneys. β-Oxidation of fatty acids takes place in the mitochondrial matrix. However, since the fatty acids, as coenzyme A esters, cannot penetrate the inner mitochondrial membrane, they are esterified with carnitine and transported across the membrane via the carnitine shuttle. As a result, loss of the shuttle proteins or available carnitine creates a metabolic block leading to fatty acid accumulation and consequent lipid storage in the tissues. All other enzymes involved in fatty acid oxidation may also be affected and may cause specific disorders. Three types are distinguished:
- Disorders of mitochondrial fatty acid transport
- Disorders of fatty acid oxidation
- Impaired coupling to the respiratory chain

In many cases, the carnitine spectrum, which can be determined by tandem mass spectrometry of blood serum, provides initial evidence of a disturbance in the breakdown of fatty acids. Generally, the presumed defects are then confirmed by enzymatic or molecular genetic testing.

A genetic defect of carnitine palmitoyltransferase may also contribute to the development of myalgia. Carnitine palmitoyltransferase (CPT) is an enzyme of the outer (CPT 1) and inner mitochondrial membrane (CPT 2). Together with carnitine, this enzyme is responsible for transporting medium-chain and long-chain fatty acids into the mitochondrion. The cardinal symptom of carnitine palmitoyltransferase deficiency is recurrent rhabdomyolysis, which may be triggered by exercise and by fasting or starvation.

Purine Metabolism Disorders, Myoadenylate Deaminase Deficiency

A lesser-known disorder of purine metabolism is myoadenylate deaminase deficiency. Transmitted as an autosomal-recessive trait, this condition is detected in 1–3% of all muscle biopsies, usually as an incidental finding. The cardinal symptom is exercise-induced stiffness of the skeletal muscles, often without a definite contracture, which may be associated with raised creatine kinase levels. Many patients with this disorder are homozygous for the C34-T mutation in the *AMPD1* gene. The definitive role of this purine metabolism disorder is not yet fully understood, however.

Mitochondrial Myopathies

Defects in the five respiratory chain complexes typically lead to multisystem disorders, as mitochondria are the power-plants for every cell in the body. Most patients manifest a variety of symptoms with muscular involvement. The dominant finding in children is a generalized muscular hypotonia, while adolescents and adults typically show exercise intolerance. Common associated findings are respiratory failure, dilated and hypertrophic cardiomyopathies, and abnormalities of cardiac impulse conduction. Neurologic examination may reveal a variety of cerebellar and cortical disorders.

Note
The symptoms of many mitochondrial disorders worsen as the body temperature rises, as in patients with a febrile infection.

Nondystrophic and Dystrophic Myotonias

Nondystrophic myotonias include genetic defects of the muscle chloride channel (Becker/Thomsen) and the muscle sodium channel (e.g., paramyotonia, sodium channel disease). The dominant feature of these disorders is abnormal muscle stiffness.

The main clinical symptoms of the two autosomal dominant forms of myotonic dystrophy (DM1, DM2) are:
- Myotonia
- Muscle weakness
- Early cataracts
- Potential for other multisystem symptoms

Curschmann–Steinert disease (DM1) is the classic form of myotonic dystrophy, characterized by an early age of symptom onset, rapid progression, and a severe course with marked cognitive impairment. "Proximal" myotonic myopathy (DM2) has a later age of onset, runs a milder course, and is characterized by proximal weakness of the limb muscles.

The genetic cause of DM1 has been identified as an abnormally expanded cytosine–thymine–guanine triplet repeat in the 3′-untranslated region of the myotonic dystrophy protein kinase gene on chromosome 19. DM2 is caused by an abnormally expanded tetranucleotide cytosine–cytosine–thymine–guanine repeat in intron 1 of the zinc finger 9 gene on chromosome 3 q.

Acquired Muscle Diseases with Myalgia

Inflammatory Muscle Diseases with Myalgia

Infectious Myositis

Infectious forms of myositis are commonly associated with myalgia. Bacterial myositis is the most prevalent inflammatory muscle disease in the world. Staphylococcal infections are the most common and have an extremely painful course. Often perceived as "body aches," the myositis that accompanies an infectious temperature rise is a very typical feature of viral infections. Causative organisms include coxsackievirus B5, as well as influenza and parainfluenza viruses. A parasitic infection such as trichinosis should also be considered in patients with blood eosinophilia. Tick-borne borreliosis (Lyme disease) may also lead to painful borrelial myositis.

Immunogenic Inflammatory Myopathies: Dermatomyositis

Acute dermatomyositis is the most important disease in the group of immunogenic inflammatory myopathies. It has a seasonal pattern, with an estimated incidence of 2–10 new cases per 1 million population per year. All other forms, idiopathic polymyositis, and inclusion-body myositis, are generally painless.

Clinical Characteristics

Dermatomyositis is a severe, acquired, acute muscle disease characterized by proximal muscle weakness, usually severe systemic symptoms, and cutaneous manifestations. A very typical finding is a reddish-purple skin rash, known as a heliotrope rash ("lilac disease"), which predominantly affects the eyelids, cheeks, and upper chest (**Fig. 9.5a**). It may also spread to other areas such as the extensor surfaces of the limbs, the nape of the neck, and lower chest. Collodion patches (Gottron sign) may appear over the metacarpophalangeal joints of the hands (**Fig. 9.5 d**). Enlarged capillaries that are tender to pressure may appear spontaneously on the nail fold (Keinig's nail sign, **Fig. 9.5c**). Some patients develop rough, cracked skin areas on the palms and fingers ("mechanic's hand," **Fig. 9.5b**). Myalgia is frequently reported in the muscles of the shoulder girdle and thighs. The quality of the pain may be described as "charley horse" soreness, burning, racking, sharp, or as a dull ache. Typically, the pain is exacerbated by exercise. Involvement of internal organs should also be considered (pharynx, lower esophagus in 50% of cases, cardiac arrhythmias in up to 40% of cases).

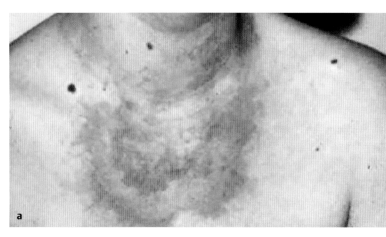

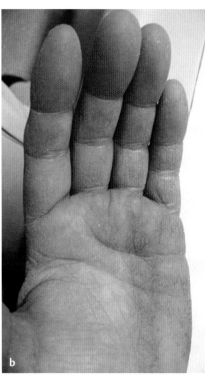

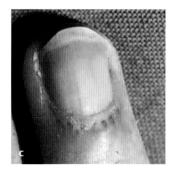

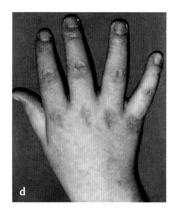

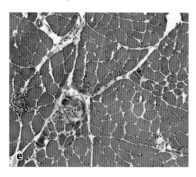

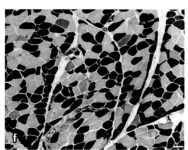

Fig. 9.5a–f   Dermatomyositis. This disease is a vessel-associated inflammation that is complement-positive and also positive for CD4 lymphocytes.

a A typical reddish-purple rash affecting the open-collar area of the neck and upper chest.
b Hyperkeratosis of the palms (mechanic's hands).
c Keinig's nail sign on the nail fold.
d Collodion patches (Gottron sign) over the knuckles.
e Perifascicular inflammation with areas of fresh necrosis (hematoxylin–eosin stain).
f Perifascicular atrophy (ATPase histochemistry pH 9.4: type 2 muscle fibers dark brown).

Differential Diagnosis

The differential diagnosis of dermatomyositis includes overlap syndromes such as progressive systemic sclerosis and Sharp syndrome. Antisynthetase syndromes such as Jo-1 syndrome are a separate clinical entity characterized by the cardinal triad of myositis, synovitis, and fibrosing alveolitis (**Table 9.4**).

Pathogenesis

Humoral factors and vasculitic processes have a key role in the pathogenesis of dermatomyositis. The vasculitis incites "pathognomonic perifascicular atrophy" in the muscle parenchyma. This atrophy is caused by inflammatory changes in the small muscular vessels, with endothelial cell proliferation and "tubuloreticular inclusions" detectable on electron microscopy. Microinfarctions with necrosis of muscle fibers are occasionally found as evidence of florid vasculitis, especially in juvenile dermatomyositis. The immunogenic and vasculitic myalgia in dermatomyositis has been attributed to the connections that exist between the free nerve endings and damaged capillaries. These C fibers show an increased expression of substance P and calcitonin gene-related peptide (CGRP), which reflects the increased nociceptor input.

Table 9.4 Clinical syndromes and autoantibody profiles of immunogenic forms of myositis

Clinical syndromes	Antibodies
Antisynthetase syndromes (joints, skin, alveolitis, myositis)	Antisynthetase antibodies: Jo-1, PL-7, PL-12
Polymyositis	Anti-SRP
Dermatomyositis	Anti-MI-2
Myositis–scleroderma overlap polymyositis	Anti-PM-Scl
Overlap, systemic lupus erythematosus, systemic sclerosis	Anti-U1-nRNP
Overlap, systemic lupus erythematosus	Anti-Ku

Note

Dermatomyositis is a common disease, the acute stage of which is associated with general malaise and myalgia.

Endocrine Myopathies

The underlying endocrinopathy initially determines the dominant clinical features of endocrine myopathies. Hypothyroidism is manifested by muscle weakness, easy fatigability, myalgia, and muscle cramps. Creatine kinase levels may be elevated. In most cases, the symptoms are gradually reversible after a euthyroid state has been restored. The variable metabolic states in autoimmune Hashimoto thyroiditis can also be a challenge. Any type of hypoparathyroidism may present with painful acute or chronic tetany caused by associated electrolyte disturbances for calcium, phosphate, and magnesium.

Toxic Myopathies with Myalgia

Skeletal muscle is characterized by its high metabolism and blood flow, making it susceptible to all kinds of circulating toxins. The clinical spectrum of toxic myopathies includes asymptomatic creatine kinase elevation, muscle pain with exercise intolerance, muscle weakness, muscular atrophy, and acute rhabdomyolysis (**Table 9.5**).

Note

Given the potential reversibility of toxic myopathy, a possible causal link should be established as quickly as possible so that the offending agent can be eliminated.

Alcoholic Myopathy

The most common form of toxic myopathy is the alcohol-induced form. Following excess alcohol consumption, an acute, painful, mostly proximal muscle swelling and weakness develops in rare cases (< 2%), with paroxysmal muscle cramps that typically affect the thighs and calves. Laboratory tests show a marked elevation of creatine ki-

Table 9.5 Causes of drug-induced toxic myopathies that are associated with muscle pain

Myopathy and neuropathy	Inflammatory myopathies	Other myopathies
Amiodarone	Cimetidine	Acetylcholine
Colchicine	D-Penicillamine	Carbimazole
L-Tryptophan	Levodopa	Clofibrate
Vincristine	Penicillin	Cromoglycic acid (cromolyn)
Heroin	Sulfonamides	
Statins	Zidovudine	Cyclosporine
	Procainamide	Enalapril
	Cocaine	Statins
	Statins	Metoprolol
		Minoxidil
		Salbutamol
		Ezetimibe
		Bisphosphonates

nase, hypokalemia, and myoglobinuria. The morphologic picture is that of necrotizing myopathy with rhabdomyolysis. Chronic alcoholic myopathy, which is more common, presents in up to 50% of alcoholic patients (persons who consume > 100 g/day for more than 10 years), usually presents clinically with painless, slowly progressive generalized muscle weakness and atrophy.

In all forms of alcoholic myopathy, lost muscle strength and mass can be restored through abstinence. Alcohol, its breakdown product acetaldehyde, and other metabolites appear to act directly on protein biosynthesis, including the synthesis of myofibrillar proteins such as myosin, titin, and nebulin. This can compromise the structural integrity of the contractile apparatus and the assembly of sarcomeric proteins. In addition to a direct toxic effect on C fibers, it is believed that a mitochondrial energy crisis and dysfunction contribute to the myalgia by reducing the production of ATP.

Steroid Myopathy

Months of continuous therapy with more than 10 mg of prednisone per day, combined clinically with Cushing syndrome and osteoporosis, will significantly increase the risk of developing steroid myopathy. A 40-mg daily dose of prednisolone for 30 days may be sufficient to induce steroid myopathy in some patients. Very rarely, steroid pulse therapy may lead to acute steroid myopathy, characterized by acute tetraparesis, diaphragmatic weakness, elevated creatine kinase, and generalized muscle pain. Fluorinated steroids such as dexamethasone and triamcinolone are considered to be associated with a greater risk for the development of acute steroid myopathy. Treatment consists of reducing the steroid dosage to the lowest therapeutically active level. Endurance training is an important known countermeasure.

Antilipemic-Associated Myopathy

Approximately 5% of patients who receive antilipemic agents experience a predominantly proximal myalgia, present at rest, that is usually associated with an elevation of creatine kinase levels. Effects may also include muscle cramps, exercise-induced myalgia, and proximal muscle weakness, with or rarely without creatine kinase elevation up to 10 times normal levels. The thighs are a site of predilection for muscle pain. In some patients, the creatine kinase levels remain elevated for more than 3 months after antilipemic therapy has been discontinued. The cause and frequency of this phenomenon are uncertain. Dermatomyositis-like and polymyositis-like symptoms, exacerbation of myasthenia gravis, and peripheral neuropathies have also been described during statin therapy. The most severe form of antilipemic-associated myopathy is rhabdomyolysis. To date, ~3350 cases of statin-associated rhabdomyolysis with acute tetraparesis, marked creatine kinase elevation (to more than 10 times normal levels), myoglobinuria, hyperkalemia, and coagulopathy have been described in the literature.

Rheumatologic Diseases

Polymyalgia Rheumatica

Polymyalgia rheumatica is a disease of unknown etiology that affects older individuals. Its pathogenesis is based on a giant cell arteritis that develops in the aortic arch or proximal limb arteries. Approximately 40%–50% of patients have coexisting cranial arteritis. The clinical hallmarks are pain, stiffness, and reflex limitation of muscular movement due to pain, chiefly involving the back of the neck, buttocks, shoulder girdle, and/or pelvic girdle (**Fig. 9.6**). The acute stage is usually marked by malaise, weight loss, and low-grade fever. Most patients also have increased inflammatory markers that show a dramatic response to steroid therapy. Up to 50% of patients have tran-

sient episodes of oligoarticular synovitis (e.g., affecting the hands, knees, and sternoclavicular joints), which have to be differentiated from rheumatoid arthritis. Headache and ocular symptoms may be present as signs of associated temporal arteritis.

Electromyography typically shows no abnormalities. Temporal artery biopsy will detect giant cell arteritis in up to 80% of cases. Muscle biopsies in polymyalgia rheumatica are negative and should not be taken (Gross and Hellmich 2003). Laboratory tests will usually show elevations of C-reactive protein (CRP), α_1- and α_2-globulins, erythrocyte sedimentation rate (ESR), and interleukin-6 (IL-6). The most sensitive laboratory parameters are CRP and IL-6. Creatine kinase levels are within normal limits.

Practical Tip

In summary, the following diagnostic tests are indicated when polymyalgia rheumatica is suspected:
- **Measurement of ESR, CRP, IL-6, α_2-globulin (electrophoresis)**
- **Creatine kinase assay (within normal limits)**
- **Temporal artery ultrasound (halo)**
- **Optional:**
  - **Temporal artery biopsy**
  - **Fluorodeoxyglucose positron-emission tomography**
- **No muscle biopsy!**

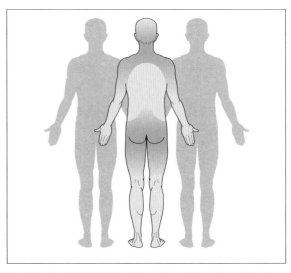

Fig. 9.6 Zonal distribution of muscle pain in polymyalgia rheumatica (color-shaded areas).

Myofascial Pain Syndrome

The German anatomist Froriep, in 1843, was the first to describe "muscle calluses" as palpable, tender areas of indurated muscle that responded well to local manual treatment. In 1919, Schade introduced the term "myogelosis" to describe a localized increase in muscle viscosity, while Lange used the term "muscle hardness" in 1925. Steindler coined now-familiar terms such as "myofascial pain" and "trigger points" in 1940. Travell introduced the term "myofascial pain syndrome" in the late 1940s. Later, Travell and Simons undertook a systematic study of trigger points, the pain arising from them, and cord-like indurations in over 130 clinically relevant muscles. Their extensive discoveries were summed up in *The Trigger Point Manual* (Travell et al. 1998).

Note

> Myofascial pain syndrome is defined as nonarticular local or regional muscle pain that is not the result of an underlying inflammatory rheumatic or neurologic systemic disease. A palpable hardening of muscle fibers, accompanied by a referred pain pattern that is familiar to the patient, is the most characteristic feature of a myofascial trigger point.

Clinical Characteristics

Physical examination reveals palpable, tender pressure points in skeletal muscle. Manipulating these elicits local and usually referred pain, which occurs in a characteristic, reproducible pattern that is recognized by the patient. These palpable spots in the muscle are called trigger points. Myofascial syndrome is usually associated with painful limitation of motion, stiffness, and subjective muscle weakness.

The clinical criteria for myofascial pain syndrome are summed up in **Table 9.6**.

Latent trigger points are clinically silent and do not cause spontaneous pain, but palpation of these points elicits clinical signs (referred pain pattern, local twitch response) similar to those produced by active trigger points.

Incidence

Epidemiologically, myofascial pain syndromes are a very frequent cause of acute as well as chronic musculoskeletal pain, but they are often missed and are rarely considered in the differential diagnosis. Up to 60% of patients with idiopathic chronic headaches and neck pain have a myofascial pain syndrome as their principal diagnosis. Approximately 80% of patients involved in a minor rear-end vehicle collision have been found to develop active myofascial trigger points. There is a slight female preponderance in myofascial pain syndrome, with a ratio of 1.5 : 1 to 3 : 1. The peak age incidence is from the fourth to fifth decades.

Etiology

Myofascial pain syndromes most commonly develop in muscles that are overused or even underused. It appears that myofascial trigger points are activated when a critical stress threshold is crossed, or possibly as a result of local myofibrillar injury. Other factors such as postural abnormalities, adverse mechanical loads, and articular dysfunction are important external influences that may affect the vulnerability of the muscle.

Table 9.6 Clinical characteristics of myofascial pain syndrome

Myofascial trigger point (essential criterion)	Hyperirritable focus of circumscribed tenderness found within taut bands of hypersensitive muscle fibers
	Palpation elicits characteristic responses such as referred pain and autonomic phenomena in the referral zone
Taut band (essential criterion)	Group of tense muscle fibers that form palpable, cord-like bands. Small contraction knots located along the band appear to be responsible for the stretched condition of the muscle fibers
Referred pain and pain recognition by the patient (essential criterion)	The stimulation of an active trigger point elicits a referred pain pattern that is specific for that trigger point. The pain may be locally confined or may radiate to distant sites (reference zone, **Fig. 9.7**). The referred pain is reproducibly related to its site or origin and rarely corresponds to the sensory distribution of a peripheral nerve or nerve root
	Causes of referred pain:
	• Regional activation of adjacent, previously silent interneurons in the posterior horn of the spinal cord in response to a peripheral stimulus
	• Central hyperexcitability
Local twitch response (optional criterion)	Stimulation of a trigger point elicits a brief contraction, or twitch, of the taut band. This local twitch response corresponds to a spinal reflex and appears to be specific for trigger points

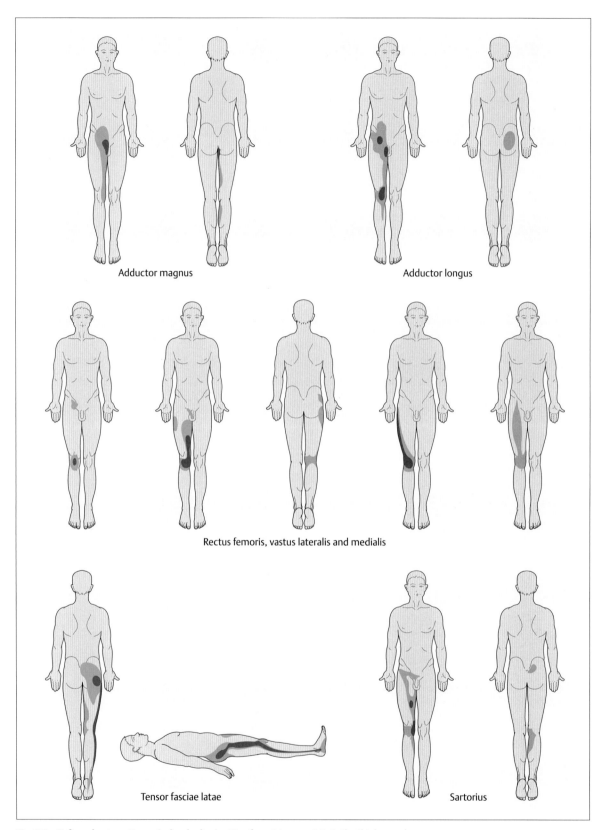

Fig. 9.7 **Referred pain patterns** (color shading) arising from trigger points in the thigh muscles.

Perpetuating factors may account for both the chronic nature of myofascial pain and the failure of established therapies in some patients. These factors include mechanical, systemic, and psychological conditions that promote the activation of myofascial trigger points and thus serve to perpetuate the syndrome. Postural guarding and immobilization with underuse often also develop secondary to an acute myofascial pain syndrome and contribute to a protracted course.

Poor nutrition, lack of sleep, electrolyte imbalances, metabolic disorders, and endocrine disorders are also recognized as systemic factors that cause muscular stress, although their contributions to myofascial pain syndrome are not yet fully understood. Additional factors are muscular aging and sarcopenia.

Pathology

Histopathologically, a trigger point is a collection of contracted sarcomere units in individual muscle fibers that cause abnormal stretching of the remaining muscle fiber segments. Electron microscopy shows a shortened distance between the Z bands in the trigger point, or even complete disruption of the Z-band structure (**Fig. 9.8**). Increased fibrotic changes are more likely to be associated with older trigger points, as are sites of individual fiber necrosis, increased lipid droplets, mitochondrial changes, and the presence of "ragged red fibers" as indicators of metabolic stress or muscular aging and sarcopenia.

Measurements of oxygen tension at trigger points in the back muscles have shown significant local oxygen depletion at these sites. The local environment in active myofascial trigger points has been investigated by microdialysis before and after eliciting a local twitch response. When active and latent trigger points were compared with control sites, significant differences were found in pH values and in the concentrations of substance P, CGRP, bradykinin, serotonin, norepinephrine, tumor necrosis factor-α (TNF-α), and interleukins IL-1α, IL-6, and IL-8. These findings led Simons to formulate an "integrated hypothesis" on the pathogenesis of myofascial pain: muscle overuse or trauma leads to dysfunction of the neuromuscular end plate, with excessive secretion of acetylcholine into the synaptic cleft. This results in postsynaptic depolarization and the release of calcium, which induces a sustained contraction of sarcomeres. This contraction in turn exerts pressure on adjacent capillaries that decreases oxygen delivery in the face of an "energy crisis" brought on by a general rise in energy demands. Another local factor is the release of neurovasoactive substances such as bradykinin and 5-hydroxytryptamine, which excite nociceptive nerve fibers, triggering the release of pain messengers such as substance P.

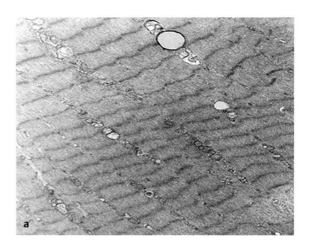

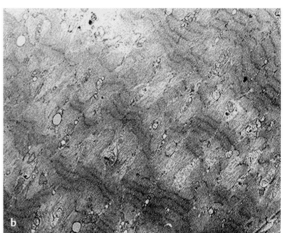

Fig. 9.8a, b Histopathology of a human trigger point (electron microscopy).

a Decreased distance between the Z bands, with "contraction disks."

b Destruction of the Z-band structure.

Relationship of Myalgia to the Classification of Muscle Injuries

A review of the classification of muscle injuries presented in this book shows several overlaps with the myalgic conditions described above. It is therefore important to explore the relationship between the myalgias discussed here and the various types of muscle injury described in other chapters (e.g., Chapter 6).

As a rule, athletic muscle injuries are localized lesions and pain syndromes, whereas most of the muscle diseases described above are manifested concurrently in several muscle groups. It is important clinically to recognize the dividing line between muscle injuries and myofascial pain syndrome with its trigger points.

Fatigue-Induced Muscle Disorder (Type 1a) Differentiated from Myalgia

In contrast to fatigue-induced muscle disorders with painful muscle firmness, the myalgias described by patients with acquired and congenital muscle diseases are usually diffusely present at rest and are not associated with local firmness in the muscle belly. These differences mainly have systemic causes (as opposed to local causes), such as changes in muscular metabolism or structural protein synthesis, as well as systemic inflammations as seen in dermatomyositis or polymyalgia rheumatica.

Spine-Related Neuromuscular Muscle Disorder (Type 2a) Differentiated from a Myofascial Trigger Point

It can be difficult clinically to distinguish a type 2a functional muscle disorder from a myofascial trigger point. There might also be some cases with overlapping syndromes, where a precise differentiation is not possible. The trigger point is usually associated with rest pain that is markedly increased by palpation or movement in the segment. This "recognition pain," along with the typical referred pain pattern for the examined muscle, are useful differentiating criteria.

In addition, spine-related neuromuscular muscle disorders are typically associated with functional or structural disorders in the lumbar spine, sacroiliac joint, or hip joints. These are common sites for lumbar multisegmental changes and proximal changes in the paravertebral muscles, which may also occur in anatomic segments located two or three levels higher or lower. This is attributable to the reciprocal intersegmental connections that exist among the intrinsic circuits of the spinal cord and span multiple segments and has been documented in model studies of referred pain.

Skeletogenic disorders of the lumbar spine, sacroiliac joint, or hip joints are usually functional in nature and are not very typical of trigger points. On the other hand, primary disorders of the lumbar spine, sacroiliac joint, or hip joints may give rise to "secondary" trigger points. These differ from primary trigger points, which are discrete, irritable foci in muscle caused by neuromuscular end plate dysfunction, not by pathology at a higher level. Secondary trigger points are activated through a projected mechanism based on disorders in the spinal column, tendons, fasciae, and presumably the muscle spindles.

Muscle-Related Neuromuscular Muscle Disorder (Type 2b) Differentiated from a Myofascial Trigger Point

The hallmark of a type 2b functional muscle disorder is escalating pain involving a relatively large area of the muscle belly, with no well-defined center. An important differentiating criterion is the presence of a palpable muscle firmness in the swollen edematous muscle belly. If a single hard spot is present, it may represent an acute trigger point. This is unlikely, however, because trigger points generally occur in groups or chains along the course of the muscle.

Partial Muscle Tears (Type 3) Differentiated from a Myofascial Trigger Point

Generally, it is easy to recognize type 3 muscle injury as a more or less discrete structural discontinuity with a tender center. The injury may consist of torn muscle fibers (type 3a) or, when findings are more pronounced, a torn muscle bundle (fascicle) (type 3b).

The latency, dynamics, intensity, and character of the pain in partial and (sub)total muscle tears are also quite different from those in other acquired or congenital muscle diseases.

Practical Tip

Differentiation is aided by noting that partial and (sub)total muscle tears are associated with typical stretch pain, whereas stretching tends to ease the discomfort of myofascial pain.

Further Reading

Cohen JA, Mowchun J, Grudem J. Peripheral Nerve and Muscle Disease. New York: Oxford University Press; 2009

Gross WL, Hellmich B. Horton's temporal arteritis (giant cell arteritis). Pioneering work and present status. [Article in German] Dtsch Med Wochenschr 2003; 128(49): 2604–2607

Pongratz D, Vorgerd M, Schoser B. Scientific aspects and clinical signs of muscle pain. J Musculoskeletal Pain 2004; 12: 121–128

Pongratz D, Schoser B. Scientific aspects and clinical signs of muscle pain – three years later. J Musculoskeletal Pain 2008; 16: 11–16

Quinlivan R, Martinuzzi A, Schoser B. Pharmacological and nutritional treatment for McArdle disease (Glycogen Storage Disease type V). Cochrane Database Syst Rev 2010; 12(12): CD003458

Schara U, Schoser BG. Myotonic dystrophies type 1 and 2: a summary on current aspects. Semin Pediatr Neurol 2006; 13(2): 71–79

Schoser B. Muskel und Schmerz – ein Leitfaden für die Differentialdiagnose und Therapie. Bremen: Unimed; 2008

Schoser B. Inflammatory myopathies. [Article in German] Z Rheumatol 2009a; 68(8): 665–675, quiz 676–677

Travell JG, Simons LS, Simons DG. Myofascial pain and dysfunction: the trigger point manual. 2nd ed. Philadelphia: Lippincott Williams & Wilkins; 1998

Udd B, Meola G, Krahe R, et al. Myotonic dystrophy type 2 (DM2) and related disorders report of the 180th ENMC workshop including guidelines on diagnostics and management; 3–5 December 2010; Naarden, The Netherlands. Neuromuscul Disord 2011; 21(6): 443–450

10

Behavioral Neurology and Neuropsychology in Sports

J. M. Hufnagl

Translated by Ruth Gutberlet

The Brain's Influence on Muscles 246
Interaction of Brain and Muscles 246
Behavioral Neurology and
Neuropsychology 246
Time, Location, and Perspective
as Pivotal Elements of the World 246

Brain Functions 247
Attention 248
Alertness 249
Memory 249
Perception 250
Thinking 250
Language and Communication 251
Autonomic Functions 251
Affects and Emotions 251
Anticipation 252
Goal Selection 252
Planning 252
Monitoring 253
Drive and the Hierarchical Relativity
of Brain Functions 253
Consciousness 253
Motor Learning 254

Motivation and Ambition 254
Motives 254
Intrinsic and Extrinsic Motivation 255

Delivering and Optimizing Performance 256
Increasing Demands Due to
Growing Complexity 256
Team Sports 257

Injuries and How the Brain Deals with Them 258

Relaxation Techniques 259
Certain and Possible Effects 259
Requirements and Mechanisms Similar
in All Techniques 259
Some Techniques in Detail 260
Applicability of Techniques
in Different Situations 261
Impact of Mental Training
on Athletic Performance 262
Mental "Doping"? 262

Examples from Soccer 263
The Penalty in Soccer—
On the Field and in the Mind 263
Cognition and Emotion as Reciprocal Processes 264

The Brain's Influence on Muscles

Interaction of Brain and Muscles

Life is motion. The brain directs and controls the muscles to execute the movements. The brain and muscles form a functional unit that most people simply take for granted. It is the muscles, in the first instance, that give us the freedom of action we enjoy. For us to be able to benefit from the potential of movement, all of the components involved in the system have to be optimized through reflection, practice, and constant adaptation to environmental conditions. Without the muscles, the brain would be powerless and weak; conversely, without the brain, the muscles would also be useless. In the Bible, it is still the flesh that is regarded as being responsible for sin, whereas nowadays we would assign full responsibility to the brain (the *flesh* is willing but the *spirit* is weak!). Among brain researchers analyzing the activity of the motor system, the freedom of the will has been the subject of controversial discussion. The significance of movement extends well beyond its spatial context; winning and losing are the effects of successful or failed movement processes.

As has been impressively demonstrated by the astrophysicist Stephen Hawking, handicapped by amyotrophic lateral sclerosis, the brain and muscles thus inseparably share a common destiny. To enable him to survive, his respiratory muscles require technological support, as does his residual motor function to enable him to communicate with others.

At the highest abstract level, the brain is always concerned with processing information and representing it. The muscles implement strength, speed, and endurance; the brain ensures precision at all times through coordinated rough-tuning and fine-tuning of the muscles with each other and through constant adaptation to changing conditions in the internal and external surroundings, consisting of the body's physiological and biochemical state and the outside environment.

Note

The brain is active not only when intentional activities are being performed, but also in most involuntary activities. It is involved imperceptibly even during spinal reflex movements and it is only during extremely rare autochthonous muscle movements that it is not involved.

Behavioral Neurology and Neuropsychology

In behavioral neurology, the relation between the brain and behavior is regarded from the point of view of the brain's influence on behavior. In neuropsychology, by contrast, the relation is seen from the point of view of behavior's influence on the brain.

The difficulty here is that behavior can only be experienced through motor function: physical and oculomotor function are recognized by an observer directly through movement effects, while the motor functions involved in speech are perceived indirectly via sound waves.

This chapter outlines the ways in which a wide variety of interacting brain functions influence behavior.

Time, Location, and Perspective as Pivotal Elements of the World

Everything we can know and observe, without exception, is subject to temporal changes. From the moment of conception to the moment when the body expires, we are moving along a timeline in one direction: always into the future. We cannot change the past, which has made us what we are and brought us to our current mental standpoint. But this standpoint should not be taken in a literal sense here to mean merely the spatial aspect, but also our (current) mental state, with all its different facets. With our knowledge and experience, we look into the world around us from the present moment. It is only very rarely that we are aware of this mental state. In terms of its significance and effect, it is enough for it to be exactly the way it is, exactly where it is, and no different.

The brain and personality are constantly changing and altering in time as a result of what we ourselves do and what we experience. No one who reads this book will be exactly the same person afterwards that he or she was before, because learning—whether it takes place actively or casually—inevitably changes our mental standpoint.

Note

The neuronal architecture of our brain is influenced and consequently changed by every flow of information. These changes are often only minimal, but at times can be dramatic.

Every scientific theory has a conceptual structure, in which a place is assigned to each cognition. From any one position the same facts can appear different and, depending on the perspective, may therefore be viewed and interpreted differently. From each position, that point of view is then decisive for every judgment made. The view may be widely or narrowly focused; clear vision and thinking develop in the dimension of depth. As Kurt Lewin states "There is nothing as practical as a good theory."

Brain Functions

The brain is in contact with the entire interior world of the body and also with the external world. The sense organs and pathways represent entrance routes, and the body's interior world can therefore be regarded as forming part of the environment around the brain in a broader sense. The exit routes consist of the motor systems involved in physical movement, eye movement, and speech. Motor systems involved in internal regulation processes essential for life, such as swallowing and visceromotor function, are also present. The overall effects of motor function are known as "behavior" (**Figs. 10.1** and **10.2**). In principle, information processing always takes place in the same control circuits. Brain functions, which are not directly accessible to observation, are therefore hypothetical constructs. They are also investigated by psychologists, and in the preexperimental and prescientific period, philosophers interpreted them in widely different ways, as objects of exclu-

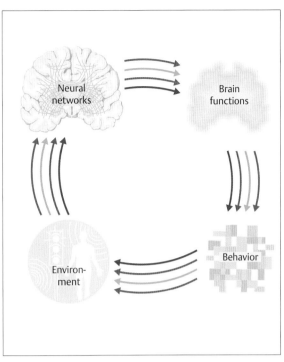

Fig. 10.1 Brain, behavior, and environment. As an anatomically structured organ, the brain gives rise to everything we call "behavior" through functions that are not directly observable. Behavior in turn has an impact on the environment. The brain itself can only function by also processing signals that originate in the environment (which in the broader sense also includes the body's internal world). This completes the cycle of information processing.

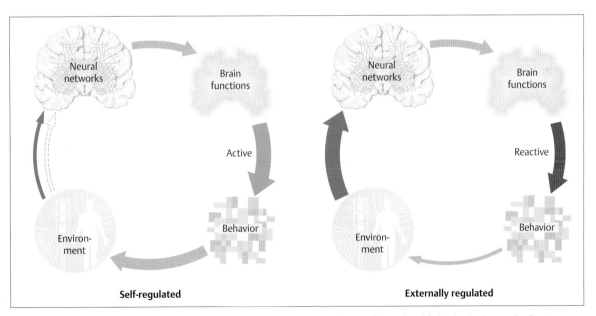

Fig. 10.2 Reciprocal influence of behavior and environment. *Autonomic (self-regulated) behavior* is characterized by the environment having a low impact on behavior, or the environment merely providing a background for otherwise independently determined actions. This makes the influence of one's own active behavior on the shaping of the environment (= situation) particularly great. *Externally regulated behavior* is the result of a strong or overly strong influence of the environment, which leaves little or no scope for any self-determined variation in responses. Consequently, reactive behavior resulting from external regulation is much more predictable and its effects on the environment (= situation) are less surprising (= less influential).

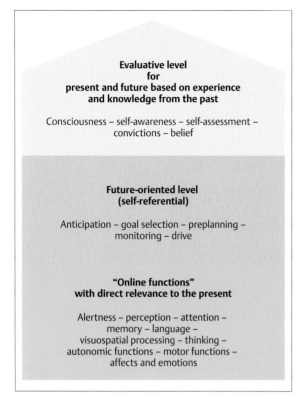

Fig. 10.3 Relative hierarchy of brain functions (adapted from Stuss and Benson 1986).

sively intellectual discourse. Today, philosophers and other humanities scholars who make purely intellectual judgments can and must be guided by the indisputable discoveries that have been made at the descriptive level. The influence of the environment on behavior is never direct, but is mediated and conveyed without exception by perception/sense organs/sensory pathways through neural networks and brain functions. Feedback mechanisms are circuits, which interact in the brain on the basis of several functional principles.

Approximately 87 billion neurons are interconnected through an estimated 10 000 contacts from each nerve cell to other nerve cells.

This is a great parallelism to data processing, with every neuron able to reach every other neuron via a maximum of four synapses. A principle of divergence is used in which the initial data are distributed to several loci—for example, for the color, shape, and position of an object. This is why strangely unreal phenomena can be observed in cases of circumscribed brain damage. Following the principle of convergence, the data are then combined again in one location. To this day, it remains a mystery how the brain integrates all the information it receives into one conscious experience. The principle of excitation is used to increase stimulation and the principle of inhibition is used to damp stimulation between the neurons. It is the spatiotemporal coordination of these extremely

complex discharge patterns that ultimately accounts for perception and also for everything else that the brain can accomplish.

On the basis of a model of brain function presented by Stuss and Benson (1986), several functional systems can be placed in a hierarchical order in which they are structurally and spatially separate but are constantly able to interact and can therefore never be viewed in isolation from one another (**Fig. 10.3**). Complementary bottom-up and top-down processing is an instructive example of the functional parallelism present in a variety of processes. In "bottom to top" processing, individual pieces of information join to form a larger whole that consequently has a new meaning. In "top to bottom" processing, by contrast, attention and perception are directed toward what is expected. When expectations are present, misinterpretations can easily take place. It is only when reality becomes irrefutable that it prevails. The brain structures involved in executing an action are also involved in the process of conceiving it.

Awareness, including self-awareness in the sense of the ability to evaluate oneself, is located at the highest level of the hierarchy. Convictions, including belief, are also located at this evaluative level. Metacognition (reflective knowledge about knowledge) also belongs in this category. All of these terms represent biological abstractions that have various different correlates. In this respect, there is no such thing as "memory," "attention," "perception," "language," etc. Instead, there are only specific memory performances, attention performances, perception performances, linguistic performances, etc.

Note

It is possible to measure selected performance aspects of brain functions in a specific way. However, it is never possible to sum these up completely and adequately in a single value.

Attention

Attention is a scarce resource, only limited amounts of which are available to us each day. Conscious acts cannot be performed without attentiveness, which is constantly required. Among the important aspects involved in attention are its intensity, which is seen in both spatial and temporal terms. Another is selectiveness, which determines how many different information sources are simultaneously kept in view. In cognitive psychology, "concentration" signifies continually focused attention. This is the opposite of multitasking—the simultaneous pursuit of several tasks involving parallel work and processing. The intensity of attention can be increased briefly through voluntary effort, but this is quickly followed by a temporary exhaustion of sorts.

We are constantly attacked by attention stealers when we try to focus totally on one subject. Both internal and external distractions, and the ability to be distracted, are a hazard. Booing from spectators has often caused athletes to lose their composure. Thoughts can become dominated by brooding over misgivings about the past or concerns about the future to such an extent that optimal performance is impaired. Thinking about previous sports events that ended in defeat can substantially reduce current performance. This phenomenon becomes acutely evident when an unlucky point lost or a goal conceded causes a player or the entire team to lose their rhythm and the game's momentum changes.

Even positive thoughts about the future can turn out to be just as detrimental if they distract us from the current situation. Anticipating an imminent victory can distract the attention to such an extent that it actually makes it possible to lose a point or concede a goal. Even a Champions League soccer final was once lost by the team that had been leading as they went into additional time.

Alertness

Typically, attention requires alertness. When we sleep we can hardly focus our attention. Even during sleep, however, there is some residual attentiveness that stays with us. The physically slight sound of an infant's whimper is capable of waking a mother, even though she could quite easily go on sleeping while a loud truck thundered past her. Psychological tension before an important game can disturb the rhythm and depth of sleep, as well as the degree of alertness the following day.

Note

There is such a thing as having too much alertness. This occurs when acute stress makes us overwrought and excessively tense, agitated, and overexcited (see **Fig. 10.5**).

Memory

We generally associate the term "memory" with thoughts about the past. Even in the scientific literature, memory is occasionally regarded as representing a kind of archive. Although looking back at what has happened in the past and what we have learned is (at least unconsciously) a constant and indispensable necessity, it is only a prerequisite for the real task: shaping the present and the future. It is only by recourse to the past that we can form ideas about how we ought to act in the present and in the future. Experience and knowledge provide the basis for predicting all our future actions. Foresight is a process that runs constantly in the present moment, usually without us being aware of it explicitly. There are evidently different types of memory.

On the highest abstract level, the philosopher Martin Heidegger describes memory as being the "gathering of thought." For those engaging with Heidegger's conceptual

and linguistic acrobatics, his line of argument is convincing.

Larry R. Squire and Eric R. Kandel begin their book *Memory: from Mind to Molecules* with the statement that "Memory pools the countless phenomena of our existence into a single identity." Neuropsychologists and molecular biologists are curious to discover—both theoretically and experimentally—which aspects of this phenomenon make which specific contributions. They agree that memory performance can be divided into declarative and nondeclarative types. The same state of affairs can alternatively be described as "explicit" and "implicit memory" or "memory for facts" and "memory for skills."

Declarative Memory

A distinction can be made in the declarative types between episodic memory and semantic memory. Experiences are stored as autobiographical as long as they belong to us. If the experiences belong to other people, we can recount them in the same way as we would re-tell the story of a novel. Retrievable information that is not related to other people (e.g., "who won a certain event in the 1960 Olympics?" or "what is the Pythagorean theorem?") is assigned to semantic memory. We speak of source memory if we can also remember the time and circumstances in which the information was obtained.

"Working memory" can be conceived of as operating at the interface between memory and attention. Today many scientists prefer this term to the less clearly definable term "short-term memory." The term "working memory" is intended to sum up the capacity for simultaneous holding and processing of cognitive material with full awareness, which is associated with limited (attention) capacity. In 1974, Baddeley outlined and later refined the first model for the functional aspects of working memory. There is extensive literature on functional circuits, using terms such as linguistic and phonological loop, visuospatial notepad, and episodic buffer. In principle, these functional circuits work in physiologically similar ways, but in different modes (and in anatomically different locations in some cases). The circuit known as the "central executive" is the one for which there is the least empirical evidence. Baddeley's cognitive model does not contain a sensorimotor working memory. The crucial feature of sensorimotor short-term memory is that when there is planned motor activity aimed at achieving an optimal result, a delay is introduced into the planned activity until the sensory input that has been stored in the buffer has been processed. There is now good experimental evidence for the existence of this type of sensorimotor working memory.

Nondeclarative Memory

Nondeclarative memory is not accessible to introspection. It works in the form of priming, perceptual learning, emotional learning, and procedural learning—which is essentially motor learning (see p. 254).

In ambiguous or complex situations that require quick decisions, we typically react intuitively. The decision is made by the sum of our represented experience based on its own independent, fast insight, without discursive examination by the conscious mind. Reflection and prolonged consideration may often be inappropriate or even dangerous in this type of situation.

Note

Intuition is often termed a "gut feeling." It usually turns out to be an appropriate basis for reacting and for justifying a decision when the data are too complex, particularly when purely rational information processing would be too time-consuming or difficult.

Perception

We perceive the world around us directly through our sensory organs. Physical energy is converted into neural discharge patterns. Our actual perception is only created after these have been conducted and have arrived in the various areas of the brain, with simultaneous linking. Proprioception, as internal perception, is also the result of the interpretation of changing discharge patterns in specialized neurons. Without visual control we perceive our position vaguely or not at all if no changes take place—for example, after prolonged motionlessness. Of all the sensory inputs, the sense of sight can be regarded as the most important. It is the sense we find most convincing, as we believe our eyes more than our ears. How much we understand what we see depends on how clear it is. This is why we admire Leonardo da Vinci's art, or an ingenious pass in a soccer match. In the process of comprehending, we cautiously and tentatively familiarize ourselves with an as yet unknown world. If we act too hastily, discovering our physical boundaries may be painful. Sounds can change our mood—such as the intonation patterns heard when someone is crying or moaning.

Hearing the chanting of "We are the champions!" after a victorious final can feel like the heights of joy. Nietzsche claimed that without music, life would be an error. What would the atmosphere be like in a stadium without the chanting? An injured player can be reassured by a hand placed on his shoulder, a slap on the back, or gentle encouragement with "You'll soon be on your feet again!" In car racing, the climax of the victory ceremony is a fizzy shower of champagne (sometimes replaced with rosewater in some countries). One way or another, the world always addresses our collection of senses and experiences.

Thinking

In its most admired form, logical reasoning, and in problem-solving in general, thinking is often equated with intelligence. The literal translation of intelligence is "reading between the lines" (Latin: *inter*, between, and *legere*, to read). Those who consider themselves intelligent and try to justify this on the grounds of their IQ demonstrate—paradoxically—that they have not penetrated the problematic aspect of intelligence. As the behavioral biologist Hassenstein has shown, cleverness or prudence ranks above intelligence. Reasoning does not require humor, but humor requires reasoning. Having a sharp mind is not a disadvantage in life, but on its own it is rather uninspiring. We should meet intellectual arrogance with poise. True intelligence is demonstrated by asking the right questions, from the standpoint and angle from which things are seen, rather than in always having the know-all answers. As Rost concludes in his book on *Intelligence: Facts and Myths* (backed up with more than 2000 literature references), even specialists in the field are not always familiar with the results of the latest research on intelligence.

Note

Creativity is a special type of thinking. It is not convergent, analytical, linear, or deductive, but rather divergent, intuitive, horizontal, lateral, and around the corner. Innovativeness is the special quality that comes to us unexpectedly and sometimes produces moments of genius.

It is often not language that enables us to perform intellectually, but the clearness of images that leave a lasting impression. Images can lead to us to fresh insights more easily than language or reasoning. Einstein hit on the theory of relativity when he imagined how the world and the universe would present themselves if he were riding on a ray of light. Was he thinking about Münchhausen's fabled ride on a cannonball? Children also learn a great deal before they are able to speak, as do animals even without speech. Symposium papers edited by Weiskrantz in 1988 entitled *Thought without Language* impressively demonstrated that it does not involve any problems. The converse—"language without thought"—can often become a problem in everyday life; from the viewpoint of the person concerned, it might be expressed as "How am I supposed to know what I think before I hear what I say?" Thinking in images and scenes can lead to clarity without language and allow communication. This can be observed in top teams, where individual players of different nationalities can otherwise only express themselves with difficulty in a foreign language.

Language and Communication

The most important means of communication across time and space is language in its verbal and written forms. A major and insurmountable drawback is the fact that words can only reflect the multiplicity of possible meanings approximately. One need only think of the more than 16 million different colors that a modern TV can display, or the variations of scent in perfumes that are sometimes composed of more than 500 individual fragrances, or the variations in wine flavors from 1000 varieties of grape grown in different locations, different climates, etc. The use of language presents a problem of the same magnitude—one and the same term may be used to refer to different objects or states of affairs, while conversely different objects or states of affairs may also be described using one and the same word. The proverbial Babylonian confusion is not limited to difficulties in communication between different languages, but has found its way into the scientific literature. The difficulty of achieving consensus on definitions that go beyond purely mathematical or natural-science terminology are a direct expression of the way in which imprecisions are dealt with—imprecisions that are continued in the form of unclear thinking. In the multilingual field, translations as well as careless usage by native speakers exacerbate this problem.

Nonverbal signs are of paramount importance for communication. Agreements and conventions rule out misunderstandings. Yellow and red cards were introduced in soccer following an incident in the 1966 World Cup, when a player dismissed by the referee pretended not to have understood him verbally or otherwise and remained on the field for an outrageous length of time.

Note

Language determines the way we think to a large degree, but the way in which spoken words are to be interpreted and what they mean can only emerge through the clarity of the terms used and their connotations in a given situation.

Autonomic Functions

In this context, the most interesting of the autonomic functions, which are also termed "vegetative" and are thus vital for life, is sleep—which entails more than the aspect of physical rest. One of the essential functions of sleep is the formation of long-term memory. For long-term storage, fresh memory traces have to be (capable of being) "solidified." This process, called "consolidation," does not consist of a passive engraving procedure, but instead involves an active process of reorganizing retained memories and their representations. The way in which existing content items are linked with new ones differs during the various stages of sleep:

- Procedural learning, including sensory and motor learning, mainly benefits from rapid eye movement (REM) sleep, which is predominant during the later part of nocturnal sleep.
- By contrast, declarative memory benefits most from delta sleep, during which slow oscillations are seen on electroencephalography (EEG). This type of sleep is predominant during the earlier part of the night.

Recent research has verified these facts, in contrast to the multitude of purely hypothetical speculations about the function of sleep and dreams.

Note

The bottom line for everyday life is that adequate sleep is beneficial for athletes and thinkers! Both sensorimotor and cognitive learning require consolidation of memory traces, which can only be achieved during sleep.

Affects and Emotions

When our feelings are stimulated by the outer world, we speak of "affects" (from Latin *affectus*, that which makes me move, from *afficere*, which is composed of *ad facere*). When our feelings originate in the inner world and are transferred to the outside, we speak of "emotions" (from Latin *emotio*, moving out). The difference between the two thus lies in their type and source, and their relation to each other is analogous to action in the sense of acting and reacting. This subtle distinction is frequently overlooked in everyday language and even in the scientific literature, but it is fundamental for the way in which actions are assessed. It is only in the case of criminal offenses based on affect (in the heat of the moment, on impulse) that it is clear that it is not emotions that are regarded as constituting mitigating circumstances, but rather that a reaction occurred that is not liable for punishment because the perpetrator's will was no longer free to intervene in a considered and moderating way.

Feelings are an indispensable part of what makes life worth living. They change our attitude toward things and the way we interpret other people's actions. When we experience a specific feeling, we want to confirm it. At times, this can cause problems, because we may be overwhelmed by a feeling to such an extent that we are no longer capable of acting in accordance with our empirical knowledge.

Note

Feelings can only be controlled to a limited extent, but they control us. When we are angry or in love, or both, we may do things (or at least tend to do things) that we will sooner or later regret.

The Limbic System

Feelings and awareness are almost always regarded as being elusive phenomena, and there is no scientific consensus on how to classify and explain them. However, there is evidence that feelings can be evoked only in a small number of areas of the brain, located beneath the outer surface of the cerebral cortex. The network or system of structures that mediate the emotional life is safely located in the depths of the brain, closer to the inner surface of the cerebral hemispheres. The early anatomists therefore called it "limbic" (= on the border). The effects of the limbic system are transmitted via two routes:

- By means of chemical molecules through blood circulation
- Through electrochemical signals along the neural pathways

The result is that the individual's overall state is changed. Antonio Damasio sums up the forms this takes by comparing feelings to actors that use the body as a stage. Feelings have an independent functional existence, which, at times, is incompatible with clear thinking. It is therefore not always we who control our feelings, but our feelings that control us. This happens when there are parallel thoughts and feelings but a simultaneous lack of coordination between them, and the feelings gain the upper hand and keep it. When something has been deeply felt but intellectually only poorly understood, if at all, then the individual may nevertheless (or precisely because of that) suppose that something wise has been learned, and this can ultimately grow into a conviction that it is true—mistakenly, because accurate conclusions have to be based on clear premises, which in this case do not exist. Esoteric teachings are concocted from a mixture of obscure ingredients of this type. Magic tricks are based on similar phenomena. As soon as we have figured them out they become explicable, of course, and no longer seem amazing—or only to those who are still seeing them naively.

Anxiety

Anxiety is the best example of the usually uneasy feeling we have in situations perceived as threatening. The anxiety is not attached to any specific object. If there is an object, then the phenomenon is known as "fear." Anxiety generally does not provide good guidance on how to act in a situation, particularly since the original biological function of anxiety—choosing between flight or fight in a given situation—is no longer present. This type of negative feeling is particularly unhelpful and can often be paralyzing when there is indecision on whether to initiate a specific action, or when disappointment and failure are anticipated. The feeling is exacerbated by the physiological side effects of anxiety, including an excessively high pulse rate, sweating, bowel movements, etc. Cognitive restructuring can be useful in these situations, but needs practice.

Despite the limited capacity of our attention functions, we have to try to eliminate the all-encompassing sense of being in a state of siege due to free-floating anxiety ("I might lose!") about the actual task ("I have to win!"). One's own resources can then be called to mind and used consistently and in a targeted way, without having anxiety as a distraction and an attention-stealer.

Anticipation

Due to phonetic assimilation, the origin of this word can easily be misconstrued. The first part of the word is from Latin *ante* (before), not from Greek *anti-* (against). The second part of the word is from Latin *capere,* to take—from which the English word "capture" is also derived, although in this case it means grasping or understanding.

Note

"Catching on" to something before it happens—that's what anticipation means, foreseeing the consequences of an action or event that might take place "if ..."

In sports, as in the rest of our life, anticipation is not primarily achieved by verbal deduction, but rather by visualizing images, scenes, and episodes that would take place "if." In the nonverbal communication that takes place between players on the soccer field, this type of predictive ability is a prerequisite for the successful actions that awaken enthusiasm in the spectators. "Communication" means to do or create something together (from Latin *communis*). It is aimed at the future. And the same also applies to the most intensive, and similarly nonverbal, form of interpersonal communication: at the moment when a new life is created.

Goal Selection

The meaning of "goal selection" is obvious. A prerequisite for it is that there must be something to select from. Selecting something from various options implies making a decision. That is what selecting a goal is about.

Planning

What does "planning" mean and how is it related to action? Planning is the mental image—that is, everything that consciously precedes the action in the form of thoughts and reflections. Planning in advance is the same as actual planning. When a plan is written down, the written record itself becomes an action, while what has not yet been carried out and is still located in thoughts and intentions continues to be a plan or planning process.

Monitoring

The purpose of monitoring is to compare the current status of our actions with the path required to reach the desired goal. It could be considered a mental navigation system. It involves determining whether we are still on track or whether we have deviated from the path. If monitoring is related not to ourselves but to events in our environment, then it typically involves noticing the difference between our own subjective expectations and actual events.

Drive and the Hierarchical Relativity of Brain Functions

"Drive" can be regarded as self-generated activity that is initiated voluntarily and is not merely a reaction. In 1964, Kornhuber and Deecke were the first to demonstrate, using a simple intentional finger movement, that motor activity is preceded by a cerebral potential, which they termed the "readiness potential" (German: *Bereitschaftspotenzial,* BP) (Kornhuber and Deecke 1965). This was the first paradigm for neurophysiological studies of the way in which the will is formed. Free will is currently a hotly debated topic, with irreconcilable opponents on each side. This shows that in the fields of medicine and biology, even undisputed facts still require interpretations that depend on the viewer's standpoint and angle.

In sports, examples of the various facets and influencing variables that affect voluntary drive can be particularly well seen. "Winning starts in the head!" is an insight that is gradually becoming more and more widely accepted. But when does it start? It starts long before kick-off or the beginning of a competition. The deliberate decision to participate in a specific sports discipline could already be described as the real starting-point. The skills required for the preferred sport should ideally also match the participant's physical constitution. The training needed to progress toward winning a competition requires consistent willpower over a long period and makes it possible to pursue ambitious, long-term goals. In the short term at least, this frequently involves coping with frustrating experiences. On a daily basis, you have to do without activities that seem more gratifying, tempting, or pleasurable, or you have to cope with setbacks in reaching your current goals. Self-discipline is another expression for the specific implementation of this type of long-term will or drive. It constantly has to prevail over challenges and obstacles, which may arise not only from external distractions, but also, for example, from temporary changes of priority or self-doubt. Verbal clashes between opponents before a competition do not only occur in boxing. The goal is to strengthen one's own willpower and positive cognitions and at the same time to weaken those of the opponent. Once the competition has begun, the sum of individual characteristics that are currently in action determines the outcome. In spite of this, verbal clashes do occur, but the will to win is an outstanding factor. However, the extent to which winning depends not on willpower alone, but on an optimal interaction between physical fitness, cognitions, emotions, and flexibility in changing conditions becomes apparent wherever strategy and tactics involving foresighted plans and actions are needed. This is true almost without exception. One exception is in 100-m and 200-m sprinting in track and field. The athletes have to go full speed from start to finish in these events, regardless of the inevitable oxygen deficit. It is a different situation in the 400-m race. The oxygen deficit that is initiated has to be carried all the way to the finishing line, which is why athletes who run too fast in the first and/or middle part typically "die" on the home straight before reaching the finishing line. The greatest willpower cannot overcome the oxygen deficit. The ability to implement voluntary drives depends on the individual's physical condition at any one time. A stitch or a sudden muscle injury can put an end to the ambitions of even the most exceptionally strong-willed athletes. Examples like these demonstrate indisputably that although willpower is generally necessary, it is by no means the only prerequisite for winning. Victory is only achieved when the finishing line has been crossed or the final whistle blown. Strategic preparation for a competition entails creating the basis for optimal physical fitness on the day of the event. During the competition itself, the challenge (particularly in sports lasting for a longer period) is to use one's own resources wisely. This optimization problem, constantly changing in multiple dimensions and multiple phases, determines relations in the hierarchy of brain functions both in sports and elsewhere.

Especially between two almost equal opponents, the ultimate victory is frequently a victory of willpower that perseveres unwaveringly to the very end. On the way to achieving that, however, one's own performance capacity must not be overestimated or overexerted—and last but not least, a little bit of luck is helpful. In soccer, if a ball bounces off the underside of the crossbar and it is difficult to see whether it is on or just behind the goal line, as happened in the International Federation of Association Football (FIFA) World Cup final in England in 1966, it is the linesman's eye or the referee's tongue that decide the outcome. Greater human stature is often seen in a sportsman-like acceptance of defeat by the losing side than in a show of superiority by the winning side. No matter how strong the will to win is, it must never be forgotten that an opponent in sports is not an enemy and that while sports events are competitive, they are never wars.

Consciousness

"Consciousness is like the Trinity: if it is explained so that you understand it, it has not been explained correctly." This statement by Joynt (1981), quoted in the volume edited by Metzinger (1996), gets to the heart of our inability to clarify the enigma of consciousness in such a way that the solution to it can be found. We focus on certain aspects that we seem to understand, but we fail to see the big picture. With cerebral functions at the middle level of the hierarchy, we are aware of their self-referential quality and subjectiveness. The level of consciousness implicitly suggests a claim to objectivity that we cannot escape from if we are not aware of it. This creates the types of paradox that arise in self-assessment: if it is adequate, then the subjectivity of the self-assessing individual ought to be reconcilable with an objective view from outside. Who would be able to judge us in an objective and completely correct way from the outside? It could only be someone with the abundance of qualities that we usually attribute to God. Claiming to be able to assess oneself with complete objectivity is like the hubris of wanting to be or feel like God, even if or precisely because we are not aware of this false conviction.

Despite this, there can be no doubt that our personal convictions, and our beliefs in things that cannot be proved and in some cases are even irrational, provide the lasting backdrop for our theater of the world.

Motor Learning

Learning is a continuous process that is constantly taking place but is not directly observable. It is only the results that are visible. In infants, motor learning takes place in a targeted way through repeated practice, but without conscious attention to the motor details needed to execute movements. When skills are being consciously acquired in a controlled way, we focus our attention on individual aspects that we control voluntarily. We can never match the complexity of the requirements involved in paying attention to everything simultaneously because our attention capacity is limited. Repeating tasks leads to increasing automation of a detail that has been noted, with the effect that less attention needs to be used up for it. The capacity now available is freed for other details.

Depending on speed and complexity, we are frequently unable to (re-)produce every detail of all the movement sequences perfectly even though we have completely mastered them in principle. Even when they have become automatic, movements all have to be created anew from motor memory. Depending on the degree of difficulty, small deviations inevitably appear that fall short of complete perfection.

The motor skills required in pole-vaulting appear to be particularly complex (**Fig. 10.4**). Apart from weather and spectators, the general conditions applying at the same height are basically static. In tennis, by contrast, every stroke except the serve starts from new basic conditions. In this respect, the serve should be the easiest stroke. In skiing, feedback information from motor learning is always immediate, for example, after edging over. In tennis or in soccer, the brain processes the extent to which the ball has hit or missed the target only after a delay, and with a detour via an explicit conscious realization.

The dynamics of constantly changing starting conditions result in varying requirements in individual sports. This is seen at the elite level when an athlete changes sport. Michael Jordan, the best basketball player of his time, was only able to play at a substandard level when he switched from basketball to the top baseball league at the age of 31—to most people's surprise, including his own. The requirements of brain performance in the two disciplines differ too much for an athlete to be equally successful at the top level. Only Fred Perry managed first to become world champion in table tennis (1929) and later to play tennis at a world-class level in the 1930s. He went down in history by winning Wimbledon three times in succession (1934–1936) and winning a total of 14 grand-slam titles (eight singles matches, two doubles, and four mixed doubles).

The extremely complex connections observed in functional neuroanatomy, with numerous and often hypothetical interactions, are discussed in detail by Grafton and Bizzi (2009).

Motivation and Ambition

Motivation is considered the key to success. However, it is not directly measurable, as it cannot be observed directly. In any case, it is indisputably one of the driving forces behind our actions. It provides the answer to the question of why we are doing something. It is no surprise, therefore, that motivation is highly contentious. Since it is not a purely on/off phenomenon, it is never a question of "being" motivated or "not being" motivated, but rather of how strong or weak the motivation is.

Motives

Another vital prerequisite is the aim that lies behind the motivation. Aims provide orientation. In the literal sense, "orientation" means knowing which direction east (the Orient) is, in order to bow one's head in the right direction during religious worship. Three basic motives, on which all other motives are based, have emerged from the plethora of possible variations:

- Achievement
- Power
- Attachment

These are known as "the Big Three." One motive does not exclude another, even a contradictory one. There are unconscious (implicit) motives and conscious (explicit) motives. Only the latter can be communicated verbally. These typically involve a mixture of all sorts of things: one's own ideals or those of others, a desire to accommodate others, genuine intentions, and many more. Many other motives guide us without our being aware of them.

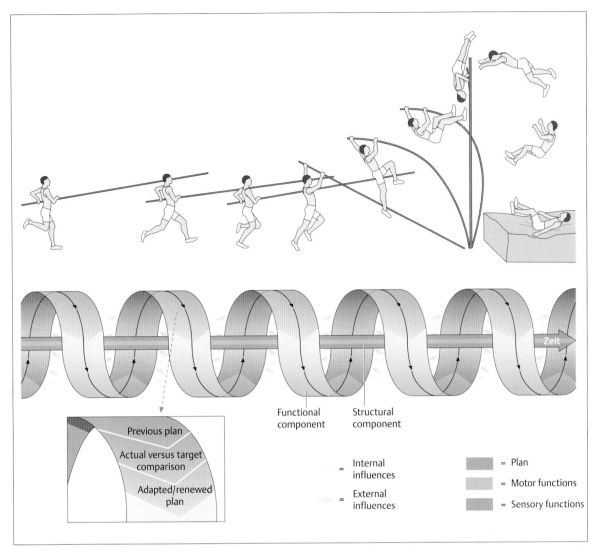

Fig. 10.4 Different phases in pole-vaulting as an example of complex interactions. The illustration is merely symbolic. The feedback circuits involved are only suggested in an extremely simplified and incomplete manner. The structural components of the anatomy that communicate functions along the time axis naturally remain constant. Only structural components that have been trained through repetitive practice can be strengthened over time. Multidirectional feedback circuits pass through them over time. With increasing complexity per time unit, fewer and fewer details can be noted with targeted attentiveness. The faster complex changes in physical posture occur, the more the sequences have to be carried out automatically.

Intrinsic and Extrinsic Motivation

Motivation that develops from within is called "intrinsic." This is when it is a matter of a cause, or doing something for the sake of a cause. Fundamentalists are an extreme example of people with intrinsic motives based on conviction. Extrinsic motivation, on the other hand, is not concerned with a cause for its own sake, but rather with the benefits arising from it, which might be money, promotion, or an advantage that distinguishes us from other people. Intrinsic and extrinsic motivations can even get in each other's way—for example, intrinsic motivation declines as a result of monetary rewards, as has been empirically confirmed in children. Amateur athletes of the past certainly put in the same effort as today's professional athletes. When highly paid professional teams are visibly reluctant (at times) to put any effort into a league match, to the extent that fans become irritated and even start booing, it is evidently due to a lack of intrinsic motivation, rather than a lack of extrinsic motivation due to underpayment.

Motivation can be directed toward actively achieving an aim (approximation) or at avoiding disadvantage and harm.

There is an old saying in soccer that "offense is the best form of defense." The state of motivation in strikers who are actively approaching the opposing goal differs from their state of motivation when defending a slight lead in front of their own goal.

Delivering and Optimizing Performance

More than 100 years ago, Yerkes and Dodson provided empirical evidence of a connection between tension and performance.

Note

The Yerkes–Dodson law, which is actually more of a rule, states that as tension increases, the performance curve initially rises to reach a peak and then drops when the tension becomes too much.

This correlation is usually illustrated in the form of an upside-down U. This U-shape may vary widely, depending on the task. Task-specific and complexity-dependent requirements have to be taken into account in order to optimize performance, and different levels of tension are also required. In physical and simpler tasks, the peak for optimal performance moves to the right, while for complex mental efforts it moves to the left in varying degrees (**Fig. 10.5**).

The important aspect shared by all possible curves is not so much achieving maximum performance with (only) moderate tension, but rather keeping the tension neither too low nor too high. Nervousness, for example, can quickly reach a level that makes reasonable performance impossible—and not just during examinations.

The goalkeeper's fear of the penalty even entered world literature in Peter Handke's novel *The Goalie's Anxiety at the Penalty Kick*, which was made into a movie by Wim Wenders (*The Goalkeeper's Fear of the Penalty*).

As a factor on the x axis, tension is certainly not one-dimensional, but performance on the y axis just as certainly involves several dimensions. Despite this, it is extremely useful to analyze performance using the Yerkes–Dodson paradigm, particularly as it is possible to consider the influencing factors on each axis separately. Factors shown on the x axis, for example, might include:

- The physical tension associated with a waking state
- The onset and extent of positive and negative emotions
- Cognitive control and familiarity with the situation
- In particular, self-confidence at the conscious level

The y axis might include:
- Power, speed, and endurance as muscle-dependent variables
- Technical precision in each individual requirement
- Strategy and tactics as control variables for the staying power required

Increasing Demands Due to Growing Complexity

As a result of a car accident in which no one else was involved, a player in a top premier-league team sustained a localized cerebral hemorrhage. After a successful rehabilitation program, the player was able to start training again, became fully physically fit and made trial appearances in league games. Despite tremendous effort and care on the part of his coaches, the player was unable to reach his previous performance level. He was therefore referred to a neuropsychology clinic for examination and treatment. Not the slightest motor abnormality was found during the neurological examination, even in difficult coordination tasks. In simple reaction-time measurements, his attention reflex performance was absolutely world class, with values better than those of anyone else at the clinic. However, as the requirements gradually increased in complexity his performance decreased in correspondence to the complexity of the tasks involved. His values declined from above-average attention reflexes to average for simple tasks, and during the same sessions, remained average for highly complex requirements involving multitasking. When more functional brain capacity was required, the effects of what was probably only a minor reduction in fiber connections (information exchange) in the neural networks became noticeable.

The challenges a soccer player faces with regard to anticipating spatially and temporally complex scenarios of play can completely exhaust the maximum brain capacity. A first-class professional soccer player differs from an amateur one in the same way that a chess champion can plan more moves ahead and has more variants in his repertoire than a proficient amateur. When the player described above was being assessed for occupational disability, it was not possible to use arguments based on pathological measurement values, but only arguments to the effect that an athlete needs 100% of his or her brain in order to compete at the top level and that even the slightest impairment prevents top performance. In the case described, the player played for a few more years in a third-class league at what was an average level there. There have been a few cases among Formula 1 racing drivers in which apparently minor brain injuries left them incapable of competing; so far as the present author is aware, there have been exceptions. The statement attributed to Einstein that human beings only use 10% of their brain capacity is factually wrong (and also inaccurately attributed to him). However, he did state that most people do not

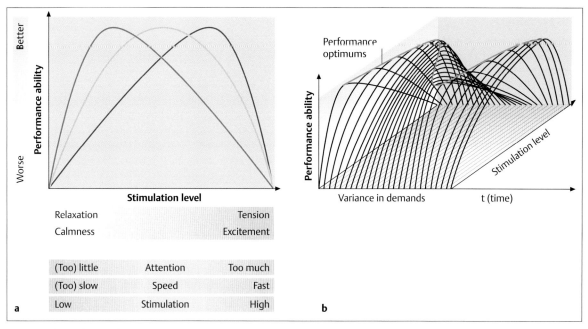

Fig. 10.5a, b Yerkes–Dodson curves.

a The most frequently illustrated Yerkes–Dodson curve is symmetrical and centered, in the shape of an upside-down U (yellow). It is idealized (for example in continuous performance), but not realistic. In long-term, vague, and/or mentally demanding tasks (e.g., during creative thinking in a state of relative relaxation), the point of optimal performance is reached quickly (blue). With simple, (usually) short-term tasks, by contrast—i.e., with clear requirements (e.g., penalty kicks, corners, or exceptionally with longer-lasting events such as motorcycle and car racing)—the point of optimal performance shifts to the right (red).

b Changes in optimal performance on the Yerkes–Dodson curve over the course of time. These changes are based on the fact that the demands do not remain constant. A Formula 1 race, for example, could hardly be completed without shifts of this type. On a long straight stretch, tension decreases slightly at least for a short time. In ice hockey, frequent interruptions by referees and due to substitutions provide intermittent relaxation.

need a brain, as they could manage with the spinal cord alone.

Team Sports

Team sports and individual sports pose different challenges for players and coaches. Getting along with yourself is difficult enough, but getting along with everybody else and yourself as well at the same time is even more difficult and can be nearly impossible. The complexity of this task grows with the number of participants involved. External factors influence the brains of individuals taking part in team sports much more than in individual sports, so much so that the outcome of a competition is (almost) always unpredictable, depending on the level of the incalculable factors involved. Top tennis players, for example, are capable of producing top performances consistently for years, whereas even top teams, including soccer world champions, can have occasionally disappointing results despite their complete superiority "on paper" against "minor" teams.

Note

A team is always more than the sum of its individual players.

In the smallest possible teams, such as doubles in tennis, there are examples of identical twins who are or have been much more successful when playing as a pair rather than singly—for example, Bob and Mike Bryan, who won 12 grand slam titles each, a gold medal at the 2012 summer Olympics, more than 80 Association of Tennis Professionals (ATP) Masters tournaments, and three ATP Masters cups. The explanation for this is that nonverbal communication is much easier for them, resulting in a low tendency to make mistakes. Any combination of equally good individual players could hardly be more successful. The Bryan brothers are "mirror twins": they mirror each other's movements, one being right-handed (Mike) and one left-handed (Bob).

The Team as a Unit

On the field, players not only have to get along with each other but also have to become a unit. The German soccer team trainer Sepp Herberger went so far as to say, "You must be 11 friends!" Commercialization has led to profound changes. Nonetheless, even today there is still absolute commitment to mutual respect off the field, particularly in public. With the inevitable rivalry that exists within a squad, it would be impossible to stick to the rules without fairness being observed both on the inside and toward the outside world. As is well known, the opposite of order is chaos. The frustration threshold is frequently put to a challenging test when teammates make the wrong move, the team starts losing, and the mood suddenly changes. Players who have to stay on the substitutes' bench in spite of their conviction that they can play just as well as the player who has taken their position need to have an extremely stable psychological balance.

Social Skills

A shared life forms common bonds; when friendly relationships develop in private life it has a positive effect on a team. There are many other aspects involved in social skills, which are the main requirement for teamwork—including communication skills, cooperativeness, empathy, considerateness, and the ability to deal with conflict. A significant prerequisite for this appears to be the proper functioning of mirror neurons in the brain, discovered by Rizzolatti et al. in 1995. He considers mirror neurons the biological foundation for compassion (Rizzolatti et al. 1996). In addition, from an intellectual perspective, there is the "theory of mind," which explains how we are conceptually capable of seeing things from another person's perspective.

Assigning the members of the team to various positions requires different characteristics both in the roles that are assigned and also in the assignment process itself. It is not possible to provide a scientific answer to the question of what the best approach is for a coach faced with these highly complex requirements. What is the maximum effectiveness in terms of positive performance development?

> *Note*
>
> **Trainers and players form a social and emotional relationship, which is often felt to be unique.**

Former Olympic gold medalists have attached tremendous importance to this relationship aspect in terms of their performance development.

Effects of Muscle Injuries on the Team

Muscle injuries only affect the person injured primarily and directly, but when an individual is part of a team, the team is also affected in a secondary and indirect way. Depending on the severity of the injury, the team's performance is always temporarily affected to some degree. If the injury is severe, the player may have to be substituted during the game, which inevitably alters the structure of the (well-coordinated) team. If the available substitutes have already been used up, the team affected by the injury may end up a man short. In the case of long-term absence due to severe muscle injuries, the team has to be (at least temporarily) restructured. This inevitably leads to complex psychodynamic processes both in the individual players and the team.

Injuries and How the Brain Deals with Them

With muscle injuries, the pathological processes take place primarily in the muscle itself. However, the brain comes into play immediately, as soon as physical contact with an opponent becomes rough and painful. Although the perception of pain is felt in the muscle, it occurs in the brain initially. The difference in pain perception, partly depending on various types of nociceptors, is discussed elsewhere. For the purpose of this discussion, the important aspects are not only that there is afferent control of pain perception (the gate control theory), but also top-down control. Strong emotions can lead to powerful suppression of pain perceptions in the same way that attention can be distracted using hypnosis. Reports on soldiers, torture victims, and also athletes show that even severe injuries are not always accompanied by pain perception. The independent cerebral representation of pain and pain memory, on the other hand, causes patients who have undergone amputation to be tormented by almost unbearable pain in limbs that are no longer there. According to the same principle, when you have a catchy tune you keep hearing in your mind, it does not need external stimulation either.

However, it is usually the case that someone who has sustained an injury feels the full force of the pain. The immediate reaction depends on the circumstances and on the individual. Previous experiences of pain can often be mentally actualized instantaneously in a condensed synopsis without use of the spoken word, with all the associated memories. Fear can also suppress pain briefly or for longer periods, depending on the motivation and prospective significance characterizing the situation. Misinterpretations can occur, for example, if momentary nerve entrapment increases the intensity of pain to such an extent that the injured person fears that the injury is much worse than it actually is. An experienced sports physician can quickly give the all-clear. Physical modalities such as applying ice to suppress afferent responses and pressure bandages to reduce secondary effects of the injury can reassure an injured person in the acute situation.

Note

If an injury is severe and protracted, the importance of adjuvant psychological supportive measures alongside purely medical treatment and physical therapy increases. This is particularly true if unforeseen complications develop, or if not even the expected values during the course of healing are achieved relative to the diagnosis.

Although everyone reacts to pain in an individualized way, a common response is that uncertainties, undecided factors, and conditions whose benign or malignant nature cannot be assessed are even harder to bear than some extremely serious diagnoses. This can be regularly observed with cancer patients. It can be explained as showing that the evaluative level—our belief in things we do not understand ourselves and can only trustingly accept from other people who do know—is suddenly put to a severe test and becomes insecure. In some circumstances, this can throw us completely off balance, and the doubts that arise can put a strain on a good physician–patient relationship. A transition into depression may sometimes be precariously close. Action is therefore needed—the stronger the self-confidence, the better the prospect of a cure. Particularly in difficult times, a stable and self-assured personality both on the part of the patient and physician can ensure hope and optimism. Optimists have better immune systems than pessimists. Self-fulfilling prophecies will have different outcomes.

Relaxation Techniques

Certain and Possible Effects

Specific types of mental activity can have a positive impact on our muscles when they are under tension. In many situations, particularly in stress, a high level of unintentional tension tends to be the rule rather than the exception, and it is counterproductive most of the time. Voluntary relaxation can solve the problem. Tensing the muscles voluntarily is relatively easy; it is significantly more difficult to relax them, but it can and must be learned—at least if the aim is to optimize performance. Simple techniques can sometimes be helpful—such as briefly taking a deep breath in an acute situation, or as a more general measure, having a sauna, daydreaming, listening to music, or whatever else helps to distract from negative thoughts. In the longer term, however, no one can fully tap their performance potential without mental

training. Relaxation techniques are never a substitute for physical modalities or physical therapy methods. In an unconventional sense, relaxation techniques can be considered a part of physical therapy in the same way as psychotherapy.

Which technique is best suited to which person depends on the individual's needs, abilities, convictions, and attitude to life. In all of the relaxation techniques, influence is exercised by changing the state of consciousness. The various techniques are not always free of ideological baggage.

Note

It is important to acknowledge that a teacher is indispensable until the specific procedures have been satisfactorily mastered.

Who would recommend a nonswimmer to make his or her first attempts to swim without the help of a swimming instructor? Wrong or wrongly applied techniques can lead to anxiety and produce the opposite of calm and relaxation. Some perseverance is always necessary until the first positive results can be noticed, and patience is also a great help. As with everything else, you can't expect to get it right first time. The positive effects produced extend beyond the actual training units not only in terms of time, but also go beyond the muscles. Heart and respiratory rate are lowered, and circulation in the skin and intestines improves. Calm rest induces a positive mood and conveys a feeling of self-control in which stress factors are viewed differently. Concentration power increases, and along with it the ability to absorb information and process it. The immune system is stimulated in a way that improves immune defenses and strengthens the capacity for self-healing. Many techniques have a positive effect on pain reduction in cases of injury, provided they are adequately mastered. However, undue expectations that relaxation techniques can be used as a miracle cure to solve all of life's problems will be disappointed.

Requirements and Mechanisms Similar in All Techniques

The involuntary reactions triggered by the autonomic nervous system are derived from ancient periods of evolution when survival meant constant danger. A flight or fight response was needed at any time as soon as the safe boundaries were crossed. When in physical danger or when noticing a danger signal, our ancestors responded by reflex with split-second mobilization of their physical reserves so that they could flee or fight. Alertness and physical arousal increased, the muscles tensed and received more blood, breathing deepened, stress hormones were released, serum lipids to supply energy were increased, and coagulation factors were raised to prevent fatal bleeding. When the danger and subsequent physical exhaustion

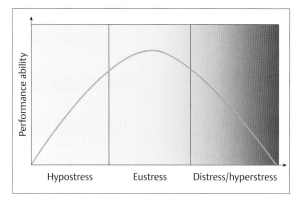

Fig. 10.6 Stress and performance.

had passed, attention returned to food, reproduction, digestion, sleep and the other forms of recovery needed. All of this inevitably determined the rhythm of ups and downs, inhalation and exhalation, tension and relaxation, in accordance with natural requirements.

In today's technological world, we face threats and dangers of an utterly different nature. They are no longer natural dangers in the true sense—although our involuntary reactions have remained the same. What an individual finds stressful depends on his or her position and perspective. Here too, the saying of Epictetus holds true: "Men are disturbed not by things, but by the views which they take of things." Stress is always a subjective experience that is impossible to quantify. However, there can be no doubt that it is real (**Fig. 10.6**). Increased muscle tension is probably the most common symptom.

Any activity that is calm, regular, and ritualized can induce a state of rest that causes relaxation. Agitating ideas and images can be deflected by a variety of attention-absorbing rituals. Calm and relaxation ensue automatically. The satisfaction and conviction that one is doing something genuinely important with perfection can lead to the phenomenon of "flow" described by Csikszentmihalyi, which he calls the "secret of happiness" (Csikszentmihalyi 2008). The German educationalist Kurt Hahn, who developed adventure-based experiential education, introduced a similar concept in 1908, which he called "creative passion."

Some Techniques in Detail

Schultz Autogenic Training

On a purely mental level, attention is diverted from everyday thoughts or distracting factors toward body sensation. There should be a pleasant feeling of warmth and heaviness first in one arm and then in the other, followed by the stomach area, and so forth, including a cool sensation on the forehead. The ability to visualize these sensations and hold them in mind is crucial to the success of this technique. The relaxation reactions that finally develop as reflexes are meant to become increasingly easier as the in-

ner images become ingrained. The basic exercises are followed by advanced exercises that include additional individually adjusted formulas for differentiation and deepening of the relaxation. At the highest level, there is a transition to autogenic training with deeper insights and motivations for personal development. Autogenic training is particularly widespread in Germany, for historical reasons.

Jacobson Progressive Muscle Relaxation

A method of progressive muscle relaxation developed in the United States at around the same time, in the 1920s, is also in widespread use. With its pragmatic and tangible quality, it is particularly suitable for beginners. The approach to relaxation is different here, focusing on the interplay and contrast between conscious sensations during tension and relaxation of muscle groups that are exercised one after the other. The active involvement this requires provides stronger stimulation for guiding and holding the attention than in autogenic training. Unsurprisingly, progressive relaxation can be learned more easily, faster, and by more people, even those who are defeated by the greater demands made in autogenic training. Scientific studies have provided evidence of this phenomenon.

Yoga

In yoga, relaxation is achieved through specific physical postures (asanas), with stretching exercises for the spine, muscles, and joints, and through controlled breathing techniques. These provide access to deep states of relaxation, with a corresponding mental state similar to that in meditation. According to the ideology, yoga is intended for spiritual development.

> *Caution*
>
> **From the neurologist's point of view, an objection must be raised to one specific yoga posture: prolonged standing on the head should not be practiced. Based on the laws of hydrostatics, this causes increased intracranial pressure. In the longer term, this might result in normal-pressure hydrocephalus, as neurosurgeons who have encountered such cases will confirm.**

Returning to the starting position has a sensual effect that is interpreted as cleansing. In principle, this is no different from the relief that follows pain as soon as the pathophysiological state is replaced with a normal physiological one.

Tai Ji and Qi Gong

Tai ji originated in the Chinese empire as a martial art in the form of shadow-boxing. It is now considered to be just a version of kinesiology or gymnastics that has become a national sport. The concept of *qi* is based on very early Chinese ideas found in the Taoist worldview, which is still held by many people in Asia. It is a complex concept of life-energy that has been very much simplified by Western adoption. The basic idea in both techniques is that the interplay between opposing forces in the body has to be brought into balance. The aim is to harmonize physical and mental processes using relaxation and energizing techniques.

Meditation

In meditation, the path is the goal. In the highly developed religions of Buddhism and Hinduism, meditation was originally a spiritual pathway rather than a technique for self-discovery. From an ideological perspective, the goal is generally to place the individual in harmony with the universe by opening up access to the inner self. This mindset is characterized by allowing things to happen, which seems passive from the Western point of view but is intended to lead ultimately to enlightenment. Meditation is certainly not suitable for everyone. Psychological health and stability are vital prerequisites. Previous experience with relaxation techniques such as autogenic training or progressive relaxation is very useful. In the Japanese Zen technique, sitting silent and motionless for at least 20–30 minutes per day is intended to promote "single-mindedness."

The German philosopher Thomas Metzinger, who specialized in consciousness research, argues for a new approach to states of consciousness. He suggests that meditation should be taught as a subject at school so that children can already safely experience altered states of consciousness without recourse to drugs or alcohol. However, he would prefer to have it taught by physical education teachers, without any bell-ringing and incense-burning and free of ideology. The crucial motivation for trying to achieve an altered state of consciousness is always the improved self-coping that follows.

Feldenkrais Technique

In the Feldenkrais technique, frequent repetition of movement exercises leads to relaxation. Individual tension patterns are dissolved and physical posture and mental attitude improve. Qualified instructors achieve surprising results in the field of rehabilitation, as well as in musicians, dancers, and athletes. The technique, which also represents a kind of whole-body therapy, is based on more than 20 years of judo practice, extensive experience of various therapists in the 1920s, and findings from manual medicine, particularly the neurological treatment methods developed in the 1940s and 1950s.

Hypnosis

The aims of hypnosis usually go beyond reaching a state of deep relaxation. It is therefore important to determine what the individual aim of hypnosis is and who to entrust oneself to. During the hypnotic trance, a state of deep in-

ner concentration, the hypnotist presents carefully chosen suggestions in a forceful manner of speaking and with regular pauses to the person undergoing hypnosis. A specific readiness to do this represents rapport. The interaction between these three elements—suggestion, trance, and rapport—may allow us to reduce or eliminate the uncertainties, doubts, and other self-obstructive ideas in normal everyday consciousness that are impediments to action. Constantly supporting an increasing belief in one's own ability to solve problems and growing confidence about imminent success is a particularly effective mechanism.

The process can ultimately merge into autosuggestion. This broadens the options available to athletes for establishing positive effects. The repeated mental visualization of a sequence of movements alone can make it possible to achieve the greatest possible concentration and lead to greater success, by autohypnotically narrowing the field of attention to the desired focus.

Caution
Reservations about the use of hypnosis are concerned in principle less with the method itself and more with the personality of the individual hypnotist.

In general, suggestions are no more dangerous than convictions acquired through a process of reasoning; in both cases, the resulting benefit and harm always depend on the content.

Applicability of Techniques in Different Situations

For the body, every muscle injury is not just a local event but affects its integrity as a whole. Injuries are typically associated with pain, which leads to functional impairment. The brain has to process sensitive feedback information in order to control the motor system. In the acute situation, abnormal signals require complete immobilization to prevent any additional tension in the injured muscle from occurring. From this moment onward, every movement has to be relearned in the altered feedback system.

Medical treatment and physical therapy are indispensable for a speedy and complete recovery. If relaxation techniques are to be used consistently in this type of situation, they have to have been previously mastered. The independent contribution of the injured individual to the process always increases the chance of the original abilities and skills being restored as quickly as possible. They cannot be restored in the same way without the use of relaxation techniques. This leads not only to an improvement in the physical state but also the mental state, both through top-down pain control and a conviction that one has had an optimal active influence on the process.

Every pain affects the emotional level. In muscle injuries, for example—particularly if caused by a third party—there is anger as well as pain and it needs to be given expression. It has in fact been scientifically proven that swearing is beneficial in certain situations. However, the swearing should not be directed in any form at the opponent, and certainly not at the referee. Smashing an innocent tennis racket, for example, can also help vent negative emotions.

Just reading the above discussion alone will not of course enable anyone to apply a professional technique immediately. The suggestions made are intended only to sow seeds that will be brought to fruition by those who practice the techniques.

Impact of Mental Training on Athletic Performance

Who benefits from mental training? The simple and conclusive answer is that in the same way as with any type of physical training, mental training can only benefit those who actually do it. And the better the training, the more useful it will be. Mental training is task-specific in the same way as physical training. A bodybuilder exercises muscles specifically for shaping and posing. A weightlifter exercises muscles for the maximum transfer of strength in clearing and jerking and/or in snatching. Although a bodybuilder's muscles superficially appear to be stronger, those of a physically comparable weightlifter are actually stronger. Sprinters, who are able to form an oxygen debt, benefit from their muscle mass. Marathon runners, on the other hand, depend on maximum energy efficiency for muscle endurance. The different physiognomy of athletes in the various disciplines reflects the anatomically and physiologically different requirements for specific types of top performance.

In the form of motor imagery training, mental training functions just as specifically as muscle training. In addition to perfecting movement sequences, it has also been shown that it is capable of increasing strength—although the explanation offered for this, that efficiency is increased through central access, is not entirely satisfactory. As an exercise method, motor imagery training directed at a specific goal can provide an ideal supplement to other types of relaxation techniques that are used for other purposes. It always improves performance, and in some cases it can even make the small difference between the winner and the runner-up.

The brain mainly uses the same overlapping structures for motor imagery as it does for the actual execution of the movement. When sleeping and dreaming, the brain normally excludes the execution of motor activities; it is solely used for memory consolidation. This process uses the same structures for practicing and learning.

In horses and other quadrupeds that are able to run off on all four legs immediately after birth, these motion patterns are not only anchored in the genes but have also been practiced countless times prenatally, as if in sleep. The degree to which individual athletes are able to benefit

from the power of their imagination probably depends, as with other characteristics and talents, on how well or poorly it has been trained.

Mental "Doping"?

The term "doping" has similarities with the term "consciousness" (see p. 253). Everyone knows all about it, although no one can give it a precise and comprehensive explanation that is free of contradictions. Whatever is written about it is merely cobbled together, because there is no cohesive and completely consistent view of the issue.

In the real world, it is not possible to achieve—even purely theoretically—either the commendable intention and reasonable aspiration not to harm oneself or others unnecessarily, or the collectively invoked consensus that genuine fairness and equal opportunity have to apply to everyone in the world of sport. A single example should suffice to illustrate the absurdity that inevitably results in some cases. The Finnish cross-country skier Eero Mäntyranta won five gold, four silver, and three bronze medals in the Olympics and in world championships during the 1960s. He was later diagnosed beyond doubt as suffering from a point mutation in the gene for the erythropoietin receptor. The word "suffering" is wrong here, as he wasn't suffering from this gene defect as if it was a disease; instead, nature had bestowed on him a gift of constant erythropoietin (EPO) doping that did not require the assistance of a physician or medication. Should he therefore have been classified as having a physical disability and sent to the Paralympics? Inequalities are seen in this world not only in relation to body weight and size, from the petite gymnast to the sumo wrestler, but in all types of possible physiological parameters and also in varying mental capacities.

The volatility of the subject is not least maintained by the ingenuity of those who work on the assumption that anything that is not forbidden is permitted. Surprises happen, even with methods that seem objectively harmless and apparently unproblematic. The winner of the Lakefront Marathon in Milwaukee in 2009 was disqualified after the race because she had used her iPod while running. She considered the disqualification ridiculous, and although many people might agree with that, her explanation that she had simply tried to push herself a little from miles 19 to 21 by listening to some rock and techno music was equivalent to admitting to the use of a performance-enhancing method (apparently successfully). People are most likely to step on the gas pedal faster and harder when there is a heavy rhythm coming from the loudspeakers inciting them to become more aggressive. They are also prepared to take more risks, compared to those who listen to soft, soothing music.

Emotional factors can have extremely performance-enhancing effects. Why else does a team that is already playing well rise to the absolute heights when the atmosphere in the home stadium comes to a boil? But emotions can also be effective when they are hidden in silence. At an awards ceremony during the 2008 Olympics, the world's strongest man, in tears, held up a photograph of his late wife, to whom he dedicated his gold medal. Many people who knew his story were moved to tears. His wife had died tragically a year before. In remembrance of her, he had not only mobilized all his physical energy but also concentrated all his emotions, hopes and wishes into the jerk of the barbell that won him the super heavyweight medal. This was certainly a form of highly specific mental doping that could not be reproduced in a different situation. In this case, however, no one raised any objection to it.

Examples from Soccer

The Penalty in Soccer— On the Field and in the Mind

The goalkeeper's fear of the penalty kick spans precisely 7.32 × 2.44 m, but the penalty taker's fears may well exceed these measurements (like the ball as well). Not converting a penalty is always blamed on the penalty taker— not without reason, because a penalty kick is normally a solvable task. The same is not true in the case of the goalkeeper if a sharp, well-placed shot is objectively unstoppable. Seen from this point of view, the goalkeeper can only win, while the penalty taker always runs the risk of losing, as everyone knows.

When the referee blows the whistle for a penalty, thoughts and emotions run through the heads of the opposing team, and can often be guessed or even read from their gestures and expressions. Who has the more difficult task? The goalkeeper can definitely influence the penalty taker nonverbally using various tricks. These might include standing off-center, giving the impression that one side is wider and therefore easier to strike, or irritating the penalty taker by making all sorts of movements on the goal line (which, incidentally, is now permitted). The penalty taker can, but need not, let himself be influenced by all this. Why? What does influence him involves two different groups of factors:

- Internal factors based in himself and his personality (see the section on the hierarchy of brain functions, p. 247)
- External factors created by the situation

Note

Every situation in life is unique, even though we may think we have experienced the same thing umpteen times before. It may help to be aware of the fact, however, that one has been successful once or even more often in comparable or similar situations before. This boosts self-confidence and can fend off self-doubts— the invisible opponents that are the strongest ones.

Even world-class soccer players fail to convert a penalty kick once in a while, sometimes in crucial situations. There are many reasons for this. The significance of the situation (e.g., the last minute of extra time, being one goal behind, the last chance to equalize) can tremendously intensify the mental stress that is involved in any case. The pressure originates partly as a result of the penalty taker's responsibility for the other players if missing the penalty will mean definite defeat and elimination of the team. Just thinking about it is enough.

Even baseline motor activities require a certain amount of attention. Parkinson patients, for example, are not able to walk and answer a question about what time it is simultaneously. They have to stop walking, look at their watch, and then answer while standing still. Once the implications of the penalty kick start to spread in the mind and push themselves to the fore, too much attention capacity is occupied and diverted from the motor action required. As a result, not only the player, but also the ball, is distracted. Even a lightning-fast thought that enters the penalty taker's mind when he is already in motion can affect him, no matter whether it is spontaneous or triggered by an external factor. An unexpected movement by the goalkeeper, getting caught on the turf, slipping on a wet spot, or anything at all surprising (i.e., extremely rapid) that may happen can have an irritating effect. Should the penalty taker change his original plan once he has begun to move toward the ball, the brain does not have enough time to adapt to a (new) motor program, under these confusing conditions, and to change and reprogram the existing movements with enough precision. The details of the predictive processes required for rough or fine coordination take time. The simultaneous quality and power of many different thoughts, emotions, desires, decisions, changes of mind, or even simply indecision, can exacerbate the acute situation and lead to overloading of the control system, which then fails. If the performance shown does not match the player's usual standard, it is due to the specific nature of the situation, the unusual combination of internal and external conditions. It is thus risky to try to do something special in a given situation, that is to deviate from the usual. But calling this merely "stress" shows that the word conceals more than it reveals.

Positive examples of determination, willpower, and concentration without being distracted by external circumstances and without hesitation—including what even seemed to be nonchalance by players totally confident of their own skills—were seen during the FIFA World Cup finals of 1974, 1990, and 2006. The missed penalty, in contrast to what would count in tennis as an "unforced error," is not entirely unforced. The pressure the athlete has to overcome lies in the mind. From this point of view, the penalty kick is not just an ordinary foot kick, but a special type of "header."

Cognition and Emotion as Reciprocal Processes

In a soccer final, a team's star striker converted a penalty by a carefully thought out process and with complete command. He was in complete control of himself despite the enormous pressure that rested on his shoulders. Later one of his opponents repeatedly held him by his shirt. He became annoyed but told him calmly that he was welcome to have his shirt, but only after the game. His opponent replied, "Then I'd rather have your sister, the whore!" Fuming with rage, the striker nevertheless initially did what every behavioral therapist would advise in the situation—he left the scene. But he was unable to get over the stinging insult against his family's honor. His brain told him that he had to control his temper, without committing a foul or doing anything violent involving either kicking or blows. But the affect, in the literal sense of the word discussed above, became so overpowering that the insulted striker turned round, walked a few meters toward the player who had insulted him, spread his arms out, and to everyone's surprise head-butted him so hard in the chest that he fell over backwards.

How can this behavior be explained from the neuropsychologist's point of view? In principle, awareness and cognitions are capable—within limits—of reflecting, classifying, and controlling affects and emotions. This is made possible by inhibitory top-down control. But it can only work as long as the intensity of the emotions does not exceed a certain limit. Once an affect has upset someone's composure, the clarity of their thoughts is clouded and their mental standpoint and angle of view are decisively altered. With the parallel processing of emotional aspects and cognition, the archaic system anchored in the limbic structures affects the more recent system in such a way that it directs attention, perception, and thoughts toward the result that is emotionally desired. In individuals who are depressive, anxious, or short-tempered, thoughts then focus on content that maintains their depression, anxiety, and anger. Every piece of information received is interpreted to favor the tendency involved. In people who are excessively—i.e., inappropriately—pleased by things, thoughts and attention become mixed up and this causes mistakes. One of the crucial tasks of thinking is to allocate emotions appropriately in order to allow optimal appropriate behavior. In turn, emotionality determines the evaluations attached to thoughts as pleasant or unpleasant and personally important or unimportant, and in the process gives them their affective hue. Over time, the conditions influencing this can vary, depending on their intensity. They can also change as a result of a shift in focus and new incoming information. Factors dynamically superior at any given moment guide the resulting actions.

In the case of the above-mentioned penalty kick, the player concerned was so self-confident that even a world-class goalkeeper was unable to distract him and he was therefore able to preserve an optimal level of excitation. Immediately after the insult, knowledge (cognition) and emotions clashed severely. Cognition was saying, no foul and no violent conduct! But the frustration on the emotional side was demanding satisfaction. In the instinct-triggered and slightly delayed reaction that followed, cognition was still effective and stopped him from using his hands or feet. Explicit information about a ban on using the head as a weapon was not in the forefront and thus had no inhibiting effect on the action. The level of excitation was overdriven by the emotions, the point of peak performance was exceeded, and the overall performance became inappropriate.

The ideal reaction would undoubtedly have been not to show any discernable reaction at all. Objectively—seen from the outside—the insult was heard by the player but by no one else. In this respect, the family's honor had not yet been outwardly violated. From a rational point of view, a reaction that would have been better and more appropriate to the overall situation would have been to pretend to be temporarily deaf and ignore the situation. Self-control might have been easier if the consequences for the team of getting a red card in a situation like this had been anticipated more clearly and cognitively weighted more strongly in comparison with the limited significance of an extremely personal insult. It might even have been sufficient to allow oneself an act of violence in thought as a mental exercise, but to have saved up the realization of the idea until after the game. On the one hand, this would have not simply suppressed the frustration, but would instead have channeled it, while on the other, the chances of reason prevailing after the game would have been greater. However, thinking through all of this in detail would probably overload the system, so that as in the case of this penalty, the best advice is to focus on what is essential and, more than anything, ignore external influences as much as possible.

However, human beings are not machines that you can just switch on and off. They are made of flesh and blood, with all the emotions that go with that. This includes people who have to take decisions about consequences during and after a game.

Further Reading

Alfermann D, Stoll O. Sportpsychologie. 4th ed. Aachen: Meyer & Meyer; 2012

Baddeley A. Working memory, thought, and action. New York: Oxford University Press; 2007

Bear MF, Connors BW, Paradiso MA. Neuroscience: exploring the brain. 3rd ed. Philadelphia: Lippincott Williams & Wilkins; 2006

Bise V. Problemlösen im Dialog mit sich selbst. Marburg: Tectum; 2008

Creutzfeldt OD. Cortex cerebri: Performance, structural and functional organization of the cortex. New York: Oxford University Press; 1995

Csikszentmihalyi M. Flow. The psychology of optimal experience. New York: Harper Collins; 2008

Damasio A. Descartes' error: emotion, reason, and the human brain. Harmondsworth: Penguin; 2005

Diekelmann S, Wilhelm I, Born J. The whats and whens of sleep-dependent memory consolidation. Sleep Med Rev 2009; 13 (5): 309–321

Eccles JC. Evolution of the brain: creation of the self. Reprint edition. London: Routledge; 1991

Ekman P. Emotions revealed: recognizing faces and feelings to improve communication and emotional life. 2nd ed. New York: Owl Books; 2007

Feltz DL, Landers DM. The effects of mental practice on motor skill learning and performance: a meta-analysis. J Sport Psychol 1983; 5: 25–57

Förstl H, Hautzinger M, Roth G, eds. Neurobiologie psychischer Störungen. Heidelberg: Springer; 2006

Gazzaniga MS. Who's in Charge? Free Will and the Science of the Brain. New York: Harper Collins; 2011

Galaburda AM, Kosslyn SM, Christen Y. The languages of the brain. Cambridge, MA: Harvard University Press; 2002

Gigerenzer G. Gut feelings: the intelligence of the unconscious. New York: Viking; 2007

Goldenberg G, Miller BL, eds. Neuropsychology and Behavioral Neurology, Vol. 88. Handbook of Clinical Neurology (Series eds. Aminoff MJ, Boller F, Swaab DF). Edinburgh: Elsevier; 2008

Goldenberg G, Pössl J, Ziegler W. Neuropsychologie im Alltag. Stuttgart: Thieme; 2002

Grafton ST, Bizzi E, eds. Motor systems. In: Gazzaniga MS, ed. The cognitive neurosciences. 4th ed. Cambridge, MA: MIT Press; 2009: 537–652

Handke P. The goalie's anxiety at the penalty kick. Roloff M, trans. New York: Farrar, Straus and Giroux; 1972

Hassenstein B. Klugheit: Bausteine zur Naturgeschichte unserer geistigen Fähigkeiten. 3rd ed. Berlin: Bucheinband.de; 2004

Hawkins J, Blakeslee S. On intelligence. New York: Times Books; 2004

Heidegger M. What calls for thinking? In: Heidegger M. Basic Writings. Rev. ed. Krell DE, trans. London: Routledge; 2009: 369–391

Hufnagl JM. Der Mensch angesichts der Anforderungen des heutigen Verkehrs. In: Bundesanstalt für Strassenwesen, ed. Kongressbericht der Deutschen Gesellschaft für Verkehrsmedizin 2007. Bremerhaven: Wirtschaftsverlag NW, Verlag für neue Wissenschaft; 2008; M195: 186–189

Humboldt W von. The limits of state action. Burrow JW, trans-ed. Cambridge: Cambridge University Press; 1969

Joynt RJ. Are two heads better than one? Behav Brain Sci 1981; 4: 108–109

Kandel E. The Age of Insight. New York: Random House; 2012

Karnath HO, Thier P. Kognitive Neurowissenschaften. 3rd ed. Heidelberg: Springer; 2012

Kogler A. Die Kunst der Höchstleistung. Vienna: Springer; 2006

Kornhuber HH, Deecke L. Changes in the brain potential in voluntary movements and passive movements in man: readiness potential and reafferent potentials. [Article in German.] Pflugers Arch Gesamte Physiol Menschen Tiere 1965; 284: 1–17

Kornhuber HH, Deecke L. The Will and its Brain: An Apraisal of Reasoned Free Will. Lanham: University Press of America; 2012

Laureys S, Tononi G. The Neurology of Consciousness. London: Academic Press (Elsevier); 2009

LeDoux JE. The emotional brain: the mysterious underpinnings of emotional life. New York: Simon & Schuster; 1998

Lewin K. Field theory in social science; selected theoretical papers. Cartwright D, ed. New York: Harper & Row; 1951: 169

Markowitsch HJ. Dem Gedächtnis auf der Spur. 3rd ed. Darmstadt: Wissenschaftliche Buchgesellschaft; 2009

Mesulam MM. Principles of behavioral and cognitive neurology. 2nd ed. Oxford: Oxford University Press; 2000

Metzinger T. The ego tunnel: the science of the mind and the myth of the self. New York: Basic Books; 2010

Metzinger T, ed. Conscious Experience. Exeter: Imprint Academic; 1995

Mielke R, Hufnagl JM, Hacke W. Von zerebralen Durchblutungsstörungen zur vaskulären Demenz. München: Hoechst Marion Roussel; 1996

Mlodinow L. Subliminal: How Your Unconscious Mind Rules Your Behavior. New York: Pantheon Books; 2012

Mlodinow L. The Drunkard's Walk: How Randomness Rules Our Lives. New York: Pantheon Books; 2008

Munzert J, Lorey B, Zentgraf K. Cognitive motor processes: the role of motor imagery in the study of motor representations. Brain Res Rev 2009; 60(2): 306–326

Nowak DA, Hermsdörfer J, eds. Sensorimotor control of grasping. Cambridge: Cambridge University Press; 2009

Pöppel E. Der Rahmen. München: Hanser; 2006

Popper KR. The logic of scientific discovery. 3rd ed. London: Hutchinson; 1968

Popper KR, Eccles JC. The self and its brain. New York: Springer; 1977

Rizzolatti G, Fadiga L, Gallese V, Fogassi L. Premotor cortex and the recognition of motor actions. Brain Res Cogn Brain Res 1996; 3(2): 131–141

Rost DH. Intelligenz: Fakten und Mythen. Weinheim: Beltz; 2009

Russell B. The analysis of mind. London: Allen & Unwin; 1921

Schacter DL. Searching for memory: the brain, the mind, and the past. New York: Basic Books; 1996

Schacter DL. The seven sins of memory: how the mind forgets and remembers. Boston: Houghton Mifflin; 2001

Squire LR, Kandel ER. Memory: from mind to molecules. 2nd ed. Greenwood Village, CO: Roberts; 2009

Stuss DT, Benson FD. The frontal lobes. New York: Raven Press; 1986

Webbe FM. The Handbook of Sport Neuropsychology. New York: Springer; 2011

Weiskrantz L, ed. Thought without language. Oxford: Clarendon Press; 1988 (Report of the Third Fyssen Symposium held at the Trianon Palace Hotel, Versailles, France, April 3–7, 1987)

Wilson FR. The hand: how its use shapes the brain, language, and human culture. New York: Pantheon; 1998

Yue G, Cole KJ. Strength increases from the motor program: comparison of training with maximal voluntary and imagined muscle contractions. J Neurophysiol 1992; 67(5): 1114–1123

Zimbardo PG, Boyd J. The time paradox: the new psychology of time that will change your life. New York: Free Press; 2008

11

Conservative Treatment of Muscle Injuries

H.-W. Müller-Wohlfahrt
L. Hänsel
P. Ueblacker
A. Binder

Translated by Terry Telger

Therapeutic Challenge of Muscle Injuries   268

Primary Care   268

Infiltration Therapy   269
Therapeutic Agents   269
Techniques   271

Monitoring Blood Parameters in Athletes   275

Physical Therapy and Physical Medicine   278

Treatment Plans for Different Types
of Muscle Injury   279
Treatment of Other Muscular Injuries   284
Treatment of Possible Complications   285

Focal Toxicosis and Interference Fields   286
Interference Fields   286
Gleditsch Functional Circuits   288
Mandel Energy Emission Analysis (EEA)   289

Therapeutic Challenge of Muscle Injuries

The treatment of muscle injuries is practiced largely as empirical medicine, due to a lack of comprehensive evidence-based studies (Järvinen 2005, Orchard et al. 2008). There are various reasons for this. One is the heterogeneity of the injuries; another lies in traditional classifications, which give only a crude depiction of muscle injuries. Another factor is that "minor injuries," consisting of *functional disorders*, are often neglected by athletes who either ignore the injury or self-prescribe some time away from their sport. Given the self-healing potential of muscle, minor muscle injuries usually do not cause significant problems for casual athletes. As a result, large numbers of these muscle injuries are not seen in every sports-medicine practice, and they are almost never seen in an orthopedic hospital.

Elite athletes tend to seek help in specialized facilities with a highly experienced staff. They "vote with their feet" by visiting facilities that seem to achieve the best and fastest results and will presumably give them the most help in recovering from their injuries. These clients are not a suitable population in which to conduct scientific studies or form control groups or placebo-treated groups. As a result, we must continue to regard empirical medicine as being equivalent to evidence-based medicine in high-performance athletes.

Most minor injuries either produce no abnormalities on diagnostic images or are difficult to identify as such. The diagnosis of these injuries is based largely on medical history and palpable impressions, with the result that inexperienced diagnosticians often do not perceive a need for treatment.

The relationships between painful muscle problems, associated "loss of function," and the underlying causal disorders involving the lumbar spine, sacroiliac joints, peripheral joints, motor and sensory nervous system, and reflex pathways at the spinal level are not widely known and are rarely mentioned in current textbooks. In many cases, therefore, therapeutic options that would address these disorders are not even considered.

Note

Practitioners who deal frequently with muscle problems or would like greater proficiency in this area should recognize palpation as an essential diagnostic tool and train their skills specifically in that direction. Palpation in sports traumatology has roughly the same importance as auscultation in cardiology.

Just as muscle injuries vary in their pathogenesis and staging, their treatment also calls for a structured, differentiated approach. Precisely defined measures should be applied, and a precise time line should be followed.

A wait-and-see approach in the hope of spontaneous recovery is not sensible from a therapeutic standpoint and will not promote rapid and effective rehabilitation (Müller-Wohlfahrt et al. 1992).

Classic textbooks list the following main principles in the treatment of muscle injuries:
- Acute care based on the RICE protocol (rest, ice, compression, elevation)
- Restriction from sports activities
- Treatment with nonsteroidal anti-inflammatory drugs

Therapists define "return to play" only in vague terms and usually leave that decision to the patient (in a symptom-oriented approach). Physical therapy is not prescribed in all cases, or often it is not specified, again leaving the therapist "up in the air." On the whole, the diagnosis and treatment of muscle injuries in both leisure sports and high-performance sports may be aptly described as non-uniform and unstructured.

Primary Care

An athlete who reports a muscle problem should be examined without delay. This is feasible only in professional sports. Prompt examination by a physician is of key importance because the postprimary care regimen and the prognosis are very different for a structural muscle injury than for a functional muscle disorder.

Following a brief examination, the area affected by a functional muscle disorder should be cooled at once by placing a sponge soaked in ice water ("hot ice") broadly over the area for ~ 20 minutes.

If a minor partial muscle tear or an even more severe structural injury is suspected, an elastic bandage soaked in ice water should be wrapped around the affected area. This pressure bandage is kept cold and wet by soaking it intermittently with ice water. The injured athlete should be placed in a position that relieves stress on the affected muscle and positions it over the center of the body. After 20 minutes, the ice-pressure bandage is removed and the injury is reexamined. This requires time, patience, and a calm atmosphere, because ideally a definitive assessment of the severity of the injury should be made during this baseline examination. A major advantage of ice-water therapy is that it produces a sustained reduction of tissue temperature. This prevents the onset of reactive hyperthermia, which may occur with classic "icing" of the injury (Müller-Wohlfahrt 2001).

The primary care provided for a minor partial muscle tear has a crucial impact on the time course of healing. Every minute wasted during primary care (for about the first 10 minutes, before autoregulation sets in) means in our experience approximately one extra day of recovery time until the athlete can return to play.

It is generally agreed that a cooling pressure bandage soaked in ice water provides a simple, fast, and convenient first-line treatment for athletic injuries and that its use is justified even in doubtful cases.

The main goal of this treatment is to control or minimize the hemorrhage and inflammatory reaction that invariably follow a structural muscle injury. Withholding appropriate primary care will not only delay the healing process but will also increase the risk that subsequent imaging will greatly overestimate the injury due to the presence of hematoma or edema.

Caution

Even today, magnetic resonance images vary widely in quality and interpretation. Because magnetic resonance imaging (MRI) is so sensitive in detecting hemorrhage and edema, examiners tend to overinterpret the injury. Only a critical combination of history, palpation, ultrasound, and MRI will allow reliable assessment of the injury.

Comprehensive experience in the treatment of muscle injuries has shown that a wait-and-see approach is not justified. It is essential, rather, to intervene in the regulation of muscle tone and regional metabolic processes by administering early, targeted injections. It is also important to provide prompt and adequate treatment for a possible causative disturbance of neural muscle control. Specific techniques of injection therapy will be described in the sections below. Patients are also treated with oral, intravenous, and locally administered agents, starting on the day of the injury.

Infiltration Therapy

Therapeutic Agents (in Alphabetic Order)

The goal of rapid hemostasis with a pressure bandage and ice is to minimize bleeding into the injured tissue and surrounding area. The intent is to limit the posttraumatic effects of potentially damaging proteolytic enzymes (local inflammatory response) to the degree that is physiologically necessary for healing. Because this can never be fully accomplished by external mechanical means, an attempt is made to control the inflammatory response more effectively by the local or systemic (oral, intravenous) administration of therapeutic agents.

Actovegin (Intramuscular)

Actovegin is a deproteinized hemodialysate from calf blood, produced by Nycomed Austria Ltd. Clinically, it is used as an intravenous infusion for several indications (Lee et al. 2011). It contains physiological components, electrolytes, and essential trace elements, with 30% organic components including amino acids, nucleosides, intermediary products of carbohydrates, and fat metabolites (Lee et al. 2011). It does not contain growth factors or hormone-like substances, as it is ultrafiltered to 6000 Da. Many studies have tried to identify the active ingredients in this mixture, but without success (Lee et al. 2011).

The present authors believe that the active ingredients include the amino acids, which are involved in both glucoplastic energy metabolism and the repair metabolism of injured muscle fiber systems. The administration of amino acids can also forestall the development of a catabolic metabolic state in damaged muscle fibers. This could promote the healing of injured cellular and fiber systems at a molecular-biologic level without the use of synthetic agents.

Current studies at the University of Hamburg using a gene-chip array in an animal model have shown that Actovegin administered by intramuscular infiltration significantly up-regulates muscle-specific genes that presumably promote muscle healing. A publication on these findings is in preparation.

Although the active ingredients in Actovegin have yet to be identified, there are many clinical studies confirming its safety and effectiveness (Lee et al. 2011). Actovegin has been used for different indications for over 60 years. Injection therapy with it appears to be safe and well tolerated (Lee et al. 2011). After administering it thousands of times, the present authors have not observed a single allergic reaction to the product.

Actovegin does not contain blood cells that are liable to increase oxygen transport and is explicitly permitted by the World Anti-Doping Agency (WADA) and the International Olympic Committee (IOC), unless it is administered by intravenous infusion. It has been tested by anti-doping laboratories, and no growth hormone or prohibited substances were found (www.wada-ama.org). However, Actovegin is not approved by the Food and Drug Administration (FDA) in the United States and not available in every country.

Arnica, Trace Elements and Minerals (e.g., Enelbin Paste; Topical)

Ointment compresses, sometimes applied as occlusive dressings with a combination of arnica preparations and mineral paste, promote the regression of inflammation and swelling in closed athletic and traumatic injuries.

Enelbin paste, which the authors commonly use, contains aluminum silicate, a special clay, and skin-soothing zinc oxide, combined with anti-inflammatory and pain-relieving salicylic acid. The special composition of the paste tends to retain a cold temperature (ideally the paste should be cooled), with beneficial effects on tissue metabolism and pain.

Discus Compositum (Epidural)

Discus Compositum is a complex homeopathic preparation, the main ingredients of which are *Kalmia latifolia* dil. D8, *Hydrargyrum oxidatum rubrum* dil. D10, and *Asafoetida* dil. D8. It is used mainly in the treatment of acute, nonbacterial inflammatory conditions of the joints and soft tissues.

Escin (e.g., Reparil) and Bromelains (e.g., Wobenzym, Phlogenzym, Traumanase; Oral)

Fibrinolytic enzymes (such as the proprietary preparations Wobenzym, Phlogenzym, and Traumanase, marketed in Germany) are administered orally at high doses. They are absorbed through the mucosa of the small intestine. This induces partial fibrinolysis and proteinolysis, which minimize the release of aggressive interleukins and phagocytic mediators from infiltrating granulocytes and macrophages, thereby shortening the duration of the inflammatory phase (Fitzhugh et al. 2008).

The aim in using Reparil, which contains escin, is similar. This product has shown efficacy in strengthening the cell membrane and reducing inflammation and edema (Wang et al. 2009).

Lactopurum (Intramuscular, Periligamentous)

Lactopurum contains dextrorotated lactic acid and is used to neutralize pH shifts in inflamed tissues.

Magnesium and Zinc (Oral, Intravenous)

Zinc and magnesium can produce a variety of effects following oral and/or intravenous administration immediately after the injury and on subsequent days.

Since the Korean War, zinc ions have been known for their ability to promote wound healing. Zinc ions are essential for protein biosynthesis from amino acids (ribosomal fiber synthesis). Zinc stabilizes synthesis-promoting RNA, acts as a free-radical scavenger in injured areas, and is involved in the phagocytic activity of granulocytes (Heyman et al. 2008, Barbosa et al. 2009).

Additionally, injuries incite the copious release of mineralocorticoids, causing electrolyte and trace-element losses that are even higher than in ordinary acute-phase reactions in sports. Thus, for example, the metabolism of muscle high-energy phosphates without magnesium replacement tends to delayed healing, while a magnesium deficiency interferes with energy storage in the cell's adenosine triphosphate (ATP) system (Hubbard et al. 2004, Watanabe et al. 2004, Iotti and Malucelli 2008).

Mepivacaine or Procaine (Intramuscular, Epidural, Perineural)

Local anesthetics block the voltage-dependent sodium channel on the axon. This keeps the nerve membrane from depolarizing at that site, temporarily blocking further conduction of action potentials past the site of action. Thus an intramuscular injection of mepivacaine or procaine will functionally block all the muscle fibers supplied by that axon (motor unit; see also Chapter 1, Functional Anatomy of Skeletal Muscle), causing the treated muscle bundle to become "unexcitable" and lose its tone (Catterall and Mackie 2005).

Nonsteroidal Anti-Inflammatory Drugs

Besides their anti-inflammatory properties, nonsteroidal anti-inflammatory drugs (NSAIDs) also suppress pain perception by inhibiting prostaglandin synthesis. The true and undistorted perception of the injured muscle by the patient or athlete is of great importance during the course of rapid or progressive rehabilitation. Also, most muscle injuries cease to be very painful even a short time after the injury is sustained. For both of these reasons, the authors generally do not recommend NSAIDs for the treatment of muscle injuries.

Indometacin is administered if there are any signs of calcification myositis ossificans, such as echo-rich particles in ultrasound with a dorsal shadow (see also Chapters 6, 7, and 16).

Platelet-Rich Plasma (PRP)

Autologous serum products have recently become a focus of growing interest in the treatment of muscle and tendon injuries. Mei-Dan et al. (2010) noted that it "is astonishing but understandable that the most influential stimulus for PRP therapy in the United States, years after the method had been popularized in Europe, was a February 2009 article in the lay press in the New York Times."

PRP is increasingly being used in situations that require a rapid return to play—which in the world of professional sports translates into fame and money (Mei-Dan et al. 2010). Several positive research reports have been published (Foster et al. 2009, Mishra et al. 2009). Hammond et al. report a faster recovery time after a "muscle strain injury" in a small-animal model with the use of locally administered platelet-rich plasma (Hammond et al. 2009).

Almost all the major manufacturers in the orthopedic and sports medicine world are now marketing various commercial kits (Mei-Dan et al. 2010). There are many different preparation protocols, with different PRP concentrations (Mei-Dan et al. 2010). Each method leads to a different product with different biological characteristics and potential uses (Dohan Ehrenfest et al. 2009). Despite its increasing use, PRP has not been systematically studied, and there is as yet no universal protocol for muscle injuries or other athletic injuries (Engebretsen et al. 2010, Harmon 2010). In a review article, Heyman et al. state that there are still serious questions regarding when and how to use PRP in muscle injuries (Heyman et al. 2008).

There are two reasons why the present authors currently cannot report on any experience of their own in the usage of platelet-rich plasma preparations in muscle-injured athletes:

- Firstly, platelet-derived preparations were still included in the Prohibited List of the World Anti-Doping Agency (WADA) until 2010 and therefore could not be administered by intramuscular injection in competitive athletes before 2011. Intramuscular administration of PRP has been permitted since January 2011. However, there are as yet no clear and standardized protocols for the treatment of muscle or muscle-tendon injuries, and the present authors therefore currently develop treatment and injection protocols for muscle injuries on an individualized basis. Further observations and research are needed on this topic.
- Secondly, platelet-rich plasma is obtained invasively, and the process is therefore more elaborate than using Actovegin, with which the authors have extensive experience. Actovegin has shown excellent clinical efficacy and is easy to obtain.

More experience is therefore needed before meaningful conclusions can be drawn about PRP and before this or other autologous serum products come into routine use in the treatment of muscle injuries in competitive athletes (Engebretsen et al. 2010).

Steroids

The authors do not use or recommend steroids in any dosage form for the treatment of muscle injuries.

Traumeel S and Zeel (Intramuscular, Epidural)

The precise mechanism of action of Traumeel S is still unclear. It has been shown, however, that Traumeel S inhibits the secretion of the inflammatory mediators interleukin-1β (IL-1β), tumor necrosis factor-α (TNF-α), and IL-8 from activated human lymphocytes by up to 70% (Porozov et al. 2004).

It has also been found that glycoproteins from certain medicinal plants (the ingredients of Traumeel S and Zeel include comfrey, *Symphytum officinale*) inhibit the influx of inflammatory cells and their mediators. Traumeel S is also used for its antiedematous and locally dehydrating effect (Schneider et al. 2008).

Vitamins A, C, and E (Oral, Intravenous)

The additional administration of antioxidants such as vitamins A, C, and E improves both local and systemic free-radical scavenging capacity. This action improves the body's ability to remove electronegative particles released in response to injury and limit the damage to cell membranes (see also Chapter 3).

Techniques

Muscle Infiltration Therapy

The aim in injecting therapeutic agents directly into the affected muscle tissue is to create the optimum conditions for rapid muscle regeneration or scar formation and to regulate muscle tone by preventing a reactive increase in tone or relieving muscle firmness (tightness) that is already present.

Muscle infiltrations are administered immediately after the injury, after the initial diagnostic work-up has been completed, and in some cases on the second and fourth days after the injury, depending on the type of muscle injury. The infiltrations can normalize muscle tone, optimize blood supply and venous drainage, support energy and structural metabolism, and inhibit the inflammatory response and edema formation. They are also helpful in preventing undesired intermuscular adhesions.

A mixture of Traumeel S and Actovegin in a ratio of 1 : 2 is infiltrated through approximately five to seven needles placed at the center of the injury and proximal and distal to that site. Approximately 1.5–2 mL of solution is injected through each needle. The needles are introduced almost painlessly into the muscle bundle by continuously infiltrating the site with local anesthetic (1% mepivacaine) during insertion (**Fig. 11.1a, b**). Only light pressure should be placed on the plunger of the syringe. High resistance to injection usually means that the needle has entered a tendinous area rather than the fleshy part of the muscle. If a circumscribed hematoma or seroma has formed (common with muscle bundle injuries), the collection should be aspirated at this time (**Fig. 11.1c**).

As in any form of medical treatment, the patient should be counseled about the nature and significance of the diagnosis and the proposed treatment. The patient should be questioned about a possible allergy to any of the agents being instilled. The authors wish to emphasize that we have not documented a single allergic reaction to Actovegin or Traumeel S in more than 30 years of using these agents. The injections are extremely unlikely to cause intramuscular bleeding, especially as the continuous instillation of local anesthetic during needle insertion will displace smaller blood vessels. A meticulous and sterile technique is used to prevent soft-tissue infection. Again, the authors have not experienced any complications of this type in decades of practice.

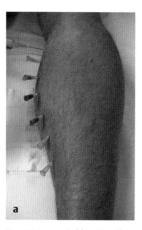
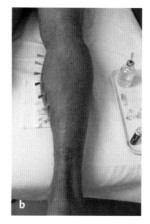
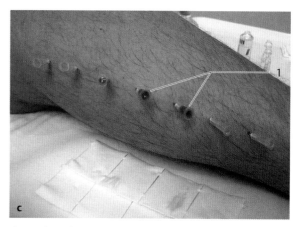

Fig. 11.1a–c Infiltration therapy for a moderate partial muscle tear (type 3b) in the right medial gastrocnemius muscle.

a Multiple needles are introduced along the injured muscle.
b Broader view for orientation.

c Spontaneous slight blood and serum drainage is noted from the center needles (1). Blood and serum collections are gently aspirated with a small syringe.

Caution

Corticosteroids should not be used for muscle injection therapy (or to promote the healing of muscle injuries in general). Local corticosteroid therapy can retard healing by suppressing the physiologic responses to injury. It may significantly increase the risk of a soft-tissue infection and/or local soft-tissue necrosis. Steroids should not be used locally or systemically in the treatment of muscle injuries.

Contraindications to muscle infiltration therapy are coagulation disorders, anticoagulant therapy (INR > 1.4), cardiac arrhythmias, or known hypersensitivity to any of the agents used.

Note

The national and international rules set out by athletic associations and anti-doping agencies take precedence in all competitive sports. Each year, therefore, the authors request written approval from the National Anti-Doping Agency (NADA) and WADA confirming the safety of Actovegin for intramuscular use. Every physician is personally responsible for following the currently applicable guidelines at all times. Particular attention should be given to the rules that apply in specific countries.

Spinal Infiltration Therapy

Spinal injections are administered when the muscle injury or disorder is considered to have a neuroregulatory cause. This applies in particular to type 2a and 2b lesions (spine-related or muscle-related neuromuscular muscle disorders; see Chapters 6 and 12).

All potential causal dysfunctions are treated, starting with infiltration therapy to mobilize spinal segments, normalize muscle tone, and relieve pain. Next, an effort is made to preserve mobility and improve stability with the aid of manual therapy, osteopathy, massage therapy, chiropractic therapy in selected cases, and therapeutic exercises.

As a peripheral motor nerve is made up of fibers from several spinal segments and a mobility disorder usually involves multiple intervertebral joints—just as splinting of the deep paravertebral muscles (especially the rotators and multifidus muscles) often spans multiple segments—the usual practice is to administer injections (epidural, paravertebral, pericapsular) over a range of two to three segments (**Fig. 11.2**).

Due to the high efficacy of infiltration therapy (e.g., in loosening tight muscles), paravertebral injections are administered bilaterally to prevent or correct for any imbalance in the affected segment.

Asymmetric loads on the sacroiliac joints lead to unphysiologic tightness of the paravertebral muscles. Because they are auxiliary joints, the sacroiliac joints cannot permanently compensate for functional deficits in the intervertebral joints of the lower lumbar spine. In this case, they create an additional problem, and like the ligaments between the spinal column and pelvis (e.g., the iliolumbar ligament), they are generally treated along with other structures. Trigger points and tender points are treated only in selected cases.

Practical Tip

The patient should be positioned for spinal infiltration therapy in a way that straightens the lordotic curve of the lumbar spine. Examination tables with a central break are particularly useful for this technique (Fig. 11.3).

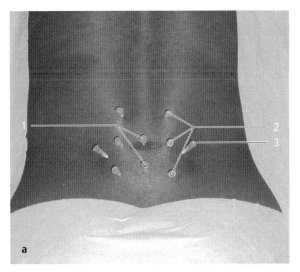 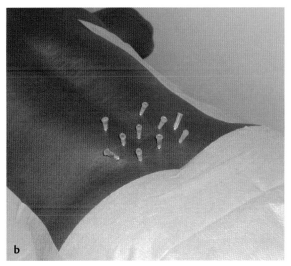

Fig. 11.2a, b **Trisegmental treatment of the lumbar spine with infiltration of the iliolumbar ligaments on both sides.**

a The needles labeled "1" have been placed epidurally at the L4–L5 and L5–S1 levels. The needles labeled "2" have been placed farther laterally to infiltrate the L3–L4, L4–L5, and L5–S1 facet joints and the paravertebral muscles on both sides. The lateral needles (3) are for infiltrating the iliolumbar ligaments.

b Therapist's view of the treatment area.

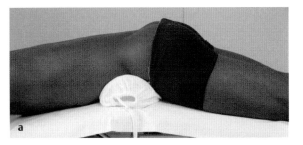 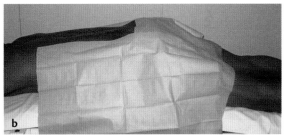

Fig. 11.3a, b **Positioning the patient for infiltration therapy of the lumbar spine.**

a The examination table is angled to straighten the natural lordotic curve of the lumbar spine.

b Appearance after sterile draping of the treatment site.

How Infiltration Therapy Works

On the basis of the hypothesis that there is a local disturbance involving the functional units of the lumbar spine, the causal disturbance may have various direct or indirect effects on the lumbar spine and dependent structures (see also Chapter 12):

- *Direct irritation of a nerve root.* This condition leads to excessive electrical stimulation of the motor units.
- *Irritation of the capsuloligamentous structures of the spine and its joints.* The body responds to this type of irritation by reactive immobilization (static contraction, splinting) of the paravertebral muscles. This firmness of the paravertebral muscles increases the compressive forces acting on the intervertebral disks and facet joints, which in turn exacerbates the mechanical causes of irritation. This sets up a classic vicious circle that has to be interrupted.

- *Blocking or down-regulation of the sympathetic trunk.* This results from the liberal use of local anesthetic, which diffuses to the sympathetic trunk and can act directly on the ventral ramus of the meningeal nerve. This effect is important in terms of improving blood flow (controlling the inflammatory reaction) and regulating lymphatic drainage.

The local, circumscribed, and temporary therapeutic action of the administered agents can interrupt the vicious circle by blocking mechanical and sensory reflex afferents. The immediate result is a reregulation or normalization of the tone of the abnormally activated skeletal muscles. The treatment temporarily and reversibly blocks nociceptive afferents (e.g., from muscle, tendons, skin, joint capsule, annulus fibrosus, and intervertebral disks) that enter the gray matter of the spinal cord through the spinal ganglia via the dorsal (sensory) root and posterior horn.

Technique of Lumbar Infiltration Therapy

In the technique described above, needle lengths of 4–6 cm (or even longer, depending on the patient) are generally used, which are appropriate for young, slender athletes.

Further information about lumbar infiltration techniques is available in Theodoridis and Krämer (2009) and other authors.

Epidural Injections

The patient is positioned prone on a table surface that is raised or angled to straighten the lordotic curve of the lumbar spine. The spinous processes are easily palpated in this position, and the interspinous spaces are identified and marked on the skin. On the basis of the clinical presentation, the therapist decides which segments require treatment. As the needle passes through the interspinal ligament, considerable resistance will be felt on the syringe plunger. A sudden loss of resistance is felt after the needle has penetrated the ligamentum flavum, confirming the epidural position of the needle tip. Placement is reconfirmed using an aspiration test, followed by epidural injection of the therapeutic agents. This is the same technique that is used thousands of times every day for epidural anesthesia. The authors recommend injecting a maximum of 3 mL of 0.5% mepivacaine, 2.2 mL (one ampule) of Traumeel S, and 1 mL (half an ampule) of discus compositum. These are empirical recommendations based on decades of experience.

Practical Tip

In patients who are sensitive to pain, it may be helpful to place the epidural needles close to the midline initially and inject the local anesthetic there (see also **Fig. 11.2b**). This can be done without causing any pain. Several minutes later, the epidural space can be entered painlessly. One side effect of this technique is that, even within this short amount of time, a marked decrease in resistance will be felt when the needle penetrates the interspinal ligament.

Periarticular Facet Joint Infiltration

The facet joints are anesthetized by introducing the needle at the level of the interspinous spaces, ~2.5 cm from the midline, and advancing the needle tip to bone. Local anesthetic is continuously instilled as the needle is advanced, temporarily relaxing the paravertebral muscles at the segmental level. A mixture of 1.5 mL Actovegin and 1 mL Traumeel S is then administered by periarticular injection.

Infiltration of the S1 Sacral Foramina

The S1 foramina are located ~2.5 cm from the midline at the level of the posterior superior iliac spine. The authors recommend using only local anesthetic and Traumeel S (which may be combined with discus compositum if desired). The direct perineural injection of Actovegin may cause severe (though temporary) irritation.

Infiltration of the Lumbar Plexus

The needle is introduced at the level of the L3 spinous process, ~4 cm from the midline and angled ~30° medially toward the vertebral body, and the tip is inserted to bone. The needle is then withdrawn a few millimeters, and a local anesthetic depot containing Traumeel S is placed to provide excellent down-regulation of the lumbar sympathetic trunk. We recommend injecting 3–5 mL of 0.5% mepivacaine on each side.

Infiltration of the Sacroiliac Joint

The needle is introduced halfway between the posterior superior iliac spine and the S1 spinous process on the affected side. From there, the needle is angled 45° laterally to infiltrate the ligaments in a fan-shaped pattern and to locate the joint space. A generous amount of local anesthetic and Traumeel S is administered.

Practical Tip

Remarkably, there are cases in which the lumbar spine may undergo significant structural changes without causing the patient any conscious pain. Some patients may describe only a history of intermittent pain, while other patients deny having any significant lumbar problems. This suggests that many patients do not mention the lumbar spine as a source of symptoms when their history is taken, and underscores the importance of routinely examining the lumbar spine and pelvic region in every patient. For the reasons stated, the authors feel that a symmetrical weight-bearing radiograph of the pelvis and lumbar spine in two-legged stance should be obtained in all patients with muscle problems involving the pelvis, inguinal region, and lower extremities (**Fig. 11.4**) (see also Chapter 12).

Clinical Effects of Infiltration Therapy in the Lumbar Spine

The clinical effects of infiltration therapy in the lumbar spine are reviewed in **Table 11.1**. For clarity, the diagrams in **Fig. 11.5** illustrate the structure of a spinal cord segment.

Practical Tip

The adductor group of muscles is innervated basically by the obturator nerve (L2–L4). The pectineus is supplied in part by the femoral nerve, and the adductor magnus by the sciatic nerve. In patients with muscle problems involving the adductor group, experience has shown that symptoms are immediately improved by concomitant treatment of the ipsilateral sacroiliac joint by injection and, if necessary, by chiropractic mobilization (next to the L2–L4 segments of origin).

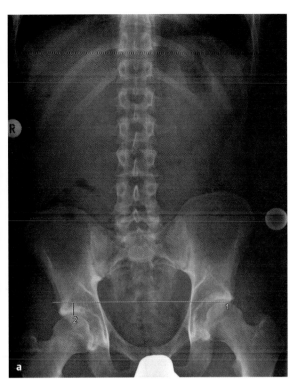
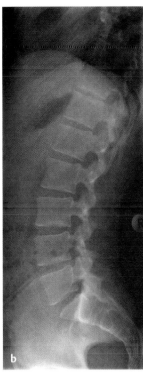

Fig. 11.4a, b   Weight-bearing radiographs of the lumbar spine and pelvis in a 23-year-old professional soccer player. The radiographs show significant true shortening of the right leg (by 14 mm), resulting in pelvic obliquity. The patient did not have any lumbar problems, but repeatedly reported muscular symptoms.

a Anteroposterior projection.
b Lateral projection.

Providing the patient with appropriate information and obtaining informed consent are essential prior to spinal infiltration therapy and should be documented in the patient's chart. Informed consent should include information on the potential risk of dural injury (cerebrospinal fluid loss, post-puncture headache, infection) and the possibility of epidural hematoma formation (neurologic complications, surgical exposure). Post-puncture headaches are observed in rare cases. In over 30 years of practicing this form of treatment, the authors have not encountered a single serious complication relating to infection or hematoma formation with a neurologic deficit that might require surgical exposure or intervention. Patients should be asked about known allergic reactions to any of the agents and about the use of hemodiluting medications.

Note

The authors do not use corticosteroids in spinal therapy.

The contraindications are the same as for peripheral muscle injections; namely, a very critical risk–benefit analysis should be carried out, especially in patients receiving anticoagulant medication.

Caution

As numerous injections are administered in the form of lumbar infiltration therapy described, very careful consideration should be given to the volume of local anesthetic injected and the contraindications to local anesthesia. In the authors' experience, 0.5% mepivacaine has proved to be a highly effective and well-tolerated local anesthetic solution.

Monitoring Blood Parameters in Athletes

Every elite athlete should have a comprehensive laboratory work-up at least twice a year. Other laboratory tests may also be advisable during periods of intense training and competition and even after strenuous travel. The authors routinely determine the laboratory parameters listed in **Table 11.2**.

Special attention should be given to thyroid dysfunction, abnormal protein metabolism (uric acid), electrolyte shifts, mineral and trace-element deficiencies, and direct or indirect signs of inflammation (leukocytes, C-reactive protein, antistreptolysin, and antistaphylolysin).

Any disorders that are detected should of course be further investigated and treated. When indirect signs of infection (antistreptolysin or antistaphylolysin) are found,

Table 11.1 Clinical effects of infiltration therapy of the lumbar spine

Infiltration site	Infiltrated agents	Effects

Epidural	Local anesthetic, Traumeel S, Discus compositum	• Temporary anesthesia:
		  ○ Meningeal nerve: supplies dura (pain on coughing may signify dural irritation), annulus fibrosus, periosteum, and posterior portions of joint capsule
		  ○ Dorsal ramus: supplies the skin (cutaneous branch), anterior facet joint capsule (articular branch), and intrinsic back muscles (muscular branch); these muscles undergo painful shortening due to dorsal ramus irritation
		  ○ Communicating branch between ventral ramus and sympathetic trunk (preganglionic): supplies vessels and connective tissue
		  ○ Gray ramus (postganglionic): innervates dermatomes, myotomes
		• Anti-edema effect on soft tissues in the spinal canal, on herniated and protruding disks, and on the nerve root itself
		• Reduce nerve root irritation
		• Relieve pain, mobilize spinal segments

Paravertebral	Local anesthetic, Traumeel S, Actovegin	• These agents quickly relax firm paravertebral muscles, block neuromuscular conduction, and increase energy metabolism • Improve blood flow • Relax firm muscles, mobilize spinal segments
Pericapsular	Local anesthetic, Traumeel S, Zeel	• Relieve facet pain (by blocking nociceptors) • Reduce swelling and inflammation in synovitis or activated spondyloarthropathy • Relieve pain, mobilize spinal segments
Periligamentous	Local anesthetic, Traumeel S, Actovegin, Lactopurum	• Reduce irritation • Normalize pH (inflamed tissue has an acidic pH) • Relieve pain
Intra-articular (sacroiliac joints)	Local anesthetic, Traumeel S, Zeel, hyaluronic acid	• Relieve joint pain by blocking nociceptors, reduce swelling and inflammation in synovitis • Relieve pain, help to mobilize spinal segments
Treatment of trigger points and tender points	Local anesthetic, Traumeel S, Actovegin	Treatment at a specific point can: • Reduce tone in shortened muscles • Reduce local or referred pain • Improve stretchability of muscle and muscle–tendon junction.

Trigger point: manifested chiefly at the neurovascular hilum. The hilum is surrounded by pressoreceptors (Vater–Pacini corpuscles), which register muscle tension. When abnormal myofascial tension acts on the receptors, the trigger point is activated. The referred pain radiates in a reproducible pattern (Simons et al. 1998; see also Chapters 1 and 14).

Tender point: located in tendinous structures near joints, interacts with up to 25 muscle fibers per Golgi tendon organ at the mechanoreceptor level. Tension on the joint capsule and intra-articular structures is registered and transmitted to the corresponding muscle. The pain at a tender point is localized and does not radiate to reference zones (Simons et al. 1998; see also Chapter 14).

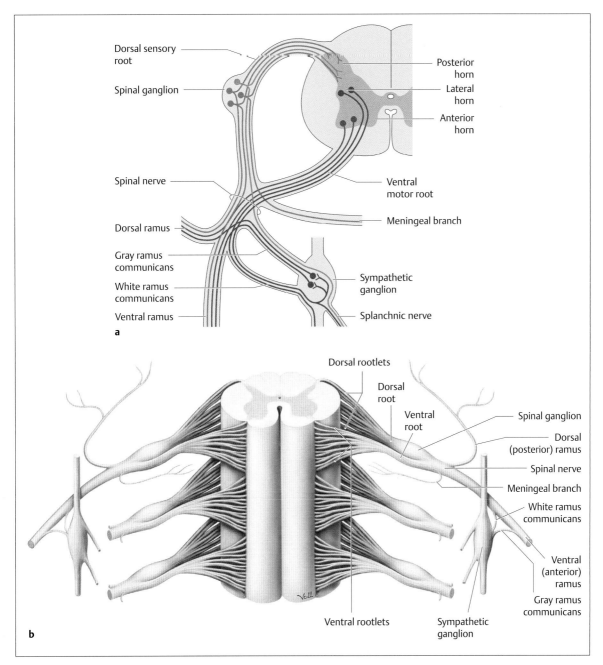

Fig. 11.5a, b Topographic and functional organization of a spinal cord segment.

a Diagrammatic representation.
b Oblique multisegmental view.

Table 11.2 Routine laboratory tests in high-performance athletes

Simple blood count

WBCs

RBCs

Platelets

Hemoglobin

Hematocrit

MCV (hematocrit/RBC count)

MCH (hemoglobin/RBC count)

MCHC (hemoglobin/hematocrit)

Blood chemistry

Calcium

Potassium

Sodium

Blood sugar (fasting)

Cholesterol

HDL cholesterol (high-density lipoprotein)

LDL cholesterol (low-density lipoprotein)

Triglycerides

IgA

IgG

IgM

Total bilirubin

Uric acid

Urea

Creatinine

CK nac (total creatine kinase activity)

CK-MB (myocardial type of creatine kinase)

GGT (gamma-glutamyl transferase)

GOT (glutamate oxaloacetate transaminase)

GPT (alanine aminotransferase)

LDH (lactate dehydrogenase)

Iron

Ferritin

Magnesium

ESR (erythrocyte sedimentation rate)

C-reactive protein quantitative

Copper

Zinc

TSH (thyrotropin)

Phosphate

Bone-specific AP (alkaline phosphatase of bone)

PTH intact (parathormone)

Vitamin D_3 (25-OH)

RF quantitative (rheumatoid factor)

ASL quantitative (antistreptolysin)

AST quantitative (antistaphylolysin)

the athlete should be examined in an attempt to locate the focus. Insidious infections in the areas of urology, otolaryngology, oromaxillary surgery, and internal medicine often go undetected and unnoticed by the patient but can be a cause of recurrent injuries and may delay the healing of injuries. More detailed information can be found below in the section on Interference Fields (see p. 286).

Practical Tip

The authors monitor the baseline zinc level of the athletes in their care. It is regularly checked and optimized. Zinc levels are known to fall sharply during the acute phase of an injury and even during extended travel (due to jet lag), and so zinc supplementation is generally advised.

Top athletes should have an aminogram analysis at least once a year. In particular, deficiencies in essential and semi-essential amino acids should definitely be corrected to create optimum conditions for fiber synthesis, collagen metabolism, and muscle healing.

Physical Therapy and Physical Medicine

In addition to medical treatments to promote and optimize healing, physical therapy and physical medicine have an equally important role in the management of muscle injuries (see also Chapter 14).

Physical medicine treatments such as pharmacotherapy are powerful tools that can be used to promote the control or rapid regression of a post-traumatic inflammatory response and stimulate physiologic healing.

Physical therapy, rehabilitative exercises, and training therapy are essential components in reconditioning an injured structure, restoring coordination and proprioception, normalizing movement patterns, preventing muscular atrophy, and recovering normal force development.

Practical Tip

In addition to having access to immediate first aid, the key advantage that professional athletes have over recreational athletes is that they have continuous, daily care by a sports physical therapist, massage therapist, and rehabilitation trainer. Physicians may need to point this out to patients who are curious about why an injury in an "ordinary athlete" takes longer to heal.

Physical therapy, physical medicine, and progressive training regimens should never be conducted on a "trial-and-error" basis and should not be self-directed by the patient. Instead, they should follow a well-structured timetable that is appropriate for the specific injury or disorder. As mentioned above, the pain caused by a structural muscle injury often subsides shortly after the injury, and this may tempt the patient to use the injured muscle at a pre-injury level. Regular follow-ups with an up-to-date assessment of healing progress are critically important for making any adjustments that may be needed in the timing and nature of proposed therapies. We again emphasize the importance of palpation and clinical evaluation. Ultrasound is a valuable imaging study that can be performed and repeated at any time, although it still requires a good deal of practical experience and interpretation skills.

The most important measures available in physical therapy and physical medicine are reviewed below. Detailed descriptions of specific measures and their mechanisms of action are given in Chapter 14. The authors have tried to formulate a treatment plan for different types of injury that will be useful for less experienced practitioners. It should always be remembered, of course, that muscle injuries and functional muscle disorders are heterogeneous conditions, and the suggested timetables should be taken as guidelines only. The physician should critically review every case several times during the course of treatment so that any necessary adjustments can be made.

Note

Treatment and rehabilitation should follow a well-structured schedule harmonized with the specific injury.

Treatment Plans for Different Types of Muscle Injury

Fatigue-Induced Painful Muscle Disorder (Type 1a)

- *Day of injury:*
  - Muscle release (contract release)
  - Strain–counterstrain
  - Spray and stretch
  - Massage for muscle relaxation
  - Low-impact aquatic exercises (water temperature 29–32°C)
  - Occlusive ointment bandage
- *First day after injury:*
  - Reciprocal inhibition, stretching by the antagonist (Sherrington I)
  - Postisometric relaxation (Sherrington II)
  - Electrotherapy force neuromuscular equilibrium
  - Classic massage to loosen the muscles
  - Thermotherapy
  - Running training at an aerobic endurance level (running training may be considered a therapeutic measure)
  - Oral preparations (e.g., magnesium)

- *Second day after injury:*
  - Status check
  - Unrestricted training is generally allowed

Delayed-Onset Muscle Soreness (DOMS; Type 1b)

- *First day after injury:*
  - Mild lymphatic drainage
  - Thermotherapy
  - Low-impact motion therapy and/or aquatic exercises (water temperature 29–32°C)
  - Oral anti-inflammatory preparations (e.g., diclofenac, profen)
- *Second day after injury:*
  - Physical modalities and physical therapy measures as above
  - Running training or cycling at a low endurance level
- *Third day after injury:*
  - Increasing training load according to clinical symptoms

Neuromuscular Muscle Disorder— Spine-Related (Type 2a)

- *Day of injury:*
  - Ice-water ("hot–ice") therapy
  - Injection therapy (lumbar; also local in selected cases)
  - Ointment bandages
  - Oral preparations (magnesium, Wobenzym, Reparil)
- *First day after injury:*
  - "Hot ice" to regulate muscle tone
  - Reciprocal inhibition, stretching by the antagonist (Sherrington I)
  - Electrotherapy to produce neuromuscular equilibrium:
    - High-voltage therapy
    - Interference current
    - Bernhard currents
  - Ultrasound for micromassage
  - Classic massage to loosen the adjacent muscles, except for the affected muscle
  - Continuous passive motion (CPM, computer-assisted motion on an isokinetic machine)
  - If possible, running training at an aerobic endurance level or adapted exercise training on an ergometer in pain-free range; the muscles are motivated, trained, and returned to their original performance capacity as soon as possible; running training may be considered a therapeutic measure
  - Low-impact aquatic exercises (water temperature 29–32°C)

Caution

Fast and explosive movements are not useful.

- *Second day after injury:*
  - Status check
  - The treatment regimen is the same as on the previous day, but with greater intensity; running training in high to medium endurance range, 20 minutes in the morning and 20 minutes in the afternoon (interval training with pauses); the second training unit is followed by active regeneration, stretching, and calisthenics
- *Third day after injury:*
  - Stretching and calisthenics
  - Training unit with variable running speeds for 20 minutes
  - Followed by regenerative physical modalities, such as:
    - Thermotherapy
    - Sherrington I and II muscle stretching techniques
    - Electrotherapy
    - Regenerative massage with firm, broad strokes, three-dimensional kneading of the muscles and surrounding tissue
  - Second training unit in the afternoon, same as morning unit
  - Followed by active regeneration, stretching, and calisthenics
- *Fourth day after injury:*
  - Generally, the patient is returned to unrestricted training
  - Medical monitoring and physical therapy during the first week

Caution

Primary massage of the affected muscle is not indicated for type 2a lesions, due to the neurogenic cause. Experience has shown that classic massage may lead to refractory nerve irritation.

Practical Tip

Type 2a lesions are caused by an abnormality in the lumbar spine; infiltration therapy is therefore generally applied to the lumbar spine rather than the muscle.
If necessary, injection therapy of the lumbar spine may be repeated on the third or fourth day. If the therapy is withheld, the muscle may remain tender and firm for weeks, making training difficult.
It should be noted that all treatments and training workouts should be conducted without pain and normally should not include the use of analgesics, as these would interfere with biofeedback mechanisms. The use of anti-inflammatory or analgesic agents is reserved for exceptional situations such as activated arthritis of the facet joints or sacroiliac joints and should be a temporary measure in which the patient should avoid progressive running and sprinting.

Neuromuscular Muscle Disorder— Muscle-Related (Type 2b)

- *Day of injury:*
  - Muscle release (contract release)
  - Strain–counterstrain
  - Spray and stretch
  - Intramuscular injection therapy (also lumbar injection therapy only in patients with functional or structural lumbar abnormalities)
  - Ointment bandages
- *First day after injury:*
  - "Hot ice" to regulate muscle tone
  - Sherrington I and II muscle stretching techniques
  - Electrotherapy to produce neuromuscular equilibrium:
    - High-voltage therapy
    - Interference current
    - Bernhard currents
  - Ultrasound for micromassage
  - Classic massage to loosen the muscles proximal and distal to the injury, including the entire kinetic chain but sparing the actual injury site
  - Continuous passive motion (CPM, computer-assisted on an isokinetic machine)
  - Running training at an endurance level or adapted exercise training on an ergometer in the pain-free range; the muscles are motivated, trained, and returned to their original performance capacity as soon as possible; running training may be considered a therapeutic measure
  - Low-impact aquatic exercises (water temperature 29–32°C)

Caution

Fast and explosive movements are not recommended.

- *Second day after injury:*
  - Status check
  - The treatment regimen is the same as on the previous day, but with greater intensity; running training in the high to medium endurance range, 20 minutes in the morning and 20 minutes in the afternoon; the second training unit is followed by active regeneration, stretching, and calisthenics
  - If sufficient tone reduction is not achieved, repeat intramuscular infiltration therapy
- *Third day after injury:*
  - Stretching and calisthenics in the morning
  - Training unit with variable running speeds for 20 minutes
  - Followed by regenerative physical modalities, such as:
    - Thermotherapy
    - Sherrington I and II muscle stretches
    - Electrotherapy

- Regenerative massage with firm, broad strokes, three-dimensional kneading of the muscles and surrounding tissue
- Second training unit in the afternoon, same as morning unit
- Then active regeneration, stretching, and calisthenics
- *Fourth day after injury:*
  - Generally the patient is returned to unrestricted training
  - Medical management and physical therapy during the first week
  - Start proprioceptive training to activate proprioceptive mechanisms and training of motor sequences, e.g., on an unstable platform (balance disc, etc.)

Practical Tip

The cause of a type 2b lesion lies in the muscle itself; infiltration therapy of the muscle is therefore indicated. One or two injection treatments are usually sufficient. The lumbar spine plays a significant role due to segmental reflex arcs and should be treated concurrently if abnormalities are present.

It should be noted that all treatments and training workouts should be conducted without pain and without analgesics. Pain relievers have no place in the framework of this type of therapy, as they would interfere with biofeedback mechanisms.

Minor Partial Muscle Tear (Type 3a)

The patient is given information about the need for physical rest and proper positioning.

- *Day of injury:*
  - First aid with a stress-relieving compression bandage, cooling with hot-ice bandage, and elevation
  - Intramuscular injection therapy
  - Oral preparations (e.g., Wobenzym, Reparil)
  - Ointment bandage (avoid heparin-containing ointments for at least 24 hours)
  - Insert an elastic heel wedge for gastrocnemius injuries
- *Phase I* (days 1–3 after muscle injury). Several measures from physical modalities can be applied, such as:
  - Electrotherapy to regulate muscle tone (not at the injury site)
  - Iontophoresis for hematoma treatment
  - Manual lymph drainage to clear the hematoma and prevent decreased blood flow due to raised tissue pressure
  - Classic massage to release reflex tension throughout the motor chain
  - No stretching!

Caution

Massage should not be applied at the injury site, as myositis ossificans might be induced.

- Therapeutic exercises (with emphasis on proprioceptive neuromuscular facilitation) to stimulate and correct pain-altered movement patterns
- Training therapy for all healthy parts of the body to prevent loss of conditioning (bicycle and arm-crank ergometry in selected cases)
- Strain–counterstrain, starting on day 3 after the injury
- Treatment of the injured muscle with "hot ice" to preempt a possible thermal reaction
- Second infiltration therapy after completion of all physical measures on day 2 after the injury
- A supportive bandage or ointment bandage is reapplied
- The intensity of exercise therapy is increased daily but is always tailored to current findings
- *Phase II* (days 4–5 after muscle injury):
  - Electrotherapy with use of muscle-activating currents
  - Ultrasound for micromassage in the injured region, plus laser therapy
  - Lymph drainage is used only if residual hematoma is found
  - The third infiltration treatment (and generally the last) is given on day 4 after the injury
  - Deep muscle layers are treated with classic massage, sparing the actual injury site (kneading technique); isolated "unwinding" treatment of the affected muscle distal and proximal to the tear site
  - Starting on day 5, light friction massage is given at the center of the injury

Caution

Early, forcible massage after a minor partial muscle tear may incite the development of circumscribed myositis ossificans (metaplasia of cells into osteoblasts).

- Change from mild passive to mild active stretching, ending with passive stretch and reaching the approximate physiologic end point
- Transition from therapeutic exercises to pure training therapy, applying sport-specific loads in a closed system
- Isolated eccentric exercise against hand-held resistance to improve muscle quality without risking pain; general conditioning is essential and is done with strict attention to hypercompensation (adapted pauses); support taping
- Motivation and training of other muscles that act in the same direction and can assume the function of the injured muscle unit that has not yet healed
- Training therapy: continuous passive motion

- *Phase III* (day 6 to approximately day 10 after muscle injury). The emphasis during this period is on training therapy.
  - Physical modalities and manual measures:
    - Electrotherapy to regulate muscle tone
    - Laser therapy
    - Massage in preparation for training therapy, also friction massage at the injury site
  - Start full training therapy on postinjury day 5 with an endurance run (~ 20 minutes) at an easy pace that does not cause muscle fatigue; early running training is beneficial for muscle regeneration (formation of new muscle fibers) and can therefore be considered a therapeutic measure (see also Chapter 4)
  - On subsequent days, workouts are increased if possible to two 20- to 30-minute runs per day at high, medium, and low endurance training levels
  - Progressive runs, sprinting, and coordination exercises are started ~ 10–12 days after the injury; when they can be performed without pain, proceed with ball training and return to team training
  - Now the athletic trainer should reassume responsibility and determine the content of training

The intensity of training always depends on how well healing of the torn muscle fibers has progressed and on the tonicity of the injured, shortened muscle band. Muscle tension is a good indicator of healing. Tone cannot be permanently reduced until the muscle has healed well enough, and tissue reactions have subsided sufficiently, that they are no longer a source of pain or irritation. If muscle tone increases again with exercise, this is a sign that the healing process has not yet progressed far enough. This underscores the need to palpate the muscle and evaluate its status each day, and also explain to the athlete how he is to train—since absence of pain is not synonymous with a healed injury, as many believe. It is imperative to avoid a recurrent tear, which would take much longer to heal than the primary injury.

Note

Pain is not a good indication for muscle healing, since it usually subsides quickly.

If the goal of full return to play at 10–14 days cannot be achieved despite adherence to the treatment plan, then additional diagnostic steps, laboratory tests, and functional diagnostic studies. For example, a focal bacterial process can significantly delay the healing process and should therefore be treated concurrently with the injury. Emotional tension associated with a general rise in muscle tone may also contribute significantly to muscle injuries in athletes and can delay healing (see also Chapter 10).

Strength training should be withheld until the injury is completely healed. Otherwise it would lead to counterproductive fatigue, shortening, or re-tearing of the muscle. Areas of shortening are palpable as firm bands just proximal and distal to the injured site, and generally result from premature muscular exertion. On the other hand, targeted strength training is essential for correcting muscle imbalances and preventing muscle injuries (Mjølsnes et al. 2004, Arnason et al. 2008; see also Chapter 15).

Therapy should include regular strengthening of the trunk and pelvic muscles. Core exercises are best for this purpose, with minimal use of specialized equipment. These exercises can simultaneously train flexibility, strength, and coordination. High coordinative and muscular stability of the trunk and pelvis can protect against adverse effects arising from the lumbar spine, sacroiliac joints, and iliolumbar ligaments (Willardson 2007, Akuthota et al. 2008, Hibbs et al. 2008) (see also Chapter 15).

Moderate Partial Muscle Tear (Type 3b)

A moderate partial muscle tear is a more serious injury than a minor partial tear. With optimum primary care and treatment, it will take at least 6 weeks for the athlete to return to sports participation. Rehabilitation may be significantly prolonged because of time lost due to delay in diagnosis or inappropriate treatment.

The rules and measures for primary care and subsequent treatment (especially injection therapy) for a type 3a lesion generally apply to a type 3b lesion as well. Due to the size of the structural defect, a large hematoma (or later a seroma) may form and should be aspirated at the time of injection therapy whenever possible.

The patient should abstain from all sports during the first week after the injury. Activities of daily living are allowed. All passive measures in physical therapy and physical modalities (see p. 281) are rigorously applied. The temporary use of crutches may be advised. The progressive therapy regimen is similar to that for a minor partial muscle tear but is more restrained.

- *First week after injury.* The principal points are as follows:
  - Lymph drainage throughout the affected limb, including the groin and lower abdomen
  - Gentle passive range-of-motion exercises
  - Electrically controlled lymph drainage at the endogenous body frequency (Lymphowave)
  - Kinesiotaping (see Chapter 14)
  - Daily sonophoresis starting on days 3 or 4 postinjury, laser therapy starting on day 5
- *Second week after injury:*
  - Ultrasonic therapy
  - Exercises resisted by body weight
  - Proprioceptive neuromuscular facilitation
  - Start careful, manually guided stretching techniques (agonists/antagonists)
- *Third week after injury:*
  - Start cycling and aquajogging
  - Neuromuscular facilitation

- Classic massage techniques proximal and distal to the injury
- Passive motion of bradytrophic tissue (tendons), avoiding traction on the injury site
- Sherrington I and II techniques, Jander technique
- *Fourth week after injury:*
  - Start treadmill exercises at reduced body weight, using an air chamber to partially offset gravity (AlterG Anti-Gravity Treadmill)
  - Aquajogging
  - Uphill treadmill walking
  - Run training and coordination, balance (running basics) including backward running and walking with eyes closed
- *Fifth week after injury:*
  - Running exercises on grass, optimization of running technique
  - Basic endurance
- *Fifth and sixth weeks after injury:* progressive sport-specific workouts

Caution

With the moderate partial tear and subtotal or avulsion injuries (type 4) described below, extensive soft-tissue trauma poses a significant risk of heterotopic ossification (myositis ossificans). For this reason, the injured region should be scrupulously protected from mechanical stresses, including massage, until the hematoma has completely resolved.

As in strength training, starting or progressing with running prematurely may cause firmness of muscle bundles proximal and distal to the injured site; this would greatly increase the inherent risk of a recurrence.

Subtotal or Complete Muscle Tear/ Tendinous Avulsion (Type 4)

A subtotal or complete tear of a muscle, or avulsion of a muscle from its bony origin or insertion, is a serious injury that forces the athlete to stop sport activity. This type of injury is generally associated with a large hematoma, and the primary measures described above are therefore of major importance. Compression, elevation, and a supportive bandage are essential. Forearm crutches can be used in some cases. A complete diagnostic work-up is usually followed by surgical reattachment of the avulsed tendon, if there is significant retraction. Avulsion injuries of the apophysis in adolescents are a special case and are almost never treated surgically. From the treatment point of view, it is important to distinguish between two types of tendinous avulsion: distal and proximal and distal.

Proximal Tendinous Avulsion

Proximal tendinous avulsions are more frequent than distal ones, and do not always undergo significant retraction or displacement from the anatomic site. Many of these cases can be managed conservatively following a detailed evaluation. With an equally good functional outcome, conservative treatment avoids the immediate risks of surgery and general anesthesia as well as the development of postoperative adhesions, which athletes often perceive as a serious limiting factor in their return to play.

An indication for surgery is certainly a complete avulsion with significant displacement of the tendon from its origin (Clanton and Coupe 1998, Cohen and Bradley 2007). Once a decision has been taken in favor of conservative (nonoperative) treatment, the injured region should be infiltrated using the same technique described for type 3a and 3b lesions.

Caution

A peritendinous injection technique should be used.
Agents should not be injected directly into the tendon.

Generally there is no need for forearm crutches or braces, but the injured athlete should be given very precise instructions on which movements and exercises are allowed and which should be rigorously avoided. This can be illustrated for the case of an avulsed hamstring tendon: since the hamstrings are typical biarticular muscles, their degree of tension is always influenced by the position of the hip and knee joints. The hamstrings shorten when the hip is extended and the knee is flexed, and they become taut when the hip is flexed and the knee is extended. Thus, hip flexion is allowed only when the knee is simultaneously flexed. Ordinary sitting is not a problem, but sitting with the legs extended is absolutely prohibited. Forces that are active during ordinary gait cause no difficulties. But stair-climbing requires active extension of the hip while the entire body weight is placed on one leg. Consequently, stair-climbing is allowed during the initial phase only if aided by a cane.

Many of the classic methods of physical therapy and physical medicine (except stretching) are applied in the immediate postinjury or postoperative period to promote rapid regression of postoperative swelling, inflammation, and hematoma formation. Suitable forms of training should be selected for the uninjured body regions to counteract general loss of condition. Approximately 4–6 weeks after the injury, the patient should start a progressive program of proprioceptive exercises and unweighted muscle exercises in the functional chain.

In athletes with severe muscle injuries, it is particularly important to conduct regular clinical examinations to evaluate the progress of healing. Only meticulous palpation by an experienced examiner can supply useful information on muscle tone. In any strengthening program, the injured muscle must gradually regain a normal functional tone without exhibiting regional or generalized protective reactions. Generally, these reactions are manifested by palpable, cordlike areas of muscle firmness and should always be taken as a warning sign. Moreover, the injured site itself (edema, discontinuity, scar tissue, retraction of the muscle bundle, etc.) should be thoroughly evaluated. Progressive exercising of the injured limb in incremental steps not only retrains the muscles in complex movement patterns but also provides valuable feedback for doctors and therapists. The patient is ready to advance to the next step only when he or she is free of pain. The authors' preferred technical tool for evaluating progress is ultrasonography. Ultrasound scans yield a wealth of diagnostic information and can be repeated as often as desired (see also Chapter 7). Although costs are rarely a priority in high-level competitive sports, it is not generally feasible to conduct weekly MRI examinations. In the authors' experience, moreover, this would also be unsettling for the patient.

Return to play in athletes with a conservatively treated complete avulsion injury will take at least 12 weeks.

Distal Tendinous Avulsion

A complete distal tendinous avulsion (e.g., of the semitendinosus or biceps femoris) is usually associated with marked retraction of the muscle belly, causing the long and sometimes slender tendons to occupy an extra-anatomic position. The only effective treatment is anatomic surgical repair that reattaches the tendon to the avulsion site.

During the perioperative period, ranging from the day of the injury to about the 10th postoperative day, we prescribe oral combination therapy to support wound healing and buffer the inflammatory tissue reaction that follows the surgery:

- *Vitamins*: A, C, E, B_1, B_3, B_6, coenzyme Q_{10}
- *Amino acids*: especially L-arginine, L-glutamine, L-lysine, and L-methionine
- *Minerals* in basic compounds
- *Trace elements*: calcium, potassium, sodium, magnesium, phosphorus, zinc, copper, molybdenum

Bracing may be prescribed after surgery, and this is done mainly to limit the active range of motion of adjacent joints. Increments in active and passive ranges of motion are prescribed and accurately charted in the postoperative care record. Under no circumstances should the athlete be allowed to return to competition before 12 weeks, as this would jeopardize the success of the repair. Meanwhile, a progressive training schedule should be very carefully formulated and instituted in close consultation with the attending surgeon. Relatively long rehabilitation periods are not uncommon.

Injection therapy is not included in the planned postoperative care for muscle repair. However, injections may be prescribed for treatment of postoperative scars and adhesions, the sensory effects of which may seriously hamper athletes in regaining their preinjury level of performance.

Muscular adhesions and scars respond very well to the intramuscular injection technique described above. The authors instill a generous amount of Traumeel S and Actovegin into the affected tissue, generally through multiple needles. Most patients report significant improvement after just a few applications. Over time, palpation will show a marked decrease in muscular rigidity and in the extent of firm scar tissue.

Treatment of Other Muscular Injuries

Muscle Contusions

A muscle contusion results from direct muscle trauma caused by a blunt external force, leading to a diffuse or circumscribed hematoma that is not necessarily accompanied by structural damage to muscle tissue. This is the definition agreed at the Munich Consensus Conference in March 2011 (Müller-Wohlfahrt et al. 2012) (see also Chapter 6).

Common examples in sports medicine occur with impact trauma, caused by colliding with an opponent or with a fixed object such as an opponent's knee.

The "blunt character" of the external force (compression) almost always contuses, rather than tears, the muscle tissue. It never tears the muscle structure in a longitudinal way, as indirect muscle injuries such as a (partial) muscle tear do. Diffuse local or regional hemorrhage is common, but does not always form an externally visible hematoma. Contusions are very often painful and may cause considerable functional disability in the affected area. In many cases, however, players become fully aware of the injury only after leaving the field. The greatest pain is felt on the day of the injury and the following day, and it subsides over the next few days. Functional capacity returns quickly, which may not be the case with significant structural injuries (tears).

From a therapeutic standpoint, it is essential to differentiate a structural injury from an indirect injury. The history provides the first clue that a direct muscle trauma (i.e., contusion) has occurred, and this impression is confirmed by palpation, function testing, and ultrasound. Deep, circumscribed hematomas in particular should be excluded, as they would require needle aspiration.

> *Note*
>
> **The physician should consider rare but possible causes of a traumatic compartment syndrome and exclude them during clinical follow-up examinations, which are initially scheduled at frequent intervals (see also Chapter 6).**

Acute care is the same as for the injuries described above. Postacute care is the unquestioned domain of physical therapy and physical medicine (Beiner and Jokl 2001). High-dose enzyme therapy is given to promote the resolution of swelling and posttraumatic inflammation.

The day after the injury, the athlete will generally be able to perform non–weight-bearing exercises such as cycling, aquajogging, and pendular movements in an exercise pool (with a water temperature of 29–32°C, wearing a compression bandage). Running at an easy pace may be started on the second day after the injury, depending on pain level. Exercises progress quickly, so that the injured athlete can return to full training and competition usually on the third or fourth day (see also Chapter 6 and Case 7 in Chapter 16).

Practical Tip

The extent of muscle contusions varies substantially. The rehabilitation plan can be based on clinical symptoms, as there is usually no underlying structural lesion in form of a longitudinal distraction.

Functional Compartment Syndrome

A functional compartment syndrome generally develops during intense training or competition, but it cannot be cured simply by restricting activity. At the very least, the compartment syndrome would recur when activities resumed. Treatment should therefore be comprehensive and causal.

The spinal infiltration therapy described earlier in this chapter (see p. 272) is indicated to reduce muscle tone and down-regulate sympathetic outflow, to improve lymphatic drainage. Enzyme preparations and nonsteroidal anti-inflammatory drugs are used. Intensive physical therapy and physical medicine treatments are indicated.

Laboratory parameters (see p. 275) should be tested for further clarification. Arterial and venous blood flow status should be evaluated. A comprehensive examination and analysis of the entire kinetic chain is essential. Any abnormalities should be corrected as needed (e.g., with orthotics, chiropractic mobilization of locked joints, etc.).

Note

All physical functions have to be taken into consideration in order to find a rapid and permanent solution to the problem.

Treatment of Possible Complications

Myositis Ossificans

Even the most sensitive treatment of a muscle injury cannot always prevent the development of myositis ossificans, although it is now considered to be a rare complica-

tion. Myositis ossificans is initially asymptomatic and is generally detected during meticulous palpation (regional inflammatory tissue reaction) or ultrasound follow-ups. Ultrasound can also accurately define the size of the heterotopic ossification and detect any changes over time (see also Chapter 7). Larger ossifications should also be documented on plain radiographs. MRI will often fail to detect smaller lesions.

The initial detection of calcific foci warrants immediate action, although treatment options are limited. Again, it is important to protect the injured area from unnecessary mechanical stresses. Indometacin is prescribed at an oral dosage of 3×50 mg/day (may require protection of the gastric mucosa). Low-dose radiotherapy is also effective for relieving pain and inflammation. Radiation is a modality used in the treatment of inflammatory and degenerative diseases of joints and soft tissues. The affected area is treated several times with low-dose radiation, each exposure lasting only a few seconds and maximally focused on the targeted site. The total administered dosage is usually ≈ 3.0 Gy, distributed over three to six sessions. The radiation induces regression of inflammatory changes, while curbing the myositic component in the affected area. It should be noted that it may take several weeks for a complete response to occur. Radiation is considered a highly effective treatment method for myositis ossificans.

Caution

A thorough risk–benefit analysis should be made before radiotherapy is performed.

If a large ossification forms despite the treatments carried out, it can be very troublesome for the affected athlete. Symptoms can include local pain, which may become lancinating during exercise, limitation of motion (e.g., loss of terminal motion in the hip joint), or a foreign-body sensation, any of which may compromise the athlete's level of performance (Engelhardt et al. 2005).

In cases in which radionuclide scans document an ossification that has become inactive, there is generally no alternative to surgical excision. It takes at least 3–6 months for progression to this state to develop. The surgeon should be highly experienced in soft-tissue surgery. Only a very meticulous, atraumatic surgical technique can prevent significant damage to surrounding tissues, eliminate the risk of recurrence, and ensure full functionality. Removal of a heterotopic ossification is not a simple operation.

The surgeon should consider the inevitable soft-tissue damage when prescribing progressive exercises after the operation.

Recurrence

Recurrence following a muscle injury constitutes a serious setback for both the athlete and the physician. Having already endured an arduous and exhausting rehabilitation process, the athlete finds that he has to go back to square one. This creates considerable emotional stress. The athlete, trainer, manager and the whole staff will immediately question the physician's competence. This loss of confidence may seriously compromise the doctor–patient relationship.

In addition, a recurrent tear also requires a considerably longer course of healing (Ekstrand et al. 2011). The rehabilitation periods for primary injuries mentioned above are then no longer valid, and sport-specific rehabilitation measures have to be carried out with greater caution.

Note

Recurrent tears are a very serious, complex problem in competitive sports. The mainstays of prevention are experience, close-interval follow-up examinations that include meticulous palpation, and providing the athlete with structured guidance in his rehabilitation plan.

Whenever a recurrence happens, a very critical analysis should be made of the findings and of the rehabilitation plan that has been followed by the team. If it has not already been done, it is also necessary to conduct a detailed analysis of all ascending and descending kinematic chains and adjacent joints, the lumbar spine, leg lengths, and sacroiliac joint function. Any abnormalities should definitely be corrected or simultaneously treated. The athlete should also be evaluated for the presence of a pathologic focus (see below).

Intralesional Cyst Formation/Seroma

Intralesional cysts can form as the result of a moderate partial or a subtotal muscle tear that was not initially recognized or treated as such. The seroma cavity cannot always be eliminated nonsurgically and generally requires multiple attempts at percutaneous aspiration.

A seroma cavity inevitably interferes with stable scar healing of the defect. There is generally a prolonged healing period until the scar tissue is stable enough to withstand functional loads. There is no universal rule on how long this may take.

Surgical treatment should be considered for patients who have large seroma cavities or inadequate functional stability and who have experienced recurrent injuries in the same region.

Focal Toxicosis and Interference Fields

A. Binder

Interference Fields

Resistance to treatment may suggest the presence of potential areas of local tissue irritation, known as interference fields, or foci. "Focal toxicosis" is the term used in holistic medicine. This term requires some explanation.

Definition

"Focal toxicosis" is derived from the words "focus," meaning the localized center of a morbid process, and "toxicosis," meaning a pathologic condition caused by poisoning. Thus, focal toxicosis denotes a process in which a local abnormality exerts adverse effects on structures that are distant from the focus (Füss 1994). In the great majority of cases, classic sepsis is not a feature of this process. Two biological principles play a central role in focal toxicosis:

- The human body is organized according to the principle of cybernetic feedback loops.
- The mesenchymal matrix or "ground regulation" system described by Pischinger (see below) plays a defining role in terms of cellular actions and information transfer.

Lechner (1993) states that the signals arising from a focus are subthreshold but permanent. This means that the focus itself is generally asymptomatic. An interference field is present "when the condition of a system at an arbitrary location determines the condition of a system at a different location" (Lechner 1993). It is the effects of the focus, then, rather than the focus itself, that produce clinical manifestations.

Note

It is usually the effects of a focus that become manifest, not the focus itself.

Kellner (1970) defines a focus as follows: "The focus is a local, nondegrading pathologic change in the soft connective tissue that is in constant, active conflict with local and systemic host defenses. It is only when local defenses collapse due to endogenous and exogenous factors that the focus begins to act on more distant structures and the focal disease becomes generalized."

Like the interference field itself, this distant effect may act at the material level (lymph, connective tissue, myokinetic chains) or it may be projected through immaterial systems (acupuncture channels, functional circuits; Füss 1994). An interference field is thus "a harmful influence that interferes with the body's system of self-regulation, especially with the control of stimuli that disturb the body's order" (Strittmatter 2003).

Typically, the body responds to cellular damage with a nonspecific mesenchymal reaction that culminates in the breakdown and removal of destroyed tissue. The basic regulation system described by Pischinger is of major importance in this regard. The connective tissue plays a key role in the regulation of pathologic processes. It is important to note that the key player is not the parenchymal cell itself, but the milieu that surrounds the cell and sustains it. This milieu delivers nutrients to the cell and eliminates waste products. It is also the medium through which all information is conveyed to and from the parenchymal cell (arterial, venous, lymphatic, neural). Pischinger himself describes the concept of the cell "as a morphologic abstraction which, in a biological sense, cannot exist without the life-sustaining milieu surrounding the cell." The ubiquitousness of this matrix underlies the potential far-reaching effects of focal processes (Füss 1994).

Note

A focus is usually based on chronic inflammatory processes that may be latent, active but unrecognized, or may be several years old.

A variety of pathologic conditions can act as interference fields:

- Otitis media
- Sinusitis (maxillary and frontal)
- Tonsillitis
- Temporomandibular joint (gnathologic interference field)
- Teeth (latent infectious foci)
- Appendicitis
- Intestinal dysbiosis or mycosis
- Cholecystitis (rare)
- Chronically inflamed hemorrhoids
- Genital interference field (chronic or old pelvic inflammatory disease, prostatitis, hysterectomy)
- Scars (traumatic, surgical, vaccination)
- Material intolerance (implants, dentures, etc.)

It should be noted that these interference fields are often not subjectively perceived as such. In many cases, functional testing has to be done to reveal a link between a hidden interference field and current symptoms.

Note

Interference fields are often not subjectively perceived as such.

In principle, a focus can act on all the regions in the body. This applies in particular to locally compromised areas in which a pathologic process may enter a chronic stage and become refractory to treatment. On the other hand, functional interrelationships may be such that interference fields become incorporated into regulatory processes,

which then create sites of predilection. These relationships can be understood only against the background of the "functional circuits" described by Gleditsch (1988) (see below).

Otitis Media

In rare cases, an acute middle ear inflammation may become an interference field. Most such cases result from childhood bouts of otitis media, which continue to irritate the mesenchyme via the lymphatic system and thus develop into an established focus.

Sinusitis

The anatomically unfavorable location of the maxillary sinuses predisposes to latent, subthreshold mucosal pathology, which often does not produce obvious clinical manifestations and may even be difficult to detect by imaging. Functional testing is often successful in identifying interference field effects of this kind. A familiarity with classic acupuncture meridians is also helpful. This system relates the frontal sinus to the colon, the right maxillary sinus to the stomach, and the left maxillary sinus to the kidney.

Tonsillitis

In addition to creating a permanent reservoir for streptococci and staphylococci, recurrent tonsillitis may also act as an interference field. Even a tonsillectomy may not eliminate the problem, as it can lead to scarring. Scars are among the most common interference fields (see below).

Temporomandibular Joint (Gnathologic Interference Field), Craniomandibular Dysfunction

Temporomandibular joint dysfunction or an unphysiologic bite may lead to positional faults in the locomotor system. The homeostasis of the myofascial function chains is impaired, and other muscle groups have to intervene constantly to correct the fault. Sustained muscular stress with persistent muscle firmness can lead to a change in physiologic movement patterns and become an interference field, quite apart from any scoliotic changes that may develop in the spinal column.

Teeth

Interference fields commonly involve the teeth. It is rare to see acute dental complaints leading to focal problems. It is far more common for interference fields to develop from devitalized teeth, chronic mandibular osteitis, periodontal disease, or other processes that are clinically occult and are usually difficult to detect on radiographs.

Appendicitis

Similarly, interference fields do not develop from acute appendicitis, with the associated symptoms and laboratory findings, but rather from a chronic smoldering inflammation that often has been present for years.

Intestinal Dysbiosis or Mycosis

Poor nutrition, medication abuse, or persistent distress often form the basis of bowel-associated dysfunctions. The symbiotic state with aerobic and anaerobic flora becomes unbalanced, leading to an increase in abnormal, dysbiotic organisms. The primary result of this process is a change in intestinal pH. This in turn creates conditions favorable for the development of mycotic infection. The mycotoxins generated by the infection can have far-reaching effects, and these processes can therefore definitely create an interference field.

Cholecystitis

Chronic, latent cholecystitis leads to disturbances in the functional circuit of the liver and gallbladder (see below). According to Traditional Chinese Medicine, the tone of muscles, tendons, and ligaments is regulated by this circuit, and so a chronic irritation in this system may predispose to injuries to these structures.

Chronically Inflamed Hemorrhoids

Like any chronic inflammation, hemorrhoids may lead to permanent mesenchymal blockage and thus acquire the character of an interference field.

Genital Interference Fields

Interference fields due to genital diseases (e.g., prostatitis, orchitis, pelvic inflammatory disease, ovarian cysts, etc.) have the greatest diversity relative to other foci and are also the most resistant to treatment. The endocrinologist Riedweg has described hormone levels as the "dimension of the formative element"—which simply means that all formative impulses in the body are controlled by hormones.

> *Note*
>
> A "genital focus" always affects the endocrine system as a whole, leading to functional disturbances in the hypothalamic–pituitary axis.

Scars

Individual cells of scar tissue often lose their capacity for active repolarization (Strittmatter 2003). They are no longer able to restore the potential of the sodium–potassium pump after depolarizing. The weakened or susceptible cell is cut off from normal information transfer to the body, and in some instances it may constantly transmit abnormal signals. Traumatic, surgical, and vaccination scars can all become interference fields.

Material Intolerance

Materials used in dentistry are mainly responsible for this type of interference field. While amalgams with their mercury toxicity have fortunately become rare, various metals can produce a galvanic effect, creating a permanent antigenic stimulus with associated effects on the oral and intestinal mucosa. Interactions between dissimilar metals often give rise to a significant interference field effect. Implants at other sites in the body, such as hip and knee replacements, can also generate electrical currents and become pathogenic foci.

Gleditsch Functional Circuits

Jochen Gleditsch, a dentist and otolaryngologist, developed the principle of "functional circuits" on the basis of the five phases of Traditional Chinese Medicine (**Fig. 11.6**). This principle states that physical and psychological aspects of human life are organized into well-defined feedback loops that function against the background of autoregulatory processes. Functional circuits are regulatory systems that display the cybernetic features of a feedback

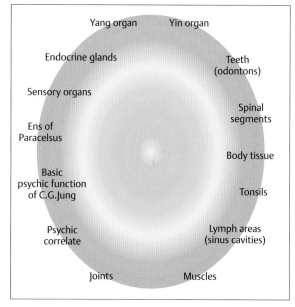

Fig. 11.6 Principle of functional circuits, after Gleditsch.

Table 11.3 Gleditsch functional circuits

Functional circuit	Teeth (odontons)	Lymph area	Tonsils	Muscles
Kidney/bladder	11, 12, 21, 22, 31, 32, 41, 42	Frontal sinus Left maxillary sinus	Pharyngeal tonsil	Iliopsoas Trapezius, descending part Peroneus longus and brevis Tibialis anterior
Liver/gallbladder	13, 23, 33, 43	Sphenoid sinus	Palatine tonsil	Pectoralis, sternal part Rhomboids Popliteus Deltoid, anterior part
Lung/large intestine	14, 15, 24, 25, 34, 35, 44, 45	Ethmoid sinus	Eustachian tube	Serratus anterior Coracobrachialis Deltoid, posterior part Tensor fasciae latae Quadratus lumborum Tibial flexors
Spleen–pancreas/ stomach	16, 17, 26, 27, 36, 37, 46, 47	Right maxillary sinus	Lymph area of larynx	Latissimus dorsi Triceps brachii Opponens pollicis Trapezius, transverse and ascending parts Levator scapulae Pectoralis major, clavicular part Brachioradialis
Heart/small intestine	18, 28, 38, 48	Middle ear, mastoid	Lingual tonsil	Subscapularis Quadriceps femoris

loop, while showing significant points of agreement with the traditional five elements in classical acupuncture (Gleditsch 1988). Vester describes this as a systemic network in which compensatory processes at the level of feedback mechanisms and interactions attempt to counteract disturbances in physiologic processes within a closed-loop control system (Vester 1999). In describing individual functional circuits, it is more important to describe functional relationships than anatomical structures (Füss 2007). A knowledge of these relationships can help us understand system-intrinsic autoregulatory resources and to include regulatory circuits in diagnostic and therapeutic considerations.

Each functional circuit has, as an integral component, a functionally linked pair of organs that give the circuit its name. These organs are linked in turn to subordinate levels, the interrelationships between which comprise another functional unit (Füss 2007). Each pair of organs corresponds to specific spinal segments, teeth, body tissues,

lymph areas in the head, tonsils, muscles, joints, sensory organs, etc. **Table 11.3** lists the teeth, lymph areas, tonsils, and muscles that correlate with specific functional circuits.

Mandel Energy Emission Analysis (EEA)

To determine whether a refractory condition actually has an interference field as its underlying cause, a diagnostic method has to be used that can detect the functional relationships described above. One option is the energy emission analysis (EEA) method described by Mandel. Based physically on the "Kirlian effect," this technique is often referred to as Kirlian photography.

The "coronas" emitted by the tips of the fingers and toes in a high-frequency field are recorded on photographic paper. A topographic and phenomenologic interpretation of these images can detect functional disturbances located anywhere in the body. As a result of

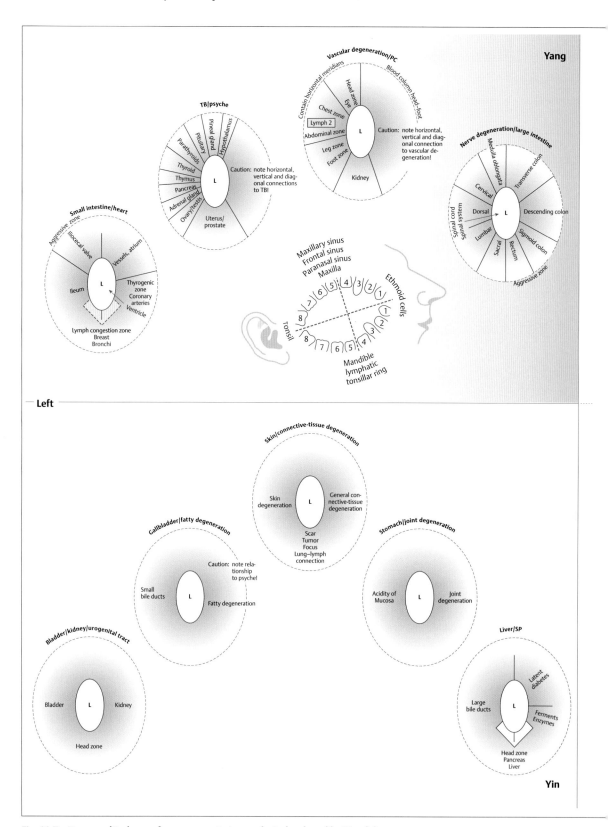

Fig. 11.7 Topographical maps for energy emission analysis developed by Mandel.
PC, pericardium; SP, spleen pancreas; TB, triple burner.

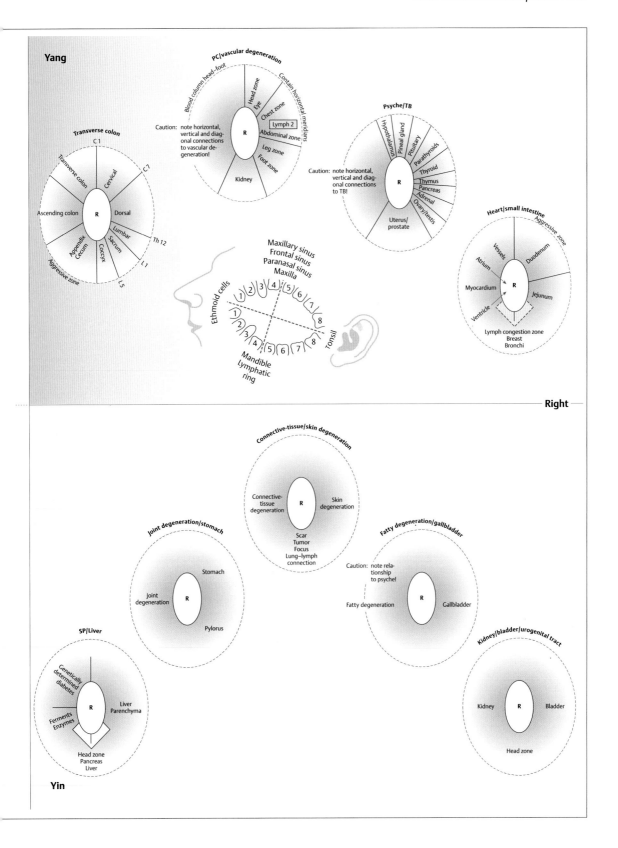

empirical discoveries and scientific studies in recent years, a reproducible diagnostic system has evolved that can supply medically relevant information based on a differentiated analysis of functional regulatory disturbances (Füss 2007).

Note

Energy emission analysis and the clinical examination are mutually supplementary modalities. EEA does not diagnose the disease itself; its main purpose is to identify the causes of a pathologic condition.

EEA is particularly helpful in understanding the gross functional structures of the body's systems and their pathogenetic relationships, especially in the search for interference fields.

Subdividing the coronal images from the fingers and toes into topographic sectors (**Fig. 11.7**) allows the above functional circuits to be analyzed in an energy emission photograph (**Fig. 11.8**)

Lung/Lymph Coronas

The emissions from the thumbs, called the "lung/lymph coronas," are centrally important in the search for interference fields (**Fig. 11.9**).

The lung/lymph coronas encompass the focal resonant zones of the head and thus cover all the lymphatic areas of the head region. This includes the tonsils, paranasal sinuses, retromolar region, and ear—all of which are potential interference fields. The thumbs also cover the entire dental system. Teeth 1–8 and the temporomandibular joint, along with their connections to the functional circuits, are related to specific quadrants in the coronal image.

Deviations from normal emissions are called phenomena. "Point protuberances" (**Fig. 11.10**) are of special interest in the present context. These outbursts provide an important clue to diseased sectors, which in turn cannot be viewed in isolation but must be interpreted within the framework of focal toxicosis as it relates to the body as a whole.

The first step in interpreting an energy emission photograph is to look for deviant phenomena in the lung/lymph corona. Working from that point, we can determine the extent to which pathogenic foci in the dental system, paranasal sinuses, tonsils, retromolar region, ears, or temporomandibular joints may be acting as interference fields.

Note

It is important to take a holistic perspective, viewing the system of functional circuits in their relationship to the body as a whole.

Colon/Nerve Degeneration Corona

Intestinal interference fields due to dysbiosis or mycosis are represented in the emissions from both index fingers (**Fig. 11.11**). The medial portions of the large intestine/nerve degeneration coronas correspond topographically to the colon, starting with the cecum and appendix at the 6-o'clock position on the corona of the right finger (note that chronic appendicitis is an interference field) and moving up the ascending colon and around to the right half of the transverse colon (**Fig. 11.11b**). The left transverse colon starts at the 12-o'clock position on the left finger, moves down to the descending colon, and terminates at the 6 o'clock position with the sectors for the sigmoid colon and rectum (**Fig. 11.11a**). The latter sector may show an interference field due to chronically inflamed hemorrhoids.

Triple Burner (TB)/Psyche Corona

Emissions from the ring fingers can be used to diagnose a genital focus (TB/psyche corona, **Fig. 11.12**). The topographic sectors for the uterus/prostate and ovary/testis occupy the range from the 5-o'clock to 7-o'clock positions. The phenomenology of these sectors supplies information on potential interference fields.

Gallbladder/Fatty Degeneration Corona

Chronic gallbladder disease and its associated effects can be diagnosed from the phenomenology of the fourth toe (gallbladder/fatty degeneration corona, **Fig. 11.13**).

Isolated Emissions below the Second and Third Toes

Isolated emissions recorded below the second or third toes on the left and right sides can be used to assess the possible pathogenic significance of scar interference fields (**Fig. 11.14**).

Note

In summary, the interference fields described above can explain why some conditions, including muscle injuries, are resistant to therapy. It is therefore important to include these foci in diagnostic and therapeutic considerations.

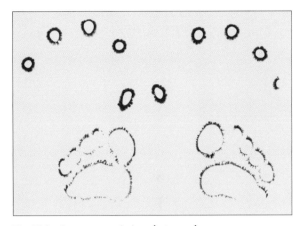

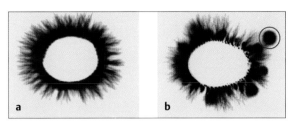

Fig. 11.10a, b   Phenomena (deviations from a normal emission pattern).

a Normal emission pattern.
b Point protuberance.

Fig. 11.8   An energy emission photograph.

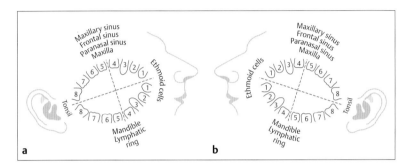

Fig. 11.9a, b   Lung/lymph topography (thumbs).

a Left thumb.
b Right thumb.

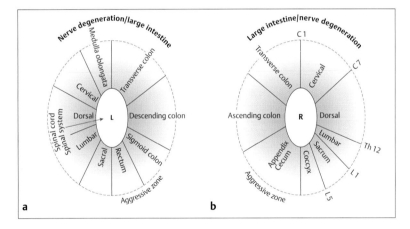

Fig. 11.11a, b   Large intestine/nerve degeneration coronas (index fingers).

a Left index finger.
b Right index finger.

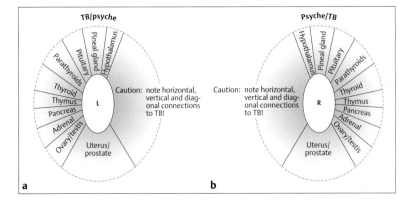

Fig. 11.12a, b   Triple burner/psyche corona (ring fingers). TB, triple burner.

a Left ring finger.
b Right ring finger.

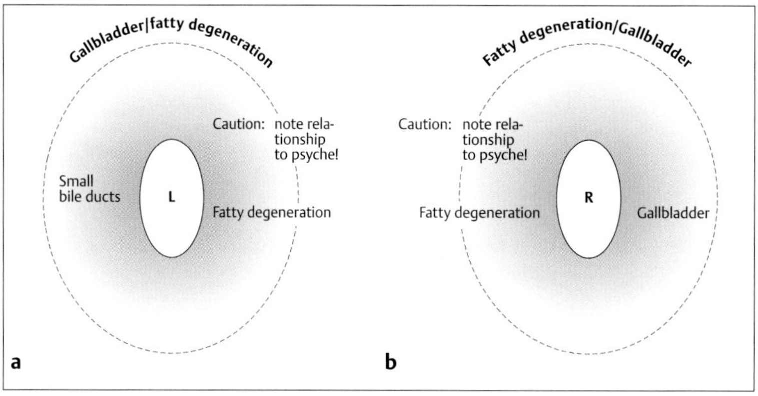

Fig. 11.13a, b   Gallbladder/fatty degeneration coronas.

a Fourth toe of the left foot.
b Fourth toe of the right foot.

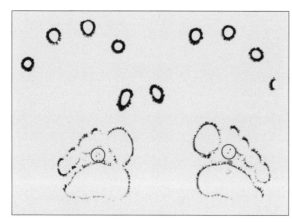

Fig. 11.14   Isolated emissions from the second and third toes of the left and right feet.

Case Report

A 24-year-old professional soccer player was experiencing frequent, recurrent muscle injuries in the legs (functional muscle disorders as well as partial muscle tears) as a result of pelvic obliquity and locking of the sacroiliac joints.

From acupuncture, the relationship between the sacroiliac joints and paranasal sinuses is known. Energy emission analysis in this patient showed irregularities at these sites. The patient was referred to an otorhinolaryngologist, who diagnosed chronic, low-grade mucosal swelling in both maxillary sinuses. Three sinus injections were sufficient to relieve the swelling. Subsequent reduction of the sacroiliac joints remained stable, and since then the patient has experienced no significant muscle injuries.

References

Akuthota V, Ferreiro A, Moore T, Fredericson M. Core stability exercise principles. Curr Sports Med Rep 2008; 7(1): 39–44

Arnason A, Andersen TE, Holme I, Engebretsen L, Bahr R. Prevention of hamstring strains in elite soccer: an intervention study. Scand J Med Sci Sports 2008; 18(1): 40–48

Barbosa E, Faintuch J, Machado Moreira EA, et al. Supplementation of vitamin E, vitamin C, and zinc attenuates oxidative stress in burned children: a randomized, double-blind, placebo-controlled pilot study. J Burn Care Res 2009; 30(5): 859–866

Beiner JM, Jokl P. Muscle contusion injuries: current treatment options. J Am Acad Orthop Surg 2001; 9(4): 227–237

Catterall WA, Mackie K. Local anesthetics. In: Brunton LL, ed. Goodman Gilman's The pharmacological basis of therapeutics. New York: McGraw-Hill; 2005

Clanton TO, Coupe KJ. Hamstring strains in athletes: diagnosis and treatment. J Am Acad Orthop Surg 1998; 6(4): 237–248

Cohen S, Bradley J. Acute proximal hamstring rupture. J Am Acad Orthop Surg 2007; 15(6): 350–355

Dohan Ehrenfest DM, Rasmusson L, Albrektsson T. Classification of platelet concentrates: from pure platelet-rich plasma (P-PRP) to leucocyte- and platelet-rich fibrin (L-PRF). Trends Biotechnol 2009; 27(3): 158–167

Ekstrand J, Hägglund M, Waldén M. Epidemiology of muscle injuries in professional football (soccer). Am J Sports Med 2011; 39(6): 1226–1232

Engebretsen L, Steffen K, Alsousou J et al. IOC consensus paper on the use of platelet-rich plasma in sports medicine. Br J Sports Med 2010; 44: 1072–1081

Engelhardt M, Krüger-Franke M, Pieper HG, Siebert CH, eds. Sportverletzungen – Sportschäden. Stuttgart: Thieme; 2005: 87

Fitzhugh DJ, Shan S, Dewhirst MW, Hale LP. Bromelain treatment decreases neutrophil migration to sites of inflammation. Clin Immunol 2008; 128(1): 66–74

Foster TE, Puskas BL, Mandelbaum BR, Gerhardt MB, Rodeo SA. Platelet-rich plasma: from basic science to clinical applications. Am J Sports Med 2009; 37(11): 2259–2272

Füss R. Die Induktionstherapie. Ganzheitliche Regulation mit den Frequenzen des menschlichen Gehirns. Sulzbach/Taunus: Energetik-Verlag GmbH; 1994

Füss R. Der Zusammenhang neurologischer Systemerkrankungen mit Befunden der Energetischen Terminalpunkt-Diagnose (E–T–D) nach Mandel/Kirlian-Fotografie. Eine Diagnose-Evaluation am Beispiel des Guillain-Barre-Syndroms und der Multiplen Sklerose. Edition COMED. Hochheim: COMED Verlagsgesellschaft mbH; 2007

Gleditsch JM. Reflexzonen und Somatotopien. 3rd ed. Schorndorf: Biologisch-Medizinische Verlagsgesellschaft; 1988

Hammond JW, Hinton RY, Curl LA, Muriel JM, Lovering RM. Use of autologous platelet-rich plasma to treat muscle strain injuries. Am J Sports Med 2009; 37(6): 1135–1142

Harmon KG. Muscle injuries and PRP: what does the science say? Br J Sports Med 2010; 44: 616–617

Heyman H, Van De Looverbosch DE, Meijer EP, Schols JM. Benefits of an oral nutritional supplement on pressure ulcer healing in long-term care residents. J Wound Care 2008; 17(11): 476–478, 480

Hibbs AE, Thompson KG, French D, Wrigley A, Spears I. Optimizing performance by improving core stability and core strength. Sports Med 2008; 38(12): 995–1008

Hubbard WJ, Bland KI, Chaudry IH. The role of the mitochondrion in trauma and shock. Shock 2004; 22(5): 395–402

Iotti S, Malucelli E. In vivo assessment of Mg2+ in human brain and skeletal muscle by 31P-MRS. Magnes Res 2008; 21(3): 157–162. Erratum in: Magnes Res 2009; 22(1): 50

Järvinen TA, Järvinen TL, Kääriäinen M, Kalimo H, Järvinen M. Muscle injuries: biology and treatment. Am J Sports Med 2005; 33(5): 745–764

Kellner G. Zum Konnex von Wundsetzung, Wundheilungsstörung und chronischer Entzündung. Oesterr Z Stomatologie 1970; 3(73): 82–89

Lechner J. Herd, Regulation und Information. Heidelberg: Hüthig Buch; 1993

Lee P, Rattenberry A, Connelly S, Nokes L. Our experience on Actovegin, is it cutting edge? Int J Sports Med 2011; 32(4): 237–241

Mei-Dan O, Mann G, Maffulli N. Platelet-rich plasma: any substance into it? Br J Sports Med 2010; 44(9): 618–619

Mishra A, Woodall J Jr, Vieira A. Treatment of tendon and muscle using platelet-rich plasma. Clin Sports Med 2009; 28(1): 113–125

Mjølsnes R, Arnason A, Østhagen T, Raastad T, Bahr R. A 10-week randomized trial comparing eccentric vs. concentric hamstring strength training in well-trained soccer players. Scand J Med Sci Sports 2004; 14(5): 311–317

Mueller-Wohlfahrt HW, Haensel L, Mithoefer K et al. Terminology and classification of muscle injuries in sport. The Munich consensus statement. Br J Sports Med 2012 (in press)

Müller-Wohlfahrt HW, Montag HJ, Kübler U. Diagnostik und Therapie von Muskelzerrungen und Muskelfaserrissen. Dtsch Z Sportmed 1992; 3: 120–125

Müller-Wohlfahrt HW. Diagnostik und Therapie von Muskelzerrungen und Muskelfaserrissen. Sportorthopädie Sporttraumatologie 2001; 17: 17–20

Orchard JW, Best TM, Mueller-Wohlfahrt HW, et al. The early management of muscle strains in the elite athlete: best practice in a world with a limited evidence basis. Br J Sports Med 2008; 42(3): 158–159

Peterson L, Renström P. Verletzungen im Sport. Cologne: Deutscher Ärzte-Verlag; 2002

Porozov S, Cahalon L, Weiser M, Branski D, Lider O, Oberbaum M. Inhibition of IL-1beta and TNF-alpha secretion from resting and activated human immunocytes by the homeopathic medication Traumeel S. Clin Dev Immunol 2004; 11(2): 143–149

Schneider C, Schneider B, Hanisch J, van Haselen R. The role of a homoeopathic preparation compared with conventional therapy in the treatment of injuries: an observational cohort study. Complement Ther Med 2008; 16(1): 22–27

Simons DG, Travell JG, Simons LS. Myofascial pain and dysfunction: the trigger point manual. Philadelphia: Lippincott Williams & Wilkins; 1998

Strittmatter B. Identifying and treating blockages to healing. Stuttgart–New York: Thieme; 2003

Theodoridis T, Krämer J. Spinal injection techniques. Stuttgart–New York: Thieme; 2009

Ueblacker P, Haensel L, Mueller-Wohlfahrt HW. Examination and treatment of muscle injuries. UEFA Manual on football/soccer injuries. 2013 (in press)

Vester F. Die Kunst, vernetzt zu denken. Munich: Deutsche Verlagsanstalt; 1999

Wang T, Fu F, Zhang L, Han B, Zhu M, Zhang X. Effects of escin on acute inflammation and the immune system in mice. Pharmacol Rep 2009; 61(4): 697–704

Watanabe M, Wu J, Li S, Li C, Okada T. Mechanisms of cardioprotective effects of magnesium on hypoxia-reoxygenation-induced injury. Exp Clin Cardiol 2004; 9(3): 181–185

Willardson JM. Core stability training: applications to sports conditioning programs. J Strength Cond Res 2007; 21(3): 979–985

World Anti-Doping Agency (WADA). The 2011 prohibited list. Montreal: World Anti-Doping Agency, 2011. Available at: http://www.wada-ama.org/Documents/World_Anti-Doping_Program/WADP-Prohibited-list/To_be_effective/WADA_Prohibited_List_2011_EN.pdf

Further Reading

Garrett WE Jr. Muscle strain injuries. Am J Sports Med 1996; 24 (6, Suppl): S2–S8

Müller-Wohlfahrt HW, Montag HJ. Diagnostik und Therapie der so genannten Muskelzerrung. [Diagnosis and therapy of "pulled muscle."] Dtsch Z Sportmed 1985; 11: 246–248

Noonan TJ, Garrett WE Jr. Muscle strain injury: diagnosis and treatment. J Am Acad Orthop Surg 1999; 7(4): 262–269

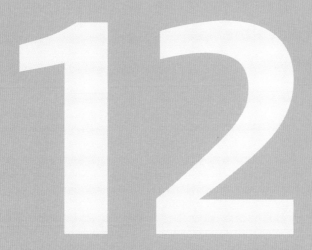

12

Role of the Spine in Muscle Injuries and Muscle Disorders

B. Schoser

P. Ueblacker

L. Hänsel

H.-W. Müller-Wohlfahrt

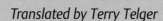

Translated by Terry Telger

Relationship between the Spine
and Skeletal Muscles 298

Functional Spinal Causes
of Muscular Dysfunction 299
Hyperlordosis 299
Locked Sacroiliac Joint 299
Functional Leg Length Difference 300
Joint Dysfunctions 300
Sacrum Acutum or Highly Curved Sacrum 300

Structural Spinal Causes
of Muscular Dysfunction 301
Pelvic Obliquity, Leg Length Difference 301
Spinal Stenosis 302

Lateral Recess Stenosis,
Foraminal Stenosis 302
Disk Bulging and Herniation 302
Spondylolysis, Spondylolisthesis 303
Lumbosacral Ligament 305

Pseudoradicular Versus
Radicular Symptoms 305
Symptom Complex of
a Pseudoradicular Syndrome 305
Symptom Complex of
a Radicular Syndrome 305
Differentiating between Pseudoradicular
and Radicular Syndromes 306

Relationship between the Spine and Skeletal Muscles

The senior author of this chapter published studies on the connection between lumbar spine pathology and muscle injuries as early as the 1980s (Müller-Wohlfahrt and Montag 1985, Müller-Wohlfahrt et al. 1992). In recent years, this concept has increasingly been addressed by other authors as well (Verrall et al. 2001, Best 2004, Orchard et al. 2004). For example, Orchard et al. (2004) write: "Theoretically, any pathology relating to the lumbar spine, the lumbosacral nerve roots or plexus, or the sciatic nerve could result in hamstring or calf pain (among other symptoms)." In his commentary on Orchard's article, Best (2004) states that "Although many of us have thought of lower lumbar pathology as a source of hamstring and calf problems, this report... certainly invites future studies aimed at risk factor detection and intervention for these kinds of problems."

Besides the peripheral muscle pain described by Orchard, we believe that abnormalities of muscle tone and other types of muscular dysfunction may be a particularly important sequel to lumbar pathology. Although greater attention has been given to the link between the spine and muscles in recent years, valid data on this subject have not yet appeared in the literature, and we must continue to rely largely on empirical data and observations.

The muscles are a target organ whose state of tension is modulated by electrical information from the motor component of the corresponding spinal nerve. When a spinal nerve root is irritated, it is reasonable to postulate that this will increase the stimulation of the muscle by nerve impulses. The result of this may be an increase in the resting tone of the muscle or a sudden, transient rise in muscle tension.

Spinal nerve irritation can have a variety of causes, ranging from transient and fully reversible functional disturbances to permanent structural changes, which may be congenital or acquired. Lumbar manifestations are not present in all cases, however, and the examiner and therapist must make a specific search for them.

The lumbar spine and pelvis form the only anatomical connection between the upper and lower body, and consequently all ascending and descending forces are transmitted across those structures. This makes them susceptible to injuries due to forces generated by the body weight as well as external weights and forces and the acceleration of body parts relative to one another.

From a neuroanatomic standpoint, the deep paraspinal back muscles, especially the multifidi, have relatively strong and/or synaptically effective connections with the central nervous system. Previously it was thought that the intrinsic back muscles, with their segmental arrangement, received their sensory supply from the corresponding spinal cord segment. But recent studies have shown that one of the most important back muscles, the erector spinae, derives its segmental sensory supply not from the spinal ganglion of the same segment but from two segments higher up the spine.

Note

The craniocaudal shift of innervation is clinically relevant in treatments involving local anesthesia, for example, or infiltration of the lumbar facet joints. Thus, the treatment of an L5 pain syndrome would require blocking the L3 and L4 spinal nerves in addition to the L5 nerve.

Painful irritation of the erector spinae or multifidus muscles can lead to increased expression of the c-Fos transcription factor via posterior horn neurons in all lumbar segments of the spinal cord. As a result, the effects of a nociceptive impulse from the lower back muscles can spread upward over numerous segments of the spinal cord. In many athletes, tonic and monotonic movement patterns will not initially trigger conscious pain even when the lumbosacral back muscles have been affected by overuse.

Competitive and recreational athletes are known to be a population at high risk for developing degenerative changes and functional problems in the lumbar spine (Ong et al. 2003). Soccer players, who perform numerous actions involving dynamic rotation, hyperflexion, and hyperextension, are at particularly high risk for injuries, degenerative changes, and functional disorders of the lower back. The most common lumbar complaints found in athletes are:

- Myofascial pain
- Ligamentous injuries
- Injuries to lumbar vertebrae
- Intervertebral disk lesions
- Foraminal stenosis
- Intra-articular disorders consisting of unilateral or bilateral pars interarticularis defects (spondylolysis), with or without associated spondylolisthesis

Note

Athletes and especially professional athletes who undergo constant, intensive training have a higher incidence of degenerative disk disease and spondylolysis. Differentiation from a congenitally narrow spinal canal may also be an important consideration in athletes.

It is not the purpose of this chapter to present a comprehensive differential diagnosis of back pain, but to focus on aspects that are relevant to sports within the overall context of this book. We have intentionally omitted rare diseases, which are addressed in specialized textbooks of orthopedics, neurosurgery, and neurology.

The intention is instead to explore the frequent association of muscular dysfunction and injuries with pathology of the lumbar spine. Frequently encountered in practice, these correlations are often missed by examiners but are essential in prescribing appropriate causal treatment. The severity may range from harmless muscle dysfunction caused by locked lumbar facet joints, for example, to recurrent structural muscle injuries based on sustained firmness of the affected muscle secondary to, say, nerve root irritation by a herniated disk.

Functional Spinal Causes of Muscular Dysfunction

We define functional disorders as dysfunctions that affect a functional unit (e.g., sacroiliac joint) or a group of functional units (e.g., facet joints and segmental paravertebral muscles) and do not have a pathoanatomic correlate or structural damage. Hence they are always reversible with proper treatment, although they do have a tendency to recur.

Functional disorders may in turn result from structural changes (e.g., locking of the sacroiliac joint secondary to a true leg length difference). Many functional disorders are self-limiting and return to normal following a variable period of dysfunction. This is not always the case, however, and persistent dysfunction requires specific therapy (e.g., medical, physiotherapeutic, chiropractic, etc.) to correct the problem and/or terminate an existing vicious cycle (see Chapter 15 for exercises for lumbopelvic stability). Many factors may interact in this vicious cycle, often making it difficult to define the actual starting point of the causal chain. Another problem is that the disorder is not always perceived in the form of symptoms.

Some possible functional disorders of the lower lumbar spine and lumbosacral junction are illustrated and described below.

Hyperlordosis

Hyperlordosis (**Fig. 12.1**) increases the axial pressure on the posterior spinal column and thus on the posterior portion of the intervertebral disks and facet joints, thereby decreasing their mobility. Effects can range from irritation of the joint capsules and ligaments to hypertrophic arthropathy. This is accompanied by an adaptation of the surrounding muscles, which attempt to immobilize the irritated joint. Hyperlordosis also reduces the diameter of the neural foramina, predisposing to mechanical irritation of the spinal nerves (especially in patients with a congenitally short vertebral arch, for example).

A hyperlordotic posture may also increase the risk of hamstring injuries (Hennessey and Watson 1993).

Locked Sacroiliac Joint

The sacroiliac joints normally have a very limited range of motion. But this slight motion still provides an important compensatory mechanism during rotary loading of the pelvic and hip region and during unilateral axial loading across the lumbar spine and sacrum. If a sacroiliac joint becomes locked in an abnormal position, it cannot move even to this slight degree, and some type of evasive, compensatory movement will take place. The iliolumbar ligaments may transmit the dysfunction to the lumbosacral junction. A locked position of the sacroiliac joints will typ-

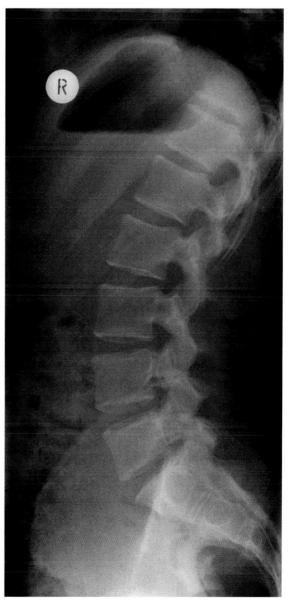

Fig. 12.1 Hyperlordosis of the lumbar spine in a 25-year-old professional soccer player with recurrent muscular dysfunction. Note also the associated steep angle of the iliac crest. Lateral radiograph of the lumbar spine.

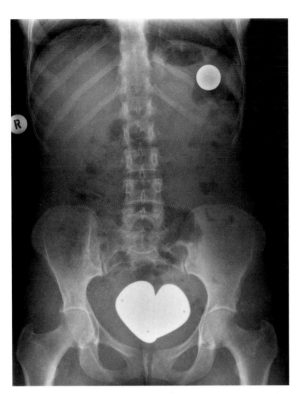

Fig. 12.2 A 23-year-old female elite marathon runner. Pelvic torsion is clearly seen, with the left iliac wing jutting out further in comparison with the right side and orthograde projection of the spinous processes of the lower lumbar vertebrae. Anteroposterior radiograph of the pelvis.

ically be found by thorough clinical and functional examination, but in some cases may also be detected on conventional radiographs (**Fig. 12.2**).

In contrast to other joints, there are no muscles that act directly on the sacroiliac joints. The lumbar multifidus muscles and the internal oblique muscle are activated by spinal motion. They help to stiffen the sacrum and reduce interspinal mobility.

Athletes in disciplines that involve forceful unilateral movements (kicking, throwing, and running disciplines like hurdles, etc.) are at particularly high risk for developing sacroiliac complaints such as:

- Unilateral pain
- Low back pain
- Sacral pain
- Gluteal pain
- Inguinal pain
- Referred pain pattern
- Piriformis syndrome
- Perianal numbness
- Pseudoradicular complaints
- Occasionally, only peripheral symptoms in the form of increased painful or painless muscle tone

Note

In most cases, muscular complaints due to locked sacroiliac joints are spontaneously reversible following mobilization or reduction.

Practical Tip

With a dysfunction in the innervation area of the obturator nerve (e.g., the adductors), it is important to exclude pathology not only in the segmental roots of that nerve, but also in the sacroiliac joints.

Functional Leg Length Difference

Pelvic obliquity or a level pelvis is recognized by the position of the posterior iliac crests. A patient with pelvic obliquity does not necessarily have a true leg length difference, however, because the tilt may have various other causes such as sacroiliac joint locking, a deformity of the ilium or lumbosacral junction, postural abnormality due to pain, etc.

Pelvic obliquity generally leads to a compensatory scoliotic posture. In turn, this postural distortion places asymmetrical loads on the ligaments and facet joints and leads to unequal paravertebral muscle tension on the right and left sides. These changes often cause multisegmental patterns of nerve irritation.

Functional causes of pelvic obliquity may be found in the lower limb (e.g., instabilities or functional disorders in the knee or ankle joints, postural distortion due to muscular imbalance, avoidance posturing due to a muscle injury that has not yet healed, etc.). A locked sacroiliac joint with malalignment of the sacrum relative to the ilium may also cause a functional leg length difference. Given the complex interaction of the ligaments and muscles that encircle and cross the lumbopelvic region, seemingly minor disturbances in this region may give rise to functional pelvic obliquity.

Joint Dysfunctions

Firmness of the pelvitrochanteric muscles often develops in response to hip problems. Sciatic nerve irritation can be caused by compression of the nerve between the piriformis and gemellus superior muscles.

Sacrum Acutum or Highly Curved Sacrum

A very upright lumbosacral junction angle due to sacral deformity causes significant shear forces to act on the intervertebral disks and secondary stabilizing structures of the L5–S1 segment (e.g., anterior and posterior longitudinal ligament, facet joints and their capsules, etc.). The result is a subthreshold or painful irritation that incites reac-

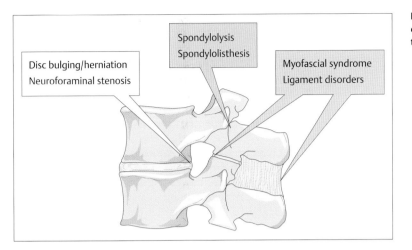

tive firmness in the paravertebral muscles. This is associated with biomechanical narrowing of the L5–S1 neural foramen.

Structural Spinal Causes of Muscular Dysfunction

Structural causes (**Fig. 12.3**) should always be sought and are usually easier to detect than functional causes, as they are generally visible on morphologic images. Imaging studies are becoming increasingly important in identifying structural causes of muscular dysfunction. Conventional radiographs and magnetic resonance imaging (MRI) are essential adjuncts to a thorough clinical examination.

Pelvic Obliquity, Leg Length Difference

Real pelvic obliquity is caused by a true leg length difference. It is most accurately measured on a standing anteroposterior pelvic radiograph that displays both femoral heads, the relative heights of which are compared (**Fig. 12.4**). Any difference in the leg length can be measured with millimeter accuracy, especially on digitally processed images. This information is useful in selecting patients for a limb length correction with orthotics, for example.

As with a functional leg length difference, the presence of true pelvic obliquity causes the body to assume a compensatory scoliotic posture. The paravertebral structures, ligaments, facets, etc. are subjected to asymmetric loads, and the muscles develop increased tone. The result is often a multisegmental disorder, which may be associated with nerve irritation.

Orthotic treatment with 5 mm of heel elevation is recommended for a symptomatic leg length difference of ≈ 5 mm or more. With a greater difference, the 5-mm insert should be worn for 3 months before another 3 mm of correction is added. An immediate, complete correction of the total difference is not advisable. We usually stop the correction at ~ 8 mm even if the leg length difference is more than 8 or 10 mm.

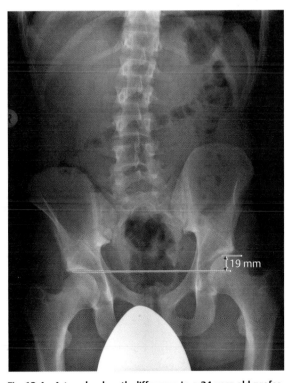

Fig. 12.4   A true leg length difference in a 24-year-old professional soccer player. Following calibration of the image, a true leg length difference of 19 mm was measured. Anteroposterior radiograph of the pelvis.

Spinal Stenosis

In athletes at a young age, stenosis of the lumbar canal can be caused by a congenitally narrow spinal canal (**Fig. 12.5**). Lumbar stenosis is classified as shown in **Table 12.1**.

The clinical presentation of lumbar stenosis is characteristic. Patients complain of decreased walking distance with "tired legs," lumbosacral pain, and pain radiating in a pseudoradicular pattern. Complaints are improved by sitting down. A burning pain may be felt in the thighs during walking. While these symptoms are rarely so pronounced in athletes, they may be latent and should be recognized.

Note

Any degree of hyperlordosis will aggravate the complaints of lumbar stenosis, whereas kyphosis of the lumbar spine tends to ease the pain.

Lateral Recess Stenosis, Foraminal Stenosis

Lateral recess stenosis (**Fig. 12.6**), as well as narrowing of the neural foramina, may irritate the corresponding nerve root or roots. This may cause pain radiating in a radicular pattern, but it is more common to find only firmness of the associated muscles and of the paravertebral muscles, usually spanning multiple segments, which may in turn cause irritation of the nerve roots.

Again, the symptoms consist mainly of peripheral muscle complaints, the lumbar cause of which has to be recognized even in patients who have mild clinical manifestations.

Disk Bulging and Herniation

An acute herniated disk—with its characteristic symptoms of acute pain, postural distortion by a reflex restriction of segmental spinal motion, and the clinical manifestations of stiff paravertebral muscles and sudden or dynamic neurologic deficits—is somewhat outside the scope of this book. The focus here is more on chronic, subclinical disk protrusions or herniations that may irritate a nerve root (constantly, or only in hyperextension or other movements) and may lead to firmness in the paravertebral and associated peripheral muscles (**Fig. 12.7**).

Obviously, subclinical symptoms of this kind are far more difficult to detect. Even magnetic resonance imaging often fails to supply definitive proof by showing disk pathology impinging on one or more nerve roots.

Note

The problem with MRI and other imaging modalities is that they cannot capture the dynamic component of high-performance sports. Disk pathology may produce relevant symptoms only in hyperextension, for example.

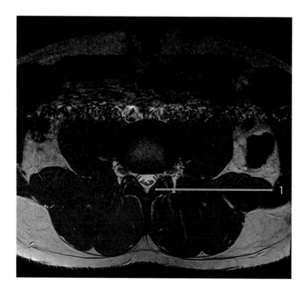

Fig. 12.5 Congenital and ligamentous (1) causes of spinal stenosis in a 20-year-old professional soccer player. The diameter of the spinal canal measures 11 mm at the L4–L5 level, indicating a relative spinal stenosis. Axial magnetic resonance image.

Table 12.1 Classification of lumbar stenosis

Central stenosis

- Primary stenosis
  - Congenital (congenitally short pedicles)
  - Developmental (idiopathic, achondroplastic)
- Secondary stenosis
  - Idiopathic
  - Degenerative
  - Degenerative spondylolisthesis
  - Postoperative (postfusion, postlaminectomy)
  - Discogenic (ruptured annulus)
- Post-traumatic
- Paget disease

Isolated lateral stenosis

Foraminal stenosis

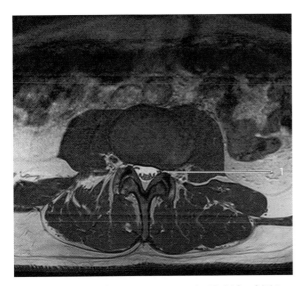

Fig. 12.6 Left lateral recess stenosis at the L3–L4 level (1) in a 45-year-old recreational soccer player with recurrent injuries of the left thigh muscles. Axial magnetic resonance image.

Spondylolysis, Spondylolisthesis

The prevalence of spondylolysis is 6.4% in the white population, 1.1% in the black population, and exceeds 50% in the Inuit (Hefti 2006). The prevalence is 15%–30% in fencers, ballet dancers, javelin throwers, weightlifters, soccer players, and swimmers (Hefti 2006). Scheuermann disease has a high statistical association with spondylolysis.

Repetitive trauma due to lumbar hyperextension or genetic factors are responsible for spondylolysis, with 95% of cases affecting the L5 segment. Most cases occur during skeletal growth. There have been only a few reported cases in which a single traumatic event caused spondylolysis (Saraste 1993), which was usually located at a level higher than L5.

Only a few patients with spondylolysis become symptomatic during their lifetime. Complaints consist predominantly of low back pain, which is usually present throughout the day, is worsened by prolonged sitting or standing, and is typically motion-dependent.

Spondylolysis (**Fig. 12.8**) may give rise to spondylolisthesis, or the slipping of a vertebra relative to adjacent vertebrae. Four grades are distinguished in the Meyerding classification (**Fig. 12.9**). Observation is indicated in adolescents due to the risk that the slippage may progress. Further progression will not occur after the cessation of skeletal growth.

Our own studies show that many athletes become symptomatic not by lumbar pain but by peripheral muscular complaints, most commonly involving the hamstrings (unpublished data). The cause lies in an increased kyphotic curve between L5 and S1, causing an anterior shift in the center of gravity. This evokes a compensatory increase in hamstring tension to correct the pelvic tilt

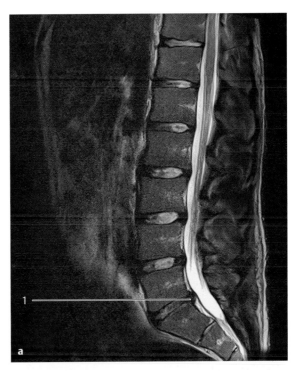

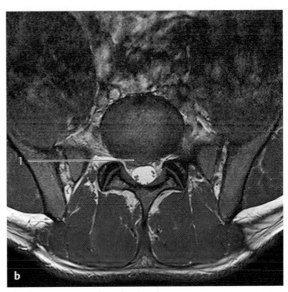

Fig. 12.7a, b A mediolateral herniated disk at L5–S1 on the right side (1), elevating and indenting the S1 nerve root, in a 24-year-old professional soccer player. The athlete reported recurrent calf muscle dysfunction, which resolved completely following lumbar infiltration therapy. Axial magnetic resonance image.

(Hefti 2006). The result is permanent firmness and shortening of the hamstring muscles. The associated instability, usually in the lumbosacral segment, leads to sustained firmness of the paravertebral muscles always extending over multiple segments. In turn, the increased paravertebral muscle tone may cause irritation of the nerve roots.

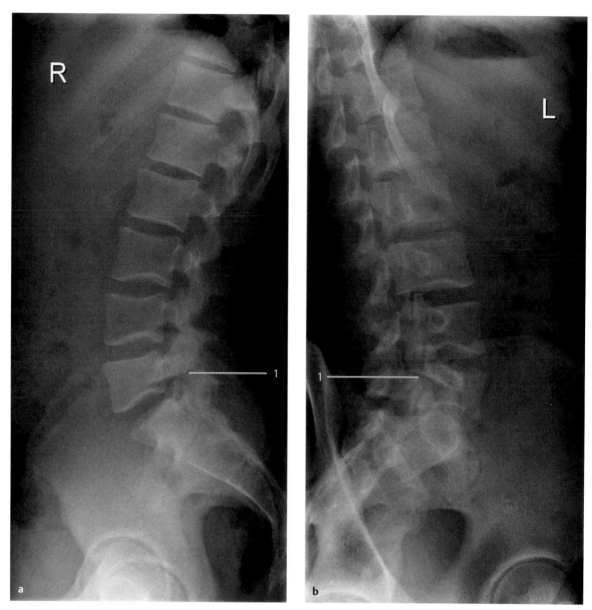

Fig. 12.8a, b   Bilateral spondylolysis at the L5 level (1). The radiographs clearly demonstrate lysis of the interarticular portion of L5 (1). Lateral (**a**) and left oblique (**b**) view. (Note: the contralateral oblique radiograph is not shown.)

Muscular complaints arising from spondylolysis and/or spondylolisthesis can be successfully managed conservatively in the great majority of cases. Conservative treatment consists of infiltration therapy of the lumbar spine (see Chapter 11) and may include local infiltration of the affected muscle, depending on muscular findings which can range from recurrent spine-related muscle disorders to structural muscle injuries.

Concomitant physical therapy is of major importance and should include a well-designed program of stabilizing and strengthening exercises for the lumbopelvic region ("core exercises"). With systematic therapy, even the stresses imposed by high-performance sports should not be a problem.

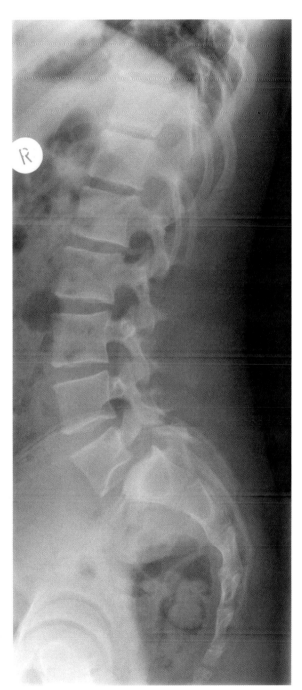

Fig. 12.9 Spondylolisthesis at the L5 level, Meyerding grade II, in a 17-year-old junior soccer player. Lateral radiograph.

Lumbosacral Ligament

Briggs and Chandraraj (1995) and Orchard et al. (2004) described another potential extraforaminal lumbar cause of muscular dysfunction, the lumbosacral ligament (an inconstant band in continuity with the iliolumbar ligament). When present, the lumbosacral ligament may become hypertrophic due to degenerative changes at the L5–S2 level and may irritate or even compress the L5 nerve root.

Pseudoradicular Versus Radicular Symptoms

Differentiation between pseudoradicular and radicular complaints is important in clinical practice.

Symptom Complex of a Pseudoradicular Syndrome

The following symptoms characterize a pseudoradicular syndrome:
• No resting pain
• Pain on muscular tension or contraction; "motion pain"
• Local tenderness at tendon attachments
• Rapid fatigability of muscle
• Local muscle firmness (trigger point)
• General muscle firmness (taut band, muscle splinting)
• Increased muscle tone in response to passive stretch
• Diffuse pain radiation or referred pain pattern
• No sensory deficits
• No muscle weakness
• No atrophy
• Autonomic disorders (sweating, vasomotor activity)

Possible causes of pseudoradicular complaints are:
• Functional disorders
• Spinal stenosis
• Spondylolysis, spondylolisthesis

Symptom Complex of a Radicular Syndrome

By contrast, the following symptoms characterize a classic radicular syndrome:
• Pain radiating in a segmental pattern along dermatomes
• Sensory deficits in the form of analgesia or hypalgesia
• Indicator muscle weakness
• Indicator muscle atrophy
• Absent or diminished muscle stretch reflexes
• Normal autonomic innervation

The classic clinical example of a radicular syndrome is a herniated lumbar disk with a compression of a nerve root.

Differentiating between Pseudo-radicular and Radicular Syndromes

What forms of diagnostic work-up are helpful for both syndromes?
- Immediate history: what, when, how, where, why?
- Evidence of trauma, fracture, or infection?
- Psychological and social history
- Clinical neurologic examination with inspection, morphologic assessment, tenderness to percussion, and limitation of spinal motion on forward bending (finger-to-floor distance)
- Additional function testing of the lumbar spine in forward and side bending, with special attention to possible blocked segments
- Function testing of the sacroiliac joints (asymmetric excursion, spine test)
- Signs of nerve stretch
- Strength testing of indicator muscles
- Search for sensory deficit in the dermatome
- Testing muscle stretch reflexes
- Neurodiagnostic studies—for example, electromyography (EMG)

Practical Tip

Indicator muscle tests should include the gluteal muscles.

Neurodiagnostic studies such as electromyography can be helpful in detecting sites of nerve root irritation. However, a negative EMG does not exclude a lumbar cause of peripheral muscle dysfunction because the examination conditions cannot reproduce the dynamic components. As a result, even this test will miss a large percentage of nerve root irritations, some subtle, caused by the large dynamic forces that are active during sports.

Practical Tip

A negative electromyogram does not exclude nerve root irritation, due to absence of the dynamic component.

References

Best TM. Commentary to: Orchard JW, Farhart P, Leopold C. Lumbar spine region pathology and hamstring and calf injuries in athletes: Is there a connection? Br J Sports Med 2004; 38: 504

Briggs CA, Chandraraj S. Variations in the lumbosacral ligament and associated changes in the lumbosacral region resulting in compression of the fifth dorsal root ganglion and spinal nerve. Clin Anat 1995; 8(5): 339–346

Hefti F. Spondylolyse und Spondylolisthesis. In: Hefti F. Kinderorthopädie in der Praxis. Heidelberg: Springer; 2006: 101–108

Hennessey L, Watson AW. Flexibility and posture assessment in relation to hamstring injury. Br J Sports Med 1993; 27(4): 243–246

Müller-Wohlfahrt HW, Montag HJ. Diagnostik und Therapie der so genannten Muskelzerrung, Diagnosis and therapy of "pulled muscle". Dtsch Z Sportmed 1985; 11: 246–248

Müller-Wohlfahrt HW, Montag HJ, Kübler U. Diagnostik und Therapie von Muskelzerrungen und Muskelfaserrissen. Dtsch Z Sportmed 1992; 3: 120–125

Ong A, Anderson J, Roche J. A pilot study of the prevalence of lumbar disc degeneration in elite athletes with lower back pain at the Sydney 2000 Olympic Games. Br J Sports Med 2003; 37(3): 263–266

Orchard JW, Farhart P, Leopold C. Lumbar spine region pathology and hamstring and calf injuries in athletes: is there a connection? Br J Sports Med 2004; 38(4): 502–504, discussion 502–504

Saraste H. Spondylolysis and spondylolisthesis. Acta Orthop Scand Suppl 1993; 251(Suppl.): 84–86

Verrall GM, Slavotinek JP, Barnes PG, Fon GT, Spriggins AJ. Clinical risk factors for hamstring muscle strain injury: a prospective study with correlation of injury by magnetic resonance imaging. Br J Sports Med 2001; 35(6): 435–439, discussion 440

Further Reading

Dejung B, Gröbli C, Colla F, et al. Triggerpunkt-Therapie. Bern: Hans Huber; 2001

Diener HC, Putzki N. Leitlinien für Diagnostik und Therapie in der Neurologie. 4th ed. Stuttgart: Thieme; 2008: 654

Foley BS, Buschbacher RM. Sacroiliac joint pain: anatomy, biomechanics, diagnosis, and treatment. Am J Phys Med Rehabil 2006; 85(12): 997–1006

Katz JN, Harris MB. Clinical practice. Lumbar spinal stenosis. N Engl J Med 2008; 358(8): 818–825

Lawrence JP, Greene HS, Grauer JN. Back pain in athletes. J Am Acad Orthop Surg 2006; 14(13): 726–735

13

Operative Treatment of Muscle Injuries

W. E. Garrett, Jr.

*My thanks go to J. R. Wittstein,
E. C. Pennington, and D. T. Kirkendall
for their great support
in putting this chapter together.*

Introduction *308*

Indirect Muscle Injuries—Muscle Tears *308*
Overview *308*
Injury Mechanisms *308*

Muscle Tears—Hamstrings *309*
Distal Injuries *309*
Proximal Injuries *309*

Surgical Treatment
of Hamstring Avulsions *311*

Quadriceps Injuries *312*
Contusions of the Quadriceps *312*
Tears of the Quadriceps *313*
Results *315*

Muscle Lacerations *316*

Conclusions *316*

Introduction

Acute injuries to skeletal muscle can be classified into direct (contusions, lacerations) and indirect injuries (partial muscle tears, (sub)total muscle tears (see also Chapter 6). Any of these can lead to significant pain and disability, with time lost to both occupational and leisure activities.

The sports physician needs to be comfortable in recognizing and treating muscle injuries, as stretch-induced injuries can account for up to 30% of the typical sports medicine practice (Krejci and Koch 1979, Peterson and Renstrom 1986).

Most muscle injuries occur in response to eccentric loading, with the resultant injury occurring near the muscle–tendon junction (Garrett et al. 1984a and Garrett et al. 1988). While the majority of muscle tears and contusions can be treated nonoperatively, some may require surgical intervention. The main focus of this chapter is on surgical treatment of muscle tears, contusions, and lacerations, with particular emphasis on quadriceps and hamstring injuries.

Note
Only a small number of muscle injuries require surgical intervention.

Indirect Muscle Injuries— Muscle Tears

Overview

Note
The term "muscle strain" can have various interpretations. Some authors interpret it to mean a functional (nonstructural) injury, but most experts define it as a structural lesion of varying dimensions. Since the term is not defined, we recommend using "tear" for structural injuries (see also Chapter 6).

There are many noncontact or indirect injuries that can disrupt muscle function. Examples include delayed-onset muscle soreness (DOMS), partial muscle tear, and a complete tear of the muscle (see also Chapter 6). These make up a continuum of injuries that have one thing in common: eccentric exercise—when the muscle develops tension while lengthening (Zarins and Ciullo 1983, Peterson and Renstrom 1986), where muscle can generate high forces with fewer active motor units (Stauber 1989).

In DOMS, eccentric loading, particularly during unaccustomed exercise, leads to microscopic damage to the contractile element, appearing as random disruptions of the Z lines (Fridén and Lieber 1992). The hallmarks of

DOMS include reversible pain, weakness, and limited range of motion. Pain typically peaks in the first 1–2 days following exercise (Clarkson and Newham 1995), while weakness and limited range of motion can persist for a week or more (Howell et al. 1985, Sherman et al. 1984). Muscle adapts very rapidly to the new exercise, as successive bouts of the same unaccustomed exercise produce progressively less soreness and less tissue damage (Clarkson and Newham 1995).

Muscle tear injury is a disruption of the muscle-tendon unit (Garrett 1990). Activity produces localized pain and general weakness of the muscle. In contrast to the protective aspects of DOMS, inadequate rest and rehabilitation of a minor muscle tear usually precedes a far more disabling injury, further increasing the time lost to work, sport, and recreation.

Injury Mechanisms

Most clinicians would agree that indirect muscle (strain) injuries occur during stretch, either passively or when activated during stretch (Krejci and Koch 1979, Radin et al. 1979, Zarins and Ciullo 1983). In addition, eccentric contraction of the muscle is a frequent occurrence (Glick 1980, Peterson and Renstrom 1986, Zarins and Ciullo 1983). Eccentric contraction is an important factor, as muscle forces can be higher during lengthening (Stauber 1989) due to more force coming from both the contractile tissue and the connective tissue (Elftman 1966). On the athletic field, muscle tears appear to occur mostly to "speed athletes" such as sprinters and participants in American football, basketball, soccer, and rugby, among others. In addition, only certain muscles appear to be highly susceptible to tearing.

In early laboratory studies on strain injury, standard techniques of muscle mechanics and electrophysiology were used on rabbit hind limb muscles, usually the tibialis anterior and the extensor digitorum longus, demonstrating that activation alone failed to produce either a partial or complete muscle tear (Garrett 1990); to obtain an injury, stretch was necessary. The forces necessary to cause muscle failure were several times the force normally produced during a maximal isometric contraction (Garrett et al. 1988), suggesting a role of passive forces.

Injury Resulting from Passive Stretch

Muscles with different architectures (pennation) or mechanical properties were stretched to failure from the proximal or distal tendon at varying rates of strain (1, 10, and 100 cm/s). Regardless of the rate of strain or architecture, muscle failed predictably at the (most frequently distal) muscle–tendon junction (MTJ), leaving a small, but variable amount of muscle tissue attached to the tendon (Garrett et al. 1984a). Thus, the site of a stretch-induced injury was predictably near the muscle–tendon junction; most often, the injury was not an avulsion, since a small and variable amount of muscle remained with the tendon.

Injury Resulting from Active Stretch

Most clinicians see patients with (partial) muscle tears that have occurred during powerful eccentric contractions. To study such injuries, a laboratory condition used to mimic the injuries involved rabbit hind limb muscles that were isolated and stretched to failure using either tetanic stimulation, submaximal stimulation, or no stimulation (Nikolaou et al. 1987). The location of tissue failure was, as expected, near the MTJ, with a similar total strain at failure among the three conditions. Interestingly, the force generated at failure was only 15% greater in the activated muscles, but the energy absorbed (the difference in strain energy between passive and active conditions) was ~ 100% greater in the activated condition.

> *Note*
>
> **It appears that muscles can protect themselves and joint structures from injury; the more energy a muscle can absorb, the more resistant a muscle is to injury.**

The data show that both the passive and contractile elements of muscle contribute to the ability of the muscle to absorb energy. The passive elements, not dependent on activation, include connective tissue and the fibers themselves. The contractile element of the muscle also participates because activation of the muscle increases the ability to absorb energy. Any condition that diminishes the ability of the muscle to contract also reduces the ability of the muscle to absorb energy, making the muscle more susceptible to injury.

Muscle Tears—Hamstrings

Hamstring injuries rarely result in the disruption of the muscle itself. Most hamstring injuries occur at the musculotendinous junction, near the origin or insertions of the muscles. Proximal injuries to the biceps femoris and distal injuries to the biceps femoris or semimembranosus are most common (Garrett et al. 1989). Hamstring injuries that involve tendinous avulsion from bone or actual tendinous disruption have to be recognized quickly and addressed without delay, as these are the ones that may need to be repaired to restore function.

> *Practical Tip*
>
> **It should be noted that hamstring tendon avulsions (as well as proximal rectus femoris avulsions), especially at the proximal level, may be associated with little retraction and respond well to conservative management.**

Distal Injuries

The distal biceps femoris may avulse from the fibular head as an isolated single tendon injury. This can occur as an isolated injury, which the authors have seen in waterskiers and American football players (Sallay et al. 1996). This produces pain and significant weakness, since both the long head and the short head of the biceps femoris lose their attachment to the fibula. The injury can be repaired by attaching the distal tendon by transosseous sutures to its anatomic location on the fibular head. More often than isolated injuries to the biceps femoris, its tendon can avulse from the fibular head as a part of a major ligamentous disruption in the lateral and posterolateral aspect of the knee.

The distal semitendinosus can also be seriously injured. This has been reported primarily in professional athletes, in whom the symptoms can be prolonged (**Fig. 13.1**)

Conway and Cooper (2007) have noted that the injury is associated with a limp, inability to fully extend the knee, and pain in the medial popliteal area. Surgery involves resecting the complete ruptured distal semitendinosus, resulting in a quicker return to sports than conservative treatment in this elite group (**Fig. 13.2**).

Proximal Injuries

Proximal hamstring tendon avulsions may be complete or partial, usually occurring in response to excessive amounts of stretch. The usual tears at the muscle–tendon junction occur in sprinters and hurdlers, while avulsions more often occur when external forces stretch the hamstrings. For example, hamstring avulsions can occur during waterskiing when the skier's knees are extended and the back and hips forced into hyperflexion over the lower extremity, which is fixed in the ski binding. Injury occurs as the pull of the powerboat forcefully accentuates this position (Sallay et al. 1996). Another mechanism of injury seen in American football occurs when a player falls to the ground with knees extended and hips flexed and another player lands on his back, forcing the hip to flex. Finally, a wet field may force a player to slide into a split position, with one side hyperextending the knee and flexing at the hip. These injuries can sometimes occur in a manner similar to the more usual hamstring tears without the external forces.

The clinical consequences of an avulsion hamstring injury can be very severe. This is especially true in athletes, who become unable to run and slide because they feel they have "no control" of their legs. The hamstring muscle serves to decelerate hip flexion and knee extension in a sprinting gait (Yu et al. 2008), so if a complete avulsion is left untreated, athletes are unable to sprint or quickly change direction. The short head of the biceps femoris is not disrupted, leaving some hamstring function, but the lack of muscle attachment to the ischium prevents high-speed running and cutting. The hamstrings exhibit less

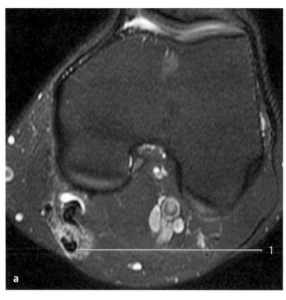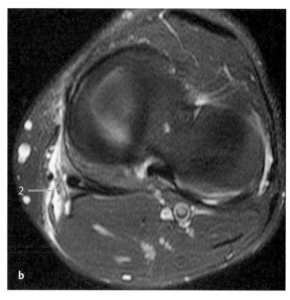

Fig. 13.1a, b Axial magnetic resonance imaging of a distal semitendinosus rupture.

a Enlarged semitendinosus at the level of the patella (1).

b Truncated semitendinosus at the level of the femorotibial joint (2). The tendon distal to this site was extensively scarred to the medial knee structures.

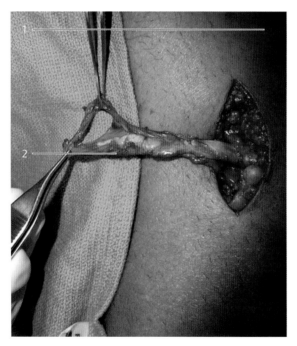

Fig. 13.2 Semitendinosus rupture. The incision is made in the long axis of the tibia over the insertion of the pes anserinus. The semitendinosus tendon has torn from the muscle. The distal tendon has been dissected from the medial structures to which it was scarred. 1, knee joint; 2, semitendinosus tendon.

power during the propulsive phase at the end of the stance phase, and at the end of the flight phase, where deceleration occurs (Yu et al. 2008).

An additional problem can be scar formation involving the sciatic nerve or one of its branches. Tension in the hamstrings can cause symptoms such as sciatica, as the adherent muscle belly pulls the nerve distally when the hamstrings move distally with either knee extension, muscle activation, or both.

Diagnosis is accomplished with a careful examination. There is tenderness at the ischium on palpation. The tendon can be palpated easily with the patient prone and the involved foot held in the air. The tendon should be palpated all the way to the ischium and compared with the contralateral side. Muscle strength is then tested, but pain can sometimes make strength testing difficult. Even with a complete avulsion of the long head from the ischium, the short head of the biceps femoris can still generate ~ 25% of the total hamstring force, so that hamstring function is not totally absent. A neurological evaluation ensures that the nerve is intact. In the supine position, there is often a remarkable increase in flexibility of the injured side. With no attachment to the ischium, there is enough of an increase in knee extension with the hip flexed to 90° to be clearly different in comparison with the contralateral extremity. In the very acute phase of injury, however, partial disruptions may be too painful to demonstrate an increase in flexibility. Magnetic resonance imaging (MRI) or ultrasound can confirm the diagnosis (**Fig. 13.3**).

Many patients who are not involved in sprinting or in other high-demand physical activities may not experience significant disability from a hamstring avulsion. However, most people who sustain this type of injury are involved with athletic activities and want to return to their former level of participation. An athlete with a partial injury may choose a certain period of rest to determine the extent of the disability associated with nonoperative treatment (see Chapter 11). If symptoms persist, surgical intervention may be performed at a later time.

Surgical Treatment of Hamstring Avulsions

Note
Complete tears/tendinous avulsions with retraction, however, should be repaired in a matter of weeks to avoid muscle retraction, fatty infiltration, and functional loss (**Fig. 13.4**).

Complete tears, i.e., tendinous avulsions, can be treated with a variety of techniques. The goal of repair procedures is to reattach the tendon of origin to the lateral wall of the ischial tuberosity (not to the most inferior portion of the tuberosity). An incision (which may be straight, or in line with the gluteal fold) is made over the lateral aspect of the ischial tuberosity. The posterior fascia of the thigh is in-

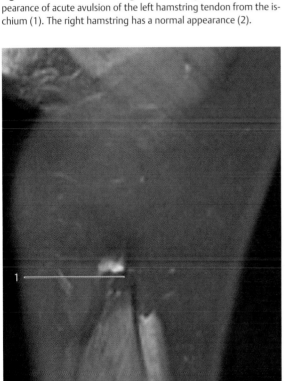

Fig. 13.3   Proximal hamstring avulsion. Magnetic resonance appearance of acute avulsion of the left hamstring tendon from the ischium (1). The right hamstring has a normal appearance (2).

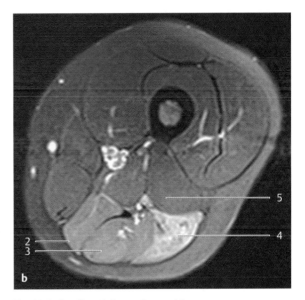

Fig. 13.4a, b   Chronic hamstring avulsion.

a Coronal magnetic resonance appearance of an avulsed and retracted hamstring common tendon 13 months after injury. There is marked displacement of the tendon. Position of proximal tendon quite distal to the ischium (1).
b Axial magnetic resonance appearance in the same patient. Changes associated with muscle atrophy can be seen in the lighter color of the injured muscles on T2-weighted sequences.
2 Semimembranosus
3 Semitendinosus
4 Biceps femoris, long head
5 Normal-appearing biceps femoris, short head

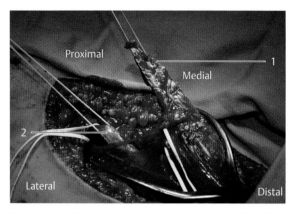

Fig. 13.5 Surgical repair of a complete proximal avulsion of the left hamstring. 1, proximal tendons; 2, sciatic nerve.

cised and, once visible, the posterior cutaneous nerve of the thigh is protected and the sciatic nerve is freed from the torn tendon stump. The tendon is sometimes retracted distal to the tuberosity, while at other times scar tissue can enclose the short distance from the ischium to the retracted tendon. This scar tissue mass may surround a small fluid-filled cavity. A whip stitch is placed in the tendon end and is used to pull the tendon proximally to its origin (**Fig. 13.5**). Next, multiple 6.5-mm corkscrew suture anchors with #2 fiber wire (Arthrex, Inc.; Largo, Florida) are placed in the tuberosity. The tendon is pulled to its proper location and the suture anchors are passed transversely across the tendon. If the lesion is over 6 months old, the tendon may reach the ischium without prolonged stretching and lysis of adhesions that may exist in the distal thigh.

> **Caution**
>
> With chronic injuries, more care is necessary to dissect the sciatic nerve past the area of obvious scarring.

The sciatic, tibial, or peroneal nerves may be scarred distal to the ischial tuberosity. When the nerves have been adequately freed, the conjoined tendon mass can be mobilized to the ischium. In some cases, it may be impossible to bring the proximal tendon to the ischium without excessive knee flexion and hip extension. In these situations, Z-lengthening of the semitendinosus and chevron lengthening of the semimembranosus and biceps femoris can lengthen the hamstring tendons distally. The hamstrings are lengthened until the tendon repair to the ischium bone is not under heavy tension when the hip is neutral and the knee is flexed to at least 70°. The knee is placed in a hinged brace, which is slowly and carefully extended over the next 2–8 weeks. Patients who have undergone an acute repair may be in the knee brace for much less time than those with more chronic injuries. A careful physical

therapy program ensures recovery of strength and motion.

Good success rates following acute repairs have been reported, and most patients have reported excellent satisfaction and strength recovery. The surgical results in more chronic cases have shown significant improvement, but still are not as successful as an acute repair (Sallay et al. 1996).

Quadriceps Injuries

Contusions of the Quadriceps

A direct blow to the anterior thigh also frequently injures the quadriceps muscles. The quadriceps contusion can cause muscle fiber disruption and may lead to a hematoma within the muscle. The muscle nearest the bone is often the most injured, typically the vastus intermedius (Walton and Rothwell 1983). There have been several clinical studies evaluating the conservative treatment of quadriceps contusions. Methods to limit the extent of hematoma formation include external compression and initial immobilization (Aronen et al. 2006). Hematomas can be limited by placing the muscle under stretch to increase the passive tension in the muscle. This stretch is usually applied by immobilization of the knee in flexion beyond 90°. This increases tension in the muscle and limits hematoma formation both within the muscle and deep to the muscle. This form of treatment is best when the immobilization is applied soon after the trauma.

Surgical Treatment of Quadriceps Contusions

There have not been many published studies of surgical evacuations of hematomas in the quadriceps. Both the evacuation of hematomas and the treatment of compartment syndrome of the thigh are controversial. There have been a few scattered case reports of hematoma evacuation, as well as fasciotomies for acute compartment syndrome following a quadriceps contusion. Diaz et al. (2003) reported on successful nonoperative treatment of professional athletes with thigh hematomas after a quadriceps contusion, and Robinson and colleagues (1992) have reported successful nonoperative management of compartment syndrome of the thigh. Other small case series have provided accounts of good results after operative treatment of both compartment syndromes and hematomas (Rööser 1987, Rööser et al. 1991). Currently, there is little evidence in the literature to support acute operative interventions for quadriceps contusion injuries.

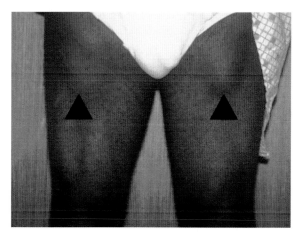

Fig. 13.6   Bilateral rectus femoris injuries in an athlete seen for a separate knee problem who had a history and physical appearance of bilateral rectus femoris injuries. The rectus injuries were asymptomatic. The retracted muscles are indicated with arrowheads.

Tears of the Quadriceps

Muscle tears involving the quadriceps usually involve the rectus femoris muscle, the only two-joint muscle in the quadriceps group. It is subject to significant stretch and possible injury with strong eccentric muscle activation when the knee is flexed and the hip is extended. These injuries are very common in the different codes of football around the world. Athletes typically experience a sudden painful episode when sprinting or kicking. Usually there is tenderness in the superficial quadriceps area over the proximal muscle and to the middle of the thigh. The pain and disability resolve over time with proper conservative treatment (Garrett 1996) (see also Chapter 11).

At times, the injury can be more severe and result in a muscle tear that creates a distinct asymmetry in the muscle when it is activated. A masslike effect may be evident, with muscle retraction upon activation resembling a complete tear from one end of the muscle (**Fig. 13.6**). The clinical explanation for this observation may be a large muscle–tendon junction tear, which can happen anywhere along the proximal tendon that extends well into the body of the muscle (see below; Hughes et al. 1995).

Although the visible asymmetry might lead one to make a clinical judgment of a complete disruption, the rectus femoris rarely loses continuity. The rectus femoris actually has two heads of origin with two distinct, separate tendons (**Fig. 13.7**; see also Chapter 1). Muscle fibers from both heads attach distally to the insertional tendon as it forms part of the quadriceps tendon. The direct head of the muscle originates from the anterior inferior iliac spine, while the reflected head originates from the posterior rim of the acetabulum. The tendon of the direct head is usually broad and flat and on the anterior surface of the muscle. The tendon of the reflected head, however, continues as a tendon that penetrates into the muscle belly

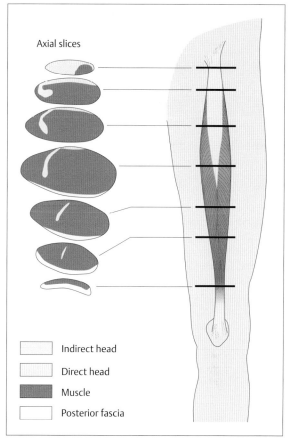

Axial slices

Indirect head

Direct head

Muscle

Posterior fascia

Fig. 13.7   The rectus femoris muscle and tendons. The anterior view on the right with axial slices shows the relative location of the two tendons at various lengths along the muscle. This anatomy is variable, but the muscle fibers from the indirect head are often surrounded by the direct head. This anatomic situation creates the appearance of a "muscle within a muscle."

(Hasselman et al. 1995). Rectus femoris tears often occur to the reflected head, where muscle fibers can be avulsed from the tendon, the tendon itself can be injured, or both.

Characteristic magnetic resonance imaging findings show edema and possibly even some fluid collection centered on the tendon of the reflected head (**Fig. 13.8**). At times the distal muscle–tendon junction may be involved, but injury to the proximal direct head is rare. The proximal head injury can range from a small amount of edema near the muscle–tendon junction to a complete disruption and distal retraction of the reflected head. A recent ultrasound study on the appearance of these injuries correlated clinical examination and time to recovery with the location of the tears and length of the indirect head (also called central tendon) that was involved (Balius et al. 2009). The longest recovery times were seen in more proximal injuries, in comparison with more distal injuries, with the mean number of days to return to sport being 45 and 39, respectively. Longer recovery was also correlated

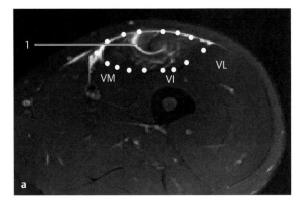

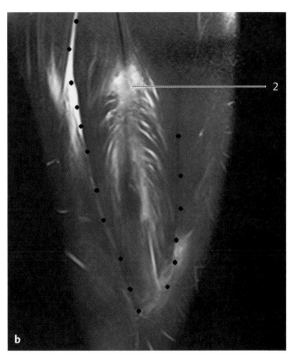

Fig. 13.8a, b   Acute musculotendinous avulsion of the indirect head of the rectus femoris.

a   An axial T2-weighted image of the left thigh of a collegiate American football player. The rectus femoris is outlined with dots.
b   A coronal T2-weighted image in the same American football player. The dots indicate the edge of the rectus femoris.

1   The injured indirect head, which is almost surrounded by fluid with a hyperintense signal in the T2-weighted image
2   The proximal edge of the retracted fibers of the indirect head, which lies inside the fibers of the direct head

VM   Vastus medialis
VL   Vastus lateralis
VI   Vastus intermedius

with involvement of a greater length of the central aponeurosis. MR imaging of chronic tears demonstrates scar tissue in the indirect head of the rectus femoris (**Fig. 13.9**). Adhesions to the vastus intermedius and distinct fluid collections also can be seen (**Figs. 13.8** and **13.9**).

Surgical Treatment of Quadriceps Tears

The majority of these injuries resolve with conservative management. Symptoms may persist, but in general are not disabling. The residual symptoms are usually an ache or some pain in the quadriceps with sprinting or powerful kicking. Surgery is indicated only in very rare cases when pain does not resolve, when athletic ability is greatly hampered, and there is a visible and palpable deformity in the activated muscle. Studies on the outcomes of surgery are lacking, and the author has limited experience with the procedure.

> *Note*
>
> These facts underscore the scarcity of effective surgical options for these relatively common injuries. It is our opinion that injuries of this kind almost always resolve with conservative treatment, whereas avulsions of the proximal rectus with relevant retraction need surgical repair.

Surgical Repair

The muscle is exposed through a straight anterior incision over the deformity, which may need to extend proximal enough to identify the femoral nerve and the branches to the quadriceps. The rectus femoris can be dissected from the quadriceps group and usually does not appear grossly damaged. When the muscle is activated by electrical nerve stimulation, the site of the disrupted muscle becomes apparent. Since the injury usually involves the deeper reflected head proximally, the surgeon can usually see the deep muscle retract distally.

To avoid a longer proximal incision, stimulating electrodes can be used to activate the muscle without actual dissection of the nerve. The anesthesiologist can stimulate the nerve proximally (catheters for delivery of local anesthetics for nerve block usually involve electrical muscle stimulation to assess proximity of the catheter to the femoral nerve). With activation, the muscle deformity is clearly identified. The muscle fibers are split proximal to the deformity. Within the muscle, an area of extensive scarring can be encountered. At times, there is a cavity with fluid and a distinct lining of the capsule, which is usually proximal to the retracted muscle and scar. The fluid-filled cavity can be seen easily on MRI (**Fig. 13.10**). The author has seen cases in which the reflected head was completely separated proximally and the reflected head of the muscle retracted distally. With activation, the detached muscle shortens and thickens, creating a mass effect in the muscle

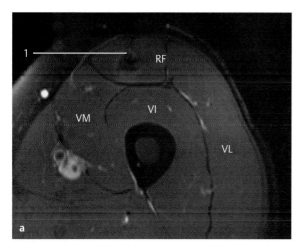
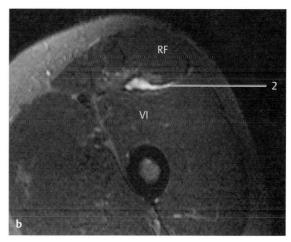

Fig. 13.9a, b   Chronic rectus femoris indirect head injury in the left thigh. The patient was an elite player in American collegiate football.

a Axial T2-weighted magnetic resonance image (MRI).
b Axial T2-weighted MRI of the rectus femoris.

1 Scar tissue with a dark appearance in the center of the rectus
2 Fluid between the rectus femoris tendon of insertion and the vastus intermedius

RF   Rectus femoris
VM   Vastus medialis
VL   Vastus lateralis
VI   Vastus intermedius

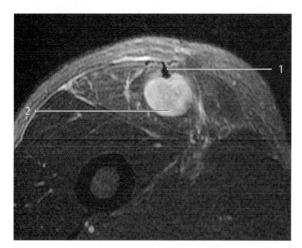

Fig. 13.10   Magnetic resonance appearance of a seroma cavity in the rectus femoris. The image shows an older chronic injury in the right rectus femoris. 1, indirect head of the rectus femoris; 2, a bright seroma in the cavity in the rectus femoris following retraction of the muscle fibers of the indirect head.

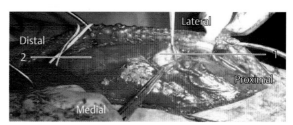

Fig. 13.11   Surgical exploration of an injury to the indirect head of the rectus femoris. 1, cavity within the rectus femoris; 2, distal rectus muscle.

belly. The scar tissue cavity is removed from the surrounding normal fibers, and the detached muscle and fibrotic scar tissue are removed (**Fig. 13.11**). Following removal of the damaged muscle, nerve activation results in what appears to be a normally contracting muscle without the formation of a mass effect centrally in the muscle. With some of the surgical explorations, there has been an extensive scarring between the posterior aspect of the muscle and the surrounding vastus muscles, usually the intermedius. This pattern was not associated with any preoperative decrease in flexibility.

Following the surgical resection and release of the rectus femoris, hemostasis is obtained and the fascia is carefully closed. Rehabilitation begins in the first few postoperative days with slight stretching, careful soft-tissue massage (caution: myositis ossificans), and early return to active motion with low intensity exercises. Most patients are able to return to play after approximately 4 months.

Results

There have been no reports on outcome studies following surgical repair of quadriceps injury. A preliminary review of eight surgical patients (unpublished observations) showed all the patients to be bothered only by intensive sports participation (five played American football and three played baseball at collegiate or professional level). Seven had experienced improvement and were able to return to participation. One patient had improvement, but was still in rehabilitation 6 months after surgery. Another patient was seen following a procedure done by another surgeon, and remains unable to return to normal sports participation after a subsequent procedure by the author. It should be emphasized that these represent only a very small fraction of the total number of patients with this injury and that the vast majority do not require surgical management.

Many patients seek a medical examination in order to rule out a tumor, because a mass is present. These patients are typically asymptomatic or minimally symptomatic and are only concerned about the mass. It should be added, however, that malignant tumors are also seen which have been assumed to be muscle injuries. Careful evaluation is necessary.

Muscle Lacerations

Direct lacerations can be difficult to repair when the zone of injury is within the muscle belly, where there is no tendon that can be sutured more easily. For some muscle architectures (e.g., pennate muscles), the tendons of origin and insertion expand over broad areas of the muscle and can be incorporated in the repair. Sutures in the tendinous expansions or the epimysium can be used to approximate the ends of the lacerated muscle.

Practical Tip

Incorporating the epimysium into the repair of lacerated muscle bellies has also been shown to increase repair strength in comparison with perimysium suturing (Kragh and Basamania 2002).

To provide a stout repair, it may be necessary to debride the zone of injury to locate and incorporate connective tissues such as tendinous expansions or epimysium.

The two options for treating muscle lacerations are operative (direct repair) and nonoperative (immobilization). A distinct advantage of repair over immobilization is that repair techniques allow early mobilization. For example, animal data suggest that lacerated muscles should be mobilized to prevent the loss of tensile properties that occurs with immobilization (Józsa et al. 1990, Järvinen and Lehto 1993). In addition, contractile strength is restored to a much greater extent after direct repair in comparison with no treatment or with immobilization (Menetrey et al. 1999).

Kragh and Basamania (2002) described the repair of acute traumatic closed transections of the biceps brachii, an unusual injury seen in paratroopers. The injury occurs when the static line (a line connecting the parachute to the airplane) gets tangled during the jump and violently strikes the anterior aspect of the arm, bisecting the biceps. In all cases, all but 5% of the muscle fibers were transected. The repair technique involved placement of absorbable perimeter sutures in a locked running fashion in the epi-

mysium as well as modified Mason–Allen sutures that crossed both the edge of the epimysium as well as the perimeter stitches. The authors reported good recovery of biceps function in the surgical cases, with twice as much contractile strength and better subjective and cosmetic outcomes. Biomechanical testing of this combined perimeter and modified Mason–Allen technique on cadavers demonstrated that combined suturing had superior pullout strength to conventional suturing (Chance et al. 2005). This technique was also used in a case report of a traumatic transection of the quadriceps, with good recovery of motion and function (Tate 2009).

Note

Other animal data suggest that identification and repair of the intramuscular nerve can improve outcomes from direct repair of muscle lacerations.

In a rabbit model, Garrett et al. (1984b) demonstrated that the tissue distal to the laceration of the extensor digitorum longus shows histologic changes consistent with denervation, such as fiber atrophy, size variability, fibrosis, and nuclear centralization. After repair, muscle bellies with complete lacerations regained 50% of their ability to produce tension and were able to shorten to 80% of normal, while the partially lacerated muscles regained 60% of baseline tension with a normal ability to shorten (Garrett et al. 1984b). These findings suggest that injury to the intramuscular nerve may diminish the results of repair. More recent animal models have demonstrated the significance of intramuscular nerve repair in the recovery of function after muscle laceration (Lim et al. 2006, Pereira et al. 2006).

Conclusions

Mechanisms of injury to skeletal muscle include most frequently tears secondary to eccentric loads, direct contusions, and (less frequently in athletes) lacerations. Some muscle lacerations can benefit from repair with combined suturing techniques and early mobilization. The majority of muscle contusion injuries appear to be amenable to conservative treatment. Most tensile injuries to the hamstrings and rectus femoris can be managed nonoperatively. Proximal hamstring avulsion injuries with relevant retraction can be particularly devastating to motor function and agility and do not have predictable outcomes when repaired in the chronic setting. An early repair should be performed in athletes or in patients who might experience functional improvement with a repair.

Injuries to the reflected head of the rectus femoris are almost always amenable to conservative treatment. Delayed excision may be considered in the rare cases in which conservative management fails.

References

Aronen JG, Garrick JG, Chronister RD, McDevitt ER. Quadriceps contusions: clinical results of immediate immobilization in 120 degrees of knee flexion. Clin J Sport Med 2006; 16(5): 383–387

Balius R, Maestro A, Pedret C, et al. Central aponeurosis tears of the rectus femoris: practical sonographic prognosis. Br J Sports Med 2009; 43(11): 818–824

Chance JR, Kragh JF Jr, Agrawal CM, Basamania CJ. Pullout forces of sutures in muscle lacerations. Orthopedics 2005; 28(10): 1187–1190

Clarkson PM, Newham DJ. Associations between muscle soreness, damage, and fatigue. Adv Exp Med Biol 1995; 384: 457–469

Conway JE, Cooper DE. Semitendinosus ruptures in elite athletes. Calgary, CA: American Orthopaedic Society for Sports Medicine; 2007

Diaz JA, Fischer DA, Rettig AC, Davis TJ, Shelbourne KD. Severe quadriceps muscle contusions in athletes. A report of three cases. Am J Sports Med 2003; 31(2): 289–293

Elftman H. Biomechanics of muscle with particular application to studies of gait. J Bone Joint Surg Am 1966; 48(2): 363–377

Fridén J, Lieber RL. Structural and mechanical basis of exercise-induced muscle injury. Med Sci Sports Exerc 1992; 24(5): 521–530

Garrett WE Jr, Almekinders L, Seaber AV. Biomechanics of muscle tears and stretching injuries. J Orthop Res 1984a; 9: 384

Garrett WE Jr, Seaber AV, Boswick J, Urbaniak JR, Goldner JL. Recovery of skeletal muscle after laceration and repair. J Hand Surg Am 1984b; 9(5): 683–692

Garrett WE Jr, Nikolaou PK, Ribbeck BM, Glisson RR, Seaber AV. The effect of muscle architecture on the biomechanical failure properties of skeletal muscle under passive extension. Am J Sports Med 1988; 16(1): 7–12

Garrett WE Jr, Rich FR, Nikolaou PK, Vogler JB III. Computed tomography of hamstring muscle strains. Med Sci Sports Exerc 1989; 21(5): 506–514

Garrett WE Jr. Muscle strain injuries: clinical and basic aspects. Med Sci Sports Exerc 1990; 22(4): 436–443

Garrett WE Jr. Muscle strain injuries. Am J Sports Med 1996; 24 (6, Suppl): S2–S8

Glick JM. Muscle strains: Prevention and treatment. Phys Sportsmed 1980; 8(11): 73–77

Hasselman CT, Best TM, Hughes C IV, Martinez S, Garrett WE Jr. An explanation for various rectus femoris strain injuries using previously undescribed muscle architecture. Am J Sports Med 1995; 23(4): 493–499

Howell JN, Chila AG, Ford G, David D, Gates T. An electromyographic study of elbow motion during postexercise muscle soreness. J Appl Physiol 1985; 58(5): 1713–1718

Hughes C IV, Hasselman CT, Best TM, Martinez S, Garrett WE Jr. Incomplete, intrasubstance strain injuries of the rectus femoris muscle. Am J Sports Med 1995; 23(4): 500–506

Järvinen MJ, Lehto MUK. The effects of early mobilisation and immobilisation on the healing process following muscle injuries. Sports Med 1993; 15(2): 78–89

Józsa L, Kannus P, Thöring J, Reffy A, Järvinen M, Kvist M. The effect of tenotomy and immobilisation on intramuscular connective tissue. A morphometric and microscopic study in rat calf muscles. J Bone Joint Surg Br. 1990; 72(2): 293–297

Kragh JF Jr, Basamania CJ. Surgical repair of acute traumatic closed transection of the biceps brachii. J Bone Joint Surg Am 2002; 84 A(6): 992–998

Krejci V, Koch P. Muscle and tendon injuries in athletes. Chicago, IL: Yearbook Medical Publishers; 1979

Lim AY, Lahiri A, Pereira BP, et al. The role of intramuscular nerve repair in the recovery of lacerated skeletal muscles. Muscle Nerve 2006; 33(3): 377–383

Menetrey J, Kasemkijwattana C, Fu FH, Moreland MS, Huard J. Suturing versus immobilization of a muscle laceration. A morphological and functional study in a mouse model. Am J Sports Med 1999; 27(2): 222–229

Nikolaou PK, Macdonald BL, Glisson RR, Seaber AV, Garrett WE Jr. Biomechanical and histological evaluation of muscle after controlled strain injury. Am J Sports Med 1987; 15(1): 9–14

Pereira BP, Tan JAC, Zheng L, et al. The cut intramuscular nerve affects the recovery in the lacerated skeletal muscle. J Orthop Res 2006; 24(1): 102–111

Peterson L, Renstrom P. Sports Injuries: their prevention and treatment. Chicago, IL: Yearbook Medical Publishers; 1986

Radin EL, Simon RM, Rose RM. Practical biomechanics for the orthopaedic surgeon. New York: John Wiley; 1979

Robinson D, On E, Halperin N. Anterior compartment syndrome of the thigh in athletes—indications for conservative treatment. J Trauma 1992; 32(2): 183–186

Rööser B. Quadriceps contusion with compartment syndrome. Evacuation of hematoma in 2 cases. Acta Orthop Scand 1987; 58(2): 170–172

Rööser B, Bengtson S, Hägglund G. Acute compartment syndrome from anterior thigh muscle contusion: a report of eight cases. J Orthop Trauma 1991; 5(1): 57–59

Sallay PI, Friedman RL, Coogan PG, Garrett WE. Hamstring muscle injuries among water skiers. Functional outcome and prevention. Am J Sports Med 1996; 24(2): 130–136

Sherman WM, Armstrong LE, Murray TM, et al. Effect of a 42.2-km footrace and subsequent rest or exercise on muscular strength and work capacity. J Appl Physiol 1984; 57(6): 1668–1673

Stauber WT. Eccentric action of muscles: physiology, injury, and adaptation. Exerc Sport Sci Rev 1989; 17: 157–185

Tate DE Jr. Use of combined modified Mason-Allen and perimeter stitches for repair of a quadriceps femoris laceration: a case report. J Trauma 2009; 67(3): E88–E92

Walton M, Rothwell AG. Reactions of thigh tissues of sheep to blunt trauma. Clin Orthop Relat Res 1983; (176): 273–281

Yu B, Queen RM, Abbey AN, Liu Y, Moorman CT, Garrett WE. Hamstring muscle kinematics and activation during overground sprinting. J Biomech 2008; 41(15): 3121–3126

Zarins B, Ciullo JV. Acute muscle and tendon injuries in athletes. Clin Sports Med 1983; 2(1): 167–182

Further Reading

Kragh JF Jr, Svoboda SJ, Wenke JC, Ward JA, Walters TJ. Epimysium and perimysium in suturing in skeletal muscle lacerations. J Trauma 2005; 59(1): 209–212

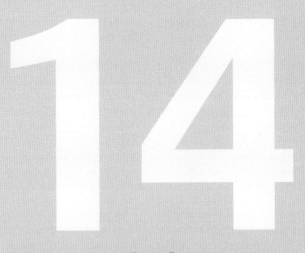

14

Physical Therapy and Rehabilitation

K. Eder

H. Hoffmann

Translated by Terry Telger

Requirements of the Care Team   *320*

Positive and Negative Influences on the Myofascial System   *321*
Sport-Specific Changes and Adaptations of the Musculoskeletal System in Soccer Players   *321*

Treatment-Oriented Assessment Strategy   *327*
Clinical Therapeutic Assessment   *328*
Clinical Motion Analysis   *329*
Methods Used in Medical Training Therapy: Rehabilitative Performance Testing   *330*

Strategies for the Treatment of Muscle Injuries   *334*
Immediate Measures   *334*
General Aspects of Therapeutic Techniques in the Treatment of Muscle Injuries   *337*

Therapeutic Techniques   *340*
Physical Modalities   *340*
Manual Therapy   *343*
Elastic Taping (Kinesiotaping)   *356*
Medical Training Therapy   *358*

Requirements of the Care Team

Regardless of the type and severity of athletic muscle injuries, all types of modern competitive sports require an optimally timed rehabilitation program that can achieve the fastest possible recovery of functional capacity and performance to the injured biological structures. Every injured athlete wants to return to training and competition as quickly as possible. Accordingly, athletes who are referred for physical therapy are generally a well-motivated population with very high level of compliance. This is certainly advantageous for implementing complex treatment strategies, but it may become a problem in "overmotivated" athletes who place unrealistic expectations on the swiftness and efficacy of the treatment they receive. While it is true that therapeutic and training aids are constantly improving, we know from previous chapters that there are underlying biological principles which cannot be violated and impose a definite timeline on the recovery of functional capacity and performance.

The makeup of the care team charged with maintaining, optimizing, and restoring the performance of the athletes in their care has changed dramatically over the years, resulting in the development of increasingly complex models of care. The goal of the care team, from both an ethical and economic standpoint, is to safeguard and ensure the success of the athlete and the team.

A variety of care concepts, each with its own history, nuances, and points of emphasis (and each influenced by geographic, legal, and monetary factors), have evolved in different sports to optimize the performance of athletes and teams. Despite their differences, all of these concepts have one thing in common: they are all based on interdisciplinary cooperation between all the professionals involved in the athletes' care. As a result, advances in medicine and physical therapy have led to growing specialization and expansion of the care staff in the various sports medicine teams and departments. This trend began in the late 1970s and early 1980s, when the typical care staff for injured athletes consisted of the team physician and a masseur. Since then, growing numbers of physical and manual therapists, aided by comprehensive continuing education and certification programs for physical therapists in sports, have been taking a more active interest in sports medicine. In turn, this has fostered the development of new therapeutic techniques, which have significantly expanded the range of treatment strategies available.

In Germany, the rehabilitation of sports-related injuries in professional athletes has been significantly advanced by the Administrative Professional Association *Verwaltungs-Berufsgenossenschaft*, VBG), a statutory accident-insurance body that extended employers' liability insurance in the mid-1980s to include professional soccer players. These athletes received the same coverage that had been made available to workers in many other industries. When a worker is injured on the job, or when a professional athlete is injured while training or competing, the VBG must provide sick pay until the player can "return to work"—that is, resume training and competition. As conventional rehabilitation methods required a very long absence from sports (leading to prolonged disability payments from the VBG) and often did not return athletes to their pre-injury level of fitness, the VBG developed and optimized an initiative for implementing complex treatment strategies in injured athletes. For the first time, specialists in training therapy (sports scientists with additional medical and therapeutic training) were added to the therapy team along with doctors, masseurs, and physical therapists. At the same time, interdisciplinary continuing education programs were mandated for the participating professional groups. Today, the health-care team for modern professional soccer teams may consist of 15–25 experts who are available on staff or as outside consultants to provide in-network care services for a roster of 20–30 professional soccer players.

In addition to these developments in medical care for athletes, escalating demands and performance levels in various sports have greatly increased the physical stresses on the musculoskeletal system—particularly the joints, ligaments, muscles, and fascia.

Note

For the purposes of physical therapy in sports, all professional groups that contribute to maintaining, developing, and optimizing the performance of individual athletes should report to the head trainer.

All care services center on the team physician, who is ultimately responsible for the health and functional status of the individual athletes. The team physician should manage and coordinate the various activities of the care providers. He assembles the "care network," ideally stays in constant contact with all the care providers, and is the person in whom the individual athletes confide. As a general rule, communication needs to be maintained among the specialists who provide different levels of care, both during routine training and especially during the treatment of muscle injuries. For example, the anti-doping manager should maintain close contact with the team physician, physical therapists, cook, and others as he addresses complex and ever-changing issues relating to individual players and the team. The equipment manager works closely with the team physician and, if necessary, with an orthopedic shoemaker and equipment suppliers. The complexity of the relationships and interactions makes it imperative to maintain strong lines of communications and establish a systemic hierarchy for assigning responsibilities and making decisions on a routine basis and especially in athletes who have sustained muscle injuries.

Positive and Negative Influences on the Myofascial System

Every sport requires its players to develop a level of conditioning and performance that are necessary for that particular sport. Players must master the techniques for executing sport-specific actions and patterns of movement, and they must acquire the tactical understanding needed to play the game. These requirements are particularly rigorous in team sports, where athletes have to plan not only their own actions (individual tactics) but also need to process the interaction and coordination of those actions with their teammates and opposing players.

Different sports and athletic disciplines are characterized by a multitude of highly specific, stereotypical patterns of movement. When the movements are performed at sufficient magnitudes for a long period of time, these sport-specific motor stimuli evoke specific responses in which certain biological structures undergo adaptations that enable the athlete to adequately "process" the loads. These changes affect bones, ligaments, and muscular structures and are characterized in all sports by an asymmetrical distribution of loads between the right and left sides of the athlete's body. Common examples are:

- Unilateral loads on the playing arm, as in racket sports
- Bilateral side-specific stick positions, as in field hockey and ice hockey
- Unilateral motion directions, as in golfers (right-handed or left-handed swing) or in sprinters who run tracks that curve in one direction
- Special side-specific loads, as illustrated by the jumping and lead legs in broad jumping and high jumping, the lead and trailing legs in hurdling, or the preferred kicking leg in soccer

Generally, the adaptations heighten the quality of the sport-specific movement patterns and thus have a positive effect on the athlete's performance in that particular sport. On the other hand, many of these adaptations cause changes in muscular loads and can sometimes lead to the overuse or unphysiologic loading of certain musculoskeletal structures. These loads may exceed the stress tolerance of the structures, resulting in all gradations of muscular injury.

An awareness of sport-specific changes in the musculoskeletal system will make it easier for the members of the sports medicine staff, especially the physical therapists and rehabilitation trainers, to evaluate the structural and functional consequences of muscle injuries and formulate appropriate, complex treatment strategies. The following discussions are intended to alert therapists to the existence and importance of sport-specific adaptations. The authors consider that an awareness of these adaptations will have a direct impact on the quality and long-term suc-

cess of therapeutic outcomes and provide the basis for an appropriate, modern, complex treatment strategy.

Note

Therapists and other members of the care team should always be able to distinguish pathologic changes from sport-specific adaptations and, if necessary, draw therapeutic conclusions that are appropriate for the individual athlete.

Sport-Specific Changes and Adaptations of the Musculoskeletal System in Soccer Players

After a sport has been practiced for some time, the active and passive elements of the musculoskeletal system undergo changes in response to the sport-specific profile of motor demands and the associated stereotypical movement patterns and mechanical loads.

Taking soccer as an example of a sport with side-specific or asymmetrical stress patterns (e.g., the soccer player has a preferred kicking side and support side), we shall look at corresponding adaptation patterns that should be noted in the evaluation of injuries. The stereotypical loads that act on certain biological structures may vary greatly in soccer, both quantitatively and qualitatively, and reflect a long-term adaptation of the musculoskeletal system to a recurring stress pattern. Players with a symmetrical kicking technique tend to be the exception in this regard. Also, the play requirements and stereotypical movement patterns vary from one playing position to the next. This difference is particularly marked between the goalkeeper and field players, but also exists among different playing positions on the field.

Sport-specific musculoskeletal adaptations are found in active soccer players, as well as in players who retired from the sport years earlier. This is particularly important in physical therapy settings (provided by a doctor, therapist, or trainer), where it is important to consider whether the adaptive changes should be prophylactically "treated" and reversed, or at least limited, with the goal of preventing future degenerative problems. There is no generally valid recommended course of action, and management decisions should be made on a case-by-case basis, depending on the extent of the changes and on individual physical factors. Finally, every care team that is aware of these potential systematic changes in the musculoskeletal system should develop the following capabilities:

- An improved ability to evaluate the history and pathogenesis of muscle injuries and identify the primary causal mechanism
- The ability to achieve the best possible recovery in the shortest possible time in the framework of a complex treatment program
- The ability to prescribe individualized measures aimed at preventing future muscle injuries

Changes Caused by Contact of the Kicking Leg with the Ball

From a mechanical standpoint, a soccer player who kicks a ball is accelerating ~ 290–450 g of air and leather (or plastic today) of a specified size and volume in a designated direction. This can be accomplished by various modes of ball contact, which impose corresponding mechanical loads on the striking area—the forehead for a header shot, the instep for an instep shot, or the inside of the foot for an inside shot. The mass (weight) of the soccer ball, the air pressure in the ball, the contact time, and the speed change at ball contact are all mechanical variables that determine the nature of the mechanical loads acting on the muscles, bones, and joints. Changing any one of these variables will alter the mechanical stress configuration, producing positive or negative effects on musculoskeletal structures.

Effect of Ball Mass, Ball Pressure, Contact Time, and Ball Speed

With regard to the mechanical stresses that are generated by striking a soccer ball, the forces transmitted by the ball that have to be "processed" by the musculoskeletal system can be calculated by assuming a given ball speed at the time of initial contact and a given ball contact time (for a given ball pressure), using the ball sizes officially approved by the International Federation of Association Football (FIFA) for junior and senior players. The maximum forces generated by a senior soccer ball during the period of ball contact are ~ 25% higher than with a junior ball. If the impact speed increases while other ball factors remain the same, the greater speed will increase the force of the impact that is transmitted during ball contact, resulting in a maximum force increase of ~ 100 N per 1 m/s of velocity increase. If the ball pressure is increased by 100 g/cm³, the mechanical behavior of the ball will more closely approximate the conditions of an "elastic collision." This shortens the ball contact time by ~ 15% and increases the maximum force of the strike by ~ 100 N.

Thus, the mechanical load transferred to the kicking foot depends in part on how tightly the ball is inflated. It is noteworthy that the soccer balls used in Germany, for example, are inflated to an air pressure 0.2–0.3 bar higher than the balls used in Brazil and other South American countries (the official air pressure of a soccer ball is 0.6–1.1 bar).

Note

Increasing the ball pressure changes the mechanical properties of the ball. The maximum force of ball contact increases by ~ 10% for each 0.1 bar of pressure added, and this will also shorten the duration of ball contact.

The ratio of ball contact time to maximum force during momentum transfer is considered to be optimal if the striking force does not reach an unphysiologic order of magnitude. At the same time, the contact time should not be too long, as this would prolong the effect of the contact on biological structures. The greater contact time would no longer have the properties of an elastic impact, and the biological structures would respond with compensatory and counteractive processes that could lead to instability of the affected joints.

Effect of the Ratio of Ball Mass to Player Body Mass and Size

The magnitude of the mechanical load also depends on the mass of the ball in relation to the player's body mass and size. The mechanical load acting on a junior player kicking a senior ball would be comparable to the load acting on an adult player kicking a ball that weighs 1.2 kg and has twice the circumference of a normal soccer ball. This is one reason why special attention should be given to the loads and stresses to which children and adolescent players are exposed in every type of sport.

Note

Because the growing musculoskeletal system in the junior age group apparently responds to mechanical stresses with increased adaptive processes, although the musculoskeletal structures are not yet fully stabilized (the muscular stabilizing component is not yet optimized), the stress levels sanctioned by FIFA should be minimized and juvenile teams should train and play only with approved junior soccer balls.

Effect of the Number of Stereotypical Loads

Besides the magnitude of the mechanical stresses associated with ball contact, the number of repetitive stereotypical loads caused by ball contact within the physiologic range will also trigger degenerative changes in the musculoskeletal system. Over the course of evolution, nature has equipped our musculoskeletal system (especially the lower limb and pelvic–leg axis) for locomotion by walking and running. Our feet have longitudinal and transverse arches designed to cushion the impact of the body weight with each step and to accelerate the body forward during the propulsive phase of gait. When the foot strikes a soccer ball, the impact exerts a force of short duration (with a ball contact time of 11–15 milliseconds, depending on ball pressure) that is opposite to the arched construction of the foot, giving rise to intra-articular shear forces. The mechanical reaction forces generated by the ball mass have a magnitude that is well within physiologic limits and generally do not exceed the stress tolerance of the biological structures. But when a large number of contacts are repeated over a long period of time, which may be measured in years, they create stimuli that act as repetitive microtrauma and will eventually evoke changes in the musculoskeletal system.

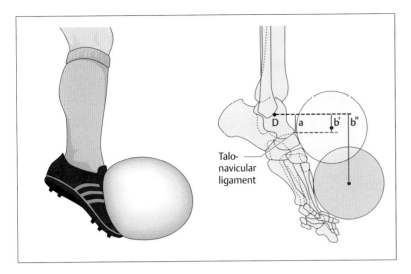

Fig. 14.1 Intra-articular loads during an instep kick.

a Distance from rotational axis to attachment of talonavicular ligament.

b′ Distance (lever length) to center of ball with correct kicking technique.

b″ Distance (lever length) to center of ball with incorrect kicking technique.

Musculoskeletal Adaptation with Talar Beak/Tibial Peak Formation

Nature tries to prepare for the sudden, brief tensile stresses caused by ball contact by strengthening the attachment sites of the talonavicular ligament. As the Sharpey fibers become stronger and more numerous, they create a mass effect that appears as a talar beak and/or tibial peak on X-ray films. This feature decreases the range of foot extension at the ankle joint. Since the early 1980s various retrospective empirical pilot studies have demonstrated that radiographically visible bone changes were noted only on the kicking-leg side in professional soccer players who had been playing for at least 3 years. The only player free of these changes was a goalkeeper who did not perform kick-offs himself. Moreover, kicking balls with a faulty, biologically unfavorable technique will quickly increase the tensile stresses on the talonavicular ligament to unphysiologically high levels that may exceed stress tolerance, resulting in an acute injury. Poor footwear can further exacerbate this adverse change in the stability of the affected joint. While the soles of soccer shoes are designed to prevent excessive arch stresses in the extended foot (plantar flexion at the ankle joint), a poor kicking technique can still produce the adverse effects shown in **Fig. 14.1**. Striking the ball with the toe of the shoe as opposed to the laces has the effect of lengthening the lever arm of the ball-strike force and will multiply the torque and tensile stress acting on the talonavicular ligament, depending on the relationship of the extended lever arm to the lever-arm length of the talonavicular ligament. Under realistic conditions, the tensile stresses generated by executing a corner kick (with an initial ball speed of 50–80 km/h) are estimated at ~ 1200 N. This load is within physiologic limits and does not exceed the stress tolerance of the ligament. But a poor kicking posture will increase the tensile stress on the talonavicular ligament to as much as 3000 N, which approaches the stress limit and poses a risk of acute injury.

Musculoskeletal Adaptation through Asymmetrical Muscular Changes

In addition to direct changes to the ankle joint in response to kicking movements, soccer players also tend to develop asymmetrical muscle changes in the kicking leg and supporting leg. From a biomechanical standpoint, the kicking movement of the leg is an "open kinetic chain" action in which the foot is moved at maximum forward speed (moving point) while the hip is relatively stationary (fixed point). At the same time, every kicking movement will impose a "closed kinetic chain" type of load on the nonkicking side. In this case, the foot is planted on the ground (fixed point), while the overlying structures of the pelvic-leg axis and torso are in motion (moving point) and therefore have to be stabilized against gravity through complex coordination. Various neuromuscular control actions, especially those that stabilize the knee joint and the entire lumbar–pelvis–hip region, initiate long-term muscular adaptations to these soccer-specific movement patterns. Current research shows that active musculoskeletal structures progressively adapt to the characteristic movements that they perform and the loads associated with those movements to develop an optimized muscular response.

Reports in the literature describe significant muscular differences between the support leg and kicking leg in soccer players. Shooting the ball is a multiple-joint movement in which an (apparently) explosive extension of the knee is combined with active flexion of the hip and extension (plantar flexion) of the foot at the ankle joint. Knebel et al. (1988) describe an increased maximum strength capacity and striking force of quadriceps muscle contraction during extension on the kicking-leg side, accompanied by an increased maximum strength and striking force of the knee flexors on the support side.

These general tendencies (quadriceps stronger on the kicking side, hamstrings stronger on the support side) vary in different playing positions according to the re-

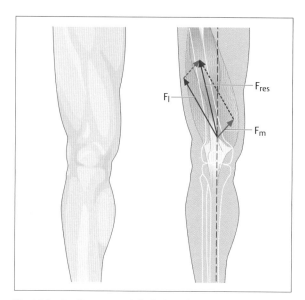

Fig. 14.2   Configuration of the kicking leg. The quadriceps muscle and lateralization. Direction of quadriceps pull.

F_{res} Resultant direction of quadriceps pull
F_l Direction of vastus lateralis pull
F_m Direction of vastus medialis pull

quirements of those positions. Goalkeepers show the greatest degree of extensor dominance. This results from their specialized ready position, in which the knees are flexed almost 90°. For biomechanical reasons, this posture inhibits coactivation of the flexor muscles to stabilize the knee joints and eliminates the contribution of the hamstrings to knee extension. This corresponds to "Lombard's paradox," which states that a contribution to knee extension is only possible at up to ~ 50–60° of knee flexion. As a result, the goalie has to rely entirely on the knee and hip extensors when initiating a jump from the ready position. This action requires considerable extensor power as a

functional response to the soccer-specific demands of training and play. Strikers, on the other hand, have to be able to react and accelerate their locomotor apparatus as quickly as possible. Their flexor–extensor ratio thus allows for very effective coactivation of the flexor muscles and closely resembles the proportions that are found in sprinters.

Musculoskeletal Adaptation through Neurophysiologic Changes

Empirical observations on the degree of quadriceps muscle development in soccer players suggest additional neurophysiologic aspects and considerations relating to long-term functional adaptations. Although soccer players have greater quadriceps strength on the kicking side than on the support side, examination of the thighs in most players will show that the thigh circumference is slightly reduced in the area where the vastus medialis muscle is most fully developed. The variable "muscular configuration" of the quadriceps appears to be an adaptive response of the musculoskeletal system to years of locally varying, stereotypical functional demands (see above). **Figure 14.2** shows the general lateralization of the quadriceps action that develops in the kicking leg of right-footed soccer players due to deficiency of the vastus medialis.

From a neurophysiologic standpoint, a "chronic" vastus medialis deficiency in the kicking leg can be explained by the reduced need for open kinetic-chain activity to stabilize the knee joint in terms of tibial rotation relative to the femur in response to gravitational effects. The innervation pattern gradually adapts and becomes optimized for kicking a soccer ball. This process alters the relative contributions of the individual quadriceps muscles to the resultant quadriceps force. Deficiency of the vastus medialis tends to lateralize the quadriceps pull on the patella, thereby altering the kinematics of the femoropatellar joint (**Fig. 14.2**). If the lateralizing effect causes patellar rotation, this will reduce the area of contact between the retropa-

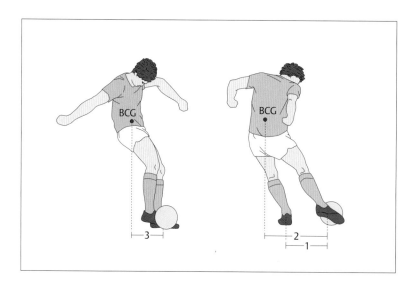

Fig. 14.3   Instep kick viewed in the frontal and sagittal planes. BCG, body's center of gravity.

1 Distance from the foot of the supporting leg to the center of the ball
2 Distance from the BCG axis to the ball center of gravity
3 Distance from the BCG axis to the foot of the supporting leg

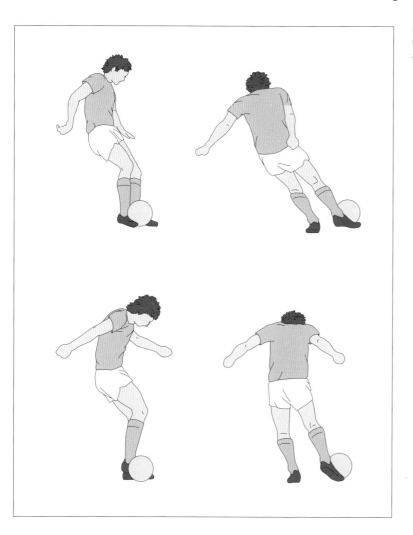

Fig. 14.4 Intraindividual differences in the position of the supporting leg for an instep kick (right-footed player).

tellar cartilage and femoral articular surface, and this could accelerate degenerative changes in the long term. By contrast, the loads on the supporting leg during running and sprinting usually do not alter the physiologic pattern of intra-articular kinematics.

Note

Degenerative changes in the femoropatellar joint are more common on the kicking side than on the support side.

More research is needed to clarify the neurophysiologic relationships.

Support Leg Changes Caused by Kicking Technique

The changes in the kicking leg described above suggest that the contralateral support leg is subjected to different loads during the kicking of a soccer ball. It is interesting that all soccer players, regardless of performance level, tend to place their support leg in a very precise position when shooting the ball (i.e., when executing an instep kick or an inside/outside kick). This causes a highly consistent pattern of stereotypical loads to act on the musculoskeletal structures (**Fig. 14.3**). To permit successful ball acceleration by the kicking leg with effective momentum transfer to the ball, the support leg must be planted next to the ball on the ground. The following observations are important in this regard:

- Soccer players plant their support leg next to the ball with remarkable consistency and precision. Tests have shown that intraindividual differences from one ball contact to the next are less than 1 cm!
- Soccer players plant their support leg level with the ball (relative to the frontal plane).
- As the foot is planted on the ground, the body's center of gravity shifts outward toward the support leg, usually moving past the left knee or even farther laterally.
- The lateral distance of the support leg from the ball can vary markedly from one player to the next. Despite

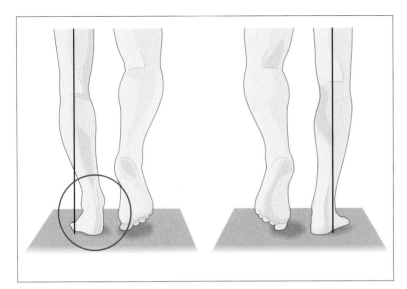

these differences, however, the individual movement patterns are performed with great precision (intraindividual consistency). However, the farther the support leg is placed from the ball, the greater the lateral shift of the body's center of gravity (**Fig. 14.4**). The joints along the left pelvic–leg axis have to stabilize and compensate for this position and adapt to it over time.

These side-specific changes are most clearly appreciated in the ankle joint. The greater the lateralization of the pelvic–leg axis, the greater the lateral and shear forces acting on the joints of the foot. These forces will evoke long-term adaptations even in the absence of trauma or injuries. These changes are reflected not just in the stereotypical kicking actions that occur during training and play, but also in ordinary walking and running. They document the overall adaptations of the pelvic–leg axis (**Fig. 14.5**).

Adaptations of the Pelvic–Leg Axis

The neurophysiologic changes described above that occur on the supporting and kicking sides in response to playing stresses also induce long-term changes in the healthy lumbopelvic–hip region. The dominance of the powerful quadriceps and hip flexors (especially the iliopsoas muscle) on the kicking side causes the pelvis to tilt posteriorly on that side. This in turn causes an anterior pelvic tilt to develop on the opposite side in an effort to stabilize the body's center of gravity. These changes are often accompanied by a decreased range of motion in the sacroiliac joint on the kicking side. The asymmetrical range of motion, combined with the twisting of the hips, causes an apparent lengthening of the support-leg axis and leads to functional pelvic obliquity. Additionally, the new stress patterns are transmitted to the structures of the lumbar spine. As a result of the posterior pelvic tilt on the kicking

side, physical examination of soccer players will often show that the lumbar spine is rotated to the right due to increased tension on the iliolumbar ligaments.

Caution
This hip torsion may adversely affect various musculoskeletal structures and should be noted and evaluated by sports physical therapists.

Adaptations in the kicking leg:
- Posterior pelvic tilt and inflare
- Decreased sacroiliac joint motion
- Iliotibial tract
- Vastus medialis atrophy
- Patellar dyskinesia
- Decreased range of plantar flexion
- Supinator weakness or endurance loss due to eccentric muscle actions
- Supinated limb position

Adaptations in the support leg:
- Upright ilium and outflare
- Normal sacroiliac joint motion
- Increased valgus angulation at the knee
- Groin problems
- Adductors? (Visceral causes)
- Increased external rotation of the foot
- Hyperpronation
- Plantar insertional tendinopathy
- Pronated limb position

It should be noted that the above listing covers expected gross musculoskeletal adaptations in soccer players. It does not provide a comprehensive differential diagnosis of sacroiliac, iliosacral, or other changes (see p. 337).

Physical Therapy Implications for the Myofascial System

Given the variety of sport-specific musculoskeletal adaptations that are induced by the stress patterns associated with stereotypical sport-specific movements (illustrated here for soccer players), it is reasonable to expect that there will also be numerous changes in the joints, ligaments, and myofascial system. This should motivate the members of sports medicine teams to familiarize themselves with the stress dimensions of the specific movement patterns that are performed in their particular sport, make an initial qualitative assessment of adaptive changes (which must be consistent with the functional demands of the sport, biomechanical dimensions, and clinical findings), and empirically determine the quantitative extent of the changes.

With regard to soccer, which we have used here as an example, we can confirm the occurrence of changes and side-specific adaptations affecting all the joints and ligaments of the lower limb, musculoskeletal and/or myofascial structures, and the entire functional unit of the pelvic–leg axis with its associated muscular chains. The changes vary in degree among different players, depending on individual predisposition and the duration (years of training) and quantity (scope of training) of the loads and stereotypical movement patterns. The changes may be a source of problems. A distinction is made between "ascending" and "descending" cause-and-effect chains, depending on the primary cause. This means that dysfunction in the joints of the foot can act through an ascending causal chain to induce changes in the joints of the pelvic–leg axis and in affected myofascial structures of the muscular chains. The body will try to engineer the changes in such a way that stereotypical movements (e.g., soccer instep kicks) can be performed economically, while adverse adaptive effects on individual joints are kept to a minimum.

When the pelvic–leg axis is considered as a whole, it is found that the lumbopelvic–hip region and the knee joint are particularly important in this regard. Owing to their ingenious design and highly complex functional capabilities, changes in both ascending and descending cause-and-effect chains are particularly likely to alter the muscular chains in these structures. This will also make it more likely that the changes will overload the biological structures in these regions. Even in the absence of trauma, the structures will be unable to return to their original "point of balanced tension." Sports physical therapists have certain techniques at their disposal that enable them to restore soccer players to their former functional capacity and performance while also minimizing or even preventing adverse changes in myofascial structures and potential muscle injuries.

Treatment-Oriented Assessment Strategy

An understanding of sport-specific adaptations makes it easier to devise appropriate strategies for the treatment of sports-related muscle injuries. When properly applied, these strategies can consistently return athletes to a normal level of muscular performance. Based on the functional relationships described above and their implications for sports physical therapy in the prevention and rehabilitation of muscle injuries, it is essential to formulate a therapeutic assessment strategy once a medical evaluation and intervention have been completed.

The responses of the myofascial system to loads and stresses, as well as reactions to injuries and insults (e.g., mechanical, chemical, emotional), are diverse and are a common predisposing factor for dysfunction.

Note

Prompt recognition of stress factors and chronic loads and the development of appropriate treatment strategies for reducing the stresses should be the first priority in sports physical therapy.

The information obtained from the medical evaluation (see Chapter 6) forms the basis for physical therapy services, and all such information should be available to the care and treatment team for muscle-injured athletes. Ideally, the attending physician or team physician will discuss this information with the team and establish the framework for a complex treatment strategy.

From the standpoint of sports physical therapy, it is helpful initially to classify the muscle injury according to the presence or absence of associated intramuscular bleeding or hematoma (**Table 14.1**). This is a pragmatic and therapeutically important criterion, based on the classification of muscle injuries described in Chapter 6. The therapeutic implications of a muscle injury will differ considerably depending on the presence or absence of hemorrhage. At the same time, the treatment techniques for muscle injuries that are associated with intramuscular bleeding are very similar to one another and generally differ only in their intensity.

Once a medical diagnosis has been established, the next step is to assess the extent of the muscle injury using the scheme described below (**Table 14.2**).

Table 14.1   Classification of muscle injuries

Structural injury with intramuscular bleeding	Structural injury without intramuscular bleeding
Minor partial muscle tear	Excessive or unphysiologic mechanical loading
Moderate partial muscle tear	Excessive or unphysiologic mechanical loading
Subtotal or complete muscle tear	Discontinuity
	Cylinder distortion
	Herniated trigger points

Table 14.2   Results of muscle function tests and their association with different types of lesion

Findings	Injury	Type of lesion
Strength ↓ **Pain** ↑	Neuromuscular dysfunction	Spine-related or muscle-related neuromuscular disorder (type 2a or 2b)
Strength ↓ **Pain** ↑	Structural muscle injury	Minor partial muscle tear Moderate partial muscle tear (type 3a or 3b)
No strength **Pain** ↑ ↑	Structural muscle injury	Subtotal/complete muscle tear (type 4)

Clinical Therapeutic Assessment

With regard to the clinical therapeutic assessment of muscle-injured athletes, it should first be noted that we cannot thoroughly explore here the fundamental aspects and principles of therapeutic assessment. Details of medical assessment, clinical examination, and palpation can be found in Chapter 6 of this book and in the specialist literature (Kaltenborn and Evjenth 1999a, 1999b; Van den Berg 2001; Eder and Hoffmann 2006). It is assumed that the reader is familiar with the practical aspects of clinical and manual therapeutic tests.

The multitude of physical therapy training curricula and continuing education programs that are available cover a wide range of approaches to clinical therapeutic assessment that are beyond the scope of this chapter. Our focus here will be limited to key aspects of assessment that will have a major bearing on treatment strategies and have proven their effectiveness in complex strategies for treating sports-related muscle injuries. Of course, other concepts and associated tests for clinical therapeutic assessment can make useful and important contributions

Practical Tip

An awareness of functional anatomic relationships and of the physiologic demands in different sports can yield important insights into the structure, extent, and quality of unphysiologic loads acting on the musculoskeletal system during an actual trauma event, which are helpful in estimating the dimensions of a potential muscle injury. It is good practice, therefore, for the sports physical therapist (ideally working with the team physician, though this is rarely the case) to be present during a match, and even during training if possible, so that he or she can closely observe the relevant events and patterns of movement. In the case of an injury, these observations can help to shape the therapeutic assessment process.

even though they are not explicitly mentioned in this chapter. Just as the authors' focus is influenced by their own training and continuing education and their personal range of experience in sports physical therapy, our readers will also draw upon their own repertoire of knowledge and experience and should view our discussions as an impetus for exploring alternative techniques and corresponding models and perhaps integrating them into their own practice.

In this regard, newer models and ways of envisioning musculoskeletal injuries have placed the myofascia in a different light. Stephen Typaldos (1999), for example, described empirically proven measures for treating myofascial changes and lesions that have influenced the way we think about myofascial relationships. In an effort to explain therapeutic phenomena, Typaldos developed a model in which the myofascial system consists partly of parallel fibers that transmit information to higher nerve centers in response to momentary forces (see also Chapter 1). According to Typaldos, the myofascial system functions as a "sensor for mechanical stresses." The individual fibers have a natural tone analogous to a stringed instrument in which each string has been individually tuned. When loaded or stressed, these structures transmit a steady flow of proprioceptive information to higher centers. Thus, a proprioceptive discharge is evoked by the tension that develops when a muscle is stretched or shortened. This concept has a direct bearing on therapeutic techniques (e.g., strain–counterstrain, spray and stretch; see pp. 349–350) that are used in the treatment of various muscle injuries (see section on "Physical Therapy and Physical Medicine" in Chapter 11) and will be described below.

The body language of the injured athlete can supply important diagnostic clues. For example, an athlete with a structural muscle injury will not only point to the injured site, but will also experience significant functional impairment. Involvement of the connective tissues will also cause autonomic dysfunction in many cases (e.g., nausea, cold sweats, etc.). Palpation reveals not only a discontinuity but also a typical "mushy feel" caused by hematoma formation, and this will suggest appropriate therapeutic measures (see the section on "Physical Therapy and Physical Medicine" in Chapter 11). Unlike a muscle injury with intramuscular bleeding, a muscle-related neuromuscular muscle disorder (type 2b lesion) with its associated dysfunction of neuromuscular control mechanisms can be envisioned as a distorted fascial band. This condition is manifested clinically by contractions that are painful, weak, and poorly coordinated.

> *Note*
>
> **Besides palpating the injury, the practitioner should also note the body language of the injured athlete, as this can be an extremely helpful diagnostic criterion.**

It should also be noted that the model used to explain and conceptualize an injury will have a major impact on subsequent treatment. The classic orthopedic model taught that traumatized tissue only needs time to heal. By contrast, the treatment strategy described by Typaldos also aims at releasing the fascial distortion, with the goal of restoring neuromuscular control mechanisms to internal fascial structures. This explains why treatment based on the fascial distortion model can yield an immediate positive result with recovery of muscle function, owing to the lack of structural damage and the absence of a true regenerative phase.

Clinical Motion Analysis

While clinical tests in the setting of therapeutic assessment can tell us what structure has been injured and the type of lesion that has occurred, techniques of clinical motion analysis can investigate the patient's current level of motor function during everyday activities and especially during sport-specific patterns of movement. Clinical motion analysis may combine objective kinematic, dynamic (or kinemetric) test procedures (quantitative aspect) with subjective observations and/or palpation (qualitative aspect).

A range of parameters can be analyzed:
- *Kinematic parameters:*
  - Point-oriented systems:
    - Ultrasound systems
    - Infrared systems
    - etc.
  - Image-oriented systems:
    - 2D/3D video systems
    - 2D/3D film systems
    - etc.
- *Dynamic parameters:*
  - Force measurement platforms:
    - 2D measurement platforms
    - 3D measurement platforms
  - Pressure measuring soles
  - Kinesiologic electromyogram
- *Palpation parameters*

> *Note*
>
> **Clinical motion analysis can be performed during the proliferative and remodeling phases (see p. 339) in the absence of pain. It cannot be performed during the acute or inflammatory phase.**

Test procedures:
- *Kinematic tests:* Two- or three-dimensional position analysis systems using image-oriented (film or video) or point-oriented recording techniques (active ultrasound markers, infrared reflective markers, etc.) are available for the qualitative and quantitative acquisition of spatial and temporal information, based on kinematic parameters such as position/joint angles, length/velocity parameters, and acceleration parameters. The frame rate should have adequate temporal resolution to supply precise information on targeted movements (faster movements require a higher frame rate).
- *Dynamic tests:* Dynamic tests can provide qualitative and/or quantitative information on the motion-producing forces acting at the periphery of the body (e.g., forces, torque, thrust, plantar pressures and distributions, etc.).

Kinesiologic Electromyography (EMG)

Recent advances in medical technology have led to greater utilization of kinesiologic EMG for recording and evaluating muscle activities in the areas of prevention, performance testing, and treatment, especially after muscle injuries. Given the inherent limitations of this modality, a critical discussion of the results and their interpretation is essential for avoiding misinterpretations. The recording of amplitude-oriented parameters can provide information on the time course of muscular activities: When is a particular muscle active during the course of a movement? With what muscles is it coordinated or coactivated?

The intensity of muscular activity can be evaluated only indirectly in relation to maximum isometric force by analyzing amplitude-based parameters under specific conditions. Frequency analysis can be used to evaluate the neuromuscular fatigue that occurs in certain muscles during contractions. This supplies information that is important in planning medical training therapy aimed at improving the neuromuscular performance of the musculoskeletal system at its current weak point (the most fatigued muscle showing decreased neuromuscular coordination and responsiveness).

Another limitation of kinesiologic EMG is its reliance on surface electrodes like those commonly used in physical therapy. These sensors can sample and analyze muscular activities only from a selected portion of the musculoskeletal system. In the treatment of muscle injuries, however, this test can provide important clues to current activity levels and neuromuscular integration in complex movement patterns—information that is useful in directing treatment.

Despite increasingly complex measuring techniques, current biomechanical methods cannot yet supply highly precise and detailed information on intra-articular kinetics and movement patterns. There is no measuring system that can quantitatively analyze the important lumbopelvic–hip region, with its small-amplitude movements, due to the presence of overlying soft tissues. The practitioner can do no more than make a qualitative evaluation of this region by palpating it during specified movements. By taking the functional consequences into account, the therapist can use this information to evaluate overall motor function following a muscle injury. The best way to obtain this information is by having the patient walk a treadmill while the therapist palpates the appropriate anatomic reference points over several strides without having to make adjustments for individual step rate. Experience has shown, however, that changes in the kinematics and dynamics of overall motor function during walking or running on a treadmill caused by the alternation of fixed and moving points, plus the resulting effects on neuromuscular control, affect only the quantitative aspects of movements along the pelvic–leg axis without altering their qualitative features.

Caution

Clinical motion analysis on a treadmill can be performed in a painless speed range following muscle injuries without intramuscular bleeding (functional muscle disorders, —that is, overexertion-related or neuromuscular muscle disorders) immediately after the acute or inflammatory phase (starting on the second or third day after the injury). In the case of muscle injuries that are accompanied by a hematoma (structural muscle injuries—that is, minor and moderate partial muscle tears, subtotal tears), clinical motion analysis at painless speeds should be withheld until the proliferative phase (not before the fifth post-traumatic day) or even later, depending on the extent of the injury.

Methods Used in Medical Training Therapy: Rehabilitative Performance Testing

Note

Rehabilitative performance testing is essential for directing the training process in competitive and professional sports, as it supplies information on the current level of an athlete's performance.

Sport-specific performance testing follows a specific rhythm and uses test procedures that yield current qualitative and/or quantitative information on a particular aspect of interest—usually the description of basic motor capabilities. The methods described below have become well established in the care of competitive athletes:

- *Lactate analysis and spiroergometry* to measure stamina and for intensity-oriented evaluation of energy metabolism
- *Force measurement techniques* to evaluate musculoskeletal performance (single- and multiple-joint forces, jump force testing, etc.)
- *Measurement techniques for assessing coordination*, for indirect evaluation of proprioceptive capacities
- *Combined measuring systems* (photoelectric sensors, contact mats, and sensing platforms) used in quickness or sprint testing to measure various *sport-specific quickness parameters*
- *Complex measuring systems for analyzing functions and movements*

Because the stress tolerance of biological structures is usually diminished after musculoskeletal injuries, all methods of performance testing that are available in sports science and medicine cannot be applied to rehabilitative performance testing without due consideration, and they cannot all be utilized to good effect within the framework of complex treatment strategies. On the other hand, the arsenal of test procedures and measuring techniques has expanded considerably in recent years, and many new types of equipment have become available.

As the "bar" for athletic performance levels has been raised over the years, the importance of rehabilitative performance testing has also increased as a means of controlling the training stimuli in medical training therapy. Starting in the 1970s, when muscle-circumference measurements and the neutral-zero method provided seemingly objective tools for documenting the results of orthopedic and trauma rehabilitation, the first true diagnostic systems were established in the mid-1980s. Today it would be unthinkable to have objective documentation without performance measurement techniques. A regular, basic conditioning assessment as well as the qualitative and quantitative documentation of the functional capacity of the musculoskeletal system allow for the rapid formulation and updating of treatment goals while also docu-

Table 14.3 Procedures used in rehabilitative performance testing

Test procedures used in physical modalities	Biofeedback documentation in electrotherapy
	Evaluation and documentation of the energy system
	Etc.
Test procedures used in manual therapy	Evaluation and documentation of joint motion ranges (goniometry)
	Evaluation and documentation of proprioception
	Evaluation and documentation of spinal column status (statics and range of motion)
	Evaluation and documentation of connective tissue status
	Etc.
Test procedures used in medical training therapy	Evaluation and documentation of selected strength parameters of the musculoskeletal system
	Evaluation and documentation of selected endurance parameters of the musculoskeletal system
	Evaluation and documentation of selected quickness parameters of the musculoskeletal system
	Evaluation and documentation of selected neuromuscular control parameters of the musculoskeletal system
	Etc.

menting the progress of rehabilitation. In this way, significant muscular imbalances and asymmetries in biologically relevant parameters can be recognized at an earlier stage and corrected without delay. As treatment progresses, the objective data should serve as indicators for controlling and adjusting the stimulus levels during therapy.

The goal of the measurements is to obtain qualitative and quantitative data of acceptable accuracy (conforming to the main quality criteria of reliability, validity, and objectivity) with respect to the following parameters:

- Stamina
- Strength
- Quickness
- Mobility
- Neuromuscular qualities (coordination)
- Functional capacity

The test procedures available for evaluating and documenting muscular performance are listed and categorized in **Table 14.3**.

Isokinetic Testing and Training Systems

Basic Principles

Isokinetic testing and training systems occupy a special place among the methods available for musculoskeletal performance testing. After more than 40 years of clinical experience and practical application in competitive sports and the rehabilitation of musculoskeletal injuries, and a multitude of scientific publications (PubMed lists over 2000 titles published in the past 20 years), isokinetic testing and training systems have become standard equipment at centers specializing in the rehabilitation of professional athletes.

> *Note*
>
> Isokinetic testing and training systems allow for isokinetic movement patterns, defined as exercises performed on an apparatus that provides maximum accommodating resistance to a movement, so that the movement takes place at a constant speed (Hollmann and Hettinger 1990).

> *Caution*
>
> Given the reduced stress tolerance of injured biologic structures and especially of the myofascial system following muscle injuries, performance tests that yield quantitative stress data should be performed with great care in rehabilitating athletes. Especially after muscle injuries, strength tests (including isokinetic strength tests) are appropriate only if the myofascial system can safely withstand the stresses imposed by the test movement without risk of reinjury, consistent with the constraints imposed by wound healing. Maximum-stress test movements in either an open or closed chain would violate this principle if done in the acute or inflammatory phase or in the proliferative phase. The potential risk of test movements involving eccentric muscular activities should be carefully decided on a case-by-case basis.

The isokinetic system thus varies the resistance to musculoskeletal effort in such a way that, no matter how much effort is exerted, the movements take place at a constant speed. The patient tries to exert a maximum force against the resistance, which is insurmountable over the whole amplitude of the movement. Isokinetic resistance has the following advantages over training with free weights and/or training apparatus with weighted resistance:

- *Muscular physiology aspect:* The performance capacity of the musculoskeletal system is length-specific, as the ability of individual muscle fibers to develop tension depends on their length and thus on the number of possible actin–myosin cross-links. On the one hand, therefore, isokinetic training can apply maximal loads to the musculoskeletal system (e.g., for performance testing). But at the same time, this type of training can help prevent overloads to injured muscles in areas with reduced stress tolerance, as the apparatus will vary the resistance according to the effort exerted by the patient.
- *Mechanical–physical aspect:* Any change in the speed of a moving mass that is accelerating or decelerating will meet with an increase or decrease in resistance as a result of inertia. This effect is eliminated or minimized in isokinetic exercises. Following (muscle) injuries, these peak loads may give rise to potentially damaging stresses during training exercises. An isokinetic system permits safer and more controlled exercising of the musculoskeletal system despite the presence of potential lesions.

During the past 40 years, the development of isokinetic testing and training systems has been marked by steady progress, with expanded capabilities for performance testing, force analysis, and therapeutic training (**Table**

14.4). These devices can analyze the performance of the musculoskeletal system, using rotary systems for jointed areas (movements in an open kinetic chain) or linear systems for a "chain-oriented" analysis (movements in a closed kinetic chain). The resultant force exerted by synergistic muscle actions can be accurately described in terms of two parameters:

- Force and/or torque
- Temporal or positional information

Corresponding data curves (**Fig. 14.6**) can be plotted to allow accurate side-to-side comparison of musculoskeletal performance and to document the progression of performance.

Interpretation of Results

The following special considerations should be noted when interpreting the test results and drawing conclusions on how to conduct medical training therapy after muscle injuries. The torque-angle curves plotted for single-joint measurements have the following characteristics:

- The shapes of the curves are synergist-specific.
- The synergist-antagonist relationships are joint-specific.
- The curve shapes and synergist-antagonist relationships have a velocity-specific character and variability.
- Typical sport-specific adaptations and changes are found.

These facts require a detailed understanding of the special characteristics and capabilities of isokinetic testing and training systems in the setting of complex treatment strategies, so that current musculoskeletal performance levels can be adequately evaluated and the proper conclusions

Table 14.4   Development and classification of isokinetic testing and training systems

Classification criterion	Classification	Type of muscular action	Integration of biodynamic parameters
Type of drive	Passive systems (since 1968)	Isometric	
		Concentric	
	Active systems (since 1983)	Isometric	
		Concentric	
		Eccentric	
Function	Rotary systems (since 1968)	Isometric	Electromyography (since 1968)
		Concentric	
		Eccentric	
	Linear systems (since 1984)	Isometric	Electromyography (since 1968)
		Concentric	Goniometer (since 1988)
		Eccentric	Sensing platform (plantar pressure; since 1990)

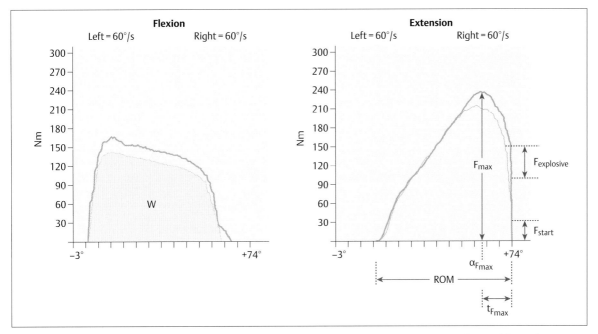

Fig. 14.6 Graphic representation of resultant joint-specific, synergistic musculoskeletal performance, illustrated for single-joint measurements with a rotatory isokinetic system. In this example, the plots for the right and left sides have been superimposed to allow side-to-side comparisons.

W	Work (thrust, area integral of the torque–time curve)
F_{max}	Maximum force
α_{Fmax}	Joint angle at which maximum torque is achieved
F_{start}	Starting force = curve rise over a specified time interval from start of movement (usually 50 ms in the literature)

$F_{explosive}$	Explosive force = force increase over a specified time interval during the steepest upslope until F_{max} is reached
ROM	Range of motion (amplitude of movement)
t_{Fmax}	Time to F_{max}

drawn for the optimum conduct of medical training therapy in muscle-injured athletes. With these factors in mind, use of the training systems in the rehabilitation of muscle injuries can achieve a very precise grading and localization of muscle tension (at least in the synergists), so that an appropriate tension stimulus can be delivered to the injured muscular structures.

An effective strategy in the rehabilitation of muscle injuries is to combine isokinetic testing and training systems with electromyographic measurements, which can provide specific information on the following parameters:

- *Coordination aspect:* post-traumatic neuromuscular integration into complex movements of the injured muscle
- *Intensity aspect:* degree of tension developed in the injured muscle during the movement
- *Energy aspect:* degree of fatigue of the injured muscle during specified motor tasks

This approach also makes it possible to exercise the muscles in any desired mode of action (isometric, concentric, and eccentric contractions) while tension and metabolism are monitored.

Regarding recent developments in isokinetic technology, purely isokinetic modes of testing and training have been expanded to produce modern system solutions in the form of neuromuscular testing and training systems. These systems offer new training capabilities for the selective recovery of musculoskeletal functions and performance, especially after muscle injuries. In the case of single-joint and/or multiple-joint exercises, even when performed from a defined starting position, special programs have been developed for selectively training and conditioning the stability of a joint by the coordinated intramuscular and intermuscular activation of the joint-stabilizing synergists and antagonists. This occurs without overloading the injured musculoskeletal structures or exceeding the current level of stress tolerance. While the training system tries to deflect the subject from a stabilized position to a destabilized position by exerting controlled forces (which are safely below the maximum isometric force), the neuromuscular system has to activate the specific muscles that can counter the destabilization. Information on the reaction time to the onset of stabilizing muscular contractions, on the time course of the activation, and on the effectiveness of the "function reversal" by a change in the direction of the deflecting forces permits an accurate evaluation of the functional capacity of the neuromuscular system and thus provides valuable guides for the further planning of medical training therapy with minimal risk of overloading the injured muscle areas.

All information from the clinical therapeutic assessment, the clinical motion analysis, and the various areas of rehabilitative performance testing based on the medical diagnosis should yield a reasonably accurate picture of the muscle injury and of the current post-traumatic status of the musculoskeletal system. Ideally, all of this information is constantly communicated within the therapy team. The team members work jointly to coordinate further measures and/or adapt them to any changes—whether in the form of progress or problems. It is important to define the necessary measures of physical therapy and physical modalities and the contents of the training therapy program, as well as revise and adapt the measures as circumstances require (see below).

Note

The selection of appropriate therapeutic measures is not sufficient in itself to achieve the desired outcome. The optimum sequencing and coordination of the individual measures and activities is also necessary to ensure a swift and efficient rehabilitation of muscle injuries with the recovery of musculoskeletal functional capacity and performance. This requires effective communication among all the professionally diverse members of the therapy team.

Strategies for the Treatment of Muscle Injuries

Immediate Measures

This section begins with a look at the initial care measures that can be rendered on site in an acutely injured athlete to prevent further harm. The goal of these immediate measures is to limit or minimize the long-term biological and functional effects of the injury without using diagnostic instruments and without making a precise diagnosis. Proper actions by the medical team (regardless of their medical and therapeutic qualifications) during this phase can significantly shorten the duration of subsequent rehabilitation for various indications and promote the functional recovery of injured muscles. Afterward, care is informed by an established diagnosis and involves the complex treatment measures that are appropriate for specific types of muscle injury.

Muscle injuries, which may also involve injuries to ligaments and/or joints, will usually present the following symptoms:
- Local pain in the joint and/or muscles
- Pain on standing, walking, and other activities
- Pain in response to muscular contraction or stretch
- Possible swelling

We should emphasize the importance of identifying the actual mechanism of the injury so that the associated kinematic and dynamic stressors and load dimensions, as well as the functional effects on injured biological structures, can be properly assessed. Certainly, the athletic trainer for a youth or senior soccer team who has no specialized medical or therapeutic training will find it harder to make such an assessment than an experienced sports medicine practitioner or physical therapist who has several years' experience working on the sidelines for a professional team. The experienced caregiver is in a much better position to judge whether the injured athlete can reasonably continue to train or compete, or whether the athlete should be removed from active training and play.

Equipment

Note

The medical team should adequately prepare for any injuries that may occur during training or competition and should maintain a first-aid kit containing all necessary supplies. The first-aid kit is the basic tool of the sports physical therapist and should be diligently stocked and replenished.

The following equipment is needed for the initial care of muscle-injured athletes:
- *Sports medicine kit* (**Fig. 14.7a**): The sports medicine kit is a full-sized case stocked with a comprehensive array of materials for first aid and injury prevention. The contents are organized so that necessary items can be quickly identified and accessed, making it easier to render care and restock the case. Tear-open packages are used to ensure that items are clean and well protected. Space is also available for adding items of personal preference.
- *Trainer's bag:* While the sports medicine kit stays in the locker room, the trainer's bag is stocked with essential supplies for rendering first aid on the playing field (**Fig. 14.7b**). The trainer's bag is kept on the sidelines and carried onto the field as needed. Designed for treating injuries sustained on the field during practice or competition, the bag contains all necessary items for rendering first aid until the athlete is either taken from the field or returned to play. The following contents have proven effective for acute use on the playing field:
  - Adhesive bandage strips in various sizes
  - Steri-Strips for closing gaping wounds, and/or Histoacryl glue
  - Sterile gauze pads
  - Hemostatic cotton
  - Cohesive (self-adhering) bandages, used for holding a dressing or pad in place
  - Denatured alcohol for cleaning the injury site

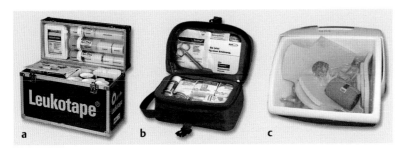

Fig. 14.7a–c Necessary first-aid equipment for sports injuries (photos **a** and **b** courtesy of BSN Medical Ltd., Hamburg, Germany).

a Sports medicine kit.
b Trainer's bag.
c Ice chest.

- Coolant spray (preferably ethyl chloride, as it rapidly cools the skin to approximately −20°C, numbing the pain nerves)
- Bandage shears
- Forceps
- Wooden blade and/or tube for intraoral injuries so that the oral cavity of an unconscious injured player does not have to be cleaned with fingers (possible foreign bodies: teeth, grass, snow, etc.)
- Elastic and nonelastic tapes in various widths
- Eyewash
- Penlight for testing pupillary reaction
- Japanese herbal oil ("second wind")
- Head bandage
- *Ice chest:* A portable cooler filled with ice water (**Fig. 14.7c**) should be available in addition to the trainer's bag. The cooler should contain prefabricated foam rubber protectors for applying cold wet compresses after blunt trauma and muscle injuries. It should also contain a sponge. One or two elastic bandages should also be stored in the ice water. The bandages should not be too old, or they may lose their compressing and hemostatic effect.

Caution

Ethyl chloride should always be sprayed over a larger area and should not be used for too long. It should not form an icy crust. Freezing of the skin must be strictly avoided!

Initial Inspection

The following priorities should be followed during initial inspection of the injury on the practice or playing field:
- Question the injured athlete about the location and quality of the pain (if present).
- Palpate the injured area to check for discontinuities, etc.
- Cool the affected limb with a coolant spray (e.g., ethyl chloride). Spray in multiple short bursts (each no more than 5–10 seconds long), keeping the nozzle at least 30 cm from the skin. Do not treat for longer than 1 minute. An ice-water–cooled sponge taken from the ice chest can also be applied to the injured site (a cloth or sock may be placed between the sponge and skin).

- Review the decision-making criteria for returning the athlete to play or continuing treatment on the sidelines or in the locker room.

Further Treatment on the Sidelines or in the Locker Room

The following measures are important in this setting:
- Cold and compression
- Elevation
- Referral to a physician

Whenever possible, the psychoautonomic state of the acutely injured athlete should be a priority concern. A calm, safe environment should be created (close the locker-room door, have all nonessential persons leave the room). This will also help to foster trust between the athlete and physician and/or therapist. Despite the unsettling nature of the situation, many athletes will benefit from a positive and calming demeanor and choice of words to ensure that mental and autonomic status will not adversely affect the injured tissues.

Cold Wet Compress

A cold wet compress is applied at a pressure of 20 MPa to suppress the exaggerated host response to injury (see p. 338). This pressure, comparable to that exerted by an elastic bandage, is high enough to limit the dilation of blood vessels, but is too low to interfere with autoregenerative processes.

To apply a cold wet compress, the therapist or physician uses a prefabricated foam-rubber protector taken from the ice chest. The purpose of the protector is to distribute the pressure evenly over a maximum area.

First, the injury site is palpated (**Fig. 14.8a**) and outlined with a marker. Next, a foam-rubber protector, previously cut to size, is taken from the ice water in the cooler and placed in a convex position over the center of the lesion (**Fig. 14.8b**). Elastic tape, also kept in ice water, is then wrapped around the pack from below upward to a tensile stress of ~ 20 MPa (**Fig. 14.8c**).

Alcohol should never be taken after an injury, regardless of the type and severity of the muscle trauma. This should be explained in particular to injured amateur athletes.

Establishing the Diagnosis

Once initial care measures have been completed, the player is referred to a physician as quickly as possible so that the injury can be competently diagnosed. If this requires prolonged transport, the cold wet compression bandage should be changed every 20 minutes to maintain a skin temperature of ~ 10°C and promote the intended physiologic effects (preventing or minimizing a potential hematoma, suppressing the host response to injury, and avoiding interference with reparative metabolic processes).

Note

An incorrect diagnosis leads to incorrect treatment!

Additional therapeutic measures for various indications are detailed in the section on "Physical Therapy and Physical Medicine" in Chapter 11.

Relieving Muscle Taping

Once initial care measures have been completed and the injury has been fully diagnosed, taping may be done to protect and support various types of structural muscle injuries, including minor and moderate partial muscle tears as well as subtotal and complete tears. When done after the acute or inflammatory phase and in the early proliferative phase after the wound has closed (see p. 338), muscle taping can help relieve tension on the injured muscle fibers and redirect tension trajectories in the affected limb.

Caution

Taping is contraindicated for complete muscle tears, as well as massive hematomas and varices.

Muscle tape should be replaced after new therapeutic measures. The tape can be worn for up to 2 days.

Key principles in muscle taping include the use of semicircular anchor strips and a symmetrical application of the support strips, as permitted by the surface anatomy of the affected area. The affected muscle area should be relaxed during the actual taping, but a static functional load should be placed on the affected limb while the final overwrap is applied. Additional general information on the methods and practical aspects of muscle taping can be found in the specialized literature (e.g., Eder and Mommsen 2007).

The technique of muscle taping can be illustrated here by describing the steps involved in taping an injured calf

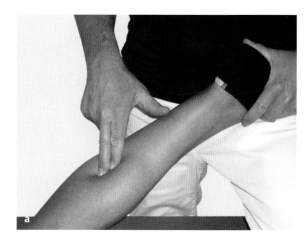

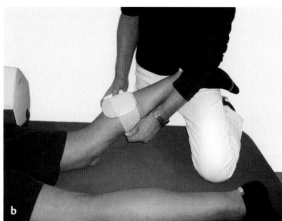

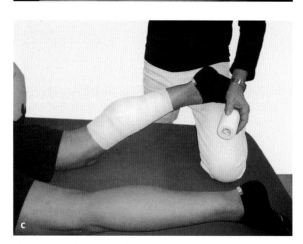

Fig. 14.8a–c   Technique for applying a cold wet compression bandage.

a The injured muscle is palpated.
b The foam-rubber protector is placed over the injured muscle.
c The protector is secured to the muscle with elastic tape.

muscle. First, the patient lies in a relaxed prone position with the knee on the injured side flexed ~ 45°. In this position, the entire lower leg is prewrapped with a suitable underlay material (**Fig. 14.9a**). Next, a distal anchor is applied above the malleoli, and a proximal anchor 3.75 cm wide is applied at the level of the upper tibia (**Fig. 14.9b**). Both anchors are semicircular strips that leave a gap over the anterior tibial margin. Next, a longitudinal anchor is applied to connect the proximal and distal anchors, again leaving the tibial margin free (**Fig. 14.9c**). The lengths of the 2-cm-wide support strips (therapy strips) are determined by measuring from the proximal to the distal anchor. The first series of support strips are applied loosely and fixed to the proximal anchor (**Fig. 14.9 d**). The medial and lateral support strips are then pulled downward and applied to the distal anchor under tension (**Fig. 14.9e**) and are secured with an additional semicircular length of tape (width 3.75 cm). Next, starting just above the ankle, transverse support strips are wrapped up the leg in an alternating medial-to-lateral and lateral-to-medial fashion, creating a criss-cross pattern in which successive strips are overlapped at an angle of ~ 45° (**Fig. 14.9 f**). It should be noted that the point at which the second ascending strip crosses the one before, is placed precisely below the injured muscle site (**Fig. 14.9 g**). Each successive strip overlaps the previous strip by ~ 2 cm, with the second, fourth, sixth, etc. support strips defining each crossing point along the way. Each strip should be applied with moderate pressure across the midline of the affected muscle. Each of the free ends is fixed to the medial and lateral longitudinal anchor, applying a slight tug on the ascending end to increase the pressure. The last ascending strip should terminate ~ 2–3 cm distal to the site of the muscle injury (**Fig. 14.9 h**). Next, the upper rows of support strips are applied down the leg in the same fashion (**Fig. 14.9i**), and the gap over the injury site is closed with semicircular strips of tape (**Fig. 14.9j**). The free ends of the support strips are secured with tape along the anterior tibial margin (**Fig. 14.9 k**). Finally, the overwrap is started with semicircular strips of tape applied from the back of the leg in the prone position (**Fig. 14.9 l**). The taping is completed by applying additional semicircular overwrap tapes from the anterior side (**Fig. 14.9 m, n**).

General Aspects of Therapeutic Techniques in the Treatment of Muscle Injuries

Regardless of the performance level of the injured athlete, no special physiotherapeutic techniques are used in the treatment of sports-related muscle injuries. The fact is that a qualified therapist can improve or relieve the athlete's complaints with his standard portfolio of therapeutic techniques. The main factors that distinguish injured athletes are their high degree of compliance and their eagerness to make a fast recovery and return to play. It is es-sential, however, to make an accurate and authoritative (sport-specific) evaluation of the athlete's individual physical capabilities and characteristics. It is also important to appreciate the special sport-specific adaptations that occur, especially in the aftermath of muscle injuries. Years of regular, active participation in training and competition, involving the repeated performance of stereotypical movement patterns that may at times have substantial magnitudes, will eventually evoke the active and passive musculoskeletal adaptations that were illustrated earlier in this chapter.

What a therapist would interpret as pathologic changes in a "normal" patient may, in the athlete, represent a sport-specific adaptation of the musculoskeletal system, which is usually both necessary and reasonable. Any attempt to alter or correct these adaptations could adversely affect the performance of the affected athlete.

Adaptations and Changes after Muscle Injuries

While sport-specific adaptations are bound to occur in the musculoskeletal system of all active athletes, muscle injuries may also induce temporary changes in the joints, ligaments, and myofascial system. This section looks at a selection of these post-traumatic reactions on the basis of several important aspects. We will consider the various biologic and neurophysiologic feedback loops and their effects on individual musculoskeletal structures. We will also explore how therapeutic interventions can influence these processes and consider their impact on biological structures.

Most sports involve typical sport-specific movement patterns with high rotatory components relative to the pelvic–leg axis. It is common for these actions to place excessive or unphysiologic loads on joints, ligaments, muscles, fascia, and neuromeningeal structures. Normally, tissue is viscoelastic, meaning that it returns to its original position after movement. But the large mechanical loads that occur in sports such as soccer, which is characterized by rapid sprints, sudden stops, and many fast cutting maneuvers (see p. 321), often cause the natural reversibility of the tissue structures to be lost.

This means that joints such as the sacroiliac joint can no longer return completely to their "resting position." Compensations of this kind are particularly frequent after muscle injuries or changes in the myofascial system. The body is forced to alter and adapt its postural pattern in a constant effort to keep movements below the pain threshold or, after muscle injuries, to unload the affected structures and avoid unphysiologic post-traumatic stresses. When an athlete injures a leg muscle, for example, he will tend to adopt a limping gait—that is, adjust the pelvic–leg axis so that he can walk with less pain. In turn, this will necessarily induce stress reactions in the structures of the pelvic–leg axis. To maintain the pain-free position,

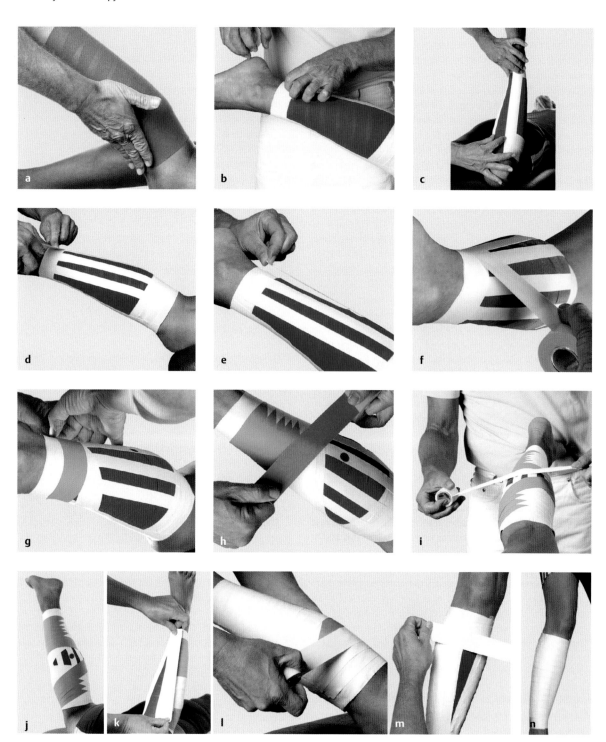

Fig. 14.9a–n   Technique of muscle taping, illustrated for a calf injury.

a The underwrap is applied.
b The proximal and distal anchors are placed.
c Longitudinal anchors are placed.
d Proximal fixation of the support strips.
e Distal fixation of the support strips.
f Additional support strips are placed in a criss-cross pattern.

g Point at which the support strips cross each other.
h Support strips below the injury are applied up the leg.
i Support strips above the injury are applied down the leg.
j Finished support strips, leaving a gap over the injured area.

k The free ends are taped to the tibial margin.
l Overwrap strips are applied from the posterior side.
m And from the anterior side.
n The completed taping.

the body has to rely on its myofascial system to exclude and protect the injured muscle areas, while "overprogramming" the muscles that enable it to move without pain. Acting in this way, the myofascial system helps to perpetuate the dysfunction. Other muscles that would be painful to move are inhibited, reflecting the principle of ascending and descending cause-and-effect chains.

With regard to ascending cause-and-effect chains, an injury to the foot or knee—the most important transverse planes in the body—can do more than cause blocks or restrictions in the limbs with associated local and systemic effects (especially fatigue-induced painful muscle disorder; see the section on "Physical Therapy and Physical Medicine" in Chapter 11). Another important aspect is the interconnectedness of the myofascial chains with one another and also with the lumbar spine (thoracolumbar fascia, gluteal fascia, fascia lata). This explains how dysfunction of the popliteal fascia can precipitate "lumbago." The lower limbs form the foundation of the trunk. If one of the pelvic–leg axes becomes altered, it can affect the entire spinal column, including the visceral structures (compare with spine-related neuromuscular muscle disorder; see the section on "Physical Therapy and Physical Medicine" in Chapter 11).

Exaggerated Host Response

When an injury is sustained, the body quickly initiates host-response mechanisms aimed at healing the injury. It dilates all blood vessels that supply the injured area so that as many "autorepair agents" (lymphocytes, granulocytes, etc.) as possible can be delivered to the affected site. The increased blood flow resulting from this "exaggerated host response" not only makes it more difficult to evaluate the injury, but also leads to unnecessary and extensive adhesions that also involve adjacent, uninjured biological structures. This can significantly delay the resumption of training and competition.

Phases of Healing

The body responds to injuries with an ordered, structured series of events aimed at achieving the fastest possible healing and recovery. Van den Berg (1999) and other authors may be consulted for a detailed description of these events. The healing of injuries to ligaments, muscles, and skin is divided into three main phases:
- *Acute or inflammatory phase.* The acute phase, known also as the vascular or cellular phase, lasts from days 1 to 4 after the trauma, depending on the extent of the injury. It may last for up to 14 days, however, if wound healing is impaired. During the acute phase, the injury incites an inflammatory reaction that initiates the necessary reparative metabolic processes.
- *Proliferative phase.* This phase starts after the wound has closed during the inflammatory phase and is marked by the formation of new connective-tissue

Table 14.5 Types of stimulus used in manual therapeutic techniques

Tissue	Therapeutic stimuli
Bone	Pressure
Cartilaginous tissue	Pressure and tension
Joint capsule	Three-dimensional tension
Ligaments and tendons	Parallel tension
Muscle	Tension-dependent adjustment

structures. This proliferative process lasts from approximately days 5 to 21 after the injury. Initially, the new connective tissue is laid down in random patterns, but physiotherapeutic techniques (mobilization and stretching techniques in the pain-free range) can actively affect the direction of the proliferation. In this way, the later functional properties of the newly formed biologic material can be positively influenced at an early stage.
- *Remodeling phase.* This phase is necessary for the further, definitive functional orientation of the healing tissues. The remodeling phase starts at approximately 3 weeks postinjury and may last for up to 1 year, depending on the necessary extent of connective-tissue development. The qualitative and quantitative tissue improvement and adaptation that occur during this phase further optimize the functional properties to meet the biological requirements of this "replacement tissue."

Besides medical treatment measures, the main therapeutic task lies in applying the correct therapeutic stimuli to the injured connective tissue and delivering those stimuli at the appropriate levels (**Table 14.5**). A trained physical or manual therapist can influence and promote the necessary tissue synthesis by applying the appropriate stimuli. The therapist can selectively apply manual techniques to exploit the stress dependence of the affected biological tissues.

Complex Treatment Strategies for Muscle Injuries

Modern complex treatment strategies for muscle injuries are characterized by an indication-specific application of various therapeutic measures and interventions that can be divided into three main areas: physical therapy, manual therapy, and medical training therapy.

Implementing complex therapeutic strategies thus clearly requires an interdisciplinary approach, with effective collaboration among various specialists from different professions. Masseurs, physical and manual therapists, and rehabilitation trainers work together under medical supervision and supported by the use of medical treatment measures. Successful treatment and rehabilitation of muscle injuries requires effective coordination of the individual interventions that are provided by doctors and therapists.

Note

It is important in this context to note that the sum total of the interventions does not automatically ensure an optimal result. The best outcome is achieved through optimal coordination and sequencing of the various interventions.

This requires ongoing expert consultations and coordination of the interventions. Additionally, all members of the interdisciplinary therapy team should have a detailed knowledge of the specific effects and modes of action of the individual measures.

Therapeutic Techniques

The methods that have proved effective in the treatment of muscle injuries, and which the authors themselves have successfully applied in the framework of complex treatment strategies for muscle-injured athletes, are described briefly below. This is not intended to be an exhaustive compilation but rather a subjective, experience-based selection that readers are free to expand on by adding their own measures. Other classification schemes based on different criteria would also be conceivable and feasible.

This section deals primarily with changes in the myofascial system that are brought about by sports-related dysfunctions of the pelvic–leg axis, including their role in the pathophysiology of muscle injuries. The selected myofascial and ligamentous articular release techniques described below should be considered in the treatment of muscle injuries, as they will help restore the functional capacity and performance of the musculoskeletal system through reorientation and reprogramming.

Physical Modalities

Electrotherapy

Electrotherapy has for many years been an essential tool in physical modalities and is used by both physical therapists and physicians in various specialties, particularly nonoperative orthopedics and traumatology. Advances in medical and biological knowledge, as well as medical technology, have expanded the traditional capabilities and application range of electrotherapy and continue to do so. However, the role of electrotherapy has declined

significantly in recent years, as most basic physical therapy curricula give relatively little attention to electrotherapy and it is not financially viable in most physical therapy centers due to high acquisition costs. Nevertheless, electrotherapeutic techniques at the right place and time can contribute to the recovery of musculoskeletal function and performance when used at the correct dosage and for specific goals.

All electrotherapy techniques are based on the external delivery of mechanical, electrical, or thermal energy to musculoskeletal structures in various forms. The energy absorbed by the structures then stimulates or induces a physiologic response. In the case of ultrasound, for example, the sound waves themselves do not alter blood flow; rather, the ultrasonic energy is absorbed in the tissue and stimulates the activation of individual cells by exciting the corresponding cell membranes. In addition to their energy effect, ultrasonic waves also produce a kind of micromassage effect in the tissue, which releases chemical transmitters that mediate a change in blood flow. This therapy, then, can stimulate normal physiologic processes that bring about the desired therapeutic result.

Some selected modern techniques are described below to illustrate the applications of electrotherapy. The section on "Physical Therapy and Physical Medicine" in Chapter 11 reviews electrotherapeutic techniques that are used for specific goals and indications in various phases of healing. The dose recommendations are empirical values that should be tailored as needed to meet patients' individual requirements.

Note

The usual contraindications to specific applications should always be kept in mind.

High Voltage

High-voltage currents consist of series of very short pulses (~ 10–50 milliseconds) that stimulate motor and sensory nerves. The pulses are too short to cause appreciable sensory discomfort. A high electrical voltage is needed to achieve the intended stimulating effect—hence the term "high voltage."

The physiologic effects can be summarized as follows:
- Stimulation of motor nerves can produce a relaxing, analgesic effect, which may be useful in the treatment of myofascial tension, for example.
- The use of low frequencies up to ~ 10 Hz has a relaxing effect on overused muscle, comparable to gentle low-amplitude shaking.

Medium Frequency

Alternating sine-wave currents at a frequency of 2500–8000 Hz have proved effective in electrotherapy. The higher frequencies are better at overcoming skin resistance, with the result that they cause almost no skin irritation and the currents are very well tolerated. With a slow sweep of the medium frequencies, the summation of multiple successive sine waves will exert a direct effect on the muscle fiber membrane. The low-frequency sweep of a medium-frequency current (amplitude modulation) can produce the effects of various frequencies that are known to occur in low-frequency electrotherapy. This technique can produce pain-free muscle stimulation.

At the physiologic level, the high intensity can overcome the cell-membrane tension and force the cell to undergo a change of state.

Microampere Currents

These currents are comparable in magnitude to the endogenous signals that occur in the body. Basically, a local injury alters the local bioelectrical activity, giving rise to currents in the microampere range. These currents produce a change in the biopotential pattern throughout the body, generating a control signal for growth and recovery. As a result of this mechanism, the biopotential returns to normal. The external application of these small amounts of energy does not overcome the cell-membrane tensions and force the cells to react, but merely excites the cell membranes. This is helpful, because excited cells work in the same way as cells in the normal state, but with greater strength and speed. A practical example of the use of microampere currents is found in biological cell regulation therapy.

Microampere currents can produce a range of physiologic effects:

- Increase adenosine triphosphate (ATP) production (by up to 500%)
- Increase membrane transport
- Increase protein synthesis
- Stimulate fibroblast activity
- Stimulate T-lymphocytes
- Stimulate lymph flow
- Promote regeneration
- Inhibit inflammation
- Relieve pain

High Frequency—Condenser Field—Deep Heat

In this technique, the tissue becomes part of the condenser, generating a vibration at a frequency of 1 MHz. The kinetic energy of this vibration is converted to heat. Transverse treatment produces a heating effect through the entire cross-section of the traversed tissue (applying a heat-transfer medium limits the penetration depth). A prolonged warming effect is also produced. The muscular effects are an increase in metabolism, increased elasticity, a change in tone, and a decrease in muscular viscosity.

Ultrasound

Sound waves in the frequency range of 0.75 to 3 MHz are transmitted to the tissue, causing it to oscillate. This excites molecular vibrations in the tissue, causing the direct generation of heat (efficient energy absorption by compact bone, periosteum, collagenous tissues, and fiber-rich muscles), and can also be regarded as a type of micromassage. Heating the tissue to 40–45°C induces a state of reactive hyperemia. Nonthermal effects result from "stable cavitation" (formation of microbubbles in the cellular fluid). The result of this energy conversion is a change in the permeability of the cell, leading to up-regulation of cellular metabolism and intracellular processes.

The physiologic effects of ultrasound include the stimulation of mast cells, platelets, neutrophilic leukocytes and macrophages, fibroblasts, and myofibroblasts.

Cryotherapy

Local Cold Application

Following decades of the indiscriminate use of ice bags and ice in physical therapy, local cold application became a topic of serious discussion in various studies and professional articles during the early 1990s (van Wingerten 1992). Apart from the benefits of pain relief, attention focused on adverse effects such as the disruption of reparative metabolic processes caused by cooling the injured site below 10°C, interruption of afferent proprioceptive input, and the local hyperemia induced by icing. These adverse factors appeared to contraindicate local cold application once the wound had closed.

Today, cold therapy for muscle injuries is being viewed and evaluated in a more deliberative way. It is now known that specific temperature ranges correlate with the therapeutic goals listed in **Table 14.6**.

These physiologic effects are based on biocybernetic feedback circuits, which maintain a biopositive temperature range that is optimal for cellular metabolic processes. Local physiologic reactions are initiated and controlled on the basis of signals arising from special subcutaneous temperature receptors.

Various media can be used for local cold application to the body surface, including water, gel, spray, and air (**Fig. 14.10**).

> ### Practical Tip
>
> While water allows for a very direct cold application to the skin, cryotherapy with cooled air has proved to be very effective owing to high patient compliance. Cold air application is particularly recommended in the rehabilitation of muscle injuries.

Whole-Body Cryotherapy

In addition to local cold therapy, "whole-body cryotherapy" has recently become a focus of interest for sports scientists and sports physical therapists. It exposes the entire body to a therapeutically active ambient temperature of −110 to −160°C for several minutes in a special enclosure called a cryochamber. Whole-body cold therapy has been known in medicine for some time and can provide a wide range of therapeutic effects for various indications (**Table 14.7**).

Table 14.6 Therapeutic goals, temperature ranges, and doses for local cold application

Therapeutic goal	Temperature range	Adverse side effects
Interruption of nociceptive impulses and reduction of pain	– 20°C or colder for 30–60 s (agent of choice: medical carbon dioxide)	• Alters afferent input for proper neuromuscular control • Tolerated only briefly by patients • Risk of skin burns
Promote reparative metabolic processes	10–15°C for 15 min to several hours (immediately after the injury, in some cases overnight)	
Reduction of pain and swelling	10–15°C for 15 min to several hours (immediately after the injury, in some cases overnight)	

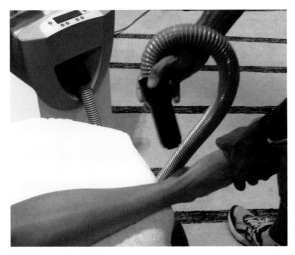

Fig. 14.10 Cryotherapy device for applying cold air to the skin. (Photo courtesy of Zimmer MedizinSystems Ltd., Neu-Ulm, Germany.)

Table 14.7 Indications and contraindications for whole-body cryotherapy (source: Papanfuss 2006)

Indications	Contraindications
• Inflammatory and degenerative rheumatic joint diseases	• Uncontrolled hypertension with pressures over 160/100 mmHg
• Fibromyalgia	• Myocardial infarction within the past 6 months
• Chronic headaches or migraines	• Cardiac arrhythmias
• Diseases with muscle firmness	• Heart failure
• Neurodermatitis	• Circulatory impairment, arterial occlusive disease
• Psoriasis vulgaris, psoriatic arthropathy	• Hypersensitivity to cold
• Hypotonic dysregulation	• Polyneuropathies
• Depression	• Kidney and bladder diseases

Different subsystems in the body are controlled via various receptors in afferent reflex pathways (similar to the afferent reflex pathway of the muscle spindles, see **Figs. 1.32, 1.33, 1.34**) that function in biocybernetic feedback loops. The results are a variety of therapeutic effects for the indications listed in **Table 14.7**. When subcutaneous arteriovenous connections are closed by vasoconstriction, this makes more blood available for muscular metabolism, resulting in positive effects on general and athletic musculoskeletal performance.

Whole-body cryotherapy is practiced in three different forms:

• *Pre-cooling:* cold application prior to athletic events. Based on the physiologic actions of whole-body cryotherapy, pre-cooling is believed to produce a temporary performance increase involving a prolongation of exercise capacity by ~ 10% at the individual anaerobic threshold and an improvement of ~ 5–7% in high-intensity performance.

• *Intermittent cooling:* applied during exercise periods in athletic activities and competitions.

• *Post-cooling.* Current studies indicate that all physiologic supply systems undergo a shortening of the regenerative phase when whole-body cold therapy is applied after exercise. Although quantitative order-of-magnitude data are not yet available for specific systems, preliminary results and study trends suggest that regeneration times are shortened by 30–40%.

The benefits of whole-body cryotherapy after muscle injuries are based on an acceleration of reparative metabolic processes, indicating that this therapy may shorten wound healing times in muscle-injured athletes (Papenfuss 2006, Banfi et al. 2009).

Manual Therapy

Covering the basic techniques of manual therapy would be beyond the scope of the present chapter; readers can consult the specialized literature (Kaltenborn and Evjenth 1999a and 1999b, Van den Berg 1999, Eder and Hoffmann 2006, Frisch 2007). The focus here is on techniques of myofascial release and ligamentous articular release. Various techniques from osteopathy have recently become established in these forms of treatment and have been successfully applied in athletes. A subjective selection of these is presented below.

Myofascial Release Techniques

In several muscular injuries and/or lesions, the dysfunction may result not only from potential mechanical disturbances, but also from a disturbance in the circulation of interstitial fluids (in addition to blood, the body is also permeated by ~14 L of interstitial fluid). Along with the arterial and venous circulation, this fluid has vital nutritional and supply functions for all tissues.

The connective tissue functions as an important interface between the capillaries (suppliers) and cells (recipients). Collagen fibers are positively charged and can bind to negatively charged proteoglycans in the extracellular matrix. This process forms a kind of gel. Additionally, proteoglycans are similar to matrix proteins in their stretchy, load-absorbing properties, which provide for the typical viscoelasticity of human connective tissue. By binding the extracellular components together, proteoglycans create a mesh or sieve for nutrients, metabolic products, bacteria, etc.

Collagen fibers are always oriented in the direction of maximum tissue stresses and therefore assume different alignments in different tissues. They also adapt qualitatively and quantitatively (function levels) to loads and stereotypical sport-specific movement patterns, for example. Unphysiologic loads or dysfunctions promote the formation of typical cross-links (pathological cross-links), due to the loss of water and glycosaminoglycans, and of typical amino acids in collagen (such as lysines and hydroxylysines), which bind chemically to other protein chains and form a lubricant that allows collagen fibers to glide relative to one another. These are the primary connective-tissue fibers from which the fascial layers are formed (see Chapter 1). The gliding ability of these collagen fibers helps maintain a critical distance between the fibers. If this distance is violated, microadhesions will develop and new collagen will form in a disordered fashion, giving rise to abnormal cross-links. Cross-links may also develop during the formation of free radicals such as hydrogen peroxide.

When a dysfunction arises, with the associated restrictions or adhesions of the connective tissue, the cells can no longer receive adequate nutrition. The individual cell within each capillary bed absorbs only the nutrients that can diffuse to it from capillaries, arterioles, and venules, and it eliminates waste products by the same route. Due to the hydrodynamic stagnation, cells in this dysfunctional area exist at a lower level of vitality than those that still have adequate extracellular fluid flow. Pain develops in the dysfunctional area due to the buildup of metabolic and waste products such as prostaglandins and nitrogenous wastes in addition to cellular hypoxia (malnutrition). By releasing the restrictions, therapeutic myofascial release techniques can restore physiologic hydrodynamic fluctuations in the area of the dysfunction.

As mentioned above, the extracellular fluid allows frictionless gliding between myofascial and neuromeningeal structures (glucosaminoglycans). The "liquid pump" is maintained by the respiratory mechanism (breathing). This circulation is impaired by the previously described firmness or adhesions in the myofascial layers or diaphragms. The cause and effect would be hypoxia, with resulting pain in the tissues. These dysfunctions are often located in the body's diaphragms, most notably the respiratory diaphragm, the pelvic diaphragm, the urogenital diaphragm (pelvic floor), the diaphragm of the knee (popliteal fascia), and the diaphragm of the foot (plantar fascia). The diaphragms also form horizontal connecting structures between the various myofascial chains. In this way, they increase the capacity for the combinations, interactions, and compensations among the different myofascial chains that are important in athletic performance.

Note

Understanding the connections that exist among the muscles, ligaments, and fascia is essential for understanding muscular treatment in sports physical therapy.

Practical Tip

Connective-tissue and myofascial restrictions can be effectively treated with "unwinding" techniques. The sports physical therapist guides the affected muscle area with his or her hands (thumbs or fingers), facilitating position changes by the athlete while following and unwinding the diminishing tension.

The following therapeutic techniques can be recommended for the various diaphragms in the body.

Cervical Fascia

The cervical fascia inserts on the skull base, mandible, hyoid, scapula, clavicle, and sternum. Its pretracheal layer is thus connected to the respiratory diaphragm via the fibrous pericardium. The cervical fascia envelops the pharynx, larynx, and thyroid gland and forms the carotid sheath. It connects the trachea and esophagus with its prevertebral layer. Owing to these relationships, the cervical fascia plays an important role in the lymphatic drainage of the head, neck, chest, and upper limb.

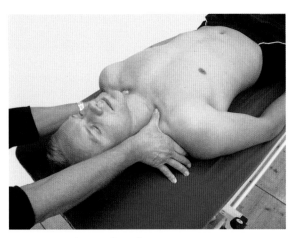

Fig. 14.11 Technique for releasing connective-tissue restrictions involving the cervical fascia.

Practical Tip

Mobilization of the cervical fascia (**Fig. 14.11**) can reduce the need for therapy to the nuchal region.

Indications for mobilization of the cervical fascia are:
- Headaches
- "Lump in the throat" sensation (globus hystericus)
- Brachalgia and/or paresthesias on the ipsilateral side
- Pain medial to the scapula
- Supraclavicular trigger-point herniation (tension in the supraclavicular fossa)

Release therapy is initiated with the patient in the supine position. With the thumbs placed in the supraclavicular fossae (lateral to the sternocleidomastoid muscle), the therapist applies pressure in the lateral and caudal direction until the tension in the cervical fascia releases. The thumbs are then allowed to "melt" slowly toward the acromioclavicular joint.

Caution

The patient's individual tolerance level should always be borne in mind! Releasing the cervical fascia also relieves firmness in the anterior scalene and omohyoid muscles.

Respiratory Diaphragm

This diaphragm is mobilized by performing a direct myofascial release with the patient in the supine or lateral position. Indications are congestion in the abdomen and inspiratory or expiratory problems. Because the respiratory diaphragm works like a piston in a cylinder, it may become fixed in a low or "inspiratory" position. In this case, the therapist contacts the diaphragm with the thenar and hypothenar eminences just above the level of the umbilicus.

Caution

The aorta must not be traumatized!

Next, the diaphragm is compressed superiorly toward the chest, causing it to reassume a "dome" shape. This technique also relieves lymphatic obstruction in the cisterna chyli (below the diaphragm), allowing it to drain through the diaphragm into the thoracic duct. If desired, the thoracic spine can be treated in the same session by placing the other hand across the dysfunctional area of the thoracic spine and the paravertebral muscles. Balanced pressure is now applied and maintained until the thoracic dysfunction releases under one hand and the "balloon" of the diaphragm releases under the other hand.

Because the interaction between the lower ribs and respiratory diaphragm can perpetuate a dysfunction in the form of an "inspiratory" or "expiratory lesion," the techniques shown in **Fig. 14.12** are helpful for treating these lesions.

Pelvic and Urogenital Diaphragm

For myofascial release of the pelvic diaphragm (**Fig. 14.13**), the patient lies supine with the knees together and flexed 90°. The feet are rotated slightly outward and placed ~ 30 cm apart. The sports physical therapist sits at the opposite side of the table, at the level of the pelvis. By palpating the pelvic floor with the thumb medial to the ischial tuberosity and working cephalad and slightly laterally along the ischial ramus, the therapist checks for a difference in resistance between the two sides. If greater resistance is felt on one side, the therapist applies tolerable pressure to the tense side until that side releases and normal resistance is restored.

Popliteal Fascia

Direct myofascial release of the popliteal fascia (the "diaphragm" of the knee, **Fig. 14.14**) is used to treat functional muscle disorders in the knee or in the popliteal fossa (often coexisting with a Baker cyst, due to the additional mass effect). The injured athlete lies supine with the knees flexed ~ 30°. The sports physical therapist shapes the fingers of both hands into a "plough" and applies them directly to the popliteus muscle. While maintaining the same finger position, the therapist applies a distally directed tensile stress to the fascia until an easing of fascial resistance is felt in the affected area.

Plantar Fascia

A direct release of the plantar fascia (**Fig. 14.15**) is used to treat pain in the sole of the foot, heel spurs, or plantar fasciitis. The patient is positioned supine. The therapist crosses the thumbs and presses the pads of the thumbs into the sole of the affected foot. The pads exert a moderate pressure directed medially and laterally upward, as shown. The therapist maintains this pressure until the fascia releases and the thumbs slide transversely across the fascia.

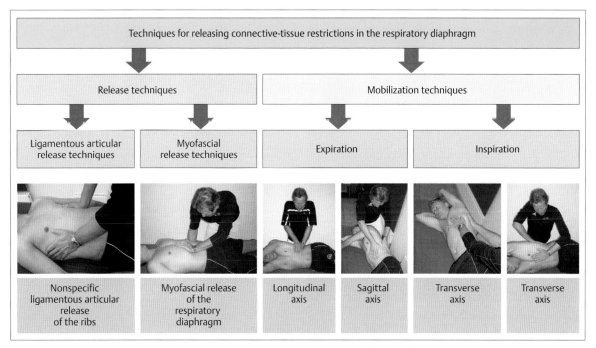

Fig. 14.12   Therapeutic techniques for releasing connective-tissue restrictions in the area of the respiratory diaphragm.

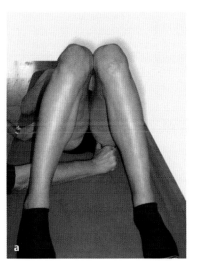

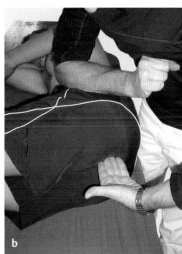

Fig. 14.13a, b   Therapeutic techniques for releasing connective-tissue restrictions in the area of the pelvic diaphragm.

a Myofascial release and mobilization of the urogenital and pelvic diaphragm.

b Alternative starting position for mobilizing the urogenital and pelvic diaphragm.

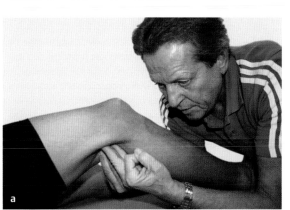

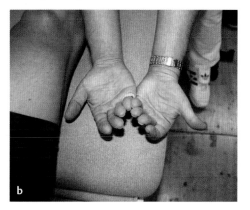

Fig. 14.14a, b   Mobilization of the popliteal fascia. Close-up of the hand position (**b**).

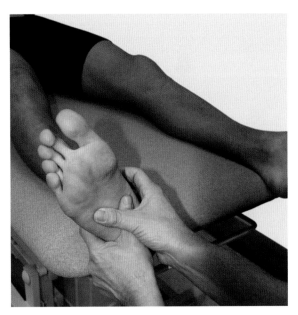

Fig. 14.15   Mobilization of the plantar fascia.

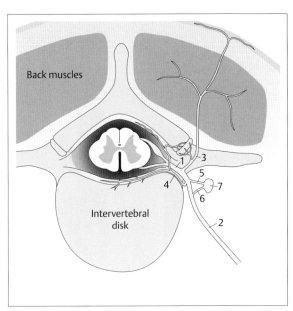

Fig. 14.16   Topographic anatomy of the spinal dorsal ramus and recurrent nerve.

1 Spinal nerve
2 Ventral (anterior) ramus
3 Dorsal (posterior) ramus. This branch innervates
   the lateral part of the joint capsule of the intervertebral facet
   joints (articular branch); the extensor muscles of the back
   (muscular branch); and the skin of the back (cutaneous nerve).
4 Recurrent meningeal nerve (recurrent nerve, sinuvertebral
   nerve). This branch innervates: the medial part of the joint
   capsule and intervertebral facet joint; the periosteum of the vertebra; the posterior longitudinal ligament; and the dura mater
   (mainly anterior).
5 White ramus communicans
6 Gray ramus communicans
7 Sympathetic ganglion

Ligamentous Articular Release Techniques

Besides pathogenic changes such as those found in fatigue-induced muscle disorders, changes in the central
and peripheral motor nervous systems can also have direct causal significance in myofascial changes. In addition
to the integrative role of the spinal cord, supraspinal levels
play a dominant role in controlling motor functions in
adults.

Particularly in high-level competitive sports, pathologic influences based on somatoemotional stress are an everyday occurrence. This stress is transmitted by tonic impulses via descending pathways directly to the muscle
spindles—the principal kinesthetic organ (gamma innervation)—and can increase muscle tone in the homonymous muscle or in entire muscle groups.

The muscle spindles contain two different types of fiber: nuclear chain fibers and nuclear bag fibers (see Chapter 1). The nuclear bag fiber is a "gamma-dynamic" muscle
fiber that is responsible for the dynamic component of the
muscular stretch reflex. This dynamic response can provide a diagnostic criterion for reflex testing and also a
therapeutic criterion to improve the coupling of eccentric
and concentric muscular activities (reflexes). The nuclear
chain fiber is a "gamma-static" muscle fiber. As the static
component of the stretch reflex, it responds for as long as
physiologic or unphysiologic stresses continue to act on it
(days, weeks, or months; see Chapters 1 and 2).

The means that signals from the nuclear chain fibers
can permanently increase the tone of the homonymous
muscle or even of the entire flexor–extensor chain on the
ipsilateral side by acting via the "2 fiber," which connects
to a reciprocal motor neuron (Mauthner interneuron).

Vertebrogenic and diskogenic dysfunctions have an effect on the myelomeres, or functional spinal cord segments (from Greek *myelo-,* medulla, marrow + *-meros,*
part). Each myelomere has three main structures:

- The *recurrent meningeal nerve* (recurrent meningeal
  branch of the spinal nerve), which innervates the medial part of the facet joint capsule, the periosteum of
  the vertebra (tenderness over the spinous process is a
  diagnostic criterion), the posterior longitudinal ligament, and the dura mater.
- The *dorsal ramus* (**Fig. 14.16**), which divides into an articular branch (zygapophyseal or facet joint) and a
  muscular branch that supplies the intrinsic musculature. The cutaneous branch provides sensory innervation to the skin.
- The *ventral ramus,* which forms a nerve plexus at the
  cervical and lumbar levels of the spine and supplies
  motor innervation to the working muscles. The intercostal nerves at the thoracic level arise directly from
  the ventral rami.

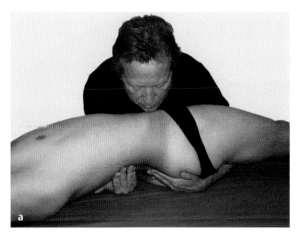 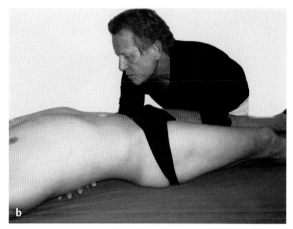

Fig. 14.17a, b   Indirect ligamentous articular release for treatment of low back pain.

a Starting position.   **b** Final position.

In sports, a range of dysfunctions may lead to spine-related neuromuscular muscle disorder that has a neurogenic (vertebrogenic and diskogenic) cause. These dysfunctions and the techniques for treating them are described below.

Ligamentous Articular Release of the Sacrum for Low Back Pain

Because of its functional anatomy, the lumbar spine is a region of key pathogenic and therapeutic importance. To perform an indirect ligamentous articular release of the sacrum for low back pain, the therapist sits at the side of the supine athlete at the level of the pelvis (right-handed therapists sit on the right side of the table, left-handed therapists on the left side; **Fig. 14.17**). The injured athlete is now asked to raise the buttocks from the table and arch the body backward or, if this movement is painful, to roll onto his or her side. The sports physical therapist places the dominant hand beneath the sacrum. The other hand contacts the vertebra in dysfunction with the ball of the thumb (thenar) and with the extended index finger, which is placed transverse to the vertebra. Next, the athlete lowers the pelvis back onto the table or rolls back to a supine position, while the therapist seeks the point of greatest relaxation by moving the sacrum superiorly or inferiorly. Meanwhile, the athlete tells the therapist which position feels the most comfortable. While holding the sacrum in that position, the therapist presses the hand proximal to the affected vertebra anterosuperiorly. This position is maintained until release of the affected structures occurs.

Ligamentous and Myofascial Release of the Iliolumbar Ligament, Erector Trunci, and Latissimus Dorsi

In addition to ligamentous articular release techniques, the corresponding myofascial release techniques must be used to relax the muscles that are perpetuating the dysfunction and relieve sites of neuromuscular muscle disorder. For direct ligamentous and myofascial release of the

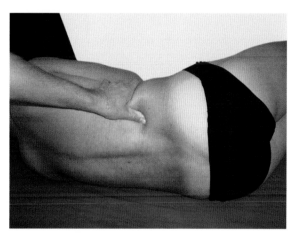

Fig. 14.18   Direct ligamentous articular release of the 12th rib and iliac crest.

iliolumbar ligament and of the erector trunci and latissimus dorsi muscles, the patient lies on his or her side with the affected side up and the hips and knees flexed 45° (**Fig. 14.18**). The physical therapist stands behind the patient at the level of the thoracic spine, facing toward the patient's pelvis. From this position, the therapist palpates the iliolumbar ligament with the pad of the thumb, locating the ligament medial and superior to the posterior superior iliac spine between the ilium and the L4–L5 vertebrae. Next, the therapist applies anteriorly directed pressure to establish contact with the ligament. For the actual ligamentous release, the pressure is increased in the anterior and inferior directions and maintained until the tension softens. This leads to relaxation of the erector spinae muscle, restoring mobility to the lumbosacral junction.

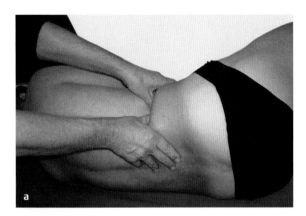

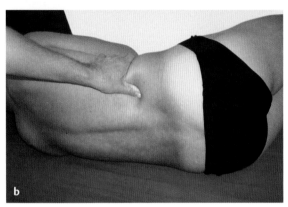

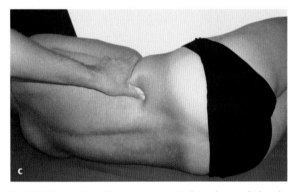

Fig. 14.19a–c **Direct ligamentous articular release of the abdominal muscles.**

a Myofascial release of the oblique abdominal muscles.
b Myofascial release of the erector trunci.
c Myofascial release of the latissimus dorsi.

Myofascial Release of the Internal and External Oblique Muscles and the Lumbar Plexus

For direct myofascial release of the internal and external abdominal oblique muscles and the lumbar plexus, the patient lies with the affected side uppermost and the hips and knees flexed 90° (**Fig. 14.19**). The physical therapist stands behind the athlete at the level of the thoracic spine,

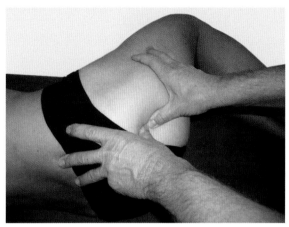

Fig. 14.20 **Myofascial release of the pelvitrochanteric muscles.**

facing toward the athlete's pelvis. After locating the painful tight zone, the therapist presses medially and slightly inferiorly on the tight internal and external oblique muscles between the iliac crest and the inferior thoracic margin (at the level of the 12th rib) until release of the affected muscular structures finally occurs.

Myofascial Release of the Pelvitrochanteric Muscles and Sacral Plexus

For direct myofascial release of the pelvitrochanteric muscles and sacral plexus (constituent muscles: piriformis, gemellus superior, obturator internus, gemellus inferior, quadratus femoris), the athlete is placed in a side-lying position with the affected side of the hip uppermost and the hips and knees flexed ~90° (**Fig. 14.20**). The sports physical therapist stands directly behind the athlete, palpates the affected tight zones, and presses each zone medially and slightly anteriorly with the thumb. At each site, the pressure is maintained at a tolerable level until the desired release occurs.

Nerve Compression Syndromes

The classic sites for nerve compression syndromes should also be taken into account. These are entrapment or impingement syndromes, characterized by the mechanical irritation of peripheral nerves at sites of anatomic narrowing. Complaints in athletes are often a result of unphysiologic loads imposed by repetitive, stereotypical movement patterns. Eventually these loads may cause nerve irritation similar to that due to "microtrauma." Nerves are most commonly affected at sites of narrowing or close to the surface of bones. A compression syndrome may also be provoked by mechanical or metabolic changes, as in spondylarthrosis or thoracic outlet syndrome. The symptoms are highly variable, depending on the site of the compression and whether predominantly motor or sensory nerve fibers are involved. Three clinical stages are distinguished in compression syndromes:

- *Stage 1.* Symptoms are limited to subjective discomfort, with no motor deficits. Findings on clinical examination are normal, resulting in a favorable prognosis.
- *Stage 2.* Subjective symptoms are accompanied by mild sensory disturbances. Motor dysfunction is usually apparent only during exercise. When present, motor deficits are mild and are confined to the actual nerve territory. This stage requires neurologic testing. The earlier sports physical therapy is initiated, the better the response.
- *Stage 3.* The motor deficits are conspicuous at this stage and are occasionally associated with muscular atrophy. As in the preceding stage, neurologic testing is essential. Laboratory tests can confirm or exclude diabetes and diabetic neuropathy.

Experience has shown that the following structures are most commonly affected in competitive athletes:

- *Upper limbs.* Upper limb tension tests are neural tension tests used to differentiate pathology and/or pain in the upper limbs from myofascial pain. They enable the physical therapist to develop an appropriate treatment strategy (**Fig. 14.21**; see Butler 1991 for details of testing techniques). Differentiation can be accomplished with the following maneuver: The muscles supplied by the nerves of interest are prestretched. If a definite aching pain is felt in the affected areas, it is then necessary to determine which structure is actually responsible for the pain. When the therapist has the patient bend the head away from the affected side, placing tension on the brachial plexus and the nerve, a marked increase in pain suggests that neuromeningeal irritation is the cause. If the pain is unaffected by the sidebend-

ing, however, it is very likely that the pain and limited motion have a myofascial cause.

- *Neuromeningeal structures.* Following the same methodologic principle, the slump test can be used to distinguish between neuromeningeal and myofascial causes of pain or limited motion (**Fig. 14.22**; technical details in Butler 1991). Therapeutic techniques are illustrated in **Fig. 14.23**.

Table 14.8 lists other common sites for potential nerve compression syndromes, based on clinical experience.

Strain–Counterstrain

Finally, peripheral motor dysfunctions may be perpetuated by the interaction of intra-articular nerves on the one hand and the peripheral muscles on the other. While type I mechanoreceptors have a direct reflexogenic connection with type I (tonic) muscle fibers, type II mechanoreceptors have reflex connections with type II (fast-twitch) muscle fibers. The type III mechanoreceptor, on the other hand, is the typical receptor of the periarticular tendons and ligaments. It interacts with 5–25 muscle and tendon fibers to directly transfer articular dysfunctions to nearby musculoligamentous structures (**Table 14.9**), giving rise to "tender points" (see p. 354).

Strain–counterstrain is the treatment indicated. It is a positional release technique in which the injured athlete is positioned in a way that moves the injured myofascial structures closer together, allowing them to relax. The patient is entirely passive in this process, and positioning by the therapist alone brings about the spontaneous release. In all muscle injuries not associated with intramuscular

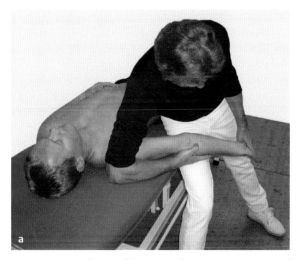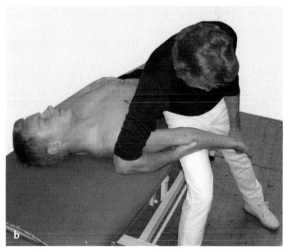

Fig. 14.21a, b   Differential diagnosis of nerve compression syndromes, illustrated for the upper limb: upper limb tension tests.

a Test phase 1: median nerve. Differentiating a myofascial from a neuromeningeal cause (starting position). Example: golfer's elbow caused by a primary lesion of the median nerve versus a primary lesion of the hand flexors.

b Test phase 3: median nerve. Differentiating a myofascial from a neuromeningeal cause (final position). On side-bending of the cervical spine, pain in the arm increases markedly with a neuromeningeal cause, but remains constant with a myofascial cause.

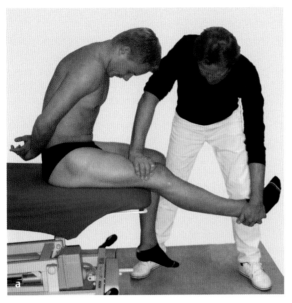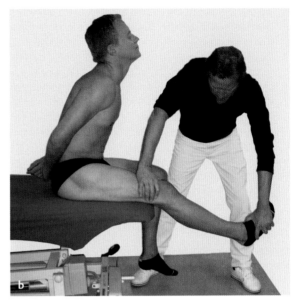

Fig. 14.22   Variations of the slump test for diagnosing a neuromeningeal source of complaints.

a Starting position for testing the sciatic nerve.   **b** Final position for testing the sciatic nerve.

bleeding, this position is held until release of the injured site occurs. The therapist supports this process by applying constant pressure to the muscle belly for ~ 30–60 seconds. The pressure is then shifted from the muscle belly to the musculotendinous junction. This can be repeated as often as needed.

Spray and Stretch

The "spray and stretch" technique has also proved effective for reducing firmness in injured muscles. The affected muscle is swept from origin to insertion for ~ 30 seconds with ethyl chloride spray or another suitable coolant medium (e.g., cold air at a temperature of −20 to −25°C) while it is passively stretched to its maximum length to release the muscle tension. Another option is to rub the affected muscle with ice cubes (e.g., in the locker room, if no other technical aids are available). The temperature reduction induces nociceptive inhibition via corresponding nerve endings in the skin.

> *Caution*
>
> **Spraying ethyl chloride in one spot for too long may freeze the skin. This must be avoided!**

Muscle Release Techniques (Neuromuscular Techniques 1–3)

The stretching techniques described below are designed to elongate the affected muscles gently without evoking an intrinsic reflex via the intrafusal fibers of the muscle spindles that would increase muscle tension. The muscle is stretched to its pain limit in a slow, controlled fashion while utilizing various neurophysiologic effects (**Fig. 14.24** and **Table 14.10**). Three main muscle release techniques are used, as described below.

Neuromuscular Technique (NMT) 1: Mobilization Using the Direct Muscular Force of Agonists

The following aspects should be considered:
- The joint is moved to the current restrictive barrier.
- The patient contracts the muscle to mobilize it past the restrictive barrier and obtain an incremental motion gain.
- Patients may have difficulty learning the movements involved in muscle release therapy. The therapist can facilitate this process by performing guided passive movements to the restrictive barrier.
- Tactile, cutaneous, and muscular stimuli in the target muscles can also help patients learn the necessary movements.

> *Note*
>
> **This maneuver should be performed several times with the therapist, and the patient should perform it independently several times during the same day.**

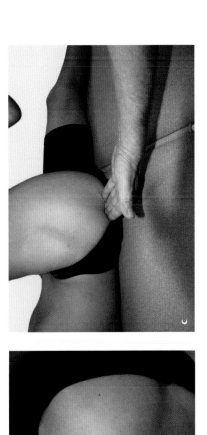

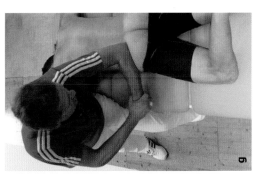

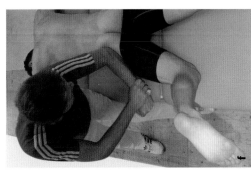

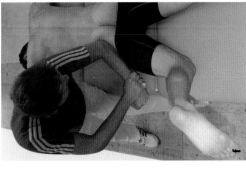

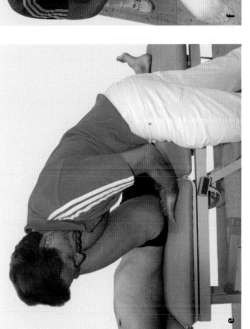

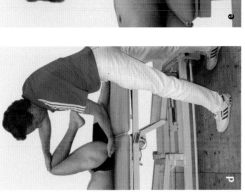

Fig. 14.23a–g   Therapeutic techniques for the sacral plexus, lumbar plexus, etc.

a Myofascial release of the pelvitrochanteric muscles.
b Myofascial release of the abdominal oblique muscles.
c Alternative hand position for mobilizing the pelvitrochanteric muscles.
d Mobilization of the pelvitrochanteric muscles (starting position).
e Mobilization of the pelvitrochanteric muscles (technique).
f Mobilization of the gluteal region including the suprapiriform foramina, myofascial release (outflare chain), mobilization of the gluteal fascia (starting position).
g Mobilization of the gluteal region, including the suprapiriform foramina, myofascial release (outflare chain), mobilization of the gluteal fascia (final position).

Table 14.8 Overview of potential nerve compression syndromes (after Barral)

Affected nerve	Location of compression site
Radial nerve	Radial groove, radial biceps groove
Median nerve	• At elbow over the ulnar epicondyle • Passage through the pronator teres and forearm flexors • Carpal tunnel at the wrist
Iliohypogastric nerve	At the level of its emergence from the inguinal canal in the transversus abdominis fascia
Cutaneous femoral nerve	Between the external inguinal ligament and anterior superior iliac spine
Saphenous nerve	Site of emergence from Hunter canal (femoral canal)
Superficial peroneal nerve	Head of the fibula
Deep peroneal nerve	Soleus arcade
Tibial nerve	Tarsal tunnel, popliteus muscle or popliteal fascia
Superior gluteal nerve	Suprapiriform foramina between the piriformis and gluteus muscles
Inferior gluteal nerve	Infrapiriform foramina between the piriformis and gemellus superior muscles
Obturator nerve	Obturator canal between the obturator externus and internus muscles
Sciatic nerve	Pelvitrochanteric muscles
Lumbar plexus	Iliopsoas muscle at muscular lacuna (inguinal ring)
Brachial plexus	Scalene interval in costoclavicular space at pectoralis minor muscle
Pudendal nerve	In Alcock canal (pudendal neuralgia)
Intercostal nerves	May be compressed by rib callus formation or fibrosis of intercostal muscles, or by vertebral or costal lesions

Table 14.9 Location and function of mechanoreceptors

Mechanoreceptor types	Location	Function
Type I	Outer layer of fibrous joint capsule	• Connects corpuscles to articular branches of spinal nerve dorsal rami • Slow-adapting receptors respond to tension in outer layers of joint capsule • Transsynaptic inhibition of stimuli arising from pain receptors • Reflex tonic effect on motor neurons of axial and limb muscles
Type II	Usually few in number, found in deeper layers of joint capsule; connected to articular branches by heavily myelinated nerve fibers	• Fast-adapting mechanoreceptors (< 0.5 s) responsive to brief stimulation or tension change in fibrous joint capsule • Phasic reflex action on axial and limb muscles • Transient inhibition of nociceptive activity of joint capsule
Type III	Typical receptors of ligaments and tendon insertions near joints; do not occur in the joint capsule	• Slow-adapting receptors with reflex inhibitory effect on motor neurons

continued next page

Table 14.9 Location and function of mechanoreceptors *(continued)*

Mechanoreceptor types	Location	Function
Type IV	Widely distributed in fibrous portion of joint capsule This receptor system is activated by depolarization of nerve fibers in response to stimuli such as: • Sustained pressure on the joint capsule • Unphysiologic position • Abrupt movement due to narrowing of intervertebral disks • Vertebral body fracture • Facet dislocation • Chemical irritation (e.g., by potassium ions or lactic acid) • Interstitial edema of the capsule due to acute or chronic inflammatory process	• Reflex tonic effect on motor neurons of axial and limb muscles • Pain induction • Reflex tonic effect on respiratory system and cardiovascular structures

Table 14.10 Nerve supply of the knee joint

Nerve	Distribution	Comments
Medial articular nerve (MAN)	• Medial fibrous capsule • Anteromedial capsule • Medial collateral ligament • Medial meniscus • Patellar ligament • Infrapatellar fat pad • Medial portion of patellar periosteum	Arises from obturator nerve and saphenous nerve Some authors doubt involvement of both nerves of origin
Lateral articular nerve (LAN)	• Capsule of superior tibiofibular joint • Inferolateral tissue of knee joint • Peroneal muscles • Lateral collateral ligament	Arises from peroneal nerve
Posterior articular nerve (PAN)	• Posterior capsule • Posterior fat pad • Posterior oblique ligament • Posterior ligamentous structures that surround the lateral and medial menisci (popliteus muscle)	Arises from posterior tibial nerve Some authors view the PAN as the largest and most constant nerve supplying the knee joint. Innervation of the popliteus muscle by the PAN has not yet been proven in humans

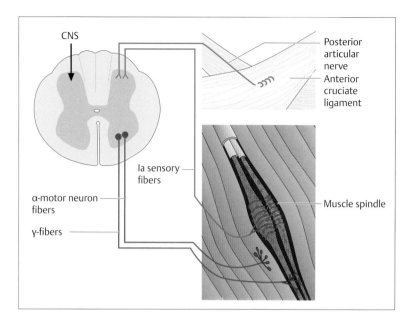

Fig. 14.24 Musculospinal reflex pathways.

CNS

Posterior articular nerve

Anterior cruciate ligament

la sensory fibers

α-motor neuron fibers

γ-fibers

Muscle spindle

NMT 2: Mobilization Using Postisometric Relaxation of Antagonists

The following considerations are important:
- First, the muscle is passively stretched to its maximum length; the patient then performs an optimum isometric contraction away from the restrictive barrier.
- The position is maintained for 3–10 seconds in the postisometric relaxation phase, or significantly longer, to improve the synthesis activity of the parallel connective-tissue structures.
- With incremental stretching, any length gain should be maintained and the muscle should be isometrically contracted to its new maximum length.
- In the great majority of cases, the patient will have to learn a stretch routine that he or she can practice regularly and independently at home.

NMT 3: Mobilization Using Reciprocal Inhibition of Antagonists

The following aspects should be noted:
- The vertebra to be mobilized is moved to engage the restrictive barrier.
- The spinal segment or joint is manually stabilized so that it cannot move.
- First the patient performs a pure isometric contraction directed toward the restrictive barrier (precise fixation, reciprocal inhibition) and maintains it for 5–10 seconds.
- The second step consists of careful passive mobilization past the restriction.

For muscle energy techniques to be effective, the muscle must have normal function and must be able to influence arthrokinematics and osteokinematics.

Tender Points and Trigger Points

Both tender points and trigger points are zones of increased tension, with tender points developing from the intra-articular nerves (proprioceptors).

Note

A tender point is a disturbance of the articular system that is projected to structures close to the joint (menisci, ligaments, tendons, and muscles). For this reason, the tender point is also called a "receptor-mediated tension zone." Most researchers agree (Travell and Simons 1998, Travell and Simons 1992) that a trigger point is manifested at the neurovascular hilum of a muscle.

The neurovascular hilum is the site where neurovascular structures enter the muscle through the myofascia. It is surrounded by tension receptors (pressoreceptors). When the tension in a muscle changes, the change is registered by the pressoreceptors—also called Vater–Pacini bodies—and a zone of increased tension called a trigger point develops around that area. The same preparatory techniques are used to treat trigger points and tender points.

First, a cold medium (ice or ethyl chloride at −18 to −20°) is applied to the tender point or trigger point for ~ 30 seconds. This is followed by a "recoil technique" in which the tissue is prestretched with two fingers or hands and then released abruptly, allowing it to recoil. Intermittent pressure is then applied to the tolerance limit until the trigger point releases. Because a tender point is recruited from the intra-articular nerves, the joint is moved to a position in which the tender point eases or disappears. To obtain optimum feedback from the patient, a

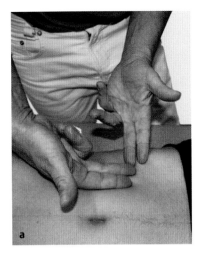
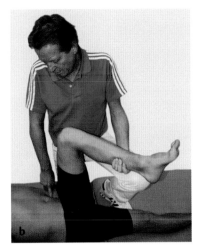
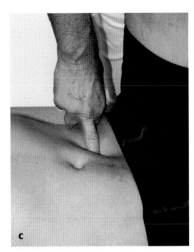

Fig. 14.25a–c Iliopsoas tender point.

a The iliopsoas muscle is located by measuring two fingerbreadths up from the anterior superior iliac spine and two fingerbreadths medially.

b Starting position and technique for tender point release in the iliopsoas muscle.
c Close-up view.

pressure of ~ 4 kg is applied to the tender point. The therapist can practice this on a portable weight scale, or he can simply apply digital pressure until the fingernail turns red. The patient is now asked to rate the pain on an analogue scale from 0 to 10, where 10 is maximum pain. While the 4-kg pressure is maintained, the joint is moved to a position in which the patient feels minimal pain. This latent position is maintained for ~ 90 seconds. If the tender point is located in a contractile structure, the structure is held in an isometric position for ~ 7 seconds at the end of the 90-second period to "reprogram" the muscle. Then the joint, limb, or trunk is passively returned to the starting position. Travell and Simons (1998, 1992) may be consulted for a detailed account of the various muscle-specific techniques for treating trigger points.

Trigger points and tender points are a common occurrence in all sports and are treated using the techniques described below. Van Assche (2001) may be consulted for more detailed descriptions of the treatment techniques.

Iliopsoas Muscle

Tender points develop in all sports that involve extreme hip flexion (kicking leg in soccer players, swinging leg in hurdlers and high jumpers, etc.). While the athlete lies supine on the table, the sports physical therapist stands next to the patient on the affected side. The leg on that side is flexed, with the foot remaining on the table surface. The therapist places one hand beneath the lower leg and positions the leg so that the hip and knee are flexed ~ 90° with the lower leg in internal or external rotation. With his or her free hand, the therapist palpates the affected area of the iliopsoas muscle with the middle finger to assess the muscular response to the position and confirm release (**Fig. 14.25**).

Piriformis Muscle

Tender points and trigger points in the piriformis muscle are particularly common in athletes whose pelvic–leg axis has been altered as a result of medium-term or long-term sport-specific changes and adaptations, or post-traumatic compensatory changes (slipping down of the ilium on one side often affects the contralateral support side). The athlete lies prone, with the affected side at the edge of the table. The sports physical therapist stands at the side of the table and flexes the athlete's leg at the hip and knee by grasping the foot with one hand and placing it on his own flexed thigh in a position of slight external rotation. The therapist's other hand palpates the affected piriformis muscle with the index and middle fingers and monitors the myofascial changes (**Fig. 14.26**).

Biceps Femoris Muscle

Myofascial changes may be caused by side-specific differences in the coactivation of all the hamstring muscles due to temporary post-traumatic changes (especially "intrasynergistic compensation" after a semitendinosus tendon reconstruction of the anterior cruciate ligament, with subsequent overloading of the biceps femoris) or by sport-specific adaptations such as reduced coactivation in soccer players when the kicking leg is in the support phase. Release is achieved by positioning the athlete supine with the affected leg flexed at the knee over the side of the table. The sports physical therapist stands or kneels next to the athlete, grasps the foot from the medial and plantar side with one hand, and holds the foot in slight external rotation while the other hand palpates the musculotendinous junction of the affected biceps femoris with the index or middle finger and monitors the progress of the re-

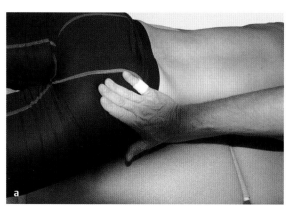

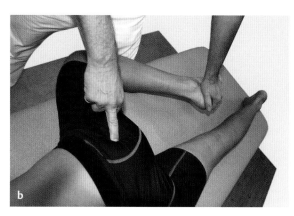

Fig. 14.26a, b   Piriformis tender point.

a The piriformis is located by placing the thenar and hypothenar over the iliac crest and then pointing the fingertip toward the ischial tuberosity.

b Final position for tender point release in the piriformis muscle.

lease (detailed description and illustrations in Van Assche 2001).

Lateral Meniscus

Long-term changes or excessive loads caused, for example, by unphysiologic tensile stresses in the iliotibial tract and/or myofascial changes in the tensor fasciae latae muscle secondary to changes in the thigh muscles after an injury (e.g., following vastus medialis atrophy) often lead to symptoms with associated joint and ligament pathology. The following technique is used to restore the "point of balanced tension." With the athlete lying supine, the sports physical therapist stands at the side of the table and grasps the patient's foot with one hand from the plantar side. He places the affected leg in a position of 90° hip and knee flexion, adduction, and slight internal rotation while the middle finger of the other hand palpates the lateral meniscal structures and monitors the release of tension (detailed description and illustrations in Van Assche 2001).

Subscapularis Muscle

The athlete lies supine with the affected side at the edge of the table and the affected arm off the side of the table. The sports physical therapist stands or sits next to the athlete, stabilizes his wrist from the lateral side, and moves the arm slightly outward while palpating the myofascial structures in the axillary region with the index or middle finger of the other hand (detailed description and illustrations in Van Assche 2001).

Elastic Taping (Kinesiotaping)

Classic athletic taping with nonelastic material has been used for many years to stabilize athletes' joints and has become an essential tool in both recreational and competitive sports (e.g., see Chapter 11). Since the late 1980s,

however, practitioners have increasingly relied on the use of colored "elastic" tapes in the treatment of various disorders. This has been happening in various areas of medicine, and especially in top-level competitive sports.

Originally conceived in Japan and based on concepts and therapeutic techniques originating in the Far East (such as kinesiology), kinesiotaping has gradually been adopted by Western physicians and therapists to promote healing and relieve pain. The elastic tape is applied directly to the skin to produce a variety of effects in different organ systems (skin, internal organs, autonomic and central nervous system, lymphatic system, etc.; Mommsen et al. 2007).

With its many different modes of application (applied with tension and in various directions), kinesiotaping after muscle injuries can selectively influence the tone of the injured muscles to either facilitate or inhibit muscular activity. The elastic tape is applied directly over the muscle from one end to the other. Tapes for muscular facilitation are applied from the origin to the insertion of the muscle, while tapes for muscular inhibition are applied from the insertion to the origin. The elastic tapes come in a range of colors, as empirical data and model concepts in color theory suggest that different colors evoke somatoemotional responses that can enhance the therapeutic effect via the visual and tactile sensors (eyes and skin). Blue is claimed to have a calming and pain-relieving effect, while red has more of a stimulating effect that can increase energy and metabolism.

Kinesiotaping can be used for all muscle injuries (see the section on "Physical Therapy and Physical Medicine" in Chapter 11) in all phases of healing (acute or inflammatory phase, proliferative phase, remodeling phase; see p. 339) to produce desired effects such as facilitation or inhibition of the injured muscle, while supporting other treatment modalities that act in the same direction. Mus-

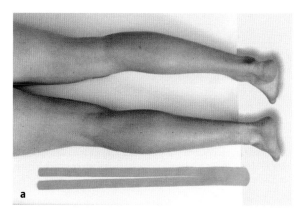

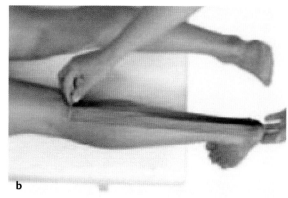

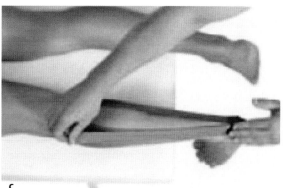

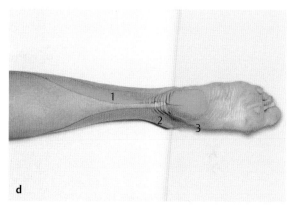

Fig. 14.27a–d   Gastrocnemius taping for muscle inhibition (photos courtesy of BSN Medical Ltd., Hamburg, Germany).

a The elastic tape is measured and precut.
b Strip placement for muscle technique.

c Taping around the calf muscle.
d Finished appearance of gastrocnemius taping.

cle techniques of kinesiotaping include blue taping from insertion to origin, with pain-dependent prestretching of the injured muscle for muscular inhibition during early rehabilitation, as well as taping from origin to insertion for muscular facilitation as therapy progresses. Fascial and lymphatic taping techniques are also used.

Several techniques for kinesiotaping of the calf muscle are illustrated below.

Taping for Calf Muscle Inhibition

To reduce gastrocnemius muscle tone (**Fig. 14.27**), blue elastic tape is applied without tension from the insertion up to the origin of the muscle. The strips are placed alongside the Achilles tendon and along the medial and lateral aspects of the gastrocnemius muscle belly.

Practical Tip

It should be ensured that the strips skirt the margins of the Achilles tendon and are not taped to the tendon itself. Higher up, the strips are shaped to the lateral and medial contours of the calf muscle and pressed into place.

The finished taping has the following characteristics:

- The strips follow the course of the Achilles tendon up to the junction of the aponeurosis and muscle.
- When the toes are pointed downward, the tape should form typical waves that do not separate from the skin and confirm tension-free application.
- The base of the tape is on the bottom of the heel.

Calf Muscle Taping Plus Lymphatic Taping over the Achilles Tendon

The muscle technique described above is sometimes combined with a fascial technique (**Fig. 14.28**). Indications for fascial taping include adhesions or restrictions of myofascial structures and tendon irritation. The elastic tape is applied under tension, causing a visible shifting of the skin. This tension should also cause the skin, subcutaneous tissue, fascia, and muscle to shift relative to one another. The base of the tape is applied in line with the intended stretch and is pulled along with the tails (the therapist does not hold it in place) to mobilize the tissue structures. The direction of the tension should be transverse to the underlying fiber orientation. When a Y-shaped tape is used, the

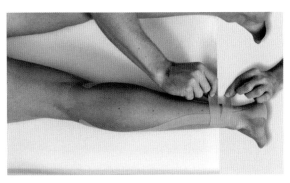

Fig. 14.28 **Combined muscle and fascial technique for the calf and Achilles tendon** (photo courtesy of BSN Medical Ltd., Hamburg, Germany).

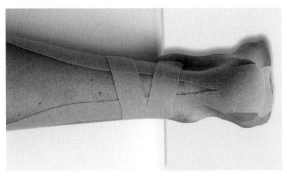

Fig. 14.29 **Final placement of the fascial strips** (photo courtesy of BSN Medical Ltd., Hamburg, Germany).

abnormal (painful) area should be located between the diverging strips.

When the fascial technique is used as an adjunct to muscle technique, a fan-shaped tape is placed transversely so that any pathology (such as an injured area) is within the fan (**Fig. 14.29**). Tapes can also be placed in multiple fan-shaped patterns, depending on the symptoms, and different colors can be used to enhance the therapeutic effect.

Combined Muscle Taping and Lymphatic Taping on the Calf

Lymphatic tapes applied without tension can be used to promote or activate the lymph system and improve lymphatic drainage. The affected area is prestretched to create skin folds. (This can be done manually by the therapist, or the patient can be placed in an initial position that stretches the area.) The elastic tape is cut into three or four strips, and the base is anchored in the area with the lowest tissue pressure (**Fig. 14.30**). The activation produced by the narrow tape strips promotes lymphatic drainage along the strips and toward the base of the tape.

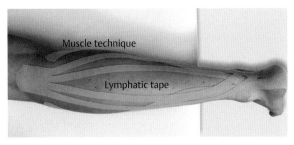

Fig. 14.30 **Technique for lymphatic taping of the calf.** The base of the tape is placed in the popliteal fossa (photo courtesy of BSN Medical Ltd., Hamburg, Germany).

Medical Training Therapy

Medical training therapy has become an integral part of complex regimens aimed at the restoration of musculoskeletal performance, both in recreational sports and especially in high-level competitive sports. In medical training therapy as in other therapeutic interventions, it is important to check for any contraindications that would preclude training activities either temporarily or generally in the rehabilitation setting, regardless of the type of muscle injury that has been sustained. Absolute and relative contraindications to medical training therapy are listed in **Table 14.11**.

> *Note*
>
> **When an injured athlete has relative contraindications, the possibility of limited or reduced training therapy should be discussed with the team physician, who evaluates this option and prescribes limitations on a case-by-case basis.**

In the setting of complex modern treatment strategies, the individual measures that are applied in physical therapy, manual therapy, and medical training therapy after orthopedic trauma are generally based on biocybernetic scientific models. Following the evolution of training science from a largely empirical discipline to a natural science with an evidence base, "training control" and "therapy control" should both be viewed as goal-directed processes that are managed within the feedback loops of a biocybernetic algorithm (**Fig. 14.31**).

This means that during or after any given training or therapeutic measures and methods, it should be determined whether or not the measures have actually produced the desired changes in the active and passive elements of the musculoskeletal system. If a measure has not yielded the intended training or therapeutic goals, prompt conclusions should be drawn that may require reorganizing the program or redefining goals. The basic tools for quantifying and/or qualifying the relevant biological parameters are the methods used in rehabilitative performance testing (see p. 330). It should be added that

Table 14.11 Absolute and relative contraindications to medical training therapy (after Seidenspinner)

Absolute contraindications	Relative contraindications
Cardiovascular diseases:	• Pain
• Acute thrombosis	• Chronic instabilities
• Thrombophlebitis	• Pregnancy
• Arterial insufficiency	• Post-traumatic reduction of stress tolerance in injured biologic structures
• Decompensated heart failure	• Osteoporosis
• Myocardial infarction	• Anemia
• Lymphangitis	• Rheumatoid arthritis
	• Chemotherapy
Skin diseases:	
• Infections	
• Tumors	
Muscle diseases:	
• Myositis	
• Myositis ossificans	
Systemic diseases:	
• Fever	
• Tumors	
Other:	
• Wound healing problems	
• Open fractures	
• Epilepsy	
• Heart failure	
• Severe peripheral occlusive disease	
• Aneurysm	
• Anticoagulant therapy	
• Severe osteoporosis	
• Malignancies in body areas selected for training	

• Assessing or discussing the previous therapy unit and its effects with the patient (feedback) and the team
• Investigating any unusual musculoskeletal symptoms that are unrelated to the actual injury
• Any physical and/or psychophysical discomfort or distress (e.g., infection)
• Fear of increased demands imposed by new, complex coordination elements
• Reevaluating the relationship between training loads and recovery
• Avoidance of overtraining syndromes by the proper grading and selection of all therapeutic and training stimuli and their evaluation as a whole

Working within this framework, we can apply all methods, tools, and contents of the sports sciences and especially of training science which can supplement the complex treatment strategies and positively influence the athlete's progress. The forms of training described below have proved to be effective in the everyday practice of medical training therapy and have become an integral part of various therapeutic strategies.

Metabolically Oriented Forms of Training

"Cardiovascular training" is a general term applied to endurance training of the cardiovascular system. The importance of this form of training and its positive effects on the functional capacity and performance of all major organ systems, and on the body as a whole, have become an established principle in sports medicine (Shephard et al. 1993, Radlinger et al. 1998a, b). A good endurance level forms the basis of all training, as it increases general exercise capacity and trainability throughout the body.

In the treatment of muscle-injured athletes, movements are temporarily constrained during rehabilitation (e.g., by taping or bracing) to rest and immobilize the injured muscle and prevent unphysiologically high levels of muscle tension. Because of these constraints, the athlete is unable to perform sport-specific endurance training. General, dynamic, and aerobic endurance training performed on a modest array of equipment (bicycle ergometer, upper arm ergometer, crosstrainer, stepper, treadmill) can selectively deliver cardiovascular training stimuli at the desired intensity while sparing the injured muscles. This makes it possible to achieve the following therapeutic goals, regardless of the specific indication:
• *Exercise below the aerobic threshold.* This can promote reparative metabolic processes during wound healing, shorten and optimize regeneration, and stimulate and support the immune system, which has been compromised as a result of the trauma.
• *Exercise above the aerobic threshold and below the individual anaerobic threshold.* This can also optimize reparative metabolic processes. Additionally, it can maintain or even improve aerobic capacity, positively affecting overall metabolic status (including the func-

the discoveries and experiences of training science and various other disciplines in the sports sciences cannot be directly applied to the requirements of medical training therapy, either collectively or on a 1:1 basis.

The cornerstones of medical training therapy are the specific indication for the therapy and the overall plan, with its various phases, that has been developed for that indication. The control of medical training therapy involves a daily evaluation of the physical and mental status of the injured athlete. Besides direct information on the current status of the injured muscle areas, this evaluation should include the following points:

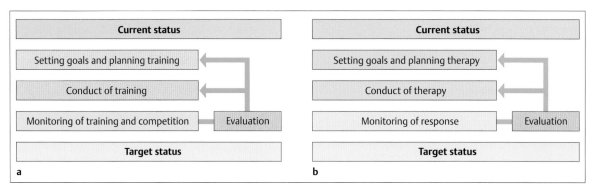

Fig. 14.31a, b   Components of medical training therapy.

a Components of performance control.   **b** Components of therapy control.

tional capacity and performance of all major organ systems) without causing further stress to the immune system, which is already compromised during this phase.

Caution

In the treatment of muscle-injured athletes, it should be noted that the many adaptations induced by intensive training in high-performance sports (cardiovascular system, muscles, metabolism, respiratory organs, and nervous system) are so pronounced that abrupt discontinuation of vigorous exercise due to the injury may lead to health problems.

Symptoms commonly associated with exercise withdrawal may include stomach problems, loss of appetite, headaches, cardiovascular complaints, and sleep disturbances. To avoid this withdrawal syndrome, the injury should be immediately followed by training measures that will either maintain cardiovascular stability or allow only a slight reduction. Despite the injury and associated disability, exercises should be developed that allow endurance training and do not harm the injured area.

Tension-Oriented and Control-Oriented Forms of Training

Note

A muscle lives by its tension—or dies by it!

The main goal of medical training therapy, especially after muscle injuries, is to restore the ability of injured myofascial structures to develop tension. This is a necessary criterion for the functional capacity and performance of the active locomotor system. To be able to perform its tasks adequately within the framework of overall motor function, a muscle that has regained its ability to produce tension also has to be quickly strengthened again so that it

can function as an effective joint stabilizer and help protect the musculoskeletal structures from unphysiologic loads.

A basic goal in medical training therapy is to develop the ability of the injured muscle to produce tension (maximum strength aspect) within the given time structure and demands (power aspect) and with the limited post-traumatic exercise tolerance of the myofascial structures during the individual phases of healing. In addition to *intra*muscular performance, it is also necessary to promote *inter*muscular coordination and integrate the tension production into complex motor programs. This can be accomplished by incorporating the training aids and various forms of training (**Table 14.12**) into tension-oriented, neuromuscular-oriented, and coordination-oriented exercises. From a methodologic standpoint, these exercises are based on the concept that the therapeutic stimulus can positively influence homeostasis in the body by utilizing the following measures:

- *Initiating adaptations:*
  - Principle of active exercise stimulus
  - Principle of progressive exercise increase
  - Principle of stimulus variability
- *Maintaining adaptations:*
  - Principle of optimum exercise and recovery planning
  - Principle of repetition and continuity
  - Principle of periodicity and cycling
  - Principle of individuality
  - Principle of increasing specialization

Medical training therapy employs various training devices and aids, which are used at different times during muscular rehabilitation. A pragmatically oriented classification is based on distinguishing between exercises in an open kinematic chain from exercises in a closed kinetic chain.

Table 14.12 Overview of the classification of training exercises in medical training therapy

Training exercises	Goals	Training parameters	Use in tension-oriented forms of training	Use in control-oriented forms of training
Neuromuscular coordination exercises (stabilization training)	Achieve neuronal training goals such as recruitment, rate coding, and synchronization	Training intensity: as tolerated Training scope: within stable limits Training density: variable	+	+++
Strength training • Multiple-joint strength training in a kinetic chain • Isolated (single-joint) strength training	Achieve muscular training goals such as muscle mass, fiber composition, metabolic capacity, etc.	Goal-oriented parameters in the form of endurance training, hypertrophic training, and maximum strength training	+++	+ ++

Single-Joint Exercises (Open Kinetic Chain) versus Multiple-Joint Exercises (Closed Kinetic Chain)

There are inadequacies in the terminology of physical therapy and training therapy, and there is a lack of clear, unambiguous definitions for classifying different aspects of the types and patterns of movements (Steindler 1973, Dillmann et al. 1994, Di Fabio 1999). For example, the following terms are used synonymously:

• Open kinetic chain = open system = single-joint movements = arthrocentric movements
• Closed kinetic chain = closed system = multiple-joint movements = chain-centered movements

It is reasonable, then, to divide potential training exercises into single-joint and multiple-joint movements. Reviewing the evolution of exercise terminology, it can be seen that Steindler (1973) emphasized the aspect of free mobility at the distal end of a body segment. Eder and Hoffmann (1992) noted the neurophysiologic difference between a fixed point and movable point, and Dillmann et al. (1994) introduced another aspect relating to a free motion segment with or without a load or external resistance. Finally, De Fabio (1999) correctly recommended avoiding the terms "open or closed kinetic or kinematic chains" in favor of stating the number of joints that are involved in a movement and the relative load that the movement places on the joints.

We consider that this is a logical approach to classifying exercises from a neurophysiologic standpoint and that it is also valid in the rehabilitation of muscle injuries:

• *Single-joint isolated movements* (such as leg extensions, arm curls, etc.). Other than stabilizing the active joint, these single-joint exercises require no further coordination to stabilize the limb chain and they allow for goal-directed intensity modulation of the synergistic muscles. They do little to train intramuscular or intermuscular coordination, however, and should never form the centerpiece of a complex rehabilitation training program.
• *Multiple-joint, partially isolated movements* (such as shoulder presses, rowing machine, etc.). These movements require minimal or partial stabilization of at least two joints in a chain and recruit neuromuscular muscle activities along the chain. But while this produces an added coordinating effect (along with the purely muscular effect), one disadvantage is that multiple-joint movements exercise a greater number of synergistic muscles in a relatively nonspecific way, so that the muscular training effects are more difficult to control.
• *Multiple-joint (semi-)free movements* (such as leg presses or squats with barbells). These are relatively free exercises that require a very high degree of stabilizing muscular activities all along the limb chain and may include active stabilization of the trunk in some starting positions. The principal training effects relate to coordination. This type of exercise has limited ability to load and activate specific (injured) muscles and induce them to generate tension.

Practical Tip

We believe that the rehabilitation of muscle injuries requires a balanced mix of isolated single-joint movements and (semi-)free multiple-joint movements to achieve an optimum result.

Figure 14.32 shows a selection of training devices that are currently used in medical training therapy.

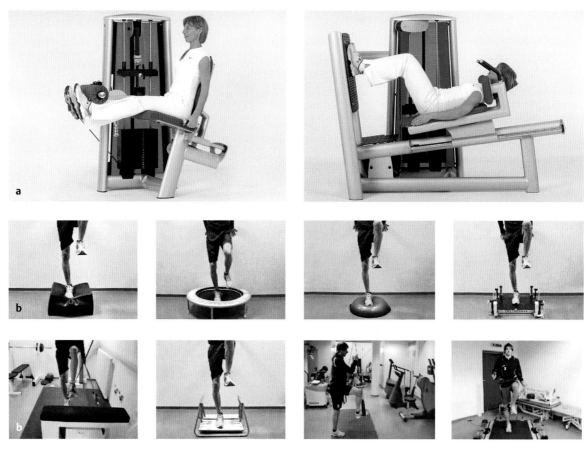

Fig. 14.32a, b Training devices used in medical training therapy (photo courtesy of gym80 International Ltd., Gelsenkirchen, Germany).

a Training devices for tension-oriented muscular rehabilitation.

b Training devices for neuromuscular coordination in muscular rehabilitation. Various types of instability are employed.

Proper Sequencing of Training Exercises

Medical training therapy employs different tools and protocols to exercise and train injured and uninjured regions. The goal is to systematically develop these regions over the course of healing (see the section on "Physical Therapy and Physical Medicine" in Chapter 11) in such a way that they regain their joint-stabilizing function as rapidly as possible. Another goal is to prevent the development of muscular imbalances with associated load and performance discrepancies, giving rise to unphysiologic loads and compensatory reactions. This goal is absolutely essential for sport-specific movement patterns and thus for a prompt and expedient return to training and competition.

In the rehabilitation of muscle injuries, restoring the tension and functional capacity of the myofascial system is certainly at the forefront of all therapeutic considerations. From the standpoint of training therapy, the selection of appropriate training aids and exercises is oriented toward the specific goal of the exercise and the mode of muscular contraction. Training exercises have proved to be most effective when prescribed in the following sequence:

- Isometric myofascial loading should precede concentric loading, before training aids that impose eccentric muscular loads are used. Eccentric and concentric series of contractions are eventually combined.
- Single-joint exercises from a defined starting position with limited and adequate tension levels should come before multiple-joint exercises that involve increasingly complex neuromuscular demands.
- Exercises performed at moderate speeds at the start of rehabilitation are increasingly supplemented by exercises performed at faster speeds.

Practical Tip

Exercising in water (aquatraining) has become an essential part of complex programs for the medical rehabilitation of muscle injuries. By relieving stress on the joints, bones, and muscles while exerting gentle pressure on the injured structures, aquatraining reduces the otherwise adverse adaptive effects that would result from immobilizing the injured area. Moreover, the basic conditioning properties of strength, coordination, mobility, and endurance can be trained with growing intensity and increasing amplitudes at a relatively early time after the injury. The water medium makes it safer for the injured patient to exercise. Additional training aids such as belts and vests provide increased buoyancy that enhances safety and enables a broader range of exercises to be performed. Initial water exercises should be geared toward the specific indication and toward the condition of the individual patient. This means giving due attention to the progress of healing for every injury, so that exercises can be conducted safely and without pain. Training units in water should be performed two to four times a week. Once sport-specific training is initiated, aquatraining may be discontinued.

Papenfuss W. Power from the cold — whole body cryotherapy at −110°C. Regensburg: Edition-K; 2006

Radlinger L, Bachmann W, Homburg J, et al. Rehabilitatives Krafttraining. Stuttgart: Thieme; 1998a

Radlinger L, Bachmann W, Homburg J, et al. Rehabilitive Trainingslehre. Stuttgart: Thieme; 1998b

Shephard RJ, Astrand PO, Rost R. Ausdauer im Sport. Cologne: Dt. Ärzte-Verlag; 1993

Steindler A. Kinesiology of the human body. Springfield: Thomas; 1973

Travell JG, Simons DG. Travell & Simons' myofascial pain and dysfunction: the trigger point manual, vol. 1: upper half of body. 2nd ed. Philadelphia: Lippincott, Williams and Wilkins; 1998

Travell JG, Simons DG. Myofascial pain and dysfunction: the trigger point manual, vol. 2: the lower extremities. Philadelphia: Lippincott, Williams and Wilkins; 1992

Typaldos S. Orthopathische Medizin. Kötzting: Verlag für Ganzheitliche Medizin; 1999

Van Assche R. AORT–Autonome Osteopathische Repositionstechnik. Heidelberg: Haug; 2001

Van den Berg F, ed. Angewandte Physiologie. Vol. 1: Das Bindegewebe des Bewegungsapparates verstehen und beeinflussen. Stuttgart: Thieme; 1999

Van den Berg F, ed. Angewandte Physiologie. Vol. 3: Therapie, Training, Tests. Stuttgart: Thieme; 2001

van Wingerten B. Eistherapie — kontraindiziert bei Sportverletzungen? Leistungssport 1992; 2: 5–8

References

Butler DS. Mobilization of the nervous system. London: Churchill Livingstone; 1991

Di Fabio RP. Marking jargon from kinetic and kinematic chains. J Orth Sports Phys Ther 1999; 29: 142–143

Dillmann CJ, Murray TA, Hintermeister RA. Biomechanical differences of open and closed chain exercises with respect to the shoulder. J Sport Rehabil 1994; 3: 228–238

Eder K, Hoffmann H. Prävention und Rehabilitation von Schäden am Bewegungsapparat. In: Steinbrück K, ed. Vol. 1: Sportverletzungen und Überlastungsschäden. Prävention, Diagnostik, Therapie, Rehabilitation. (Series: Rheumatologie – Orthopädie). Wehr: Ciba-Geigy; 1992: 79–87

Eder K, Hoffmann H. Verletzungen im Fussball – vermeiden – behandeln – therapieren. Munich: Elsevier; 2006

Eder K, Mommsen H. Richtig Tapen – Funktionelle Verbände am Bewegungsapparart optimal anlegen. Balingen: Spitta; 2007

Frisch H. Programmierte Untersuchung des Bewegungsapparates. 9th ed. Berlin: Springer; 2007

Hollmann W, Hettinger T. Sportmedizin — Arbeits- und Trainingsgrundlagen. 3rd ed. Stuttgart: Schattauer; 1990

Kaltenborn FM, Evjenth O. Manuelle Therapie nach Kaltenborn — Untersuchung und Behandlung. Teil 1: Extremitäten. 10th ed. Oslo: Olaf Norlis Bokhandel; 1999a

Kaltenborn FM, Evjenth O. Manuelle Therapie nach Kaltenborn — Untersuchung und Behandlung. Teil 2: Wirbelsäule. 10th ed. Oslo: Olaf Norlis Bokhandel; 1999b

Knebel KP, Herbeck B, Hamsen G. Fussball Funktionsgymnastik. Reinbek bei Hamburg: Rowohlt Taschenbuch; 1988

Mommsen H, Eder K, Brandenburg U. Leukotape K — Schmerztherapie und Lymphtherapie nach japanischer Tradition. Balingen: Spitta; 2007

Further Reading

Banfi G, Melegati G, Barassi A, et al. Effects of whole-body cryotherapy on serum mediators of inflammation and serum muscle enzymes in athletes. J Therm Biol 2009; 34(2): 55–59

Banzer W, Pfeifer K, Vogt L. Funktionsdiagnostik des Bewegungssystems in der Sportmedizin. Heidelberg: Springer; 2004

Barral JP, Croibier A. Manipulation peripherer Nerven. Osteopathische Diagnostik und Therapie. München: Elsevier; 2005

Bennett JG, Stauber WT. Evaluation and treatment of anterior knee pain using eccentric exercise. Med Sci Sports Exerc 1986; 18(5): 526–530

Bizzini M. Sensomotorische Rehabilitation nach Beinverletzungen. Stuttgart: Thieme; 2000

Brown LE, ed. Isokinetics in human performance. Champaign, IL: Human Kinetics; 2000

Burstein AH, Wright TM. Fundamentals of orthopaedic biomechanics. Baltimore: Williams and Wilkins; 1994

Dvir Z. Isokinetics – muscle testing, interpretation and clinical applications. London: Churchill Livingstone; 1995

Ekstrand J, Gillquist J, Liljedahl SO. Prevention of soccer injuries. Supervision by doctor and physiotherapist. Am J Sports Med 1983; 11(3): 116–120

Ellenbecker T, De Carlo M, DeRosa C. Effective functional progressions in sport rehabilitation. Champaign, IL: Human Kinetics; 2009

Engelhardt M, ed. Sportverletzungen – Diagnose, Management und Begleitmassnahmen. Munich: Elsevier; 2006

Enoka RM. Neuromechanics of human movement. 4th ed. Champaign, IL: Human Kinetics; 2008

Fridén J, Sjöström M, Ekblom B. Muscle fibre type characteristics in endurance trained and untrained individuals. Eur J Appl Physiol Occup Physiol 1984; 52(3): 266–271

Froböse I. Isokinetisches Training in Sport und Therapie. St. Augustin: Academia; 1993

Fröbose I, Nellessen G, Wilke C, eds. Training in der Therapie – Grundlagen und Praxis. Munich: Urban & Fischer; 2003

Gardiner PF. Advanced neuromuscular exercise physiology. Champaign, IL: Human Kinetics; 2011

Gibala MJ, Interisano SA, Tarnopolsky MA, et al. Myofibrillar disruption following acute concentric and eccentric resistance exercise in strength-trained men. Can J Physiol Pharmacol 2000; 78(8): 656–661

Grounds MD, White JD, Rosenthal N, Bogoyevitch MA. The role of stem cells in skeletal and cardiac muscle repair. J Histochem Cytochem 2002; 50(5): 589–610

Hislop HJ, Perrine JJ. The isokinetic concept of exercise. Phys Ther 1967; 47(2): 114–117

Hoffmann H. Biomechanik von Fussballspannstössen. Unveröffentlichte Examensarbeit. Frankfurt am Main: Johann-Wolfgang-Goethe Universität; 1984

Hoffmann H, Brüggemann P, Ernst H. Optimales Spielgerät: der Ball — biomechanische Überlegungen zum Einfluss der Ballmechanik auf die Belastung des Körpers. Der Übungsleiter 1982; 3: 18–21

Kamen G, Gabriel DA. Essentials of electromyography. Champaign, IL: Human Kinetics; 2010

Komi PV. Kraft und Schnellkraft im Sport. Cologne: Dt. Ärzte-Verlag; 1994

Kunz HR, Schneider W, Spring H, et al. Krafttraining. Theorie und Praxis. Stuttgart: Thieme; 1990

Latash ML. Neurophysiological basis of movement. Champaign, IL: Human Kinetics; 2008

Lephart SM, Henry TJ. The physiological basis for open and closed kinetic chain rehabilitation for the upper extremity. J Sport Rehabil 1996; 5: 71–87

MacIntosh BR, Gardiner PF, McComas AJ. Skeletal muscle – form and function. 2nd ed. Champaign, IL: Human Kinetics; 2006

Meert GF. Das Becken aus osteopathischer Sicht. Munich: Urban & Fischer; 2003

Mitchell FL, Mitchell PKG. The muscle energy manual. Vol. 1: Concepts and mechanisms, the musculoskeletal screen, cervical region evaluation and treatment. Vol. 2. Evaluation and treatment of the thoracic spine, lumbar spine, and rib cage. Vol. 3: Evaluation and treatment of the pelvis and sacrum. East Lansing, MI: MET Press; 1995, 1998

Myers TW. Anatomy trains: myofascial meridians for manual and movement therapists. 2nd ed. London: Churchill Livingstone; 2008

Perrin DH. Isokinetic exercise and assessment. Champaign, IL: Human Kinetics; 1993

Perry J, Burnfield JM, Cabico LM. Gait analysis: normal and pathological function. 2nd ed. Thorofare, NJ: Slack; 2010

Pfeifer K. Bewegungsverhalten und neuromuskuläre Aktivierung nach Kreuzbandrekonstruktion. Neu-Isenburg: Linguamed; 1996

Schünke M, Schulte E, Schumacher U, et al. Thieme Atlas of Anatomy. Vol. I: General Anatomy and Musculoskeletal System. Stuttgart–New York: Thieme Publishers; 2010

Speeche CA, Crowe WT, Simmons SL. Osteopathische Körpertechniken nach WG. Sutherland – Ligamentous Articular Strain (LAS). Stuttgart: Hippokrates; 2003

Spring H, Dvořák J, Dvorák V, et al. Theorie und Praxis der Trainingstherapie. 2nd ed. Stuttgart: Thieme; 2008

Steinbrück K. Sportverletzungen und Überlastungsschäden. Wehr: Ciba-Geigy; 1992

Strobel M, Stedtfeld HW, Eichhorn HJ, eds. Diagnostik des Kniegelenks. 3rd ed. Berlin: Springer; 1995

Ückert S, Joch W. Effects of warm-up and precooling on endurance performance in the heat. Br J Sports Med 2007; 41(6): 380–384

Van Cranenburgh B. Neurorehabilitation-Neurophysiologische Grundlagen, Lernprozesse, Behandlungsprinzipien. Munich: Elsevier; 2007

Van den Berg F, ed. Angewandte Physiologie. Vol. 5: Komplementäre Therapien verstehen und integrieren. Stuttgart: Thieme; 2005

Watson T. Elektrotherapie. In: Van den Berg F, ed. Angewandte Physiologie. Vol. 3: Therapie, Training, Tests. Stuttgart: Thieme; 2001

Whiting WC, Zernicke RF. Biomechanics of musculoskeletal injury. Champaign, IL: Human Kinetics; 1998

Wilmore JH, Costill DL, Kenney WL. Physiology of sport and exercise. 4th ed. Champaign, IL: Human Kinetics; 2008

Wirhed R. Sport — Anatomie und Bewegungslehre. Stuttgart: Schattauer; 1984

Zichner L, Engelhardt M, Freiwald J, eds. Neuromuskuläre Dysbalancen. 4th ed. Nuremberg: Novartis; 2000

15

Prevention of Muscle Injuries

A. Schlumberger

Translated by Terry Telger

Mechanisms of Muscle Injury   *366*

Preventive Training Strategies   *367*
Training Measures for Preventive Optimization
of Neuromuscular Function   *367*
Optimizing Basic Fitness   *372*

Muscle injuries are among the most common injuries sustained in sports that involve rapid and explosive actions (e.g., sprints and jumps). As a result, they are particularly common in team sports and in track and field disciplines. With regard to the incidence of muscle injuries in team sports, researchers have noted a trend toward a relatively high number of hamstring injuries in soccer, for example (Sherry and Best 2004, Verall et al. 2009) (see also Chapter 5).

The specific muscles that are susceptible to injury depend on the type of sport, the typical sport-specific actions involved, and the muscles used in performing those actions. Hamstring injuries predominate in team sports like soccer or rugby, and in sprinting. Team sports are also associated with more frequent injuries to the rectus femoris muscle (e.g., while kicking a soccer or rugby ball) and to the adductors. The specific actions in tennis predispose to injuries of the gastrocnemius ("tennis leg") and the abdominal muscles (e.g., overhead smashes) (see also Chapter 6).

Muscle injuries are a serious problem for athletes, teams, trainers, and medical care staff for several reasons:
- *Missed playing time.* Because of their frequency, muscle injuries are a major reason for longer absence from training and competition. Missed training time and in particular missed match-playing time can adversely affect the athlete's development.
- *Impact on the team.* Sidelining one or more injured athletes will temporarily compromise team performance.
- *High reinjury rate.* Reinjuries are relatively common after muscle injuries. For example, hamstring injuries have a recurrence rate of 12%–55% during the first year after the injury (Comfort et al. 2009).

The relatively high reinjury rates alone suggest that (beside a correct evaluation and diagnosis) current rehabilitation programs after muscle injuries are in need of improvement. Recent scientific findings indicate that optimum rehabilitation results require very comprehensive and multimodal treatment strategies (Sherry and Best 2004, Croisier et al. 2008). A major objective of the medical care team in this regard is to develop effective, safer, and relatively rapid treatment protocols.

Note

In addition to optimal rehabilitative strategies, special emphasis should be placed on taking specific measures to prevent or reduce the risk of sports-related muscle injuries.

The results of recent studies confirm that preventive training measures can reduce the risk of muscle injuries (survey in Engebretsen and Bahr 2009). Knowing that a prior injury increases the risk of subsequent muscle injuries, we may conclude that injury prevention programs should be designed both to prevent the initial injury and to reduce the risk of reinjuries (see also Thelen et al. 2006). Accordingly, one goal of prevention programs is to implement measures specifically designed to prevent reinjuries that may occur when athletes with a prior muscle injury are returned to training and competition before they have been adequately rehabilitated from the initial injury (see Devlin 2000).

Various aspects should be considered in planning strategies to reduce the risk of muscle injuries. In addition to making a direct analysis of training effects on injury risk (as documented in longitudinal studies), it is also important to understand the factors that lead to injury. These include neuromuscular factors, as well as factors related to training methods. Familiarity with the causal mechanisms that underlie muscle injuries will also influence the design of preventive measures.

This chapter explores these issues and considers their relevance in the planning and implementation of preventive training programs and strategies. Special emphasis is placed on the prevention of hamstring injuries. There are two main reasons for this:
- Hamstring injuries are common in many types of sport.
- Very comprehensive and detailed research results are available on the hamstring muscle group (e.g., Comfort et al. 2009). The hamstrings serve as an example to illustrate the basic principles involved in active injury prevention.

It is likely that findings on the hamstring muscles and associated training strategies can also be applied to the prevention of other muscle injuries.

Mechanisms of Muscle Injury

In developing preventive strategies and programs, it is essential to consider the mechanisms that cause muscle injuries. These mechanisms are illustrated below for the hamstring muscles.

Hamstring injuries most commonly occur during explosive activation of the hamstring group. Accordingly, hamstring injuries are common in team sports that require fast action, and in track and field events that involve sprinting. From the standpoint of muscle work, these injuries appear to occur most often during eccentric contractions—that is, when the contracting muscle is lengthened (Proske et al. 2004). In the sports mentioned above, the hamstrings are exposed to this eccentric load when the athlete initiates a sprint, is at maximal sprint, kicks the ball, and picks up the ball from a fast run (e.g., in rugby) (Proske et al. 2004). These are the actions that appear to have the highest association with hamstring injuries (Arnason et al. 2008).

Note

Muscle injuries most commonly occur during eccentric muscle loads.

Analyzing the mechanisms of injury involved in sprinting reveals two movement phases that are critical in producing injuries: firstly, the late swing phase, at which time the hamstrings actively slow the forward motion of the leg; and secondly, the late stance phase, in which many hamstring injuries appear to occur.

Yu et al. (2008) found that the hamstring muscles undergo eccentric contractions during the late stance phase and also during the late swing phase of sprinting. It is also suggested that muscle injuries in the late swing phase may occur not only during the purely eccentric phase, but also during the transitional phase from eccentric to concentric muscle work (Petersen and Hölmich 2005; see p. 370).

Hamstring injuries may be precipitated by another mechanism as well. They occur in ballet dancers, who perform very large-amplitude movements with a high static component (Verall et al. 2009). This shows that slow stretching movements at a very large amplitude can also cause hamstring injury.

Note

Muscle injuries can result from fast actions or from slow movements with a large amplitude.

A muscle is injured when it is subjected to loads that exceed the mechanical limit of the muscle tissue (Verall et al. 2009). In theory, then, an important goal of preventive training measures is to raise this mechanical limit by increasing the load tolerance of the muscle. Reports on the mechanisms of muscle injuries consistently show that preventive training programs should be geared toward optimizing muscle function under eccentric conditions.

Preventive Training Strategies

The goals of active preventive measures are derived from the various factors that predispose to muscle injuries. A general distinction can be made between neuromuscular factors and factors related to training methods. The considerations on the mechanisms of muscle injuries (see above) suggest that neuromuscular factors play a crucial role in the prevention of muscle injuries. We will begin, then, by reviewing active preventive measures that can optimize neuromuscular function.

Training Measures for Preventive Optimization of Neuromuscular Function

Flexibility and Stretching

It is widely believed that a lack of flexibility increases the risk of muscle injuries. It is also assumed that regular stretching exercises can reduce the risk of muscle injury by improving flexibility. Recent research results have shed new light on the importance of flexibility deficits and their relationship to stretching exercises.

Research Results

Several studies have shown that insufficient flexibility increases the relative risk for sustaining muscle injuries. In a study of Belgian professional soccer players, Witvrouw et al. (2003) found that players with lower flexibility in the hamstring and quadriceps muscles during the preseason had an increased risk of injury to both muscle groups. These findings were supported by Bradley and Portas (2007), who found that a deficit in preseason lower-extremity range of motion correlated with an increased risk for injuries of the hip or knee flexors during the competitive season in soccer players. From the standpoint of reducing reinjuries, it should also be noted that flexibility may be decreased due to a previous muscle injury. For example, a significant loss of hamstring flexibility was observed in sprinters with previous injuries in comparison with uninjured sprinters (survey in Devlin 2000).

Note

Flexibility training can reduce the risk of muscle injury.

Published data vary with regard to the direct effect of stretching exercises on the reduction of muscle injury risk. Dadebo et al. (2004) analyzed the use and preventive benefits of stretching on hamstring injuries in English professional soccer clubs. They found that hamstring stretching could significantly reduce the incidence of these muscle injuries. The stretching volume applied was isolated as an important training factor (see Practical Tip below).

A very comprehensive study by Arnason et al. (2008) in professional soccer players from Iceland and Norway yielded important findings. These authors found that flexibility training alone was not effective in reducing hamstring muscle injuries, but that adding an eccentric training program did correlate with a reduced incidence of those injuries.

Both of these studies suggest that flexibility training can be effective in preventing muscle injuries, but that stretching by itself is not effective in all cases.

Another aspect of the possible influence of stretching on muscle injury prevention concerns the effect of stretching on the compliance of the tendons and musculotendinous system (Witvrouw et al. 2004, Thelen et al. 2006). On the basis of biomechanical considerations in the pathogenesis of muscle injuries, it was theorized that lengthening of the muscle fibers may exceed the critical limit faster in critical eccentric situations (see above) when tendon compliance is poor. This suggests that flexibility training can help reduce the risk of muscle injuries by increasing tendon compliance (Witvrouw et al. 2004, Thelen et al. 2006).

On the basis of the results presented in this section, stretching aimed at increasing joint flexibility and improving muscle lengthening behavior may be an effective measure for preventing muscle injuries. On the other hand, stretching alone does not appear to be sufficient to reduce the risk of muscle injuries. In addition, stretching can help prevent muscle injuries by increasing tendon compliance.

Preventive Stretching Program

In the practical application of stretching programs, joint flexibility generally serves as a major criterion for exercise selection. Since the improvement of joint flexibility has major importance from a preventive standpoint (see above), it is recognized as an important training goal.

However, using stretching in a discriminating way as a preventive measure also makes it necessary to include muscle-specific criteria in exercise selection. Three-dimensional positioning has to be taken into account in order to deliver a selective stretching stimulus to specific muscles. For example, the hamstrings are stretched most effectively by extending the knee joint while the leg is maximally flexed at the hip. Adding rotation at the hip will deliver the stretch stimulus more selectively to the lateral hamstrings (biceps femoris, internal hip rotation) and medial hamstrings (semi group, external hip rotation; see **Figs. 15.6** and **15.7**).

A preventive stretching program is presented below, illustrated here for a soccer player (**Figs. 15.1, 15.2, 15.3, 15.4, 15.5, 15.6, 15.7**). This program stretches all the lower extremity muscles that are known to be at risk for injury in soccer players.

> *Practical Tip*
>
> To achieve a preventive effect, stretching exercises should be performed in two or three repetitions, each with a holding time of 30 seconds. This routine should be repeated two or three times a week.
>
> For professional athletes, it is recommended that stretching exercises should regularly be included as separate training units—that is, units that are separate from sport-specific training units. In amateur athletes, regular stretching can be practiced in both the warm-up and cool-down phases of training.

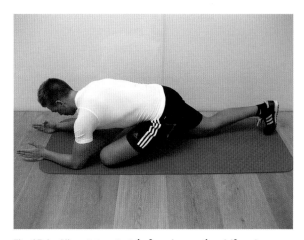

Fig. 15.1   Hip rotator stretch, focusing on the piriformis.

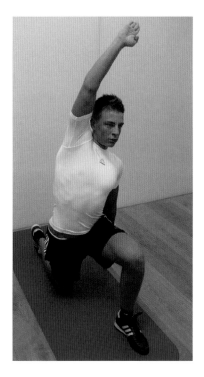

Fig. 15.2 Stretching the psoas major.

Concentric Muscle Function and Concentric Training

It is widely believed that muscle strength deficits can promote muscle injuries. Orchard et al. (1997) found in a prospective study that soccer players with deficits in the maximum concentric strength of the hamstrings were at greater risk for muscle injuries ("concentric" means that the muscle shortens during exercise; see the section on "Isotonic versus Isometric Contraction" in Chapter 1). A maximum strength deficit was defined as a low hamstring–quadriceps strength ratio and a low strength ratio between the subsequently injured leg and the healthy leg. In a more recent study, Yeung et al. (2009) found that a reduced hamstring–quadriceps strength ratio in sprinters could be a predisposing factor for hamstring injury.

> *Note*
>
> **Maximum concentric strength deficits can predispose to muscle injuries.**

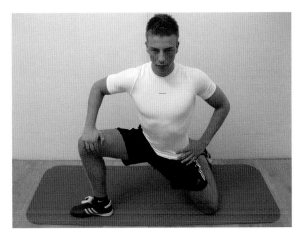

Fig. 15.3 Stretching the adductors with the knee flexed.

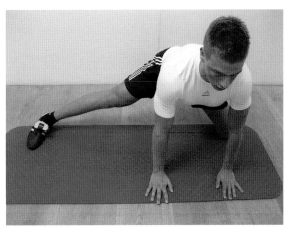

Fig. 15.4 Stretching the adductors with the knee extended.

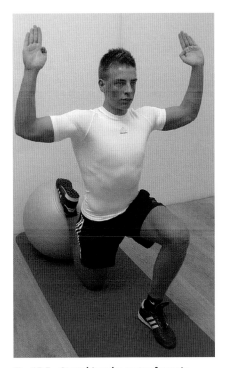

Fig. 15.5 Stretching the rectus femoris.

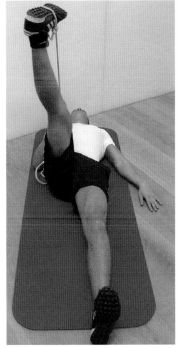

Fig. 15.6 Hamstring stretch, focusing on the biceps femoris.

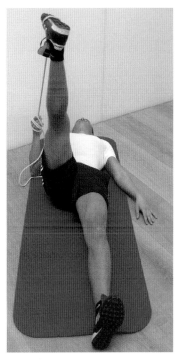

Fig. 15.7 Hamstring stretch, focusing on the semitendinosus and semimembranosus muscles.

Eccentric Muscle Function and Eccentric Training

The results of various recent studies show that the incidence of hamstring injuries can be reduced by improving eccentric muscle function.

Askling et al. (2003) found that eccentric strength training on a special device could lead to a significant reduction of injuries in professional soccer players. Subsequently, various studies investigated the effects of eccentric hamstring exercise without special equipment. Requiring only a floor mat, the "Nordic hamstring" is easier to implement in practical conditions (the technique is shown in **Fig. 15.8a–c**). The studies clearly show that this type of eccentric training can have a significant preventive effect (survey in Arnason et al. 2008). These studies recommend performing the Nordic hamstring exercise once or twice a week in three sets of 8–12 repetitions with 2–3 minutes rest between sets.

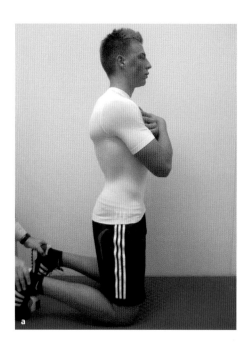

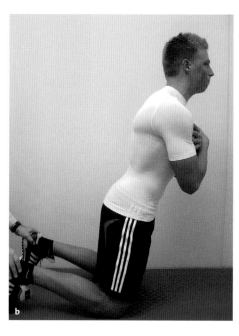

Fig. 15.8a–c
Nordic hamstring exercise.

a Starting position.
b Lowering to the mat.
c End position.

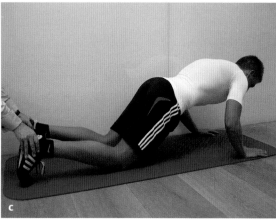

Practical Tip

Eccentric exercises such as the Nordic hamstring should be regularly included in training programs to reduce the risk of hamstring muscle injuries.

Prospective analyses of eccentric strength characteristics validate the importance of eccentric muscle function in the prevention of hamstring injuries. For example, deficits of maximum eccentric strength in the knee flexors of soccer players (Croisier et al. 2008) and of sprinters (Sugiura et al. 2008) have been linked to an increased risk of hamstring injury. With regard to the prevention of hamstring injury recurrence, Croisier et al. (2002) also found that an eccentric strength deficit may be a predisposing factor for hamstring reinjury. These findings highlight the importance of optimizing or normalizing eccentric muscle function and strength for preventing hamstring injuries. They also show that regular assessment of eccentric muscle strength is an important screening tool for identifying muscular deficits that predispose to muscle injuries and reinjuries. It should be emphasized that deficits in maximum eccentric strength not only increase the risk of injury, but can also compromise competitive performance (Croisier et al. 2008).

Force–Length Relationship

Another apparently important factor in assessing the risk of hamstring injuries is the hypothesis advanced by Proske et al. (2004) on the optimum angle for generating muscle torque. Athletes who develop maximum torque at a shorter muscle length are more prone to sustaining eccentric microtrauma to the muscle. Because muscle injuries are most often sustained during eccentric exercise (see above), this change in the optimum angle for torque may pose an increased risk for muscle injuries. Previously injured muscles were found to be at greater risk for reinjury when the optimum angle for torque occurred at shorter muscle lengths. Accordingly, athletes with a history of muscle injuries appear to be more susceptible to eccentric microtrauma and therefore more prone to muscle injuries (Proske et al. 2004).

Note

A change in the optimum angle for eccentric torque production increases the risk of sustaining a muscle injury.

Eccentric training appears to be a possible way of normalizing the force–length relationship (Proske et al. 2004). In addition, findings in strength training research suggest that isometric or strength training in the range of optimal joint angles should be able to normalize the angle for gen-

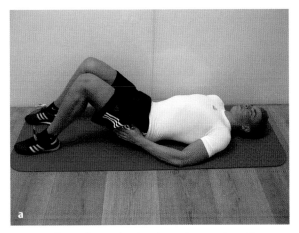 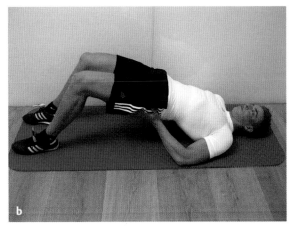

Fig. 15.9a, b Bridging. The gluteal muscles are voluntarily contracted before the hips are lifted from the ground.

a Starting position.   **b** End position.

erating maximum torque, thereby reducing the incidence of hamstring injuries.

Intermuscular Coordination

Another presumably important risk factor for hamstring injuries is a change in intermuscular coordination between the hamstrings and gluteus maximus (Devlin 2000). This phenomenon is common during or after back pain, for example. One result of this change in muscular coordination may be increased stiffness combined with a deficit in flexibility. The increased stiffness appears to result from an altered synergistic relationship between the hamstrings and gluteus maximus—that is, hyperactivity of the hamstrings accompanied by hypoactivity of the gluteus maximus (see also McGill 2007). Accordingly, exercises that improve intermuscular coordination between the hamstrings and gluteus maximus could be an important preventive measure. One such exercise, bridging, is illustrated in **Fig. 15.9a, b**. A study by Sugiura et al. (2008) confirms the importance of the functional state of the gluteus maximus. These authors found that a strength deficit in the hip extensors was a predisposing factor for the occurrence of hamstring injuries.

In summary, it has been found that optimizing local neuromuscular muscle function is an important preventive measure for reducing muscle injuries. The scientific data suggest that effective prevention programs should not focus on a single muscular factor (e.g., flexibility or lengthening characteristics), but should take into account various aspects of muscular function. Accordingly, it is not enough to apply stretching as a general measure for injury prevention. Besides improving flexibility, a comprehensive program should include measures to improve concentric and eccentric muscle strength, optimize the force–length relationship, and improve the intermuscular coordination of synergists such as the hamstrings and gluteals. Moreover, acute preventive measures should preferably

be applied on an individual basis, especially in professional athletes. Muscle function tests should be performed regularly in professional sports to establish the necessary basis for individualized programs. These tests may include:

- Flexibility tests
- Isokinetic maximum strength tests in concentric and eccentric conditions, performed at various test speeds and including the force–angle relationship
- Tests to evaluate the intermuscular coordination of synergists during a particular movement

Practical Tip

Regular tests of joint and muscle function (flexibility, eccentric strength, force–length relationship in concentric and eccentric conditions) provide an important basis for designing individualized preventive training programs.

Training to Improve Lumbopelvic Control and Stability

Core exercises to stabilize the trunk have become increasingly popular in recent years for general injury prevention in high-level sports. This appears to be an important preventive measure from a physiologic standpoint, as deficits in the neuromuscular control of the entire lumbopelvic region (called also the lumbopelvic–hip complex or "core") are considered an important predisposing factor for muscle injuries.

Note

Deficits in the neuromuscular control of the lumbopelvic–hip region increase the risk of muscle injuries in the lower extremity.

From a functional standpoint, the basic idea of training to improve lumbopelvic control is to create a stable base for the dynamic actions of the lower extremity during sport-related movements (i.e., without unphysiologic compensatory movements of the ilium or lumbar motion segments, for example). A stable lumbopelvic base appears to be an important precondition for optimal leg muscle function, in terms of better force development in the leg extensor chain and a normal force–length relationship of the participating muscles.

Research Results

We conducted a pilot study to investigate the importance of lumbopelvic stability and strength for force development in the leg extensor chain (Hajduk and Schlumberger 2010). The effects of 6 weeks of combined leg and trunk strength training were compared with an equal period of leg strength training alone. It was found that the maximum strength gain in the leg extensor chain (dynamic maximum strength in squats) was significantly greater with combined leg–trunk strength training (+15.9%) than with leg strength training alone (+7.5%). A study by Kuszewski et al. (2009) further documents the importance of training for improvement of lumbopelvic control. These authors found that lumbopelvic stability training for several weeks was effective in reducing the stiffness of the hamstrings.

> #### Note
>
> **Training to improve lumbopelvic control can increase muscle activation while also reducing the tension of certain muscles.**

Observations on the predisposing factors for muscle injuries have yielded other important discoveries on the importance of training in improving lumbopelvic stability and control. For example, Hennessey and Watson (1993) found that a hyperlordotic posture of the lumbar spine correlated with an increased risk of hamstring injuries in athletes. Because the abdominal muscles have an important function in the active control of lordosis, abdominal muscle training aimed at improving lumbar postural control could make a significant contribution to the reduction of hamstring injuries. This presumed effect of abdominal muscle function on hamstring injury prevention is supported by observations that the risk of hamstring muscle injuries rises with increasing fatigue of the abdominal muscles (Devlin 2000). These discoveries underscore the importance of optimum abdominal activation for lumbar postural control in the sagittal plane. Optimizing the fatigue resistance of the abdominal muscles also appears to be an effective means of injury prevention.

Discoveries on the rehabilitation of muscle injuries yield further clues on the importance of lumbopelvic stability. Sherry and Best (2004) found that a rehabilitation program emphasizing trunk stabilization led to a significant reduction in reinjury rates in comparison with a training program based entirely on classic strength training and stretching.

In summary, the findings and considerations reviewed in this section show that training to improve lumbopelvic stability and strength can significantly influence the function of the lower extremity muscles. This type of training thus also appears to be able to make an important contribution to the prevention of muscle injuries by optimizing the function of the lower extremity muscles.

Preventive Exercises to Improve Lumbopelvic Stability

An exercise program for improving lumbopelvic stability and strength is described below. It is significant that these exercises always involve optimal activation of important target muscles, combined with a postural or motor control task. The aim is to train important target muscles in the lumbopelvic region in their functional task of carrying out sport-related movements. Additionally, the overall program should include exercises with sport-specific upright positioning along with exercises that involve horizontal positioning. From the point of view of motor control, the upright exercises will help ensure that the effects of lumbopelvic stability training can be transferred to the sport-specific actions that the athlete has to perform (e.g., sprinting or kicking a ball; Schlumberger 2009).

The program illustrated in **Figs. 15.10, 15.11, 15.12, 15.13, 15.14, 15.15, 15.16, 15.17, 15.18** can serve as a general exercise program for many types of sport that require a high degree of lumbopelvic stability. In sports that have an increased risk of lower extremity muscle injuries, it can also provide an effective injury prevention training program to reduce the incidence of muscle injuries in the leg, hip, and pelvic region.

Optimizing Basic Fitness

Optimizing basic fitness is an important training component for reducing the risk of injuries. Basic fitness in this context encompasses endurance and motor coordination (i.e., sport-specific techniques and coordinating ability) in a particular type of sport. Both of these factors are particularly important in team sports.

Endurance

Good endurance is synonymous with good general exercise tolerance and is therefore essential for the successful completion of demanding training and competition units. Good endurance will enable athletes to sprint more often and recover more quickly between sprints (Glaister 2005). Endurance is also an important factor in achieving high total running distances in soccer, for example (the international average for midfielder players is 12–15 km per match).

> #### Note
>
> **Good endurance is essential for tolerating the stresses of training and competition.**

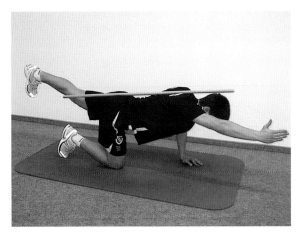

Fig. 15.10 Quadruped position, with alternate arm/leg raises, for local lumbar stabilization and lumbopelvic control.

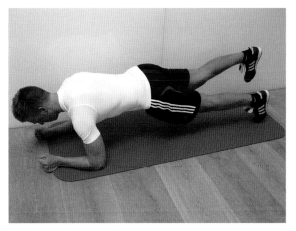

Fig. 15.11 Prone plank, with alternate leg raises for abdominal–lumbar coactivation and three-dimensional lumbopelvic control.

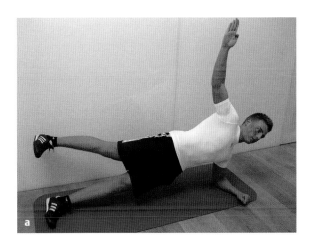

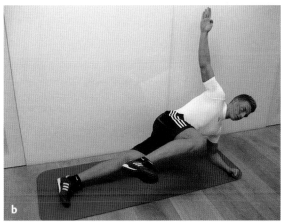

Fig. 15.12a, b Side plank, with runnerlike raising and flexion of the swing leg to activate the whole lateral stabilization chain and for three-dimensional lumbopelvic control.

a Starting position.

b End position.

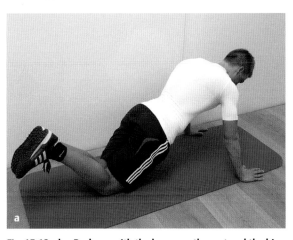

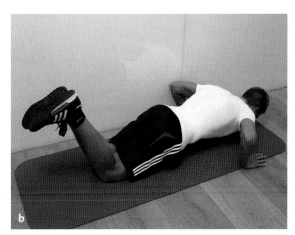

Fig. 15.13a, b Pushups with the knees on the mat and the hips extended for abdominal–lumbar coactivation and lumbar control in the sagittal plane.

a Starting position.

b End position.

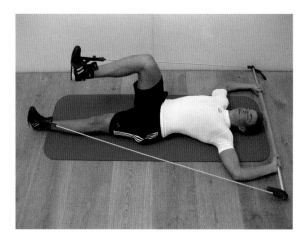

Fig. 15.14   Lumbar control in the sagittal plane, with eccentric abdominal work and alternating unilateral leg extension.

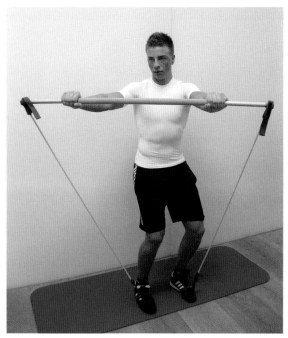

Fig. 15.15   Pelvic–trunk rotation control in two-legged stance.

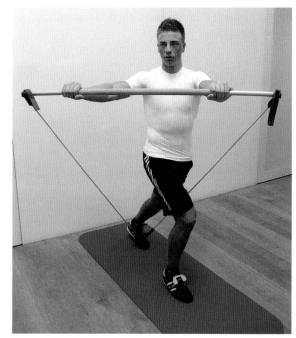

Fig. 15.16   Pelvic–trunk rotation control in a moderate lunge position.

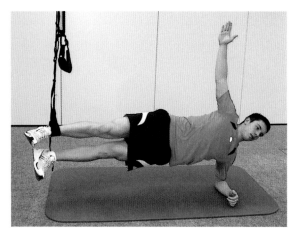

Fig. 15.17   Sling exercise for three-dimensional lumbopelvic stabilization, with enhanced activation of the hip adductors (left leg).

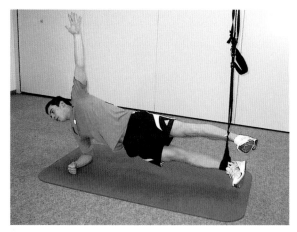

Fig. 15.18   Sling exercise for three-dimensional lumbopelvic stabilization, with enhanced activation of the hip abductors (right leg).

Effect of Fatigue

Endurance is a key factor for preventing injuries in sports in which fatigue affects the occurrence of muscle injuries. This is particularly true in team sports. In soccer, for example, the incidence of muscle injuries was found to be highest at the end of the two 45-minute halves (Hawkins and Fuller 1999; see also Chapter 5). Soccer is a sport in which more or less pronounced fatigue effects are expected to occur toward the end of each half. The heightened susceptibility to injuries due to fatigue may be explained by the fact that fatigued muscles have a reduced capacity for energy absorption (Mair et al. 1996). This assumption is indirectly supported by the study by Greig and Siegler (2009), who had soccer players perform treadmill exercises simulating the conditions of a soccer match. The authors found that eccentric hamstring muscle strength declined with increasing fatigue near the end of the simulated match, indicating a greater risk of injury from eccentric loads at those times (see p. 369). It is also possible that deficits in intermuscular coordination within the hamstring group (e.g., caused by the dual innervation of the two biceps heads) may predispose to injury (Devlin 2000).

It can be assumed, then, that factors which delay fatigue can make a significant contribution to reducing the risk of muscle injuries. From the physiological point of view, improvement in endurance appears to be an effective means of helping athletes to play longer without undue fatigue. Good endurance enables a player to recover quickly from the repeated explosive actions (especially sprints) that are characteristic of soccer play (Glaister 2005). The player can then perform successive sprints with better performance and without significant fatigue. This in turn should help reduce the risk of muscle injuries associated with repetitive sprints. Optimal endurance for better recovery between repeated sprints is particularly important for the relatively higher load intensities that are experienced during play, as opposed to training. It is known that muscle injuries are more likely to occur during play than during training (see Chapter 5). In terms of injury prevention, endurance training should be geared toward the relatively higher load intensities that occur during play and the associated importance of rapid recovery.

Improvement of Endurance

Although no research findings have yet been published on the specific endurance requirements for reducing the risk of injuries, practical experience at the elite soccer level can still provide us with guidelines for optimizing player endurance. **Table 15.1** lists position-specific endurance guidelines that were developed for professional soccer players in the German National League. These guidelines take various factors into account, including the position-specific requirements for total running distances. For example, midfield players generally have the longest running distances in high-level national and international competition. Optimizing endurance at the performance

levels shown in **Table 15.1** should have a positive effect on reducing the risk of muscle injuries in soccer.

From the point of view of training techniques, similar endurance gains can be achieved with endurance runs, as well as interval exercises (Faude et al. 2009). In the recent past, interval training has very often been preferred in team sports based on sport-specific considerations. While classic extensive/intensive interval training and modern intermittent interval training are useful for direct conditioning, continuous endurance training is still a valuable adjunct for promoting (basic) endurance while also stabilizing overall performance.

In the selection of endurance training methods, it should be noted that continuous training with interval-like units of higher intensity is unlikely to provide the training scope that is necessary for comprehensive endurance gains. Experience from classic endurance sports clearly shows that a more comprehensive program is needed to achieve peak performance. This means that goal-directed endurance training in sports such as soccer should always include an adequate combination of interval and continuous exercises.

Note

Effective, lasting endurance gains are always achieved by a combination of continuous and interval training methods.

It should also be noted that the continuous method is not limited to endurance runs alone, and that run training can be combined with training in soccer techniques. Again, a combination of continuous and interval methods is always desirable for the optimization of endurance. A key function of the continuous training method is to develop and maintain endurance on a long-term basis.

Note

Improved endurance leads to higher exercise tolerance and improved fatigue resistance, which help reduce the risk of injuries.

Table 15.1 Endurance guidelines: individual anaerobic thresholds in m/s (after Stegmann) recommended for various soccer positions in the German National League

Position	Individual anaerobic threshold (m/s)
Goalkeeper	3.7–3.9
Central defender	4.0–4.1
Outer defender	4.1–4.2
Central midfielder	4.2–4.4
Outer midfielder	4.1–4.3
Forward	4.0–4.2

In sports that involve intervals of intense activity, continuous methods of endurance training may still be a useful adjunct to interval methods. Even in classic sports that require explosive strength, endurance gains from continuous training can help to optimize exercise tolerance and recovery. In martial arts such as wrestling and judo, for example, the fighter must be able to recover as quickly as possible between individual bouts and between explosive actions during a bout. This underscores the importance of developing endurance in classic sports that require explosive strength.

Coordination

A factor that is often overlooked in active prevention programs is the development of specific motor coordination for a particular sport. Good coordination is characterized by optimal muscle use, which basically means optimal intermuscular coordination for executing the target movements in a given sport (see Schlumberger 2009). Optimal muscle use in this context refers to the coordinated interaction of the prime movers, antagonists, and stabilizing muscles. Less-than-optimal muscle use would be characterized by hyperactive muscles acting in an uncoordinated way. This increased muscle tension may be a contributing factor to muscular and joint injuries.

Practical training experience and scientific studies have both shown that specific coordination training helps athletes to move more skillfully and economically (Schlumberger 2009). Besier et al. (2003) made an important observation in this regard; they found that making a cutting maneuver from a linear run has optimal muscular control when the athlete knows the direction of the cutting maneuver in advance. But when the cutting maneuver is cued by a visual signal just moments before it is performed, the intermuscular coordination of the prime movers and stabilizers is less favorable. This means that the prime movers become hyperactive in unanticipated situations, undergoing a general co-contraction, while the stabilizing muscles do not show a physiologically selective activation pattern. Three conclusions can be drawn from this regarding the prevention of muscle injuries:

1. Increased activity of the prime movers, in terms of relatively greater muscle loading, is an ineffectual solution. This relative increase in muscle effort may lead to earlier onset of muscle fatigue, resulting in a greater risk of muscle injury, since preliminary fatigue in itself appears to increase the activity of injury-prone muscles like the hamstrings (Greig and Siegler 2009).
2. This unfavorable activation pattern may also reflect a lack of coordination among the prime movers (e.g., coordination deficits between the heads of the biceps femoris; see p. 377).

3. The findings reported by Besier et al. (2003) suggest that regular training in sport-specific movement patterns with realistic spatial and temporal constraints, variable external stimuli, and multiple possible solutions will train athletes to move with greater skill and economy. Specific coordination training to optimize muscle use should be of general benefit for reducing injury rates.

Training sport-specific movement patterns in specific spatial and temporal conditions is important for preventing excessive muscular activation.

Warming Up: Importance and Techniques

It is widely recognized that an adequate warm-up can reduce the risk of sports-related injuries. As far as muscle injuries are concerned, several physiologic mechanisms can be used for an "injury prevention" warm-up. It has been claimed that inadequate warm-up routines fail to reduce muscular viscosity, resulting in insufficient elastic compliance in the muscle tissue. Moreover, an inadequate warm-up cannot raise neuromuscular coordination (both intramuscular and intermuscular) to the necessary level. In both cases, the result may be an increased risk of injury. Since coordination deficits are considered a potential predisposing factor for muscle injuries (see above), optimum coordinative preparation of the muscles appears to be an important part of warming up. Thus, a brief practice of relevant sport-specific movement patterns is necessary during warm-up in order to retrieve and activate the automatisms that are involved in sport-specific coordination processes.

Practicing the movement patterns that are typical of a given sport is an important, specific preventive measure during warm-up.

In understanding the importance of warm-up for preventing muscle injuries, it is helpful to recognize that the primary goal of warming up is to generate a starting condition that is optimal for performance. The content of the warm-up routine should be geared strongly toward that goal. With detailed planning, measures that help prevent injuries can be combined with short-term performance-increasing measures without compromising the quality of the warm-up. In soccer, for example, including exercises in the pregame warm-up that will help to promote performance and prevent injuries results in the three-phase warm-up routine outlined in **Table 15.2**.

Table 15.2 Three-phase warm-up routine before a soccer match

Phase 1	Running and moving at moderate intensity
Phase 2	Specific preparation of muscles and joints important for soccer movements
Phase 3	Preparation of all soccer-related specific movement

Phase 1: Optimizing Core Temperature, Muscle Temperature, Blood Flow, and Neuronal Activation

The emphasis in phase 1 is on optimizing core and muscle temperature, improving blood flow, and promoting effective nervous system function. This is achieved by moderate exercise in a predominantly aerobic range. Running at an easy pace can be safely combined with variable movements with and without a ball. For injury prevention, it is important to avoid explosive actions and large changes in muscle length during this initial warm-up phase. Negative examples of this would be unprepared kicking at goal (risk to the hamstring group and rectus femoris) and fast cutting maneuvers with or without a ball (risk to the adductors).

Phase 2: Preparation of the Muscles and Joints

The emphasis in phase 2 is on specific preparation of the muscles and joints important for the soccer player. The joints are moved through a greater (not necessarily maximal) range of motion, and key soccer-specific muscles are prepared in a way that presets them for the muscle lengths that will be used later during play. This phase also increases local blood flow to essential muscles. Active length preparation also appears to induce optimal α–γ co-activation, which is an important factor in regulating the sensitivity of the muscle spindle system.

Note
Adequate "length preparation" of the muscles is an important part of warming up.

Static stretching is traditionally used to achieve this goal. Studies indicate, however, that this type of stretching reduces muscle tone and thus causes a short-term reduction of rapid force generation in the muscles. This would seem to be counterproductive before a soccer match, where players are required to perform fast and explosive actions. Dynamic preparation or activation exercises would seem to be more favorable in this setting. **Figures 15.19, 15.20, 15.21, 15.22, 15.23, 15.24, 15.25** illustrate the dynamic activation exercises that are important during phase 2 warm-up. Integrating these exercises into a complex warm-up routine can specifically prepare the muscles and joints for rapid and explosive actions (Little and Williams 2006).

Dynamic activation exercises have two advantages over classic static stretching exercises:
1. They are performed in an upright position that conforms to actual play. This should allow better coordinative transfer to the specific motor actions in soccer.
2. The lumbopelvic–hip region is actively stabilized during all exercises. Active stabilization of the lumbar and thoracic spine and pelvis is believed to be an essential precondition for optimal length control of the dynamically activated hip and leg muscles.

These exercises are generally performed from a walk rather than a stationary start. Five to 10 repetitions are recommended for each exercise to achieve optimal warm-up effects.

It should be added, however, that the frequently-cited adverse effects of static stretching on athletic quickness in complex warm-up routines are not as negative as many believe (Little and Williams 2006). Moreover, dynamic activation exercises are not technically easy to perform. There is even a risk that dynamic activation may not produce important short-term gains in muscle flexibility during the warm-up.

Caution
When performed by less practiced individuals, dynamic activation exercises may sometimes miss the goal of selective muscle preparation due to their technical difficulty.

This is a good reason to include classic static stretching in the warm-up routine, especially for young and amateur athletes who have limited training opportunities (e.g., twice a week). Static stretches are technically easier to perform, and the short-term flexibility gains are easier to control in terms of muscle length preparation.

Practical Tip
Static stretching should not be categorically rejected during warm-up. It is an effective measure for muscle preparation in many athletes, owing to its technical simplicity.

It should also be noted in this regard that individualized static stretching may be advantageous during warm-up. For example, O'Sullivan et al. (2009) found that static stretching of the hamstrings in players with a previous muscle injury increased hamstring flexibility whereas dynamic activation techniques did not. These findings support the empirical observation that players with varying degrees of shortening or prior muscle injuries will benefit from individualized static stretching before the actual warm-up. These players can perform their individual exercises in the locker room just before joining the complete team warm-up (which includes dynamic activation techniques).

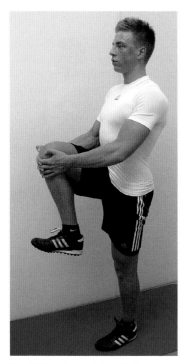

Fig. 15.19 Dynamic hip flexion.

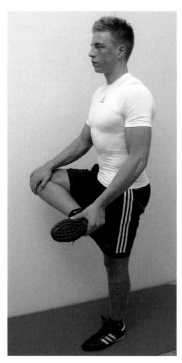

Fig. 15.20 Dynamic external hip rotation.

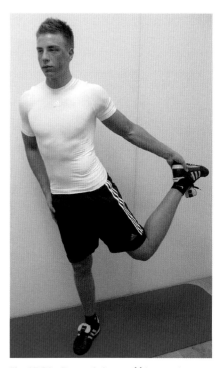

Fig. 15.21 Dynamic internal hip rotation.

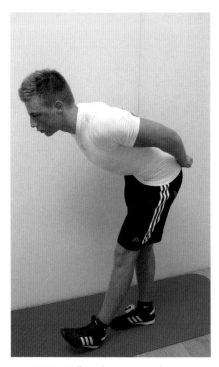

Fig. 15.22 Walking hamstrings (dynamic length preparation of the hamstrings).

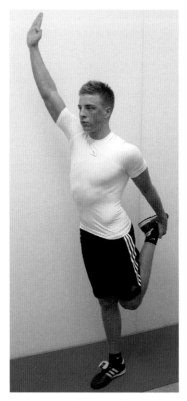

Fig. 15.23 Walking quadriceps (dynamic length preparation of the quadriceps).

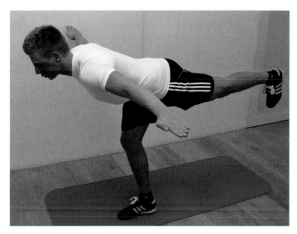

Fig. 15.24   One-legged balance stance from a walk (dynamic length preparation of the hamstrings of the support leg and the hip flexors of the swing leg).

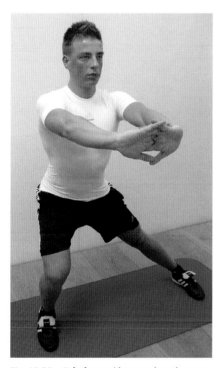

Fig. 15.25   Side lunge (dynamic length preparation of the adductors).

Practical Tip

Athletes with muscle shortening should do individual static stretching exercises prior to warm-up.

These strategies require close cooperation within the medical care team (doctors, physical therapists and athletic trainers) to allow for optimum individual work. These individualized strategies are best implemented in professional sports, therefore.

Phase 3: Playing Actions Performed at High Intensity

Phase 3 is characterized by successive playing actions performed at high intensity (shooting and passing, accelerating and full-out sprinting, specific actions involving paired opponents—e.g., five-versus-five drills). These exercises are important for retrieving motor automatisms and preparing for optimal muscular coordination.

Practical Tip

The temperature should also be taken into account when planning the warm-up routine. A longer and more intensive warm-up is recommended at low ambient temperatures (see also Devlin 2000).

Note from the Editors: The editors would like to take this opportunity to specifically recommend the "11+" prevention program, developed by the International Federation of Association Football's Medical Assessment and Research Center (F-MARC), which provides excellent videos and illustrations. Details are available at: http://f-marc.com/11plus/about/11plus/.

References

Arnason A, Andersen TE, Holme I, Engebretsen L, Bahr R. Prevention of hamstring strains in elite soccer: an intervention study. Scand J Med Sci Sports 2008; 18(1): 40–48

Askling C, Karlsson J, Thorstensson A. Hamstring injury occurrence in elite soccer players after preseason strength training with eccentric overload. Scand J Med Sci Sports 2003; 13(4): 244–250

Besier TF, Lloyd DG, Ackland TR. Muscle activation strategies at the knee during running and cutting maneuvers. Med Sci Sports Exerc 2003; 35(1): 119–127

Bradley PS, Portas MD. The relationship between preseason range of motion and muscle strain injury in elite soccer players. J Strength Cond Res 2007; 21(4): 1155–1159

Comfort P, Green CM, Matthews M. Training considerations after hamstrings injury in athletes. Strength Cond J 2009; 31: 68–74

Croisier JL, Forthomme B, Namurois MH, Vanderthommen M, Crielaard JM. Hamstring muscle strain recurrence and strength performance disorders. Am J Sports Med 2002; 30(2): 199–203

Croisier JL, Ganteaume S, Binet J, Genty M, Ferret JM. Strength imbalances and prevention of hamstring injury in professional soccer players: a prospective study. Am J Sports Med 2008; 36(8): 1469–1475

Dadebo B, White J, George KP. A survey of flexibility training protocols and hamstring strains in professional football clubs in England. Br J Sports Med 2004; 38(4): 388–394

Devlin L. Recurrent posterior thigh symptoms detrimental to performance in rugby union: predisposing factors. Sports Med 2000; 29(4): 273–287

Engebretsen L, Bahr R. Why is injury prevention in sports important? In: Bahr R, Engebretsen L, eds. Sports injury prevention. Oxford: Wiley-Blackwell; 2009: 1–6

Faude O, Schnittker R, Müller F, et al. Similar effects of high-intensity intervals and continuous endurance runs during the preparation period in high level football. In: Loland S, Bo K, Fasting K, et al., eds. 14th Annual Congress of the European College of Sports Science. Book of Abstracts; 2009 June 24–27; Oslo, Norway, p. 490

Greig M, Siegler JC. Soccer-specific fatigue and eccentric hamstrings muscle strength. J Athl Train 2009; 44(2): 180–184

Glaister M. Multiple sprint work: physiological responses, mechanisms of fatigue and the influence of aerobic fitness. Sports Med 2005; 35(9): 757–777

Hawkins RD, Fuller CW. A prospective epidemiological study of injuries in four English professional football clubs. Br J Sports Med 1999; 33(3): 196–203

Hajduk K, Schlumberger A. Effects of core stability exercises on maximum force and postural control of the lower extremity during 1RM squat performance. In: Hamar D, ed. 7th International Conference on Strength Training. Book of Abstracts; 2010; Bratislava, Slovakia. p. 109–110

Hennessey L, Watson AW. Flexibility and posture assessment in relation to hamstring injury. Br J Sports Med 1993; 27(4): 243–246

Kuszewski M, Gnat R, Saulicz E. Stability training of the lumbo-pelvo-hip complex influence stiffness of the hamstrings: a preliminary study. Scand J Med Sci Sports Exerc 2009 (2); 19(2): 260–266

Little T, Williams AG. Effects of differential stretching protocols during warm-ups on high-speed motor capacities in professional soccer players. J Strength Cond Res 2006; 20(1): 203–207

McGill S. Low back disorders. Champaign, IL: Human Kinetics; 2007

Mair S, Seaber AV, Glisson RR, Garret WE Jr. The role of fatigue in susceptibility to acute muscle strain injury. Am J Sports Med 1996; 24(2): 137–143

Orchard J, Marsden J, Lord S, Garlick D. Preseason hamstring muscle weakness associated with hamstring muscle injury in Australian footballers. Am J Sports Med 1997; 25(1): 81–85

O'Sullivan K, Murray E, Sainsbury D. The effect of warm-up, static stretching and dynamic stretching on hamstring flexibility in previously injured subjects. BMC Musculoskelet Disord 2009; 10: 37

Petersen J, Hölmich P. Evidence based prevention of hamstring injuries in sport. Br J Sports Med 2005; 39(6): 319–323

Proske U, Morgan DL, Brockett CL, Percival P. Identifying athletes at risk of hamstring strains and how to protect them. Clin Exp Pharmacol Physiol 2004; 31(8): 546–550

Schlumberger A. Aufbau der sensomotorischen Leistungsfähigkeit nach Verletzungen am Beispiel der Sportart Fußball. In: Laube W, ed. Sensomotorisches System. Stuttgart: Thieme; 2009: 600–617

Sherry MA, Best TM. A comparison of 2 rehabilitation programs in the treatment of acute hamstring strains. J Orthop Sports Phys Ther 2004; 34(3): 116–125

Sugiura Y, Saito T, Sakuraba K, Sakuma K, Suzuki E. Strength deficits identified with concentric action of the hip extensors and eccentric action of the hamstrings predispose to hamstring injury in elite sprinters. J Orthop Sports Phys Ther 2008; 38(8): 457–464

Thelen DG, Chumanov ES, Sherry MA, Heiderscheit BC. Neuromusculoskeletal models provide insights into the mechanisms and rehabilitation of hamstring strains. Exerc Sport Sci Rev 2006; 34(3): 135–141

Verall GM, Arnason A, Bennell K. Preventing hamstring injuries. In: Bahr R, Engebretsen L, eds. Sports injury prevention. Oxford: Wiley-Blackwell; 2009: 73–90

Witvrouw E, Danneels L, Asselman P, D'Have T, Cambier D. Muscle flexibility as a risk factor for developing muscle injuries in male professional soccer players. A prospective study. Am J Sports Med 2003; 31(1): 41–46

Witvrouw E, Mahieu N, Danneels L, McNair P. Stretching and injury prevention: an obscure relationship. Sports Med 2004; 34(7): 443–449

Yeung SS, Suen AM, Yeung EW. A prospective cohort study of hamstring injuries in competitive sprinters: preseason muscle imbalance as a possible risk factor. Br J Sports Med 2009; 43(8): 589–594

Yu B, Queen RM, Abbey AN, Liu Y, Moorman CT, Garrett WE. Hamstring muscle kinematics and activation during overground sprinting. J Biomech 2008; 41(15): 3121–3126

16

Special Case Reports from High-Performance Athletics

P. Ueblacker
L. Hänsel
H.-W. Müller-Wohlfahrt

Translated by Gertrud G. Champe

Introduction *382*

Cases 1–8 *382*

Introduction

In high-performance sports, the health-care team for the top athletes involved is faced with a variety of problems that players have every day. Usually, the real challenge is not how to interpret a complex, serious injury (such as an anterior cruciate ligament rupture); instead, the problem lies in recognizing and evaluating the almost daily disorders or small injuries that cause athletes pain and difficulties and possibly a significant sense of insecurity.

Since not every player can be provided with a comprehensive diagnosis, the physician or physical therapist has to be able to rely in most cases on the history and a confident clinical examination (see Chapter 6). The related questions are:

- Is additional imaging needed for the diagnosis?
- Can the player continue to train or play?
- From the medical point of view, is there a danger that the injury could get worse?
- Or are these symptoms with which the player can continue to play or train without medical consequences?

It is the team physician's duty to inform the trainer about the injury and to provide answers to the above questions. It is up to the physician alone, in consultation with the physical therapist, to decide whether the player can take part in a game. But particularly in the case of muscle injuries, because they vary so widely, there are borderline cases that are initially difficult to evaluate. Extensive experience, a detailed examination, and further accurate clinical checks, especially palpation, are helpful in reaching the best possible evaluation.

> *Note*
>
> Like other injuries, muscle lesions can sometimes have a surprising course. Not every assessment is correct; there are "outliers" in both directions, with more rapid or slower progress to healing.

Both high-performance and amateur athletes must be given an expected time frame for the healing process, according to which they can plan. The first estimate of the extent of the injury is the decisive one; examinations during the course of healing may show slightly different responses to the recommended and administered therapy. Selected cases from high-performance and amateur sports, illustrating typical and atypical courses of muscle injuries, are described below.

Case 1

Five months previously, a 26-year-old professional soccer player in the First Division in Germany had suffered an injury to the middle third of the left rectus femoris that was surgically treated at an external institution by the team physician responsible. Four months after that, during a league game, the player had suffered a painful event proximal to the operated region in the rectus femoris. Despite this, the medical department approved the player for training and play.

The player presented with persistent symptoms of pain in the ventral, proximal thigh. Palpation detected firmness of individual muscle bundles in the rectus femoris and a suspicion of an extensive fluid accumulation in a defect in the muscle structure. Scars were palpated in the operated area of the muscle. Sonography and the latest magnetic resonance imaging (MRI) examination established the diagnosis of a subtotal muscle tear (**Fig. 16.1**).

Appropriate therapy was prescribed for the player. The seroma was aspirated (30 mL of bloody fluid). The presence of blood in the fluid led to the suspicion that during training, in addition to an extensive earlier injury, the player had suffered further tearing in an injured zone that had not yet healed.

The entire length of the rectus femoris was then infiltrated for tension relief and to support the healing process (see also Chapter 11). Indometacin was prescribed for prophylaxis against myositis ossificans, and in addition, zinc and enzymes. A compression bandage was applied, and physical modalities and physical therapy treatment were administered (see Chapters 11 and 14).

When the player returned 2 weeks later, he was already reporting considerable symptomatic improvement; he no longer had a feeling of pressure in the muscles. An ultrasound check showed that the seroma was now very thin (**Fig. 16.2**); on palpation, the rectus femoris was still distinctly firm and partially indurated. The circumference of the affected thigh was 2 cm less than contralaterally.

MRI 6 weeks after the first visit showed adaptation of the muscle fibers in the area of the former rupture and the subfascial seroma, which was now flat. In addition, only discrete intramuscular fibrosis was detectable (**Fig. 16.3**).

Four weeks later, after intensive rehabilitation with running and muscle building, palpation detected a distinct improvement in the muscle tone; no structural defect could now be palpated. The muscle circumference was almost that of the other side. MRI now showed only discrete edema at the former tear, and there was only a small amount of scar formation after this previously extensive muscle injury (**Fig. 16.4**).

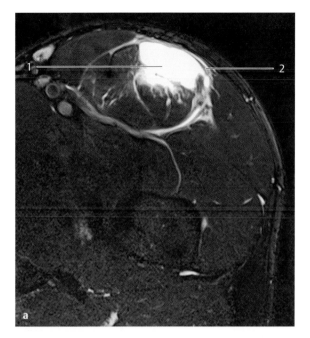

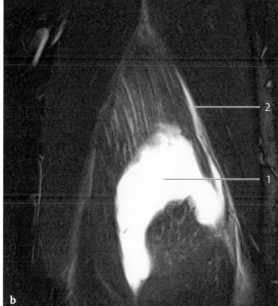

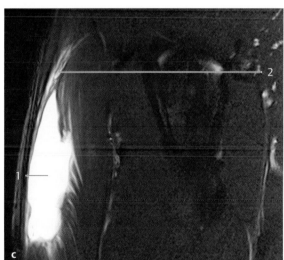

Fig. 16.1a–c High-resolution magnetic resonance imaging of the left rectus femoris muscle (at the first visit). At (1), there is a distinct seroma measuring 65 × 44 × 16 mm, with an extensive (subtotal) muscle tear (40% of the muscle cross-section) in the rectus femoris, 6 cm distal to the origin, with a dehiscence of ≈ 5 cm. Ventrolaterally, the muscle is separated from the fascia (2).

a Axial section.
b Coronal section.
c Sagittal section.

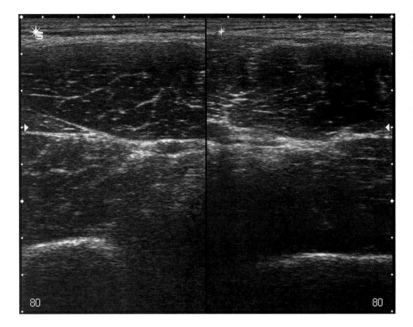

Fig. 16.2   Sonographic control with contralateral comparison (2 weeks after the first visit; injured side on the right in the image). Only a thin seroma, no longer representing an intramuscular mechanical impediment, is left. The muscle structure is loosened and is starting to show cicatricial changes.

Ten weeks after the start of treatment for this large, partly older and originally inappropriately treated injury, the player was able to take part in team training and has since been playing at a high level without recurrences or symptoms.

Critical Issues

- Was the indication for surgical treatment of the muscle lesion in the middle third of the rectus femoris correct, or might conservative therapy perhaps have led to a better result?
- Could the subsequent injury proximal to the operated injury have been avoided?
- Why did the medical department consider the player, with such an obvious finding and persistent symptoms, fit for unrestricted training and play?
- Would appropriate therapy, administered earlier, have led to a faster return to play?

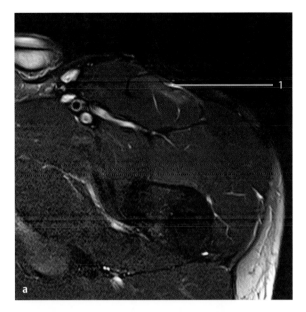

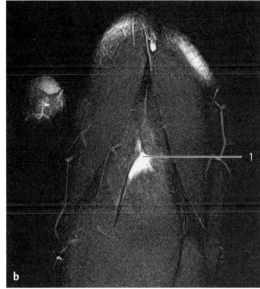

Fig. 16.3a–c   Follow-up MRI (6 weeks after the first visit).

a Axial section.
b Coronal section.
c Sagittal section.

1 Site of the previous tear with seroma

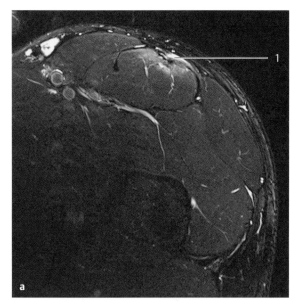

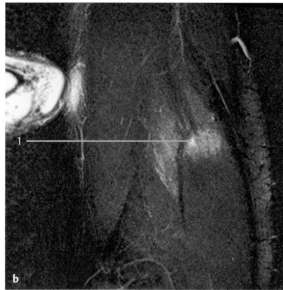

Fig. 16.4a–c   Follow-up MRI (10 weeks after first visit).

a Axial section.
b Coronal section.
c Sagittal section.

1 Site of the previous rupture

Case 2

On his first visit to our center, a 28-year-old professional soccer player in the English Premier League reported a sudden, painful injury that had occurred 6 days earlier without external impact on the right thigh, in the 60th minute of a soccer game, forcing him to retire from the game. Since then, he had been unable to train; he had had daily physical therapy without any significant improvement in the persistent symptoms.

Examination detected firm muscle strands in the rectus femoris in the ventral thigh and a structural defect in the medial third, as well as a swollen tendon structure. MRI demonstrated, as suspected from palpation, an extensive (subtotal) muscle tear in the proximal rectus femoris with a maximal axial extension of 25 × 25 × 60 mm (**Fig. 16.5**).

In view of these serious findings, appropriate treatment was started immediately, with puncture of the hematoma, infiltration therapy of the rectus femoris, and supportive drug treatment (see also Chapter 11).

One week later—that is, barely 2 weeks after the injury —the athlete reported significant subjective improvement; the rectus femoris had become firmer and the swelling had receded markedly.

Intensive therapy was continued, and 4 weeks after the trauma, palpation detected an almost normal muscle tone; only a small structural defect could be felt. A follow-up MRI confirmed the distinct improvement. Only a minimal amount of fluid was detected; the defect was significantly smaller (**Fig. 16.6**).

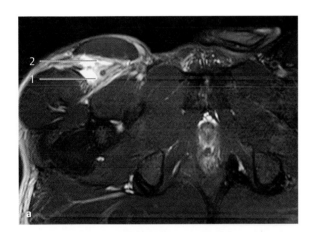

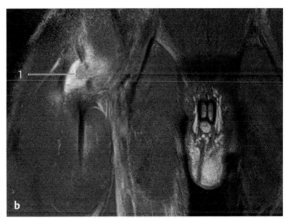

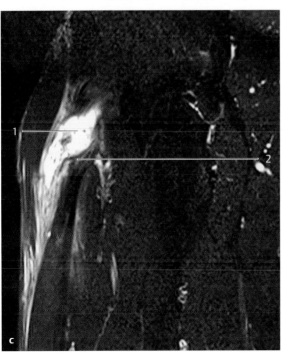

Fig. 16.5a–c High-resolution MRI of the right rectus femoris (at the first visit). The images show an extensive (subtotal) muscle tear, with partial rupture of the intramuscular tendon of the rectus femoris in the proximal medial aspect, with maximum dimensions of 25 × 25 × 60 mm (1). Correspondingly, there is a signal abnormality on the dorsolateral aspect of the sartorius (2).

a Axial section.
b Coronal section.
c Sagittal section.

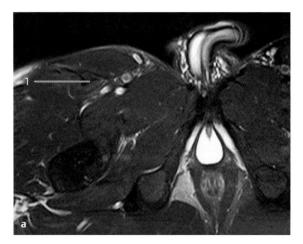

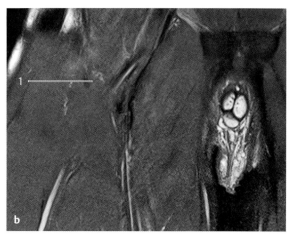

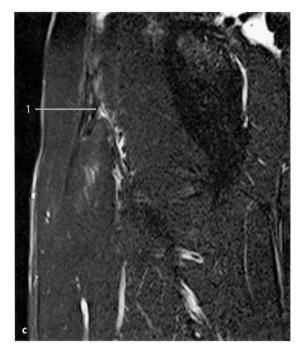

Fig. 16.6a–c   Follow-up MRI (3 weeks after the first visit).

a Axial section.
b Coronal section.
c Sagittal section.

1 Site of the previous rupture

Because of the rapid course of healing, running training was permitted 4 weeks after the injury and 3 weeks after the start of the appropriate therapy. Six weeks after the injury, the player returned to team training and since then he has been playing in the Premier League again without symptoms or recurrences.

Case 3

A 35-year-old soccer player in a First Division team in Germany felt a sudden piercing sensation in the right ventral thigh when kicking the ball. The next day, the symptoms were considerably worse, causing the player to come to our center.

Palpation showed a clearly palpable interruption of the fibrous structures along the rectus femoris within a firm muscle band. The subsequent MRI demonstrated the injury (**Fig. 16.7**). A diagnosis of a moderate partial muscle tear of the right rectus femoris was made, and treatment with muscle injection, lymphatic drainage, manipulation, and oral medications was started (see Chapter 11). A 7-day absolute interruption of training for the right lower extremity was prescribed.

After 1 week, the patient was free of pain. After a further 2 weeks, a follow-up MRI showed almost complete resolution of the diffuse intramuscular bleeding and edema formation. The injured muscle bundle demonstrated only a minimal, unproblematic retraction (**Fig. 16.8**).

After 4 weeks, training was permitted in the long-term endurance range. Ball training, high speeds, explosive

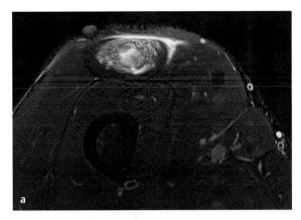
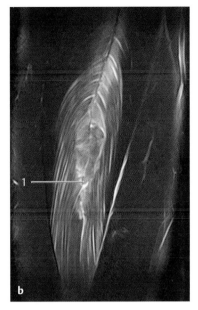
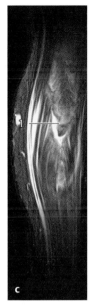

Fig. 16.7a–c High-resolution MRI of the right rectus femoris muscle (at the first visit). The images show a moderate partial muscle tear (bundle/fascicle tear) in the mid-section of the muscle, which can be easily recognized, particularly in the sagittal plane (1).

a Axial section.
b Coronal section.
c Sagittal section.

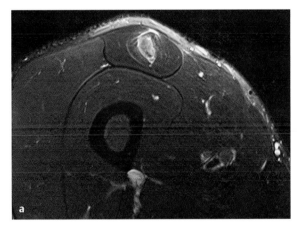
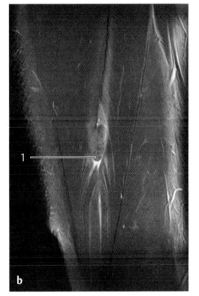
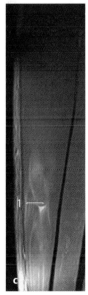

Fig. 16.8a–c Follow-up MRI (3 weeks after the first visit).

a Axial section.
b Coronal section.
c Sagittal section.

1 Site of the previous tear

stress, and passive stretching, however, were strictly forbidden.

On the basis of the good clinical findings and complete absence of pain, the situation was underestimated by the club's rehabilitation and fitness department—the player was exposed to greater stress, against what had been prescribed. One aspect of rehabilitation was force-loaded knee bends > 90°, as well as passive stretching of the rectus femoris.

After another week, a control MRI showed distinct retraction of the muscle bundle, an indication that the fibrous stabilization of the defect was not yet sufficient for the exercises performed (**Fig. 16.9**).

The deterioration in the imaging appearance was not reflected by a corresponding clinical deterioration. Nevertheless, a reduction of stress was definitely called for. Two weeks of pure running training without explosive stress and stretching was prescribed. Because of the complica-

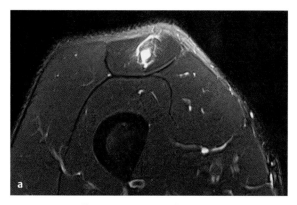
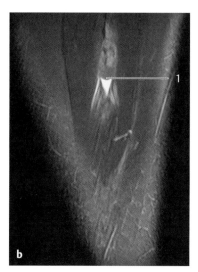
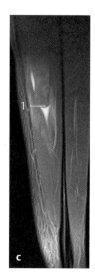

Fig. 16.9a–c   Follow-up MRI (5 weeks after the first visit, 1 week after premature start of high-effort rehabilitation exercises).

a Axial section.
b Coronal section.
c Sagittal section.

1   Site of the previous tear

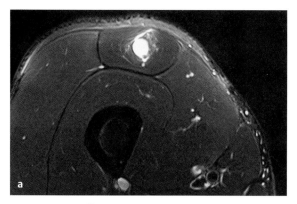
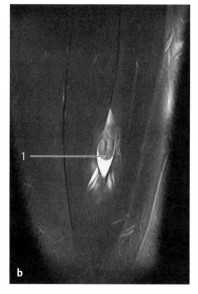
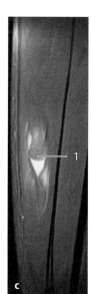

Fig. 16.10a–c   Follow-up MRI (7 weeks after the first visit).

a Axial section.
b Coronal section.
c Sagittal section.

1   Site of the previous tear

tion that had occurred, control MRIs were performed. These conclusively documented the fact that very distinct muscle bundle retraction had taken place, with formation of a seroma cavity ≈ 10 × 10 × 12 mm (**Fig. 16.10**).

After this, and assumed scar stabilization without further tearing, it was possible to increase the stress in a sport-specific manner over a period of 3 weeks. With the passage of time, there was no additional deterioration of the findings. Eight weeks after diagnosis, the player was approved for unrestricted team training. He has remained free of symptoms or recurrences up to the present.

Critical Issues

- Was the existing injury aggravated by continued training and passive stretching?
- Why was the player subjected to excessive stress in spite of clear orders from the physician responsible?
- Did the new deterioration and protraction of the healing process with resulting healing of the defect result from this?

Case 4

A 25-year-old professional soccer player in a national league team was referred by the team physician treating him. About 7 weeks previously, during a league game, he had suffered a muscle injury in the left adductor that was diagnosed as a moderate partial muscle tear. Images of the injury were not available. He had been treated with physical therapy and rehabilitation, acupuncture, laser treatments, and oral enzymes and nonsteroidal anti-inflammatory drugs.

After 4 weeks, the player was approved for team training, but had to drop out again immediately because of recurrent symptoms in the same location without a new trauma. The MRI taken at this time is shown in **Fig. 16.11**.

When a more detailed patient history was taken, firm questioning elicited the information that over the course of his career, the player had frequently reported muscle problems, such as recurrent partial muscle tears. There were repeated and sometimes long absences from play. The player reported no lumbar symptoms.

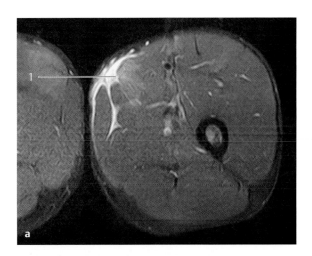

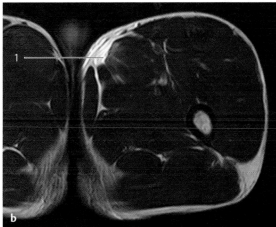

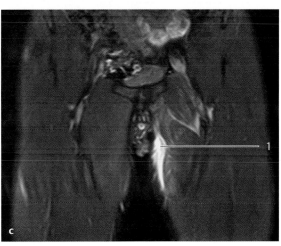

Fig. 16.11a–c **Magnetic resonance images (from an external facility, 4 weeks after trauma)** at low resolution demonstrate a lesion in the adductor muscles, with a local fluid accumulation (1).

a Axial section.
b Coronal section.
c Sagittal section.

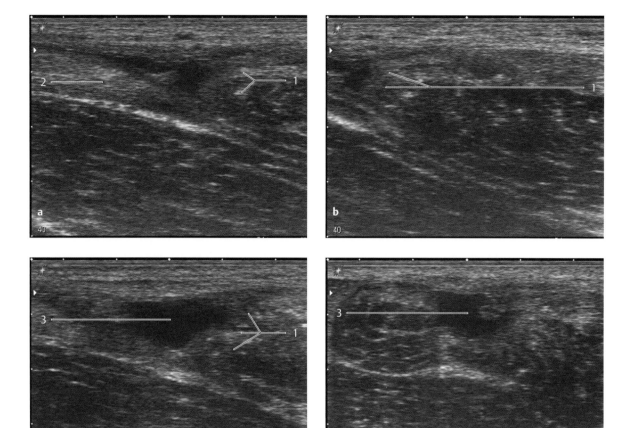

Fig. 16.12a–d   Sonography of the left adductor longus (at the first visit, ~ 4 weeks after trauma). Images **a–c** show in different longitudinal sections, the proximally ruptured muscle bundle, which is retracted by 2 cm distally (1). The echo-dense elongated structure on the left edge of the image is the proximal stump of the adductor longus (2). Image **d** shows a representative cross-section. The fluid-filled cavity of the defect (a hematoseroma) is clearly visible (3) in **c** and **d**.

On palpation, a defect zone in the proximal adductor longus as well as reactive muscle firmness in the distal adductor longus were observed. There was significant local pain on pressure. Examination of the lumbar spine showed a distinct right pelvic obliquity, with lumbar scoliosis and limitation of flexion. There was significant functional muscle shortening of the iliopsoas on both sides.

The quality of the MRI brought by the patient was poor, especially due to the low resolution of detail.

The authors carried out an ultrasound examination, which clearly visualized the actual extent of the injury. An extensive partial muscle tear in the adductor longus was seen, with distinct retraction of the affected muscle bundle and a fluid-filled defect area (**Fig. 16.12**). The diagnosis was clear, and another (high-resolution) MRI was not necessary.

Because of the findings in the lumbar examination with restricted motion in individual segments, a conventional radiograph of the lumbar spine in the standing position was requested (**Fig. 16.13**; see also Chapters 11 and 12). Despite the patient's unremarkable history of back problems, the radiograph revealed a surprising collection of pathological changes and variants from normal conditions.

On the day of the patient's first visit with the authors, multisegmental injection treatment of the lumbar spine was administered (see also Chapter 11). In addition, the left iliosacral joint (the functional connection between the iliosacral joint and the distribution area of the obturator nerve) was infiltrated, and local infiltration of the point of injury and the distal firm muscle band was administered. At the same time, the hematoseroma was aspirated. The injections were repeated twice, and in each case it was possible to drain the seroma (**Fig. 16.14**).

An ultrasound check-up 2 weeks after the start of treatment (**Fig. 16.15**) showed almost complete reduction of the seroma and a growing scar tissue bridge over the defect.

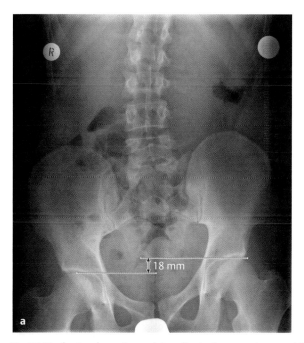
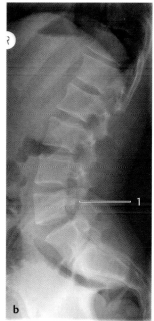

Fig. 16.13a, b   Lumbar spine–pelvis radiography (with the weight equally placed on both legs, with special attention to the knee joints being completely extended bilaterally), revealing a leg length difference of ~ 18 mm on the right, a resulting pelvic obliquity on the right and a compensatory right convex lumbar scoliosis. In addition, there is defective closure of the vertebral arch at S1 (possibly also at S2), a lumbosacral transition vertebra S1, and a spondylolysis at L5. Distinct formation of a gap in the vertebral arch (1) and initial spondylolisthesis (Meyerding grade I) can be seen. In addition, considerable hyperlordosis with early osteochondrotic changes at T12/L1 and formation of slight wedging vertebrae from T12 can be detected.

a   Anteroposterior radiograph.
b   Lateral radiograph.

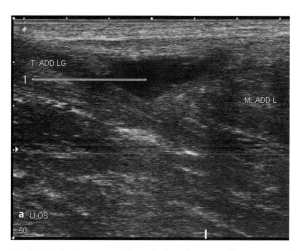
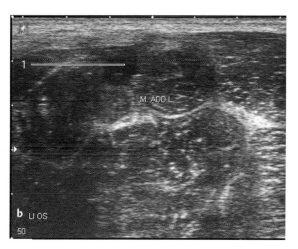

Fig. 16.14a, b   Ultrasound 1 week after the start of treatment, still demonstrating a distinct residual seroma cavity (1).

a   Longitudinal section.
b   Cross-section.

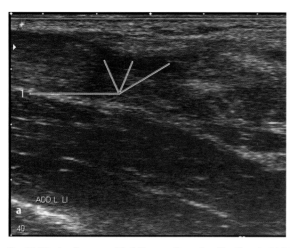
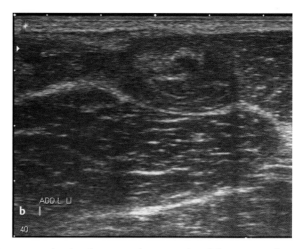

Fig. 16.15a, b   Sonographic follow-up 2 weeks after the start of treatment, showing almost complete resorption of the seroma and increasing fibrous bridging of the defect area (1).

a Longitudinal section.   **b** Cross-section.

With regard to training, only bicycle riding was allowed for 1 week; aerobic running was then started. Increased running speed and changes of velocity were permitted after 14 days. At the same time, the physical therapy and physical medicine measures described in Chapter 11 were administered. In the fourth week after the patient came to our center, he was able to take part in team training. Since then, he has been playing without recurrences or symptoms.

Medium-Term and Long-Term Treatment Plan

- Optimized orthotic inserts for normal, running, and soccer shoes, and initially a 5-mm and after 3 months an 8-mm leg length correction on the right side.
- Regular and independent stretching exercises for the ischiocrural, iliofemoral, and pelvitrochanteric muscles, especially the iliopsoas.
- Regular and independent core exercises to eliminate lordosis and gain stability.
- In case of lumbar or muscular complaints, multisegmental injection treatment of the lumbar spine.
- Lateral radiographic check-up in the lumbar spine to detect possible progression of the spondylolisthesis.

Case 5

A 24-year-old attacking midfield soccer player in the First Division in Germany was considered to be one of the team's key players and held a particularly important place in the team.

During the final training session before a league game, the player noticed a "pulling sensation" in the middle of the left dorsal thigh. However, he delayed informing the trainers of this. He was sent into the game on the Saturday.

He felt that the problem had improved and was able to play without pain. However, the "pulling sensation" returned during training sessions on Sunday and Monday. In the evening, he went to the team physician. A detailed examination with palpation found normal tone in all the posterior thigh muscles. There was no indication of a structural problem. The pain was interpreted as a neurogenic radiation and the player was informed of this. He was known to have some degenerative changes in the lumbar spine. However, a disk prolapse was ruled out with an MRI (**Fig. 16.16**). The lumbar spine was treated with injections.

During training the next day, after a center pass with hip rotation, he experienced a shooting pain in the same spot. Training was interrupted. The head physical therapist examined the muscle again, but with no remarkable findings. He undertook a chiropractic mobilization of the iliosacral joints, the lower lumbar spine, and the lumbosacral junction.

Immediately after this, the team traveled to a national Cup game. At the hotel, the team physician examined the muscle again and could not find any sign of a structural injury of the ischiocrural muscles. However, the player continued to lack confidence. The physician and the physical therapist were not able to clear up the player's uncertainties. Although he had been approved by the medical department, the player refused for this reason to play in the Cup game.

He was sent to our center the next day, either to rule out or confirm a muscle injury definitively by means of a technical examination. The MRI (high resolution with contrast and use of a surface coil) showed completely normal muscles in the left thigh (**Fig. 16.17**).

After repeated assurances that there was no danger to the muscle, the player was sent back to team training and given further intensive physical therapy.

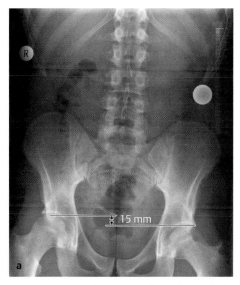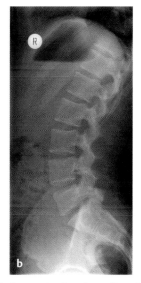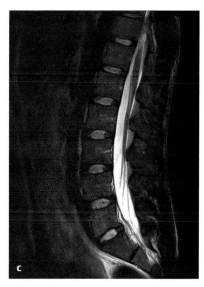

Fig. 16.16a–c Lumbar spine–pelvis radiography (with the weight placed equally on both legs), demonstrating a considerable real leg length difference of 15 mm on the left, with resulting pelvic obliquity and compensatory lumbar scoliosis. There is also considerable hyperlordosis, with a dorsally shifted center of gravity in the body (**a, b**). Magnetic resonance imaging shows only minor degenerative changes (**c**).

a Anteroposterior image.

b Lateral image.

c MRI of lumbar spine T2.

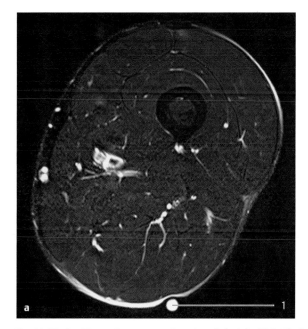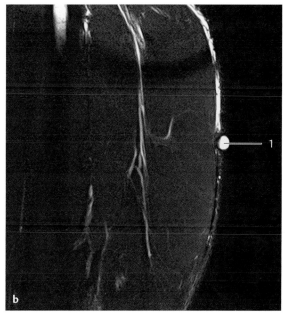

Fig. 16.17a, b Magnetic resonance imaging of the left thigh. The light spot on the surface (1) is caused by an attached liquid capsule and corresponds to the location of the maximum pain reported by the athlete. All sequences, as well as bilateral comparisons, showed completely normal muscles.

a Axial section.

b Coronal section.

Three days after the above-mentioned Cup game, the player returned to training for the first time without any muscle symptoms. Continuing specific increases in stress proceeded without problems. Six days later, the midfield star was assigned to the next important league game. He no longer reported muscle problems.

Critical Issues

The case described is meant to indicate how seriously a person, especially an athlete, experiencing pain can misinterpret it. The player was firmly convinced that he had suffered a muscle injury and saw participating in a game as being a serious threat to his health.

In this case, not even a functional muscle disorder (such as a fatigue-induced or neuromuscular muscle problem), which can cause serious pain, muscle firmness, and prevent an athlete from taking part in sports, was found on clinical examination. The muscle tone was always normal and back-related pain was excluded by clinical and radiological examinations.

The case also shows how difficult decision-making can be for the physician responsible. A physician accompanying a team can only rely on his or her experience and the clinical assessment, especially with palpation. A mistaken evaluation of the situation could mean a risk for a relevant injury, with a considerably longer recovery time.

Case 6

The following case is not from professional sport, but because of its dramatic course it is highly instructive.

A 25-year-old recreational athlete presented at an external clinic following a prolonged (but customary) jogging session with intense pain in the right calf. The clinical examination (according to the medical reports) revealed muscle firmness and pain on pressure in the tibialis anterior, with intact circulation and sensorimotor function. After an outpatient examination, the patient was discharged with a diagnosis of "muscle spasm in the tibialis anterior" and was recommended to stretch and take a muscle relaxant.

Because of persistent pain, he returned several times as an outpatient. Eight days after the start of the symptoms, he noticed weakness in the dorsal flexors of the foot. Three days later he returned to the same clinic; in the meantime, an increasing pretibial redness was visible, with complete paresis of the dorsal flexors of the foot. On the basis of a clinical suspicion of compartment syndrome, the fascia of the tibialis anterior and the peroneal compartment were immediately surgically split. Intraoperatively, a grayish discoloration with decreased circulation in the tibialis anterior muscle was seen.

After two further revisions with debridement, resection of muscle necroses and tenodesis of the tibialis anterior tendon in neutral position of the foot, secondary closure of the fascia 11 days after splitting of the compartment was performed. The tibialis anterior was resected in large part because of extensive necroses. A peroneal splint was fitted, and the patient was completely mobilized with intensive physical therapy.

Three months later, the dorsal flexors of the foot were still paralyzed; foot raising could be functionally compensated in part, using the peroneal group, by means of pronation. The circumference of the calf was 5 mm smaller in comparison with the contralateral side. The range of motion in the upper ankle, at 5/0/15°, was limited in comparison with the contralateral side. A neurological examination revealed a complete lesion of the peroneal nerve, with paralysis of the dorsal flexors of the foot. Electromyographically, stimulation of the nerve did not elicit a motor or sensory response potential either proximally or distally. MRI showed extensive destruction of the tibialis anterior, the extensor digitorum longus, and the extensor hallucis longus (**Fig. 16.18**).

Functional compensation for this considerable and potentially avoidable damage to the extensor compartment muscles was good, and continued treatment with physical therapy was advised, especially to maintain the range of motion of the ankle as well as to improve the gait. The only surgical intervention that might be considered would be tendon transposition, but even after this, the functional benefit would be uncertain.

Critical Issues

This case is presented to illustrate the dramatic course of a functional (and later structural) compartment syndrome in the calf, with disastrous consequences. The special feature of the case is that the initial cause was purely functional, without trauma, simply involving a sports activity. The drama of the case certainly lies in the late intervention by means of splitting the compartment. In this context, the symptoms of a compartment syndrome must once again be clearly emphasized: massive pain is the first symptom. At this point, it is essential to respond with therapy—that is, rest, measures to reduce swelling such as elevating and cooling the limb, hospital admission, detailed clinical check-ups, and readiness to operate in case of deterioration. If the circulation or sensorimotor function are damaged, it is usually too late, as the muscles have then already suffered considerable necrotic damage.

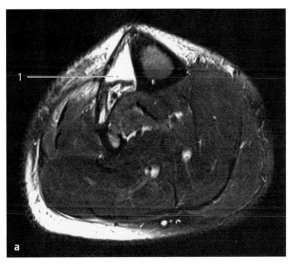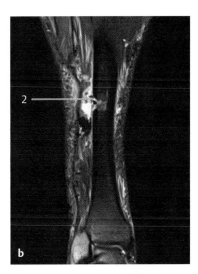

Fig. 16.18a, b   The muscles of the extensor compartment of the tibialis anterior, extensor digitorum longus, and hallucis longus show almost complete liquid and atrophic changes (1). There is a significant decrease in volume, retraction of the thickened muscle fascia, and secondary forward curvature of the posterior tibial and peroneal muscles toward the extensor compartment. The earlier keyhole surgery is evident in the tibia, during which the tendon of the tibialis anterior was attached (2).

a Axial section.
b Coronal section.

Case 7

A 34-year-old midfielder in the "Series A" top division in Italian soccer suffered a kick to the left calf from a player in the other team. Two days later, he started to experience swelling and pain, to the extent that training was no longer possible. The team physician sent the player (without clinical examination) for an MRI. After examining the images, he ordered a break from sports lasting "up to 8 weeks" due to a large "hole" in the muscle measuring 50 × 15 mm. Treatment consisted of massage, but this resulted in more swelling.

Ten days after the injury, the player came to our center. The clinical examination revealed firmness in the calf, specifically in the area indicated for the injury, which was painful to pressure, as were the surrounding muscles. The circumference of the calf was slightly increased in comparison with the contralateral side.

Sonography showed a distinct increase in volume (measured by comparison to the contralateral side) in the soleus muscle, directly under the distal aponeurosis of the lateral gastrocnemius, caused by a previous contusion hemorrhage that had a largely hyperechoic appearance and was therefore organized. Small hypoechoic liquid areas were only seen centrally, with small, diffuse foci of calcification (circumscribed hyperechoic inclusions with a dorsal acoustic shadow) (**Fig. 16.19**).

An MRI was taken, which showed a partially organized and thrombosed hematoma measuring 53 × 15 × 15 mm in the center of the lateral aspect of the soleus muscle (**Fig. 16.20**).

The liquid central portions of the hematoma, with a total of 10 mL of old blood, were therefore punctured and drained, and adjacent portions of the muscle were carefully infiltrated (see Chapter 11) to relax the muscle and promote muscle healing. Treatment over the next few days consisted of lymphatic drainage and aquatic exercises. Massage was avoided. Indometacin was prescribed for prophylaxis against ossification, as small foci of ossification were already visible on sonography (which is particularly sensitive to this process).

Only 2 days later, the player reported significant improvement of his problems, saying he was able to walk normally without pain. The clinical findings showed resolution of the muscle firmness; sonography demonstrated increasing dispersion of the organized hematoma.

Two days later, with continuation of the measures mentioned above, training runs at endurance speed were started, which the player was able to tolerate without problems.

Instead of the originally predicted break from sports of "up to 8 weeks," the player made a problem-free comeback 8 days after the start of the appropriate treatment, in a game that was important for his national team. Three days later, he played again for over 90 minutes.

At a follow-up visit 15 days after the start of treatment, the clinical examination showed at most a moderate, circumscribed firmness in the calf, and sonography demonstrated only a diffuse loosening of the muscle structure at the site of the former hematoma, without organized or

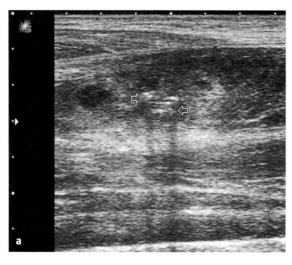

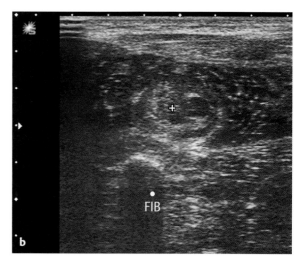

Fig. 16.19a–c Ultrasound imaging of the injured soleus muscle under the distal aponeurosis of the lateral gastrocnemius reveals calcifications—i.e., small hyperechoic areas with acoustic shadowing (arrows in **a**). The hematoma is largely hyperechoic (+) and thus organized, with only small central hypoechoic areas (**b**). An increase in volume (measured by comparison with the contralateral side) in the soleus muscle can be detected.

a Longitudinal section.
b Cross-section.
c Longitudinal section (in comparison with the contralateral side, shown on the left in the image)

FIB   Fibula

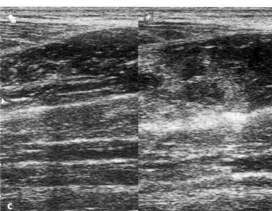

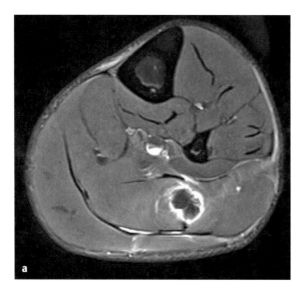

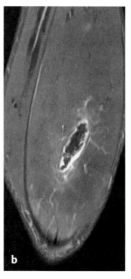

Fig. 16.20a, b Magnetic resonance imaging of the calf, showing a partly organized and thrombosed hematoma, 53 × 15 × 15 mm in size, at the center of the lateral aspect of the soleus muscle.

a Axial section.
b Coronal section.

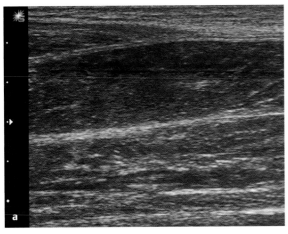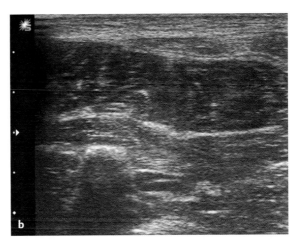

Fig. 16.21a, b   Follow-up ultrasound 15 days after the start of appropriate treatment, showing only diffuse bulking of the muscle structure at the site of the previous hematoma. Organized or thrombosed portions and ossifications are no longer visible.

a Longitudinal section.   **b** Cross-section.

thrombosed portions. A slightly increased diameter of the soleus muscle in comparison with the contralateral side was still detectable (**Fig. 16.21**). Ossifications were no longer visible.

Regular relaxation massage for the calf was prescribed, and the player was cleared for normal training and play; indometacin was discontinued. Since that time, the midfielder has been playing in "Series A" games in Italy without problems.

Critical Issues

- A fresh injury site with hematoma, whether caused by distraction or contusion, may not be massaged at first. Otherwise, the risk of calcifications and the onset of myositis ossificans is significantly increased.
- The muscle injury was incorrectly evaluated and not seen in context with the mechanism of injury. The "large hole measuring 5 cm" recognizable on the MRI was created by a partially thrombosed hematoma that was displacing the muscle structure. The muscle bundles were compressed by contusion, not torn by distraction. If the latter had been the case, a longer break from playing of ≈ 6 weeks would have been necessary.
- This case shows how important it is to differentiate between distraction and contusion as the cause of injury, moreover, how important it is to include medical history in the assessment of a muscle injury. Contusion injuries involve compression of the muscle structure by hematomas of varying extent and are tolerated much better, as there usually is no longitudinal tear. They can be subjected to a load much earlier without risk.

Case 8

A player in a First Division team in Germany suffered a muscle injury while playing in another country's national team in a preliminary match for an international tournament. Examinations by the foreign national team's medical staff, including MRI, identified a muscle injury with a structural defect extending for 18 mm (**Fig. 16.22**), as described in the written report by the foreign radiologist (corresponding in size to a moderate partial muscle tear).

Treatment by a therapist who was not part of the national team's medical staff consisted of "no heat, but extreme stretching," as the practitioner himself expressed it. The player experienced this treatment as being very painful; pain medication was administered several times.

Seven days later, the player returned to the national team. The national team's medical staff drained 20 mL of blood from the distal thigh several times. Twelve days later, the player was sent into two games in the international tournament, and 4 days after that, he played for 90 minutes. He played in two more tournament matches, in one of them for more than 120 minutes.

According to his own report, he received pain medications repeatedly for training and match play, and 20 mL of blood was "pulled out of the muscle" several times.

After a vacation 3 weeks later and 8 weeks after the injury, the player was examined before the start of training by his German club's team physicians. On inspection, palpation, and sonography, changes corresponding to a (sub)-total tear in the distal biceps femoris were immediately noticeable. On inspection, the muscle belly was proximalized, and there was a defect formation distally (**Fig. 16.23**). On palpation, the gap could be clearly felt as a seroma cavity, which was confirmed on sonography, with a fluid-filled cavity 50 mm long and 20 mm wide (**Fig. 16.24**). A

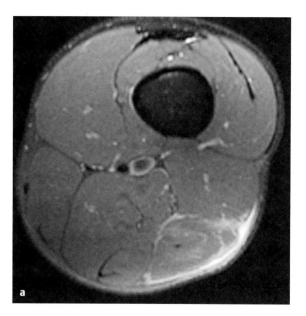

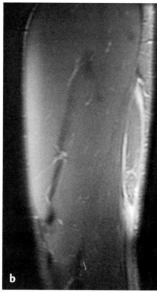

Fig. 16.22a, b Magnetic resonance imaging (carried out at an external facility) of the left hamstrings 1 day after injury, showing a partial muscle tear in the biceps femoris, with a structural defect 18 mm in size (which was described in the written report by the external radiologist) and intermuscular edema extending along the fascia of the whole muscle.

a Axial section.
b Sagittal section.

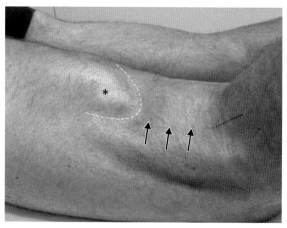

Fig. 16.23 Clinical image of the injured muscle 8 weeks after trauma. The muscle belly is retracted and proximalized (asterisk; comparable to a rupture of the long head of the biceps brachii at the shoulder, with distalization of the biceps on the arm). A defect zone is visible distally (arrows).

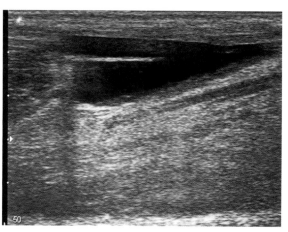

Fig. 16.24 Ultrasound of the left biceps femoris 8 weeks after trauma. At first sight, a subtotal tear of the muscle, with proximal retraction of the muscle and a subsequent seroma in a defect zone 50 × 20 mm in size, are clearly visible (longitudinal section).

subsequent MRI revealed a subtotal tear in the long head of the biceps femoris, except for a continuous cordlike strip of muscle 5 mm wide, with the formation of a gap in the muscle belly measuring 50 mm on the craniocaudal plane, 50 mm on the coronal plane, and 26 mm on the sagittal plane, with an intrafascial seroma and avulsion of the distal tendon of the muscle, ~ 70 mm proximal to the fibular attachment (**Fig. 16.25**).

Immediate treatment was started: 20 mL of serous fluid (not bloody, indicating that this was not a fresh injury) was drained from the seroma cavity, the thigh was wrapped in compression bandages to above the knee joint, and a break from training and play was prescribed. In ad-

dition, appropriate medications were prescribed (see Chapter 11).

The player was seen every 2–3 days for detailed clinical and sonographic check-ups; therapy consisted of passive measures such as lymphatic drainage, compression, and later, water therapy in the form of pool walking, followed by undemanding bicycling to improve drainage but without any training effect.

Repeated punctures were necessary in the weeks that followed, until the seroma was finally no longer visible. After each drainage procedure, a special compression bandage was applied that the player had to wear constantly.

Three weeks after the first drainage procedure, an 8-mL seroma was still visible (**Fig. 16.26**); 9 weeks after the

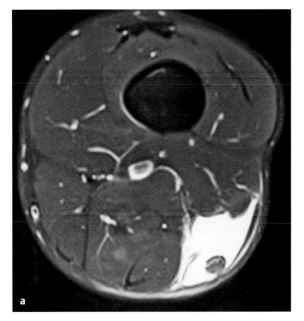

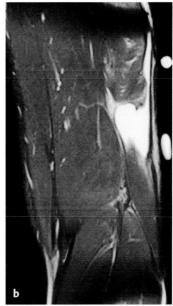

Fig. 16.25a–c Magnetic resonance imaging of the left biceps femoris, 8 weeks after the trauma (and at initial visit for diagnosis), revealed a subtotal tear of the long head of the biceps femoris, except for a continuous cordlike strip of muscle 5 mm wide, with formation of a gap in the muscle belly measuring 50 mm on the craniocaudal plane, 50 mm on the coronal plane, and 26 mm on the sagittal plane, with an intrafascial seroma and avulsion of the distal tendon of the muscle, ~ 70 mm proximal to the fibular attachment. (Note: massive aggravation of the initial injury is clear when these images are compared with the initial MRI in **Fig. 16.22.**)

a Axial section.
b Coronal section.
c Sagittal section.

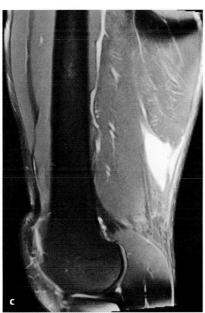

first drainage procedure, a small border of 2 mL of fluid was observed, until finally healing with scar formation ensued. (It should be noted that any collection of fluid after a muscle injury has to be removed, as the fluid is a mechanical barrier in the muscle tissue that must be healed. Healing—and possibly scarring—can only take place in "dry conditions.") Concurrent infiltration treatment (see Chapter 11) was performed when the seroma was no longer detectable.

From that point, light strength training was permitted and the scar was massaged, as the distal stump of the tendon proved to be hardened. Ten weeks after diagnosis,

light endurance running was started and gradually increased to a 20-minute effort without fatigue or pain.

Eleven weeks after diagnosis, the difference in circumference between the thighs was 1.5 cm at 10 cm above the patella and 2.0 cm at 20 cm above the patella. Five weeks later, as a result of training, the difference in circumference was reduced to only 5 mm.

Sixteen weeks after diagnosis, the player had no difficulty in performing any aspect of training runs, including sprinting, so that individual training with the ball was permitted. Two weeks later, he was allowed to take part in team training. The previous final MRI findings showed a developed scar plate in the long head of the biceps femo-

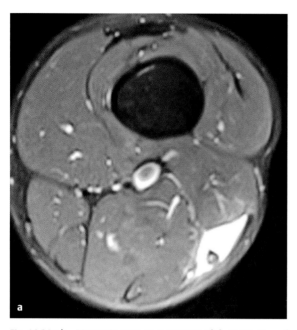
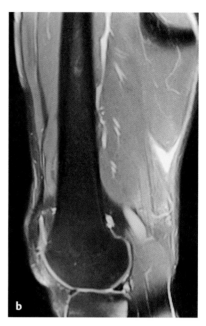

Fig. 16.26a, b   Magnetic resonance imaging of the injury 3 weeks after diagnosis and the start of appropriate treatment, again showing the muscle retraction and a residual seroma of ~ 8 mL.

a Axial section.

b Sagittal section.

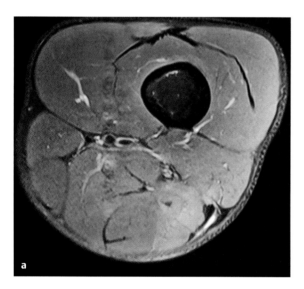
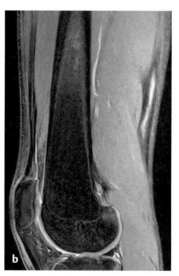

Fig. 16.27a, b   Magnetic resonance imaging 18 weeks after diagnosis and the start of appropriate treatment, demonstrating a scar plate in the long head of the biceps femoris at the former injury site, as well as increasing closure of the musculotendinous separation of the long head from the distal tendon of the short head. Only discrete, residual intramuscular and musculotendinous signal changes in the distal long head, as well as a very slight seroma, are still visible.

a Axial section.

b Sagittal section.

ris, as well as increasing closure of the musculotendinous separation of the long head from the distal tendon of the short head. In comparison with the preliminary examinations, there were also only discrete residual intramuscular and musculotendinous signal changes in the distal long head (**Fig. 16.27**).

The player made his comeback 31 weeks after the initial injury, i.e., 23 weeks after correct diagnosis and the start of appropriate treatment. Since then, he has played without any recurrent problems of the healed muscle injury. A further MRI examination 8 months after his return to play showed complete scarred healing of the biceps ten-

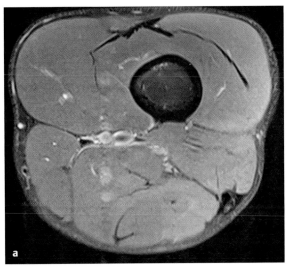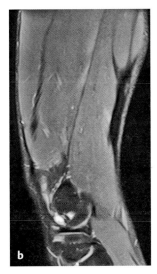

Fig. 16.28a, b   Magnetic resonance imaging 8 months after the player's return to play, showing complete scarred healing of the biceps tendon without any further structural damage, signs of inflammation, or seroma. (Note: due to the slightly different plane of the section in the MRI, the bony structures of the knee joint have a different appearance from that in **Fig. 16.28b**. Both images show the region of the previous musculotendinous injury.)

a Axial section.

b Sagittal section.

don, with no further structural damage or signs of inflammation (**Fig. 16.28**).

Critical Issues

- If the original injury had been correctly diagnosed, with appropriate treatment and interruption of athletic performance, the healing phase would not have taken 31 weeks (or 23 weeks), but probably only 6 weeks.
- As a result of the (painful) stretching (partly with administration of pain medication) as part of the treatment, a moderate partial muscle tear was extended to become a (sub)total rupture of the biceps femoris. It is absolutely necessary not to apply stretching when there is structural damage (i.e., a tear injury) because this causes the tear in the muscle to open up further (stretching a muscle that has a structural injury can be compared with pulling on a hook and loop fastening).
- Administering pain medications is contraindicated, because these suppress the (protective) perception of pain on exertion.
- Bloody fluid from a muscle puncture is always an indication of extensive structural injury.

- How was the player able to continue high-level play despite such an extensive muscle injury? The answer can only be that the maximally trained surrounding muscle was able to compensate for the (sub)total rupture of the long head of the biceps femoris. The low degree of pain toward the end can be explained by the fact that the muscle was torn across its diameter, so that there was no longer a painful pull on the structures. The paradox is that a complete rupture can consequently be less painful than a partial rupture, in which the surrounding muscle fascicles transmit a steady pull to the area of the tear.
- Continuing athletic performance without treatment would very probably have entailed a risk of sports invalidity due to increasing failure of the compensating muscles. The first result of failing function in the biceps femoris would probably have been lateral instability in the knee joint.

Subject Index

Page numbers in *italics* refer to illustrations or tables

A

abdominal wall muscles   9, *9, 10*
   myofascial release   *348, 351*
abductor muscles   5
accessory nerve   52
acetylcholine (ACh)   49, 61, 62
acetylcholine receptor (AChR)   49, 62
acetylcholinesterase   62
Achilles tendon   37
   lymphatic taping   357–358, *358*
acidosis   95, *95*
   muscle fatigue and   83
acoustic enhancement   171
acoustic shadow   171, *172*
actin   60
actin filaments   29–31, *29, 30*
   function   64
   structure   *60*
action potential   62
   frequency   67
   superposition   65–66, *66*
Actovegin   269, 272
adductor muscles   5, *16, 17, 18, 55, 183*
   adductor brevis   *16, 18, 177, 183*
      tendinous avulsion   *214*
   adductor longus   *16, 18, 173, 177, 183,* 220
      minor partial muscle tear   *206, 209*
      moderate partial muscle tear   *209,* 393, *393–394*
      tendinous avulsion   *212, 213, 214*
   adductor magnus   *8, 16, 18, 56, 173, 177, 180, 183*
   adductor minimus   *183*
   preventive stretching   *370*
   ultrasonographic appearance   179, *182*
adenosine triphosphate (ATP)
   hydrolysis   95
   resynthesis   83, 86
aerobic metabolism   79–80
afterloaded contraction   *68,* 69, 70
age
   influence on muscle regeneration   120–122, *121*
      antioxidative capacity   122
      extracellular matrix   122
      growth factors   122
      phagocytosis   121
      signaling pathways   121–122
   muscle injury relationships   144
      soccer injury risk   131, *131*
   ultrasonographic appearance and   *175*

alanine   94–95
alcoholic myopathy   237
alertness   249
alkalosis   83
alpha–gamma coactivation   74
amino acids   92–95, *93*
   demand in athletes   93–95
      alanine   94–95
      carnosine   94–95
      creatine   94
      glutamine   94
      taurine   94
   essential amino acids   92
   metabolism   *94, 96*
   supplementation   96
AMP-activated protein kinase   87
amyotrophic lateral sclerosis   232
anaerobic alactacid energy production   78
anatomic nomenclature   3–5, *4*
anatomic profile   25, *26*
anconeus   *11, 13*
angulation of fascicles   24–25
ankle
   injuries   19
   segmental innervation and movements   *54*
ansa cervicalis profunda   50
anticipation   252
antilipemic-associated myopathy   238
antioxidants   84, 96–98, *97*
   function   96
   importance in athletic activity   96–98
   intake   96
   mechanisms of action   *97*
   muscle healing and   120
   therapy   271
anxiety   252
aponeurosis   23, 37
apophyseal avulsion   162–163, *163*
appendicitis   288
aquatraining   362–363
arm
   agonist versus antagonist muscles   *23*
   muscle compartments   11–14, *11, 13*
   tension tests for compression syndromes   349, *349*
arnica   269–270
articularis genus   *17, 183*
atrophy   175, *175*
attention   248–249
attenuation   172
autogenous inhibition   75
autonomic functions   251
auxotonic contraction   *68,* 69

B

basal lamina, synaptic   43
behavior   247
   environment interactions   247–248, *247*
behavioral neurology   246
Bessman cycle   79, *79*
biceps brachii   5, *11, 13, 55*
   fascia   *36*
   insufficiency   42
   laceration repair   316
biceps femoris   *8,* 17, *19, 55, 56,* 179, *183*
   injuries
      intramuscular tendinous rupture   *211*
      partial muscle tears   *152, 187, 189, 206, 210, 219*
      soccer players   133, *152*
      subtotal tear, case study   400–404, *401–404*
      tendinous avulsion   309
   long head   *177, 180, 182*
   preventive stretching   *370*
   short head   *177, 182*
   tender points   355–356
   ultrasonographic appearance   *175*
biopsy indications   229, *230*
blood flow
   after exercise   86
   warm-up and   81, 378
blood parameters   275–278, *278*
body axes   *3*
body language   328–329
brachial artery   11
brachial plexus   50, *51,* 52
brachialis   *3,* 5, *11, 13*
   fascia   *36*
brachioradialis   *2,* 5, *13, 55*
bracing   283
brain   48–50, *49*
   functions   247–254
      affects and emotions   251–252
      alertness   249
      anticipation   252
      attention   248–249
      autonomic functions   251
      consciousness   253–254
      drive   253
      goal selection   252
      hierarchy   *248*
      language and communication   251
      memory   249–250
      monitoring   253
      motor learning   254

brain, functions
    perception   250
    planning   252
    thinking   250
    motor cortex   48–49
        somatotopic organization   49
    muscle injuries and   258–259
    muscle interaction   246
    sensory cortex   50
bridging exercise   372, *372*
bromelains   270
bursa   40
buttock muscles   14–15, *14, 15*
    see also specific muscles

C

calcineurin/nuclear factor of activated
    T cells (NFAT)   87
calciol   101
calcitriol   101
calcium   98
    concentration   *61*, 62, *63*, 65
    disturbed homeostasis during muscle
        injury   110
    supplementation   102
calcium adenosine triphosphatases   65
calf muscle compartments *see* lower
    leg muscle compartments
capillaries   32–33, *34*
carbohydrates
    metabolism   80
    muscle healing and   120
cardiomyocytes   28
cardiovascular training   359–360
care team   320
carnitine palmitoyltransferase
    (CPT)   234
carnosine   94–95
cauda equina   53
cauda syndrome   54
cervical fascia release   343–344, *344*
cervical plexus   50–52, *51*
cholecalciferol   101
cholecystitis   288
closed kinetic chain   361
closed muscle chain   2
clubfoot   18
coenzyme Q10   97
cognition   264
cold wet compress   335, *336*
collagen fibers   34, 343
    formation   116–117
    Golgi tendon organ   45
    tendons   36
collodion patches   235, *236*
colon/nerve degeneration corona
    292, *293*
communication   250, 251
compartment syndrome   18, 154
    acute   7
    case study   397, *398*
    chronic   7

functional   162, 397, *398*
    physical therapy   285
    MRI appearance   216
    traumatic   165
    ultrasonographic appearance
        198, *199*
    see also muscle compartments
complex regional pain syndrome
    (CRPS)   48
compression therapy   125
concentric contraction   70
concentric training   369
connective tissue   34
consciousness   253–254
contraction *see* muscle contraction
contracture   228
contusion injuries   108, 153–154
    case study   398–400, *399–400*
    MRI appearance   *193*, 211
    physical therapy   284–285
    quadriceps   312
        surgical treatment   312
    ultrasonographic appearance
        190, *192–194*
conus syndrome   54
cooling   82
coordination   377
    assessment   330
coracobrachialis   *11, 13*
corticospinal tract   48–49
corticosteroids   272
coupling artifact   171, *171*
cramps *see* muscle cramps
cranial sutures   2
craniomandibular dysfunction   287
creatine   94
    supplementation benefits   95–96
creatine kinase   95
    diagnostic significance   228–229, *230*
    in healthy individuals and ath-
        letes   229
    macro-creatine kinase   229
    rhabdomyolysis and   229
creatine kinase reaction   78, 79
creatine phosphate   78, 79
    resynthesis   86
creativity   250
cryotherapy   124–125, 341–342
    ice-water therapy   268–269
    local cold application   341, *342*
    whole-body cryotherapy
        341–342, *342*
Curschmann–Steinert disease   235
cytokine release   111, 112, *113*
cyst   163–165
    intralesional cyst formation   286
    MRI appearance   215
    ultrasonographic appearance   195

D

declarative memory   249
decorin   118
delayed-onset muscle soreness
    (DOMS)   70, *142*, 147
    findings on examination   160
        MRI examination   208
        ultrasonographic appearance   185
    physical therapy   279
deltoid   3, *55*
dermatomes   54
dermatomyositis   235–237, *236*
    clinical characteristics   235
    differential diagnosis   236
    pathogenesis   236
desmodromic contraction   26
diagnosis *see* differential diagnosis;
    examination
diaphragm   33, *55*
    innervation   52
    mobilization   344, *345*
    pelvic   344, *345*
differential diagnosis
    acquired muscle diseases   235–241
        endocrine myopathies   237
        inflammatory muscle dis-
            eases   235–236, *236, 237*
        myofascial pain syndrome
            239–241, *239, 240*
        rheumatologic disorders   238
        toxic myopathies   237–238, *237*
    creatine kinase as laboratory marker
        228–229, *230*
    hereditary muscle diseases   233–235
        degenerative myopathies
            233–234
        hereditary metabolic myopathies
            234–235
        nondystrophic and dystrophic
            myotonias   235
    MRI application   216
    muscle biopsy indications   229, *230*
    myalgia versus muscle injury   242
    neurologic disorders   230–233
        clinical syndromes   230, *231*
        first or second motor neuron
            lesions   232
        lesion location   230–231
        muscle cramps   232–233, *233*
        peripheral nerve lesions   232
    specific diagnostic issues   228
digital arteries   14
dihydropyridine receptors   62
Discus Compositum   270
disinhibition   75
dorsal ramus   346, *346*
drive   253
drug therapy   123–124
    glucocorticoids   124
    new approaches   124
    nonsteroidal anti-inflammatory drugs
        (NSAIDs)   123–124
dynamic tests   329

E

eccentric contraction 70
eccentric training 370–371, *371*
elbow, agonist versus antagonist
   muscles *23*
electromechanical coupling 62
electromyography (EMG) 67, *67*
   kinesiologic 329–330
electrotherapy 125, 340–341
   high frequency–condenser field–deep
      heat 341
   high voltage 340
   medium frequency 340–341
   microampere currents 341
emotions 251–252
   cognition and 264
   muscle injuries and 258
endomysium 29, 34
endoneurium 42
endurance 373–377
   fatigue effects 376
   guidelines *376*
   improvement 376
Enelbin paste 269–270
energy emission analysis (EEA)
   289–295, *290–291, 293*
   colon/nerve degeneration corona
      292, *293*
   gallbladder/fatty degeneration corona
      292, *294*
   isolated emissions below second
      and third toes 292, *295*
   lung/lymph coronas 292, *293*
   triple burner (TB)/psyche corona
      292, *294*
   see also interference fields
entheses 38
enthesopathy 38
environment, behavior interactions
   247–248, *247*
epicondylus lateralis 5
epicondylus medialis 5
epiconus syndrome 53
epidural injections 274, *276*
epimysium 29, 34, 174
epineurium 42
episodic memory 249
erector spinae 2, 5, 11, *11, 12*
   innervation 298
erector trunci, myofascial release
   347, *348*
Escin 270
ethyl chloride spray 350
eversion 2
examination 156–159
   diagnosis establishment 336
   findings 160–162
   initial inspection 335
   laboratory diagnosis 159
   palpation 157–158, *158*
   see also magnetic resonance imaging
      (MRI); ultrasound
excitability *see* muscle excitability

excitatory postsynaptic potential
   (EPSP) 49
exercise
   extracellular matrix responses 123
   muscle growth and 123
   muscle injury treatment
      122–123, *124*
extension 2
extensor carpi radialis *55*
   brevis 5
   longus 5
extensor carpi ulnaris *55*
extensor digitorum 2, 17, *20, 55*
   longus *21*
extensor hallucis longus 17, *20, 21,
   55, 56*
extensor muscles 5
   arm *11*
   back *12*
   calf *21*
   knee *16, 17*
   see also specific muscles
extracellular matrix
   age influence 122
   exercise effects 123
   formation 116–118
      collagen formation 116–117
extrafusal fibers 44–45, *45*, 72
extraocular muscles 2, 43

F

facet joint infiltration 274
facial expression muscles 2
fascia 7, 34, 35–36, *36*
   thoracolumbar 11
fascicles 36
   angulation 24–25
   primary 36, 150, 174
   secondary 36, 150
fasciculations 228, 230
   benign 231
   diagnostic significance 230–231, *232*
fasciotomy 7
fast-twitch muscle fibers 5, 6, 65, *66*
fat metabolism 80
fatigue effects 376
fatigue-induced muscle disorder
   142, 146–147
   differentiation from myalgia 242
   findings on examination 160
      MRI examination *207*, 208
      ultrasonographic appearance
         184–185, *185*
   physical therapy 279
   see also muscle fatigue
fatty acid oxidation disorders 234
feelings 251–252
Feldenkrais technique 261
femoral artery 15, *177*
   deep 17
femoral nerve 15, 42, 50, 53, *56*, 274
femoral vein *177*

fibroblast growth factor (FGF) 115
   basic (bFGF) 119
fibroblast migration 116
fibronectin 117
fibrosis 99, 101, *117*, 165
   following minor muscle tears 151
   MRI appearance 215, *215*
   ultrasonographic appearance
      195, *196*
fibular artery 18
fibular nerve 18, 53
   common 53
   deep 50
   superficial 50, 53
fibularis brevis *185*
fibularis longus *185*
first aid equipment 334–335, *335*
flexibility training 368–369
flexion 2
flexor carpi radialis 2, *55*
flexor digitorum 18, *55, 56*
   longus *20, 22, 185*
   profundus 3
   superficialis 3
flexor hallucis longus 18, *20, 22, 185*
flexor muscles 2, 5
   abdominal wall *10*
   arm *11*
   calf *22*
   see also specific muscles
flexor retinaculum 53
fluid intake 86
focal toxicosis 286–288
   definition 286–287
foot, segmental innervation and
   movements *54*
foraminal stenosis 302
force measurement techniques 330
   see also muscle forces
free radicals 96
   muscle fatigue and 84
functional circuits 288–289, *288, 289*
functional compartment syn-
   drome 162
   case study 397, *398*
   physical therapy 285
functional muscle disorders
   107, 141–144, *142*, 145–149, *150*
   neuromuscular muscle disorder
      147–149
      muscle-related *143*, 148–149, 160
      spine-related *142*, 147–148, 160
   overexertion-related muscle disorder
      108, 146–147
      delayed-onset muscle soreness
         (DOMS) 70, *142*, 147, 160
      fatigue-induced muscle disorder
         142, 146–147, 160

G

gallbladder/fatty degeneration corona 292, *294*
gamma-aminobutyric acid (GABA) 74
ganglion nodes 41
gastrocnemius 18, *20, 22, 55, 56, 184, 184*
  infiltration therapy *272*
  injuries 220
    contusion injury *193*
    partial muscle tears 152, *189, 223, 224*
    tendon rupture *223, 224*
    lateral head *180, 185*
    medial head *180, 185*
    taping 357, *357*
gemellus *15*
  inferior *180*
  superior *180*
genital interference fields 288
genitofemoral nerve 53
ghost images 172
Gleditsch functional circuits 288–289, *288, 289*
glucocorticoids 124
glutamine 94
gluteal arteries 15
gluteal muscles 15, *15*
  gluteus maximus 2, 3, *14, 15, 55, 56, 180*
  gluteus medius 3, *14, 15, 55, 56, 180, 183*
  gluteus minimus 3, *14, 15, 180, 183*
gluteal nerves 15, 50
glycogen
  deficiency, fatigue and 84
  metabolism 80
    breakdown activation 78–79
    replenishment after exercise 86
glycogen storage diseases 234
gnathologic interference field 287
goal selection 252
Golgi tendon organ (GTO) 45–46, *45, 75, 76*
  architecture 45–46
  function 46
Golgi tendon reflex *48*
Gottron sign 235, *236*
gracilis 3, *8, 16, 18, 56, 173, 177, 180, 183*
granulation tissue 117
Guillain–Barré syndrome 232

H

hamstrings 2, 17, *19*
  injuries 220, 309–312
    distal injuries 309, *310*
    mechanisms 367–368
    MRI appearance 220
    partial tear 152

    proximal injuries 309–311, *311*
    soccer players 133, *133*
    stiffness relationship 145
    surgical treatment 311–312, *312*
    tendinous avulsion 162, *162, 309–310, 311*
  injury prevention
    bridging exercise 372, *372*
    eccentric training 370–371, *371*
    intermuscular coordination 372
    length–force relationship and 371–372
    stretching 368, 369, *370*
  pennation angle 25
  ultrasonographic appearance 179, *181, 182*
healing phases 339
  see also muscle regeneration
heart muscle 27, 28
heel foot position 19
heliotrope rash 235, *236*
hematoma 116–117
  case studies 199, *200–201*, 398–400, *399–400*
  contusion injuries 153, 190–192, *193, 194*, 211
  MRI appearance 209, *209, 210*
    differential diagnosis 216
  partial muscle tears 151, 161, 188, 209, *209, 210*
  ultrasound examination 170, 190–192, *193, 194*, 199, *200–201*
hemorrhoids 288
hepatocyte growth factor (HGF) 115
herniation
  disk 302, *303*
  muscle 165
    MRI appearance 213
heterotopic ossification *164*, 165
  MRI appearance 215
  ultrasonographic appearance 198, *198*
hip
  muscles 14–15, *14, 15*
    see also specific muscles
  preventive stretching 369, *369*
  segmental innervation and movements *54*
histology
  heart muscle 27, 28
  skeletal muscle 27, 29
  smooth muscle 26–28, *27*
homeostasis *90*
host response 339
hyperlordosis 299, *299*
hypertrophy 175
hypnosis 261
hypoparathyroidism 237
hypothenar muscles 14, *55*
hypoxia-inducible factor (HIF) 87

I

ice chest 335
ice-water therapy 268–269
  see also cryotherapy
iliacus *14, 56, 173, 183*
iliocostal nerves 9
iliohypogastric nerves 50, 53
ilioinguinal nerves 9, 50, 53
iliolumbar ligament release 347, *347*
iliopsoas 14, *14*, 15, *55, 173, 183*, 220
  tender points 355, *355*
iliotibial tract 23, *173, 177, 180, 183*
indometacin 270
infectious myositis 235
infiltration therapy 269–275
  Actovegin 269, 272
  arnica 269–270
  bromelains 270
  contraindications 272
  Discus Compositum 270
  Escin 270
  Lactopurum 270
  magnesium 270
  mechanisms 273
  Mepivacaine 270
  NSAIDs 270
  platelet-rich plasma (PRP) 270–271
  spinal infiltration therapy 272, *273*, 274–275, *275*
  steroids 271
  technique 271–272, *272*
  Traumeel S 271
  vitamins A, C, and E 271
  Zeel 271
  zinc 270
  see also drug therapy
inflammation 95, 107, 110, 119
  age influence 121
  antioxidant benefits 120
  cytokine release 111, 112, *113*
  inflammatory muscle diseases 235–237, *237*
    dermatomyositis 235–237
    infectious myositis 235
  macrophage migration 112
  neutrophil migration 112
infraspinatus 55
inguinal ligament *56, 173*
injury prevention *see* muscle injury prevention
insulin-like growth factor-1 (IGF-1) 87, 115, 122
intelligence 250
intercostal arteries 9, 11
intercostal nerves 9, 50
intercostales muscles 3
interdigitations 38, *39*
interference fields 286–288
  appendicitis 288
  cholecystitis 288
  genital interference fields 288
  hemorrhoids 288
  intestinal dysbiosis or mycosis 288

material intolerance   288
otitis media   287
scars   288
sinusitis   287
teeth   287
temporomandibular joint   287
tonsillitis   287
see also energy emission analysis (EEA)
interleukin-6 (IL-6)   80
intermuscular septum   23, 35–36, *36*
   lateral   *177*
   medial   *177*
   posterior   *185*
   transverse   *185*
interosseous ligament   2
interosseous muscles   *55*
intervertebral disks   2
intestinal dysbiosis or mycosis   288
intrafusal fibers   44, *45*, 72
inversion   2
iron deficiency   100
ischemia   33, 109
ischial nerve   152
isokinetic contraction   26
isokinetic testing and training systems
   331–334, *332*
   interpretation of results
      332–334, *333*
   principles   331–332
isometric contraction   25–26, *68*, 69
isotonic contraction   25–26, *68*, 69

J

Jacobson progressive muscle
   relaxation   260

K

Keinig's nail sign   235, *236*
kicking a ball, musculoskeletal
   adaptations   322–325, *323, 324, 325*
   support leg changes   *324*, 325–326,
      325, 326
kinetic chain   24
   closed   361
   open   361
kinematic tests   329
kinesiologic electromyography
   (EMG)   329–330
kinesiotaping   356–358
   calf muscle   357–358, *357, 358*
Kirlian effect   289
knee
   adductor muscles   *16*
   extensor muscles   *16, 17*
   innervation   *353*
   patella   40–41, *41*
   patella tendon reflex   46, *47*
   segmental innervation and
      movements   *54*

L

laboratory diagnosis   159
lacerations   211
   surgical repair   316
lactate
   analysis   330
   production   79
Lactopurum   270
lacuna
   muscular   53
   vascular   53
language   250, 251
large intestine/nerve degeneration
   corona   292, *293*
latent period   65
lateral articular nerve (LAN)   *353*
lateral cutaneous nerve of the thigh   53
lateral meniscus   356
lateral recess stenosis   302, *302*
latissimus dorsi   2, 11
   myofascial release   347, *348*
learning   254
leg
   innervation   *54, 56*
      movements and   *54*
   length difference   300, 301–302, *301*
      case study   393, *394, 396*
   lower leg muscle compartments
      9, 17–19, *20, 21–22*
      injuries   18–19
   thigh muscle compartments   *7*
      anterior   15–16, *16, 17*
      medial   *16,* 17, *18*
      posterior   17, *19*
length–force diagram   67–70, *68*
leukocyte inhibitory factor (LIF)   115
ligamentous articular release techniques   346–347, *347*
      abdominal muscles   *348, 351*
      iliolumbar ligament   347, *347*
      sacrum   347, *347*
lilac disease   235, *236*
limbic system   252
load–velocity relationship   70–71, *70*
local muscles   24
locked sacroiliac joint   299–300, *300*
lower leg muscle compartments
   9, 17–19, *20, 21–22*
   injuries   18–19
lumbar plexus
   infiltration therapy   274
   myofascial release   348, *351*
   see also lumbosacral plexus
lumbar scoliosis, case study   392–395,
   393–396
lumbar spine   274, *275*, 298
   functional causes of muscular
      dysfunction   299–301
      hyperlordosis   299, *299*
      locked sacroiliac joint
         299–300, *300*
      sacrum acutum   300–301

infiltration therapy   272, *273,*
   274–275, *275,* 280
   clinical effects   274–275, *276*
   involvement in injuries   153, *154,*
      274, *275*
   ligamentous articular release
      347, *347*
   structural causes of muscular
      dysfunction   301–305, *301*
      disk bulging and herniation
         302, *303*
      lumbosacral ligament   305
      spinal stenosis   302, *302, 303*
      spondylolisthesis   303–304, *305*
      spondylolysis   303–304, *304*
   see also spine
lumbopelvic stability training   372–373,
   374–375
lumbopelvic–hip complex   372
lumbosacral ligament   305
lumbosacral plexus   50, *51,* 53
   see also lumbar plexus; sacral plexus
lumbrical muscles   2
lung/lymph coronas   292, *293*
lymphatic taping   357–358, *358*

M

M line   60
McArdle myopathy   234
macro-creatine kinase   229
macrophage growth factor (MGF)   87
macrophages
   migration   112
   muscle fiber regeneration and   114
magnesium   99
   therapy   270
magnetic resonance imaging
   (MRI)   159, 204
   contusion injuries   *193,* 211
   differential diagnosis   216–217
      fatty atrophy pattern   216
      muscle edema pattern   216
      tumor, hematoma, bony avulsion
         pattern   216–217
   examination technique   204–205
      pulse sequence selection   205, *206*
      spatial resolution   205, *206*
   normal muscle   205, *207*
   pathological conditions   208–220
      compartment syndrome   216
      cyst   215
      delayed-onset muscle soreness
         208
      fatigue-induced muscle disorder
         207, 208
      fibrosis/scar   215, *215*
      heterotopic ossification   215
      minor partial muscle tear
         206, 209, *209*
      moderate partial muscle tear
         209, *209, 210, 219, 223, 224*
      muscle denervation   213

magnetic resonance imaging,
  pathological conditions
    muscle herniation   213
    muscle-related neuromuscular
      muscle disorder   208, *208*
    myositis ossificans   215
    seroma   215
    spine-related neuromuscular
      muscle disorder   208
    subtotal/complete muscle
      tears   *207,* 211, *212, 213, 218*
    tendinosis   213
    tendinous avulsion   211, *212, 213,*
      214
    tendon rupture   *211,* 213, *221, 222,*
      223, 224
  prognostic criteria   217
  proton density-weighted images
    205, *206*
  relevant anatomic microstructure
    204
  risk factors for repeated injury   217
  soccer injury examination   132
  specific muscle injuries   217–220
    adductus longus   220
    gastrocnemius   220
    hamstrings   220
    quadriceps   217
  T1-weighted images   205
  T2-weighted images   205, *206*
mammalian target of rapamycin
  (mTOR)   87, 123
Mandel energy emission analysis
  see energy emission analysis (EEA)
manual therapy   343–356
  ligamentous articular release
    techniques   346–347, *347*
    iliolumbar ligament   347, *347*
    sacrum   347, *347*
  muscle release techniques   350–354
  myofascial release techniques
    343–349
    cervical fascia   343–344, *344*
    erector trunci and latissimus
      dorsi   347, *347*
    lumbar plexus   348, *351*
    oblique muscles   348, *349, 351*
    pelvic diaphragm   344, *345*
    pelvitrochanteric muscles
      348, *348, 351*
    plantar fascia   344, *346*
    popliteal fascia   344, *345*
    respiratory diaphragm   344, *345*
    sacral plexus   348, *351*
  spray and stretch   350
  strain–counterstrain   349–350
  tender points and trigger
    points   354–356
    biceps femoris   355–356
    iliopsoas   355, *355*
    lateral meniscus   356
    piriformis   355, *355*
    subscapularis   356
  see also physical therapy

massage   125, 280, 281
masseter   2
material intolerance   288
mechanical syncytium   26
mechanic's hand   235, *236*
mechanoelectrical syncytium   28
mechanogram   65, *66*
mechanoreceptors   349, *352–353*
medial articular nerve (MAN)   *353*
median nerve   11, 42, 50, 52
medical training therapy   358–363
  components of   *360*
  contraindications   358, *359*
  devices   *362*
  metabolically oriented training
    359–360
  sequencing of training exercises
    362–363
  single-joint versus multiple-joint
    exercises   361
  tension- and control-oriented
    training   360, *361*
meditation   261
memory   249–250
  declarative   249
  nondeclarative   250
mental position   246
mental training   262–263
  mental doping   262–263
Mepivacaine   270
metabolism *see* muscle metabolism
metalloproteinases   99, 101
microampere currents   341
microtears   26, *27*
microvasculature   32–33, *34*
minerals   98–99
  disturbances   98–99
    spasms   98–99
    therapy   99
  functions in muscle   98–99
mirror-image artifact   172, *172*
mitochondrial myopathies   234–235
mobilization
  neuromuscular techniques
    (NMT)   350–354
    NMT 1: using direct muscular force
      of agonists   350
    NMT 2: using postisometric
      relaxation of antagonists   354
    NMT 3: using reciprocal inhibition
      of antagonists   354
  with minor partial muscle tears
    122–123
  with muscle firmness   122
  see also exercise; manual therapy
mobilizer muscles   24
monitoring
  blood parameters   275–278, *278*
  brain functional role   253
monosynaptic reflex   46–47, *47, 48*
motion analysis   329
  kinesiologic electromyography
    (EMG)   329–330
motion patterns   23–24, *23*

motivation   254–256
  intrinsic and extrinsic   255–256
  motives   254–255
motor cortex   48–49
  somatotopic organization   49
motor end plate   43, 61
motor learning   254
motor points   42–43
motor units   43, *43,* 61
  as target for neuromuscular
    regulation/control   72
multi-joint muscles   2
multifidus muscle   298
multiple-joint movements
  partially isolated   361
  (semi-)free   361
muscle *see* skeletal muscle;
  specific muscles
muscle adaptations *see* musculoskeletal
  adaptations
muscle biopsy indications   229, *230*
muscle compartments   7, *8*
  abdominal wall   9, *9, 10*
  arm   11–14, *11, 13*
  hip and buttocks   14–15, *14, 15*
  lower leg   9, 17–19, *20, 21–22*
  posterior trunk   11, *11, 12*
  thigh   *8*
    anterior   15–16, *16, 17*
    medial   *16, 17, 18*
    posterior   17, *19*
  see also compartment syndrome
muscle contraction   25–26, 62
  initiation   62–64, *63*
  regulation   62, *63*
    see also neuromuscular control
  shortening velocity   70–71
    load–velocity relationship
      70–71, *70*
  spatial summation   67
  striation changes   31, *32*
  temporal summation   66–67
  time course   65
    single twitch   65, *66*
    superposition   65–66, *66*
  types of   67–71
    afterloaded contraction   *68,* 69, 70
    auxotonic contraction   *68,* 69
    concentric contraction   70
    contraction against a stop
      68, 69–70
    desmodromic contraction   26
    eccentric contraction   70
    isokinetic contraction   26
    isometric contraction
      25–26, *68,* 69
    isotonic contraction   25–26, *68,* 69
    length–force diagram   67–70, *68*
  see also muscle length
muscle cramps   228, 232–233
  differential diagnosis   *233*
muscle excitability
  muscle fatigue and   84, *85*
  warm-up effects   81, *85*

muscle fatigue   31, 82–86
  ATP resynthesis   83
  causes   83
    acidosis   83
    excitability decrease   84, *85*
    free radicals   84
    glycogen deficiency   84
    phosphate effects   *83*, 84
    temperature   86
  central fatigue   83, 86
  definitions   82
  peripheral fatigue   83
  recovery   86
  see also fatigue-induced muscle
    disorder
muscle fibers   5–6, *6*, 29, *35*, 36
  fast-twitch (type II) fibers   5, 6, 65,
    66, 77
    transition forms   6, *6*
  fiber chimerism   110
  pennation angle   24–25
  regeneration   114–116, *115*
    satellite cell division   114, *114*
    satellite cell regulation
      114–116, *116*
  slow-twitch (type I) fibers   5, 6, 65,
    66, 77
  tears *see* muscle injury
  types of   77, *78*
    training effects   86–87
  see also fascicles; sarcomere
muscle forces   60
  control of   75, *76*
  force–length relationship   371–372
    length–force diagram   67–70, *68*
  gradation during voluntary
    movements   66–67
  motile force production   62–64
  shortening velocity relationship
    70–71, *70*
muscle function tests   *328*
muscle growth
  exercise effects   123
  see also muscle regeneration
muscle healing *see* muscle regeneration
muscle injury   90, *90, 91*, 106–107, 367
  adaptations after   337–339
  age and   144
  brain responses   258–259
  classification   *106*, 137–145, 327, *328*
    current systems   138–139
    fundamentals   137–138
    location of injury   144
    need for new classification
      136–137
    new system   141–145, *141–143*
  clinical approach   *108*
  complications   163–165, *164*
  contusions   108, 153–154
  current literature   137
  delayed-onset muscle soreness
    (DOMS)   70, *142*, 147, 160
  direct injuries   106, 141,
    142–143, 153

epidemiology in sports
  see specific sports
fatigue-induced muscle disorder
  142, 146–147, 160
fibrosis   99, 101
functional muscle disorders
  107, 141–144, *142*, 145–149, *150*
healing phases   339
  see also muscle regeneration
host response   339
indirect injuries   106, 141, *142*,
  149–150
inflammation   95, 107, 110
ischemia   109
lacerations   211, 316
longitudinal distraction injuries   108
mechanisms of damage   108–110,
  367–368
  cellular mechanisms   109
  dependence on contraction
    and fiber types   109–110
  extracellular mechanisms   109
  impaired neuromuscular
    regulation   110
metabolic effects   90
muscle-related neuromuscular muscle
  disorder   *143*, 148–149, 160
neuromuscular muscle disorder
  147–149
nutrient relationships   90
  amino acids   95–96
overexertion-related muscle disorder
  108, 146–147
pathobiological approach   *108*
prevention *see* muscle injury
  prevention
recurrence   163, 286, 367
secondary phase of injury   110
spine-related neuromuscular muscle
  disorder   *142*, 147–148, 160
structural muscle injuries   *143*, 144,
  149–153, *150*
  see also muscle tears
team level effects   258
terminology   137, 139
  consensus conference
    139–141, *140*
therapy   96, 268
  complex treatment strategies
    339–340
  drug-based therapy   123–124
  exercise   122–123, *124*
  infiltration therapy   269–275
  nutrients   120
  physical methods   124–125,
    268–269
  primary care   268–269
  see also specific therapies
  see also specific injuries and muscles
muscle injury prevention   95–96, 367
  optimizing basic fitness   373–378
    coordination   377
    endurance   373–377
    warming up   377–380, *379–380*

training measures   368–373
  concentric training   369
  eccentric training   370–371, *371*
  flexibility and stretching   368–369
  intermuscular coordination
    372, *372*
  lumbopelvic control and stability
    372–373, *374–375*
muscle insertion   2, 5
muscle insufficiency   42
  active   42
  passive   42
muscle length
  length–force diagram   67–70, *68*
  regulation   72–75, *73*
    alpha–gamma coactivation   74
    muscle spindles   44–45, *45*,
      72–75, *73*
    reciprocal inhibition   74
    Renshaw inhibition   *73*, 74
  see also muscle contraction; stretching
muscle metabolism   78–81
  aerobic metabolism   79–80
    fat or carbohydrate metabolism   80
  anaerobic alactacid energy
    production   78
  basal metabolic rate   90
  glycogen breakdown activation
    78–79
  lactate production   79
  metabolic disturbance   95–96
  phosphofructokinase activation
    78, *79*
muscle origin   2, 5
  number of origins   5
muscle pain
  acquired muscle diseases   235–241
    endocrine myopathies   237
    inflammatory muscle diseases
      235–236, *236, 237*
    myofascial pain syndrome
      239–241, *239, 240*
    rheumatologic disorders   238
    toxic myopathies   237–238, *237*
  hereditary muscle diseases
    233–235
    degenerative myopathies
      233–234
    hereditary metabolic myopathies
      234–235
    nondystrophic and dystrophic
      myotonias   235
  myalgia versus muscle injury   242
  neurologic disorders
    first or second motor neuron
      lesions   232
    peripheral nerve lesions   232
  pain history   228
  perception of   258
  referred pain   *239, 240*
  shoulder   232
  special diagnostic issues   228
muscle plasticity   6, *6*
muscle reflexes *see* reflexes

muscle regeneration 90–91, *92*, 111–119, *111*
  age influence 120–122, *121*
  destruction phase 111–112, *113*
    macrophage migration 112
    neutrophil migration 112
  exercise effects 122–123
  laboratory markers 119
  nutrition influence 90–91, 120
    antioxidants 120
    carbohydrates 120
    proteins 120
  remodeling phase 111
  repair phase 111, 112–119
    extracellular matrix formation 116–118
    muscle fiber regeneration 114–116, *115*
    neovascularization 118–119
    reinnervation 119
    scar formation 118, *118*
muscle relaxation 65
  relaxation time 65
muscle shortening *see* muscle contraction; muscle length
muscle spasms *see* spasms
muscle spindles 44–45, *45*, 72–75, *73*
  afferents and their connections 73–74
  density 45
  discharge pattern 72–73
  efferent innervation 72
  muscle spindle reflex *48*
  reciprocal inhibition 74
  Renshaw inhibition *73*, 74
muscle strain 137, 139
  see also muscle injury; muscle tears
muscle taping 336–337, *338*
  elastic taping 356–358
    calf muscle 357–358, *357, 358*
muscle tears 36, 99, *106*, 139, 308
  mechanisms 308–309
    active stretch 309
    passive stretch 308–309
  microtears 26, *27*
  minor partial muscle tear 107, 122, *143*, 150–151, 161
    MRI appearance *206*, 209, *209*
    physical therapy 281–282
    ultrasonographic appearance 186–188, *187*
  moderate partial muscle tear 108, *143*, 151–152, *151, 152*, 161–162
    case studies 383–385, *384–387*, 388–392, *388–391*, 393–395, *393–394*
    MRI appearance 209, *209, 210, 219, 223, 224*
    physical therapy 282–283
    ultrasonographic appearance 188–190, *188–189*
  partial tears 149–152
    anatomic background 150

findings on examination 161–162, *161*
    myofascial trigger point differentiation 242
    see also specific types
  recurrence 163, 286
  subtotal/complete muscle tears/tendinous avulsion 108, *143*, 152–153, 161–162
    case study 400–404, *401–404*
    MRI appearance *207*, 211, *212, 213, 218*
    physical therapy 283–284
    ultrasonographic appearance 190
  see also muscle injury; *specific muscles*
muscle tension *see* muscle force
muscle warm-up *see* warm-up
muscle-related neuromuscular muscle disorder *143*, 148–149
  findings on examination 160
    MRI examination 208, *208*
    ultrasonographic appearance 186
  myofascial trigger point differentiation 242
  physical therapy 280–281
muscle-tendon interface 38, *39*
muscular dystrophies 233–234
muscular work 70
musculocutaneous nerve 11, 52
musculoskeletal adaptations 86–87
  after muscle injuries 337–339
  physical therapy implications 327
  soccer players 321
    changes caused by contact with ball 322–325, *323, 324, 325*
    pelvic–leg axis adaptations 326
    support leg changes *324*, 325–326, *325, 326*
myalgia *see* muscle pain
myelin sheath 42
myelomeres 346
myoadenylate deaminase deficiency 234
myofascial pain syndrome 239–241, *239*
  clinical characteristics 239
  definition 239
  etiology 239–241
  incidence 239
  pathology 241
  referred pain *239, 240*
myofascial release *see* manual therapy
myofascial system 34
  influences on 321
    see also musculoskeletal adaptations
myofibrils 29, *29, 35, 60*
myoglobulin 95
myokinase reaction 78
myokymia 228
myomuscular junctions 38
myopathies *see specific disorders*
myosin 60
  heads 30, 31, 60, *60*

motile force production 62–64, *63*
  heavy chains 60
    heavy-chain (MyHC) proteins 6
  isoforms 64
  light chains 60
myosin filaments 29–31, *29, 30*, 60
  structure *60*
myositis ossificans 154, *155–156*, 165
  MRI appearance 215
  physical therapy 285
  ultrasonographic appearance 197, *197*
myostatin 122
myotactic reflex 46–47, *47*
myotendinous junction 38, *39*
myotomes 54, *55*
  lower extremity *56*
myotonia 228
myotonic dystrophy 235

N

nebulin 29, 31, *31*
neck muscles, deep 11, *12*
neovascularization 118–119
nerve compression syndromes 213, 348–349, *352*
  differential diagnosis *349*
  stages 349
  tibial nerve compression 19
nerve point 50, 52
nerves 42
  see also specific nerves
neuraxis 50, *51*
neurologic disorders 230–233
  clinical syndromes 230, *231*
  first or second motor neuron lesions 232
  lesion location 230–231
  muscle cramps 232–233, *233*
  peripheral nerve lesions 232
neuromuscular control 71–77
  force and tension control 75
  impairment 110
  muscle length regulation 72–75, *73*
  rhythmic movement patterns 75
  spinal cord level 75–77
  voluntary movement hierarchical organization 71–72
    fine control of motor activity 71
    motor units as target for regulation/control 72
    preprogrammed movement patterns 71–72
neuromuscular end plate 61
neuromuscular junctions (NMJs) 43, 49
neuromuscular muscle disorder 147–149
  myofascial trigger point differentiation 242
  see also muscle-related neuromuscular muscle disorder; spine-related neuromuscular muscle disorder

neuromuscular signal transduction
61, 62
neuromuscular spindle *see* muscle spindles
neuromuscular synapses 43, *44*
neuromuscular techniques (NMT)
350–354
NMT 1: using direct muscular force
of agonists 350
NMT 2: using postisometric relaxation
of antagonists 354
NMT 3: using reciprocal inhibition
of antagonists 354
neuromyotonia 232
neuropsychology 246
neurovascular hilum 354
neutrophil migration 112
nomenclature 3–5, *4*
nonsteroidal anti-inflammatory drugs
(NSAIDs) 123–124, 270
nondeclarative memory 250
nondystrophic myotonias 235
Nordic hamstring exercise 370, *371*
Notch signaling pathway 121
nuclear bag fibers 44, *45*, 72, 346
nuclear chain fibers 44, *45*, 72, 346
nucleus donation 32
nutrients 90–103
amino acids 92–95, *93*
demand in athletes 93–95
essential amino acids 92
metabolism *94, 96*
supplementation 96
antioxidants 84, 96–98, *97*
function 96, *97*
importance in athletic activity
96–98
intake 96
muscle healing and 120
carbohydrates, muscle healing
and 120
minerals 98–99
function in muscle 98
muscle regeneration and 90–91, 120
protein, muscle healing and 120
trace elements 99–101, *100*
function 99–100
deficiencies 100
importance in athletic activity 101
intake 100–101
vitamin D 101–103
importance in athletic activity 103
intake 102–103
metabolism 101, *102*

O

oblique muscles 5
external 5, 9, *9, 10*
internal 5, 9, *9, 10*
myofascial release 348, *348, 351*
oblique capitis 11
inferior *12*
superior *12*

obturator artery 17
obturator muscle
externus *18, 183*
internus *15, 180*
obturator nerve 17, 42, 53, *56*, 274
occipital artery 11
open kinetic chain 361
orientation *3*
otitis media 287
overexertion-related muscle disorder
108, 146–147
delayed-onset muscle soreness
(DOMS) 70, *142*, 147, 160
fatigue-induced muscle disorder
142, 146–147, 160
oxygen deficit 80, *80*, 81

P

pain *see* muscle pain
painful insertion tendinopathy 16
palmar muscles 14
palmar interossei 2
palpation 157–158, *158*, 328–329
Parkinson syndrome 232
passive length–tension curve 67, *68*
passive stretching *see* stretching
patella 40–41, *41*
patella tendon reflex 46, *47*
patellar ligament *173*
patient history 155–156
pectineus *16, 18, 56, 173, 183*
pectoralis major *55,* 220
pelvic diaphragm release 344, *345*
pelvis 299
obliquity 300, 301
case study 392–395, *393–396*
pelvic girdle muscles 14–15, *14, 15*
torsion *300*
pelvitrochanteric muscles, myofascial
release 348, *348, 351*
pennation angle 24–25
perception 250
pain 258
performance 256–258
complexity and 256–257
mental training impact 262–263
rehabilitative performance testing
330–334, *331*
team sports 257–258
tension relationships 256, *257*
periarticular facet joint infiltration 274
perimysium 29, 34, 36
perineurium 42
peritendineum 37
peroneal artery 18
peroneal nerve 42
common 53, *56*
deep 18, *56*
superficial 18, 53, *56*
peroneus fibularis
brevis 3, 18, *20, 21*
longus 3, 18, *20, 21, 55, 56*

perspective 246
phagocytosis, age influence 121
Phlogenzym 270
phosphocreatine shuttle 79, *79*
phosphofructokinase activation 78, *79*
phrenic arteries 33
phrenic nerve 50–52
physical therapy 124–125, 278–279,
320, 340–342
assessment 327–334
clinical motion analysis 329–330
clinical therapeutic assessment
328–329
initial inspection 335
rehabilitative performance testing
330–334, *331*
strategy 327, *328*
see also examination
cold wet compress 335, *336*
compression 125
contusion injuries 284–285
cryotherapy 124–125, 268–269,
341–342
delayed-onset muscle soreness 279
electrotherapy 125, 340–341
equipment 334–335, *335*
fatigue-induced painful muscle
disorder 279
functional compartment
syndrome 285
immediate measures 334–337
intralesional cyst formation 286
massage 125
medical training therapy 358–363
components of *360*
contraindications 358, *359*
devices *362*
metabolically oriented training
359–360
sequences of training exercises
362–363
single-joint versus multiple-joint
exercises 361
tension- and control-oriented
training 360, *361*
minor partial muscle tear 281–282
moderate partial muscle tear
282–283
muscle taping 336–337, *338*
calf muscle 357–358, *357, 358*
elastic taping 356–358
lymphatic taping over the Achilles
tendon 357–358, *358*
muscle-related neuromuscular muscle
disorder 280–281
musculoskeletal adaptation
implications 327
myositis ossificans 285
recurrence 286
spine-related neuromuscular muscle
disorder 279–280
subtotal or complete muscle tear/
tendinous avulsion 283–284
therapeutic stimuli 339, *339*

physical therapy
  ultrasound   125
  see also manual therapy
physiological profile   25, *26*
piriformis   *15, 173, 180, 183*
  preventive stretching   *369*
  tender points and trigger points
    355, *356*
planning   252
plantar fascia release   344, *346*
plantaris   *20, 22, 180*
plasticity   6, *6*
platelet-rich plasma (PRP)   270–271
platysma   *3*
plexuses   50–53
  brachial plexus   50, *51*, 52
  cervical plexus   50–52, *51*
  lumbosacral plexus   50, *51*, 53
pole-vaulting   254, *255*
polymyalgia rheumatica   238, *238*
polyradiculitis   232
polysynaptic reflex   47, *47*
Pompe disease   234
popliteal fascia release   344, *345*
popliteus   *8, 18, 19*
post-stress muscle imbalance   163
posterior articular nerve (PAN)   *353*
posterior trunk muscle compartment   11, *11, 12*
preloaded contraction against
  a stop   *68*, 69–70
prevention *see* muscle injury prevention
profile   25, *26*
pronation   2
pronator muscles, calf   *21*
pronator teres   2
protease activation   112
protein, dietary
  muscle healing and   120
  see also amino acids
pseudoradicular syndrome   305
  differentiation from radicular
    syndromes   306
psoas
  major   *14, 56, 173, 183*
    preventive stretching   *369*
  minor   *14*
punctum nervosum   50, 52
purine metabolism disorders   234
pyramidal cells   48
pyramidal tract   48–49, *49*
  lesions   *232*
pyramidalis   10
pyruvate   79
pyruvate dehydrogenase   79, 80

qi gong   260–261
quadratus femoris   *56, 180*, 220
quadratus lumborum   *9, 9, 10*
quadriceps femoris   2, 15, *15, 16, 17, 55, 177, 183*

injuries   217, 312–428
  contusions   312
  soccer players   133, *133*
  surgical treatment   312, 314–316
  tears   313–316, *313*
muscle fibers   5
ultrasonographic appearance   *174*

radial artery   14
radial nerve   11, 42, 50, 52
radiation therapy, myositis
  ossificans   285
radicular syndrome   305
  differentiation from pseudoradicular
    syndromes   306
radiculopathy   *232*
Randle cycle   80
reactive oxygen species   96
rectus abdominis   5, 9, *9, 10*, 23
rectus capitis   11
  major   *12*
  minor   *12*
rectus femoris   *8, 17, 56, 173, 177, 179, 183*, 217, *313*
  fibrosis   215
  injuries   313–314
    apophyseal avulsion   *163, 212*
    case studies   383, *384–387, 388–392, 388–391*
    MRI appearance   217, *314*
    muscle tears   *161, 188, 196, 207, 218, 219*, 313, *313*, 315, 383–392, *384–391*
    surgical treatment   314–315, *315*
    tendinous avulsion   *153, 164, 190*, 313, *314*
    tendon rupture   *221, 222*
  preventive stretching   *370*
  seroma   *161*
  tendon   *178, 313*
rectus sheath   23
recurrent meningeal nerve   346, *346*
reference muscles   54, *54*
reflection artifact   171, *171*
reflexes   46–47, *47*
  monosynaptic (myotatic) reflex   46–47, *47, 48*
  musculospinal reflex pathways   *354*
  polysynaptic reflex   47, *47*
  spinal reflexes   71–72
  stretch reflex   47, *48*, 72–75, *73*
  withdrawal reflex   47, *47*
regeneration *see* muscle regeneration
rehabilitation   320
rehabilitative performance testing   330–334, *331*
reinnervation   119
relaxation techniques   259–262
  applicability   261–262
  effects of   259
  Feldenkrais technique   261

hypnosis   261
Jacobson progressive muscle
  relaxation   260
meditation   261
requirements and mechanisms   259–260, *260*
Schultz autogenic training   260
tai ji   260–261
yoga   260
Renshaw cells   *73*, 74
Renshaw inhibition   *73*, 74
Reparil   270
reverberations   172, *172*
rhabdomyolysis   229
  antilipemic-associated   238
  causes   *231*
rhomboids   11, *55*
rhythmic movements   47
  regulation   75
ryanodine receptors (RyR1)   62

S1 sacral foramina infiltration   274
sacral plexus   *15*, 50
  myofascial release   348, *351*
  see also lumbosacral plexus
sacroiliac joint   299–300
  infiltration therapy   274, *276*
  locked   299–300, *300*
sacrotuberous ligament   *180*
sacrum
  ligamentous articular release   347, *347*
  sacrum acutum   300–301
saphenous nerve   *56*
sarcolemma   *30*, 43
sarcomere   6, 60
  contraction   31, *32*
  microarchitecture   29–31, *29*
  see also muscle fibers
sarcoplasm   *61*
  calcium ion concentration   *61*, 62
sarcoplasmic reticulum (SR)   *30, 30, 61*
sarcous fibers   36, 150, 151
sartorius   2, 15, 16, *16, 17, 56, 173, 177, 183*
satellite cells (SC)   32, *33*, 114
  division   114
  exercise effects   123
  regulation   114–116, *116*
scalene gap
  anterior   52
  posterior   52
scars
  as interference fields   288
  formation   118, *118*, 165
    following minor muscle tears   151
    mobilization and   122
    MRI appearance   215, *215*
    sciatic nerve involvement   310
    ultrasonographic appearance   195
  rectus femoris   314–315

scatter 171
Schultz autogenic training 260
Schwann cells 42, 43, *44*
sciatic nerve 42, 50, 53, *56, 177,* 274
  compression 300
  scar formation and 310
  slump test *350*
semantic memory 249
semimembranosus *8,* 17, *19, 55, 56, 177,* 179, *180, 183*
  moderate partial muscle tear *223*
  preventive stretching *370*
  tendinous avulsion *162*
  tendon rupture *223*
semitendinosus *8,* 17, *19, 55, 177,* 179, *180, 183*
  injuries 309, *310*
    partial muscle tear *187*
    tendinous avulsion *191,* 309
  pennation angle *25*
  preventive stretching *370*
  tendon 179, *181*
sensory cortex 50
seroma 161, *161,* 163, 286
  case studies 383, *384–385,* 392, *393–394,* 400–402, *401, 403*
  MRI appearance 215
  rectus femoris *315*
  ultrasonographic appearance 195, *195*
serratus
  anterior 3
  inferior 11
  superior 11
sesamoids 40–41, *41*
short-term memory 249
shoulder
  innervation 52
  pain 232
silicium deficiency 100
single twitch 65, *66*
single-joint isolated movements 361
single-joint muscles 2
sinusitis 287
skeletal muscle
  adaptations in *see* musculoskeletal adaptations
  histology *27,* 29
  innervation 42
  motor units 43, *43*
  spine relationships 298–299
  structure 35–36, *35, 36*
  support structures 38–41, *41*
  see also specific muscles
sleep 251
slow-twitch muscle fibers 5, 6, 65, *66*
slump test 349, *350*
smooth muscle 26–28, *27*
soccer
  complexity 256
  musculoskeletal adaptations in players 321
    changes caused by contact with ball 322–325, *323, 324, 325*

pelvic–leg axis adaptations 326
  support leg changes *324,* 325–326, *325, 326*
penalties 263
soccer injuries
  case reports 383–404
  data evaluation 134
  examination procedures 132–134
  hamstring injuries 133, *133*
  incidence 130, *130*
  injury risk 131–132
    age and 131, *131*
    contact situations and foul play 132
    variation during matches 131, *131*
  localization 129, *129*
  partial muscle tear *152, 153, 161*
  quadriceps injuries 133, *133*
  recurrent injuries 132, *132*
  severity 132, *132*
  study design 128–129
    definitions 129
social skills 258
sodium chloride replacement 86
sodium-potassium ATPase 81
soleus 18, *20, 22, 56,* 184, *184, 185*
  muscle cramps 232
  muscle fibers 5
  muscle-related neuromuscular muscle disorder *208*
spasms 98–99, 228
  at rest 99
  during exercise 99
spatial summation 67
spinal canal 53
spinal cord 48–50, *49,* 53, *277*
  lesions 232, *232*
  neuronal circuit regulation 75–77
spinal infiltration therapy *272, 273,* 274–275, *275*
spinal muscular atrophy 232
spinal nerves 11, 42, *51, 277, 346*
  irritation 298
spinal reflexes 71–72
spinal stenosis 302, *302, 303*
spinal syndromes 53–54
spine, skeletal muscle relationships 298–299
  see also lumbar spine
spine-related neuromuscular muscle disorder *142,* 147–148
  differentiation from a myofascial trigger point 242
  findings on examination 160
    MRI examination 208
    ultrasonographic appearance 186, *186*
  physical therapy 279–280
spinocostalis muscles 11
spiroergometry 330
spondylolisthesis 303–304, *305*
spondylolysis 303–304, *304*
  case study 393, *394*
sports medicine kit 334, *335*

stabilizer muscles 24
stapedius 2
sternocleidomastoid 5
  innervation 52
sternocostal joints 2
steroids 271
  steroid myopathy 238
stiff-person syndrome 232
strain–counterstrain treatment 349–350
stress 260
stretch reflex 47, *48,* 72–75, *73*
stretching 81–82
  injury prevention 368–369
  injury relationships 145
  muscle release techniques 350–354
  warm-up 378
striated muscle *27,* 28–29
striations 30
  changes during contraction 31, *32*
structural muscle injuries *143,* 144, 149–153, *150*
  see also muscle injury; muscle tears
subclavian artery 11
subcostal artery 9
subcostal nerves 9, 50, 53
suboccipital nerve 11
subscularis 356
superposition 65–66, *66*
supination 2
supinator 2
supraspinatus *55*
surface changes 144–145
symphysis 2
synaptic cleft 61, 62
synchondrosis 2
syndesmosis 2
synostosis 2
synovial joints 2
syringomyelia 232

T

T tubules 30, *30,* 62
Tai Ji 260–261
talar beak formation 323
taping *see* muscle taping
taurine 94–95
team sports 257–258
  injury effects on the team level 258
  social skills 258
  team as a unit 258
tears *see* muscle injury; muscle tears
teeth 287
temperature
  muscle fatigue and 86
  thermal effects on muscle 81
temporal summation 66–67
temporomandibular joint 287
tenascin C 117
tender points 354–356
  biceps femoris 355–356
  iliopsoas 355, *355*

tender points
  lateral meniscus 356
  piriformis 355, *356*
  subscapularis 356
tendinosis 213
tendinous avulsion *143*, 152–153,
  161–162
  adductor brevis *214*
  adductor longus *212, 213, 214*
  hamstring 162, *162*, 309–310, *311*
    surgical treatment
     311–312, *312*
  MRI appearance *212, 213*
    differential diagnosis 216–217
  physical therapy 283–284
    distal tendinous avulsion 284
    proximal tendinous avulsion
     283–284
  rectus femoris tendon *153, 164,*
   190, 313, *314*
  semimembranosus *162*
  ultrasonographic appearance
   190, *190, 191*
tendon organs 46
tendon rupture 213
  biceps femoris *211*
  gastrocnemius *223, 224*
  rectus femoris *221, 222*
  semimembranosus *223*
tendon sheaths 38–40, *41*
tendons 36–38
  architecture 36–37, *37*
  function 37–38
tendon–bone junction 38, *40*
tennis leg 152
tensor fasciae latae (TFL) *14*, 15, 23,
  173, 180
terminal cistern 30, *30*
terminology
  muscle injury 137, 139
    consensus conference
     139–141, *140*
  myology *28*
tetany 228
thenar muscles 14, *55*
theory 246–247
thigh muscle compartments 7
  anterior 15–16, *16, 17*
  medial *16*, 17, *18*
  posterior 17, *19*
thinking 250
tibial artery, anterior 18
tibial nerve 17, 42, 50, 53, *56*
  compression 19
  injury 17
tibial peak formation 323
tibialis
  anterior 17, *20, 21, 55, 56*
    contusion injury *194*
    ultrasonographic appearance
     175, 194
  posterior 18, *20, 22, 55*
time 246
time gain compensation (TGC) 171

titin 29, 31, *31*, 60, 65
tonsillitis 287
trace elements 99–101, *100*
  deficiencies 100
  function 99–100
  importance in athletic activity 101
  intake 100–101
trainer's bag 334–335
training adaptations 86–87
transcutaneous electrical nerve
  stimulation (TENS) 125
transforming growth factor beta
  (TGF-beta) 115, 118, 119
transverse tubules (T tubules)
  30, *30*, 62
transversus abdominis 5, 9, *9, 10*
trapezius 3, 5, 11
  innervation 52
Traumanase 270
traumatic compartment syndrome
  165
Traumeel S 271
triad 30, *30*
triceps brachii 2, *11, 13, 55*
  fascia *36*
triceps surae 2, 18, *20, 22*
trigger points 42–43, 239, 241, *241,*
  354–356
  neuromuscular muscle disorder
    differentiation 242
  partial muscle tear differentiation
    242
  piriformis 355
triple burner (TB)/psyche corona
  292, *294*
tropomyosin 29, 30–31, 60, *60*, 62,
  63, 64
troponin 29, 30–31, 60, *60*, 62,
  63, 64
two-joint muscles 2

U

ulnar artery 14
ulnar nerve 11, 42, 50, 52–53
ultrasonography
  artifacts 170–171
    coupling artifact 171, *171*
    mirror-image artifact 172, *172*
    reflection artifact 171, *171*
  examination 159, 170
    adductors 179, *182*
    anterior thigh 177, *177, 178, 179*
    calf 185, *185, 186*
    criteria for interpretation 174
    hamstrings 179, *181, 182*
    protocol *174*
    skeletal muscle 172–174, *174*
    soccer injury 132
  normal findings 174–177
    factors influencing imaging
     175, *175*
  pathological conditions 184–190

compartment syndrome
  198, *199*
  cyst 195
  delayed-onset muscle soreness
    185
  fatigue-induced painful muscle
    disorder 184–185, *185*
  fibrosis/scar 195, *196*
  heterotropic ossification
    198, *198*
  minor partial muscle tears
    186–188, *187*
  moderate partial muscle
    tears 188–190, *188–189*
  muscle-related neuromuscular
    muscle disorder 186
  myositis ossificans 197, *197*
  seroma 195, *195*
  spine-related neuromuscular
    disorder 186, *186*
  subtotal/complete muscle
    tear 190
  tendinous avulsion 190, *190, 191*
physical phenomena 170–172
  absorption 171
  acoustic enhancements 171
  acoustic shadow 171, *172*
  attenuation 171
  reflection 171
  reverberations 172, *172*
  scatter 171
  technique 176–177, *176*
ultrasound therapy 125, 341
upper limb tension tests 349, *349*
uric acid 95
urogenital diaphragm release 344

V

varicosities 42
vascular endothelial growth factor
  (VEGF) 119
vastus intermedius *8, 17, 56, 177,*
  179, 183
  contusion injury *192*
vastus lateralis *8, 17, 56, 173, 177,*
  179, 183
vastus medialis *8, 17, 56, 173, 177,*
  179, 183
  myositis ossificans *155–156*
ventral ramus 346
vertebral column muscles 11, *11, 12*
vitamin A therapy 271
vitamin C 97, 98
  therapy 271
vitamin D 101–103
  biosynthesis *102*
  importance in athletic activity 103
  intake 102–103
  metabolism 101
  toxicity 103
vitamin E 96–98, *97*
  therapy 271

voluntary movements   71
  gradation of muscle forces   66–67
  hierarchical organization   71–72
    fine control of motor activity   71
    motor units as target for
      regulation/control   72
    preprogrammed movement
      patterns   71–72

W

warm-up   81–82, *82*, 377–380,
  379–380
  active methods   81

blood flow   81
excitability and   81, *85*
injury relationships   145
passive methods   81
thermal effects   81
three-phase warm-up routine
  378–380, *378*
withdrawal reflex   47, *47*
Wnt signaling pathway
  121–122
Wobenzym   270
work   70
working memory   249
wound healing   118, *118*
  see also muscle regeneration

Y

Yerkes–Dodson law   256, *257*
yoga   260

Z

Z-disk   29, *29*, 30, 60
Zeel   271
zinc
  deficiency   100
  monitoring   278
  therapy   270